third edition

Financial Management *for* Nurse Managers

Merging the Heart with the Dollar

Edited by

Janne Dunham-Taylor, PhD, RN

Joseph Z. Pinczuk, MHA

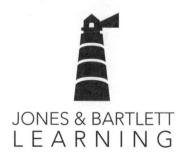

JONES & BARTLETT
LEARNING

World Headquarters
Jones & Bartlett Learning
5 Wall Street
Burlington, MA 01803
978-443-5000
info@jblearning.com
www.jblearning.com

Jones & Bartlett Learning books and products are available through most bookstores and online booksellers. To contact Jones & Bartlett Learning directly, call 800-832-0034, fax 978-443-8000, or visit our website, www.jblearning.com.

The content, statements, views, and opinions herein are the sole expression of the respective authors and not that of Jones & Bartlett Learning, LLC. Reference herein to any specific commercial product, process, or service by trade name, trademark, manufacturer, or otherwise does not constitute or imply its endorsement or recommendation by Jones & Bartlett Learning, LLC and such reference shall not be used for advertising or product endorsement purposes. All trademarks displayed are the trademarks of the parties noted herein. *Financial Management for Nurse Managers: Merging the Heart with the Dollar, Third Edition* is an independent publication and has not been authorized, sponsored, or otherwise approved by the owners of the trademarks or service marks referenced in this product.

There may be images in this book that feature models; these models do not necessarily endorse, represent, or participate in the activities represented in the images. Any screenshots in this product are for educational and instructive purposes only. Any individuals and scenarios featured in the case studies throughout this product may be real or fictitious, but are used for instructional purposes only.

The authors, editor, and publisher have made every effort to provide accurate information. However, they are not responsible for errors, omissions, or for any outcomes related to the use of the contents of this book and take no responsibility for the use of the products and procedures described. Treatments and side effects described in this book may not be applicable to all people; likewise, some people may require a dose or experience a side effect that is not described herein. Drugs and medical devices are discussed that may have limited availability controlled by the Food and Drug Administration (FDA) for use only in a research study or clinical trial. Research, clinical practice, and government regulations often change the accepted standard in this field. When consideration is being given to use of any drug in the clinical setting, the health care provider or reader is responsible for determining FDA status of the drug, reading the package insert, and reviewing prescribing information for the most up-to-date recommendations on dose, precautions, and contraindications, and determining the appropriate usage for the product. This is especially important in the case of drugs that are new or seldom used.

Production Credits
Executive Publisher: William Brottmiller
Senior Editor: Amanda Martin
Editorial Assistant: Rebecca Myrick
Associate Production Editor: Sara Fowles
Senior Marketing Manager: Jennifer Stiles
VP, Manufacturing and Inventory Control: Therese Connell
Composition: diacriTech
Cover Design: Scott Moden
Photo Research and Permissions Coordinator: Joseph Veiga
Cover Image: © Psycho/ShutterStock, Inc.
Printing and Binding: Edwards Brothers Malloy
Cover Printing: Edwards Brothers Malloy

Library of Congress Cataloging-in-Publication Data
Financial management for nurse managers (Dunham-Taylor)
  Financial management for nurse managers : merging the heart with the dollar / [edited by] Janne Dunham-Taylor, Joseph Z. Pinczuk.
  — Third edition.
      p. ; cm.
Includes bibliographical references and index.
ISBN 978-1-284-03103-4 (pbk.)
I. Dunham-Taylor, Janne, editor of compilation. II. Pinczuk, Joseph Z., editor of compilation. III. Title.
  [DNLM: 1. Economics, Nursing. 2. Nursing Services—economics. 3. Nursing Services—organization & administration. WY 77]
  RT86.7
  362.1068'1—dc23
                        2013043621

6048

Printed in the United States of America
18 17 16 15 14   10 9 8 7 6 5 4 3 2 1

BRIEF CONTENTS

CONTENTS

Part II   **Providing Value-Based Service**

Chapter 4   **Providing Patient Value While Achieving Quality, Safety, and**
                  Cost-Effectiveness 167

Sandy K. Diffenderfer, PhD, MSN, RN, CPHQ,
   Janne Dunham-Taylor, PhD, RN, Karen W. Snyder, MSN, RN,
   and Dru Malcolm, DNP, MSN, RN, NEA-BC, CPHRM

Part IV   Health Care and the Economy

Paul Bayes, DBA Accounting, MS Economics, BS Accounting, is formerly Chair and Professor of Accountancy at East Tennessee State University. Dr. Bayes earned his bachelor and doctorate degrees in accounting from the University of Kentucky. He also holds a master's in economics from Indiana State University. Dr. Bayes has published and presented over 50 articles for both practitioner and academic organizations and has published an accounting information systems case textbook with co-author Dr. John Nash.

Sandy K. Diffenderfer, PhD, MSN, RN, CPHQ, is an assistant professor in the graduate program at East Tennessee State University (ETSU) College of Nursing. Her research focus is related to her dissertation topic, *Overcoming: A Theory Of Accelerated Second-Degree Baccalaureate Graduate Nurse Transition To Professional Nursing Practice*. She plans to extend her substantive theory to different, but similar social structures in populations that are not well understood including male and minority student populations. Dr. Diffenderfer has 38 years of nursing experience with concentrations in nursing administration, leadership, quality management, risk management, and education. She teaches undergraduate and graduate students in the classroom, online, in Second Life, and clinical.

Janne Dunham-Taylor, PhD, RN, Professor and Graduate Coordinator of Nursing Administration, teaches nursing administration graduate courses at both master's, PhD, and DNP programs at East Tennessee State University College of Nursing. She has been a head nurse, nursing supervisor, and director of nursing in a teaching hospital, a university hospital, and a state hospital. She has been an assistant dean, chair, and has held two acting dean positions in university settings. She has taught nursing administration courses for 35 years. Her research has been concerned with transformational leadership at the CNO level nationally. She has numerous publications on various nursing administration topics. Dr. Dunham-Taylor is a co-author of this book and has previously co-authored the first and second editions of *Health Care Financial Management for Nurse Managers: Merging the Heart with the Dollar* (Jones & Bartlett Learning); and *Health Care Financial Management for Nurse Managers: Applications in Hospitals, Long-Term Care, Home Care, and Ambulatory Care*, published by Jones & Bartlett Learning in 2006.

Joellen Edwards, PhD, RN, FAAN, is Associate Dean for Research and Professor at East Tennessee State University College of Nursing. Dr. Edwards' program of research centers on the health status and clinical outcomes of rural populations. She focuses on improving the health of rural women through adherence to recommended health screenings and healthy lifestyle. Health policy implications and health care system issues are integral parts of her work. Her research has been funded by NIH (NCMHD); DHHS, HRSA, Office of Rural Health Policy; DHHS, HRSA, Office of Women's Health (subcontract); DHHS, HRSA Division of Nursing; and others. She publishes widely in journals such as *Journal of Professional Nursing, Women's Health Issues, Journal of Rural Health*, and many others; and presents nationally and internationally. Dr. Edwards is a member of the Editorial Board of the *Journal of Rural Health*, and a Fellow in the American Academy of Nursing. Dr. Edwards teaches quantitative research methods and health policy in the PhD program and health policy in the MSN program.

Patricia A. Hayes, PhD, RN, is an Associate Professor of Nursing at East Tennessee State University. Dr. Hayes is an American Foundation Virginia Stone Scholar. In 2010, she received a Health Resources and Service Administration grant to deliver primary care and in-home case management to public housing residents. She teaches philosophy of nursing science, as well as theory and research.

Catherine B. Leary, MSN, RN, CNAA, works as an independent nursing consultant. She is the co-author of *A Charge Nurse's Guide: Navigating the Path of Leadership*, published by the Center for Leader Development Press in Cleveland, Ohio. While with the Regional Cleveland Clinic hospitals, she held many leadership positions, including Charge Nurse, Nurse Manager, Chief Nurse Executive, Vice President of Patient Care Services, and Chief Operating Officer. Ms. Leary holds a master of science in nursing degree, a nursing diploma, and a bachelor of arts degree in psychology. In addition, she has completed numerous graduate semester hours in the areas of education and business. She holds nursing licenses in Ohio and Wisconsin and is a member of Sigma Theta Tau International honorary nursing society. She is board certified as a Nursing Executive, Advanced. Ms. Leary is a nurse who is very proud of her profession. Experience has taught her that effective nursing leaders are the key to high-quality health care.

Kelly Loyd works in the areas of Circulation and Interlibrary Loan at the East Tennessee State University (ETSU) Quillen College of Medicine Library. In a former life she was an English instructor. She has a BA in English from ETSU and currently is a student in the School of Information Studies at the University of Tennessee, Knoxville.

Lois W. Lowry, DNSc, RN, ANEF, is Professor Emerita at East Tennessee State University. She was rewarded for 30 exemplary years of teaching students from associate, baccalaureate, master's, and doctoral degree programs by induction into the inaugural class of the Academy of Nursing Education in 2007. Dr. Lowry was director of the DNS program at East Tennessee State University for its first 6 years. Her greatest expertise is in the area of theory development in which she publishes extensively. Further, Dr. Lowry has been instrumental in designing interdisciplinary courses for students within the health care profession in the areas of law and ethics. Currently, she is engaged with nurses in Magnet hospitals as they seek to apply ethical principles in nursing practice.

Dru Malcolm, DNP, MSN, RN, NEA-BC, CPHRM, is currently Chief Nursing Officer and Assistant Administrator at Johnston Memorial Hospital, a facility of Mountain States Health Alliance. She celebrates 35 years of nursing experience with a focus in emergency nursing, emergency preparedness, quality, risk management, and administration. She holds a doctorate of nursing practice from Old Dominion University, master of science in nursing administration, certification as Nurse Executive Advanced (NEA-BC), Certified Professional Healthcare in Risk Management (CPHRM), and a Fellow in The Advisory Board.

Kathy Malloch, PhD, MBA, RN, FAAN, is a recognized expert in leadership and the development of effective evidence-based processes and systems for patient care. Her uncanny focus on accountability and results is the hallmark of her practice.

Her expertise has been useful to many organizations across the country.

A nationally known writer and speaker, Dr. Malloch has been a registered nurse for 40 years. Kathy has published extensively in proctored health journals. She is a frequent presenter and author on leadership topics, healing environments, professional nursing practice, and patient classification systems. Kathy and Tim Porter-O'Grady, her writing partner, have published five textbooks on leadership. The textbook "Quantum Leadership" co-authored with Tim Porter-O'Grady is a best seller and is currently used in over 220 graduate programs.

Most recently, Dr. Malloch has served as the first program director for the Arizona State University, College of Nursing and Health Innovation, Master's in Healthcare Innovation program. This innovative, multidisciplinary program is the first of its kind in the country.

Dr. Malloch is a graduate of Wayne State University, College of Nursing, received an MBA from Oakland University and a PhD in nursing from the University of Colorado. She is a member of the American Academy of Nursing.

Currently Dr. Malloch also serves as:

- Member and Current Vice-President of the Arizona State Board of Nursing
- Associate Professor, Arizona State University, College of Nursing and Health Innovation
- Clinical Consultant, API Healthcare, Inc. Hartford, Wisconsin
- Area I Director, National Council of State Boards of Nursing Board of Directors
- Senior Consultant for Tim Porter-O'Grady Associates

R. Penny Marquette, DBA, presently retired, was a KPMG Peat Marwick Faculty Fellow in Accounting and a Professor in Accounting at the University of Akron, Akron, Ohio. She has also taught at Cleveland State University in Cleveland, Ohio and at Kent State University in Kent, Ohio. She has a DBA in accounting with a finance minor at Kent State University, an MBA at the University of Akron in accounting, and a BS in journalism and English from the University of Florida in Gainesville. She has authored numerous publications.

Jo-Ann Summitt Marrs, EdD, RN, is presently a professor in Graduate Programs at East Tennessee State University College of Nursing. She holds a doctor of education in public health and a master of science in nursing from the University of Tennessee. She acquired her family nurse practitioner certificate from Pittsburg State University and is presently practicing in one of the College of

Nursing's nurse managed clinics for Hispanic women and children. She served in an administrative capacity from 1987 to 2007. Her main interest is in the area of moral turpitude and licensure for nurses. She has led a national campaign for background checks and fingerprinting to be a requirement for admission to nursing schools.

Joseph Z. Pinczuk, MHA, presently retired, held executive positions overseeing finance, administration, and operations for 29 years. He has a master of professional management in hospital administration from Indiana Northern University and a bachelor of business administration in accounting from Cleveland State University. He has been a Chief Financial Officer (CFO) in hospitals ranging in size from 55 beds to serving as the CFO of the Tri-County Hospital Group in Ohio consisting of 3 hospitals with a total of 254 beds. He also served as CFO of a Continuing Care Retirement Community consisting of 285 resident units, 75 skilled nursing, and 24 assisted living beds. He has served as Director on the Board of the Healthcare Financial Management Association Northeast Ohio Chapter and received the Follmer Bronze, Reeves Silver, and Muncie Gold Awards for his contributions to the organization. A former Adjunct Professor of Nursing, College of Nursing, University of Akron and a co-author of an article "Surviving Capitation," *American Journal of Nursing* (March 1996), Mr. Pinczuk is a co-author of this book and has previously co-authored three books: *Health Care Financial Management for Nurse Managers: Merging the Heart with the Dollar*, first and second editions. (Jones & Bartlett Learning); and *Health Care Financial Management for Nurse Managers: Applications in Hospitals, Long-Term Care, Home Care and Ambulatory Care*, published by Jones & Bartlett Learning in 2006.

Susan R. Rasmussen, PhD, RN, ACNS-BC, is an Assistant Professor of Nursing at East Tennessee State University. Having worked in cardiovascular and rehabilitation nursing, her research interest is chronic nonmalignant pain. Experience in discharge planning and rehabilitation supports the chapter on case management.

Mary Anne Schultz, PhD, MBA, MSN, RN, is nurse-scientist, formerly a faculty member of the Nursing Department at California State University, Los Angeles. Her specialties are Nursing Administration, Nursing Economics, and Nursing Informatics. She holds a master of nursing degree from Case Western Reserve University in Cleveland, Ohio and an MBA degree from the Peter Drucker Management Institute of the Claremont Graduate University in Claremont, California. In her doctoral work at the UCLA School of Nursing, she examined economic factors of California hospitals impacting adverse patient outcomes such as unexpected death and complications.

Frances W. "Billie" Sills, MSN, RN, ARNP, LNC, received a diploma from St. Mary's School of Nursing in Rochester, Minnesota; a bachelor of science degree in nursing at the University of Miami, Coral Gables, Florida; and a master of science degree in nursing as a clinical nurse specialist/advanced registered nurse practitioner with a double major in administration and education at the University of Alabama. She is a retired Air Force Flight Nurse and has held nursing administrative positions at various settings including a 1,200-bed teaching hospital, a 180-bed comprehensive freestanding rehabilitation hospital, and a 120-bed long-term care facility. She has met the challenges, the rewards, and the multiple changes that have occurred in health care over the last few decades first hand. She is very active in professional organizations, having held several positions in state nursing associations, Sigma Theta Tau, Association of Rehabilitation Nurses, Case Management Association, and was past president of the American Association of Neuroscience Nurses. She served on the American Hospital Association Council for Rehabilitation and Long-Term Care. As an Assistant Professor at the University of Texas, Houston, she was responsible for undergraduate and graduate courses and served as the Director of Student Affairs. She has presented both nationally and internationally on advanced practice, leadership, case management, and gerontology. She presently teaches in the College of Nursing at East Tennessee State University and serves as an expert witness for nursing practice in the areas of neuroscience, orthopedics, rehabilitation, and long-term care. She is the President of the Tennessee Nurses Association.

Karen W. Snyder, MSN, RN, is currently working in the role of Quality Improvement Specialist for Integrated Solutions Health Network, a subsidiary of an 11 hospital system. ISHN is a care management company and Accountable Organization. Her 31 years of nursing experience include critical care, active duty time in the U.S. Army Reserve, staff development, Education Coordinator for rollout of the electronic health record across an 11 hospital system, and Director of Clinical Education. She holds a Master of Science in Nursing Administration.

Norma Tomlinson, MSN, RN, NE-BC, FACHE, is a registered nurse with over 30 years of professional nursing experience. As a staff nurse, her practice included medical-surgical and orthopedic nursing, children's psychiatric nursing, and geriatric skilled nursing. She has been a staff development instructor in a general hospital and developed and administered a Medicare-certified, hospital-based home health agency. She has experience as the Director of Medical-Surgical Nursing in both a large urban hospital as well as in a hospital system. She has served as the Vice-President of Clinical Services in hospitals in Ohio, Michigan, and Tennessee. She is currently the Associate Vice-President, Associate Executive Director, at University of Toledo Medical Center in Toledo, Ohio. She holds an associate degree in nursing from Purdue University, a bachelor of science degree in nursing from Youngstown State University, and a master of science degree in nursing from the University of Akron. She is a fellow in the American College of Health Care Executives, a member of Phi Kappi Phi, Sigma Theta Tau, and is currently past president for Zeta Theta Chapter, AONE, and OONE. She served for several years as the president of the Akron-Canton Regional Organization of Nurse Executives and on the Board of OONE.

Patricia M. VanHook, PhD, MSN, RN, FNP-BC, has 25 years of nursing management experience in acute care, specifically critical care. She has managed in rural and urban community hospitals. She served as the Magnet coordinator for the first hospital in Tennessee to be designated as Magnet. She is active in state and national efforts to reduce stroke through evaluation of systems and design of systems to improve access and the delivery of care across the continuum. She currently is Associate Dean of Practice at East Tennessee State University's College of Nursing.

Rick Wallace, MA, MDiv, MAOM, MSLS, EdD, AHIP, is the Assistant Director for the Quillen College of Medicine Library. The library provides services to hospitals, clinics, and public health departments in 48 Tennessee counties.

Nakia Joye Woodward, MSIS, AHIP, is a Clinical Reference Librarian at East Tennessee State University Quillen College of Medicine Library. She attends clinical rounds with Family Medicine, Pediatrics, and Surgery. She coordinates the Medical Library's Database Instruction/Evidence-Based Medicine Classes, along with working in Consumer Health, Reference, and Outreach. Her research interests are evidence-based practice, clinical use of health information, and consumer health. Nakia is currently working on her master's in public health with an emphasis in epidemiology.

Janne and Joe have been working together for years, and remain friends through this third edition. It all started when the CNO at Joe's hospital invited Janne (an experienced nurse administrator teaching at the local university) to work with the hospital's nurse managers to enhance their knowledge about budgeting. When Janne met Joe (the CFO), she realized that he was an unusual CFO because he both understood and supported the "care" side of health care. She found out that he was a former respiratory therapist and married to a registered nurse. Joe thought that Janne's information for the nurse managers was important, and it was evident that the CNO and CFO worked well together.

Then Joe began to regularly come to talk to graduate nursing administration students in Janne's fiscal course. He could clearly explain financial terms, the way the finance department worked, and the future implications of reimbursement and how it would affect the healthcare organization, nurses, patients, and community.

Gradually, the ideas for this book began to take root and blossom. Janne and Joe knew they did not want to create the typical financial book that kept finances in a silo. Instead, they wanted to present finances in the larger dimension—as a part of a greater whole. They also both felt strongly that regular dialogue and respect between finance and nursing were critical to the success of a health care organization. Their goal was to provide nurse administrators with information so they can be more effective in their roles.

This book has been a labor of love. This book is made richer by the many contributors who have shared their expertise on certain subjects. Joe and Janne thank them for all their time, knowledge, and dedication, once again, to this book.

Every Management Decision Has Financial Implications— Every Financial Decision Has Management Implications!

Janne Dunham-Taylor, PhD, RN, and

Joseph Z. Pinczuk, MHA

This text addresses healthcare financial management issues for nurse managers. In many cases, this information is also helpful for chief nursing officers and other nurse administrators. Nurse managers and nurse administrators work in a variety of healthcare settings such as hospitals, ambulatory/ outpatient clinics and centers, long-term care facilities, and home care. This text is written to provide helpful, evidence-based information that pertains to each of these settings.

To be successful in financial management, nurse administrators must understand, regardless of setting, what affects the healthcare environment and the financial implications that result from these forces. The nurse administrator must express what needs to happen for good nursing practice and also must be able to articulate the financial aspects involved. Understanding the organization's finances is not sufficient. A nurse administrator must be able to anticipate actions in response to a changing financial environment and to encourage staff to do the same.

This text covers a wide range of financial information, including evidence, in healthcare finance, economics, budgeting, comparing reimbursements with cost of services provided, accounting, and financial strategies. Concepts are presented followed by examples. At times, we make suggestions for actions that we have found to be helpful. Although many of the examples have an inpatient focus, many examples are provided from other healthcare settings such as ambulatory care, home care, and long-term care.

Even though this book has a financial title, there is more included here than just the financial part of health care. This is because everything in health care is *interrelated/interconnected/interwoven* with finances. For example, when nurse administrators discuss budgeting, they must also be concerned with staffing, patient acuity, and productivity of staff as well as quality standards. We cannot ignore leadership in an organization because if that is broken, everything else is.

This interconnection demands coverage of the broad range of topics in this book that influence each other, including the finances. Chapters discuss quantum leadership, organizational issues, workload management, quality and safety, evidence-based practice, ethics, legal responsibilities, and strategic planning. Case management, predominantly used in hospitals, is discussed because it is needed to achieve continuity of care across all settings including the home.

It is important to note here that every financial decision we make has management implications. And the same is true in reverse: Every management decision has financial implications. So, we cannot ignore the additional aspects we have included in this book because they are all interwoven and, if one is ignored, such oversight can negatively affect the bottom line.

The bottom line should *never* be the primary focus in a healthcare organization. *When the bottom line is most important, the organization will lose money.* Many in the organization will have forgotten that our reason for existence is to *serve patients*. That is our primary focus. As long as we stay in touch with this truth, we will thrive.

This is not to say that we can ignore the financial implications. As mentioned later, no margin, no mission. We cannot exceed the budget we have—if we do, we must have another area in the budget that we can draw from to counter the overspending. The bottom line must remain solvent. However, the patient *always* comes first.

We have entered into a new *value-based reimbursement environment* that demands different approaches for healthcare organizations to stay solvent. Our old volume-based reimbursement environment of the previous century is outdated. Healthcare organizations cannot continue to survive unless we change and create a value-based environment. This text outlines what is needed to achieve this objective.

We emphasize the importance of *giving the patient what is valued*. Many in health care do not fully understand this concept. Whereas we have been good about measuring patient satisfaction (although these data are often collected only after the experience), many times we miss the most important point: We have not *listened* to the patient. We have not involved the patient in making the decisions about care. To do this we need to stay updated on the evidence and pay attention to individual patient differences. Many times after care has been given, we find that the patient did not receive what he or she actually wanted! Sadly, often we do not realize that this is the case.

How do we turn this situation around? For value-based reimbursement, the American Hospital Association advocates nurse and physician leadership at the point of care and making decisions with the patient about that care within the available finances. Administrators' roles need to change to support the point-of-care leaders. Teamwork and interdisciplinary shared governance are necessities. Everyone—from the board/CEO/CNO/CFO to nurse aides/house-keepers—needs to be doing regular rounds listening to patients. This needs to replace some of the meetings, especially ones where administrators have no perception of what is going on at the bedside. Patients are more likely to get what they value when the whole thrust of the organization is toward finding out this information, and then providing it as much as possible. This creates messy communication, conflicts that lead to better solutions, and messy flat structures as well as better reimbursement.

In the value-based environment, we need to examine current practices. For instance, we burden RNs with a lot of paperwork and non-valued-added activities that take them away from the bedside for more than 50% of their time. We understaff units, which creates negative environments for everyone, yet we expect staff will do the care to achieve reimbursement. Evidence shows that missed care is occurring and this may cause side effects for the patient, such as pressure sores and infections that will not be reimbursed. Yet we do not pay attention to these issues. Instead, we allow these issues to continue and fester. We need to start valuing the staff nurse at the bedside, encouraging staff to lead and make changes as they do their work. In fact, 90% of the decisions about their work needs to be made by staff as they take care of patients each day.

An enormous challenge in the current healthcare climate is achieving quality care and safety while keeping expenses down. This is especially important now that reimbursement depends on appropriate, timely care and does not cover errors. The patient has always suffered from poor care, but now with value-based reimbursement, healthcare organizations are penalized as well with lower reimbursement.

The healthcare environment is complex and continues to increase in complexity. This causes increased bureaucracy, more errors, and more expense. Complexity and chaos are constantly changing the environment and affecting our work organizationally. We need to strive to involve all stakeholders, including those at the bedside, physicians, and patients and families to simplify the environment. What we do today will be outdated tomorrow, so we need to continually stay tuned into the new evidence. This is interwoven with ethical and legal implications that cannot be ignored.

Last, the financial aspects cannot be ignored. To respond effectively in this complex healthcare environment and to work successfully with the financial arm of the healthcare entity, nurse managers must understand financial concepts such as staffing, budgeting, identifying and analyzing variances, measuring productivity, costing, accounting, and forecasting as well as the strategies that achieve a positive bottom line. Although finance and accounting terminology is used throughout the chapters, chapters focused specifically on accounting and assessing financial performance are included.

This text provides nurse managers with an interconnected view of the nursing and financial sides of health care and suggests methods nurses can use to successfully integrate these viewpoints.

This realistic integration of nursing and finance (along with all the other departments and professions) enhances nurse manager effectiveness.

A critical element for success is the ability of nurse managers to interface effectively with finance department personnel. An unusual feature of this book is that it contains both typical nursing administration terminology and financial accounting terminology. Suggestions are made for nurse managers on how to communicate with and maximize understanding of concepts and issues by financial personnel, who may come from different backgrounds and attach different meanings to the same terms.

The problem with the financial aspect of health care is that it is often viewed as a separate silo—a silo where nurses do not enter and where financial personnel reside. Meanwhile, nurses are in their own silo, and financial personnel are not found there. As coauthors of this book, we, a nurse administrator and a chief financial officer, believe that it is time to break down and end this silo mentality. Our effectiveness in health care demands that *nursing and finance interface regularly* and truly have dialogue about the issues. We are most effective if we can face these issues *together* using the strengths of both our professions.

Nurses need to express themselves more effectively using financial principles and data; financial personnel need to more effectively understand the care side of health care. Because this book is written for the nurse administrator, we emphasize the first. We hope this book will be helpful for finance personnel as well.

A problem that occurs when nurses and financial people try to talk together is that financial officers often think in a linear way. When they talk to each other, they talk about numbers, ratios, and stats. On the other hand, nurses think in an abstract, interpersonal way. When nurses talk to each other, they talk about how someone feels, how someone will be affected by a certain treatment, or whether tasks have been accomplished.

The breakdown in communication occurs when nurses talk to financial people using abstract language and financial people talk to nurses using linear language. The conversations run parallel to each other, with both sides not understanding what the other side is talking about. Nurses complain that financial people never think about anything but the bottom line; financial people complain that all nurses do is whine about quality. True dialogue and communication do not occur.

This book gives examples that nurses can use to better communicate with financial personnel, as well as with other linear-thinking administrators. In addition, we recommend that if a nurse administrator really wants to talk effectively with financial administrators, he or she should be able to *express/communicate the abstract information using linear language* (i.e., numbers that will be affected by something that has or has not occurred or that is being planned, including specific amounts of money needed to implement a project, and so forth).

Abstract thinking is effective in communication between nurses and physicians. However, it is often ineffective when communicating with the finance department. For example, concepts such as "care" might not have meaning to a finance officer. *Caring* is an abstract term. Exceptions occur when a financial person experiences a serious illness or when the financial officer previously worked as a healthcare professional.

At times, this communication problem can be compounded by simple differences in male and female communication techniques (remember *Men Are from Mars, Women Are from Venus*

[Gray, 1992]), especially if the chief financial officer is male and the chief nursing officer is female. This is changing with less gender-specific roles in the workplace. In the past, a male chief nursing officer often had an edge because he could be "one of the boys." This is also slowly changing with more males in nursing and more females in finance.

Properly prepared nurse managers and nurse administrators can successfully provide an interface between finance and nursing, making decisions based on *both* clinical and financial perspectives. A nurse manager, as well as financial personnel, cannot make the mistake of ignoring the whole while dealing with the individual parts.

This interconnection goes beyond just nursing and finance. In this book, we strongly encourage every person and every department and profession to collaborate as they provide what the patient values. Because of this interconnection there is a ripple effect. What one person or department does affects all the others. Yet some of us cling to the old silo mentality.

Another financial silo exists when the organization's mentality is that staff are not leaders and should not be involved with financial information. We are in the Information Age. Transparency is best. Because we are all interconnected, every task a staff member does has financial implications. It is critical to *involve all staff and nurse managers with the finances*—payment structures and how much is actually received; reimbursement that is lost when timely, appropriate care is not given; costs of technology and supplies; staffing costs; quality and safety costs; costs incurred with safety or quality issues; and legal costs. They should understand the impact their actions have on the bottom line.

Staff need to be making 90% of the care decisions right at the bedside. We administrators only *serve* the staff and help facilitate them to do their best work for the patients. We need to create positive environments because the evidence shows that these environments have the best outcomes—including for the bottom line. We need to empower staff, but more than that, we need to support them being leaders in their work and need to support patients being leaders in what care they choose to receive.

Solutions are always better when the people directly involved are involved in the process of devising the solutions. Therefore, we advocate that *staff and patients, as well as administrators, come to the table on issues and decide on the best way to accomplish the work through **interdisciplinary shared governance**.* This gets rid of another silo—the one where administrators make all the decisions and do not delegate to others—which is a leftover from the previous century.

We will have small successes we can celebrate, and we will have failures. Failures are natural, a fact of life. As they occur we need to learn from each one and figure out better ways or changes to make to simplify the environment. Many errors are actually caused by a series of events—because we are all interconnected. Dealing with failures goes beyond being blame free. We must make incremental changes that will simplify processes that have become cumbersome.

We have written this book in interesting times. The U.S. economy has slowed down as many jobs were outsourced to other countries. Weather events are getting more severe. Can you imagine experiencing no electricity—or worse yet, no home, and yet still taking care of patients? This has happened in a number of places right here in our country. We have pulled together in such times of crisis, and, hopefully, we can pull together in fixing our healthcare system. It takes each of us. We are all interconnected.

Discussion Questions

1. How does understanding complexity break down silos?
2. What silos exist in your workplace? In your own thinking? How will you contribute to breaking down these silos?
3. What actions further the silo concept?
4. Give an example where a nurse administrator effectively expresses a need to the finance department using numbers and dollars.
5. State an administrative decision and explain its financial implications.
6. Describe a financial decision, giving the administrative implications of this decision.
7. Describe an administrative or financial decision and map out the ripple effect of this decision.

Reference

Gray, J. (1992). *Men are from Mars, women are from Venus*. New York, NY: HarperCollins.

Necessary Essentials for Financial Viability

Some may wonder why we have included the chapters in Part I in a financial management book. After all, why aren't we getting right into finances and budgeting? Actually, we start with these chapters for a very specific financial reason. As will become clear later, any time we make the finances, or bottom line, come first, we create more financial problems—things become more expensive. So, for the most effective bottom line, the bottom line cannot be first priority! It has to become second behind some *very* important issues.

Part I is given first placement in this book because the issues discussed are basic and when broken result in serious financial issues. If we do not pay attention to every aspect discussed in Part I, we will lose money! However, when these aspects are functioning well, we have the foundation in place to realize financial success.

Part I starts with a letter to nurses about doing what is right for patients, written by a hospital chief operating officer who is also a nurse. The message behind the letter is, if we do what is right for the patient (more about this in the next section), the money will follow. We found this letter to be energizing and personally moving. We hope you do too.

The second chapter is concerned with quantum leadership. Leadership is what happens between two or more people as they interact. *Staff need to be leaders. Patients need to be leaders in determining their care.* Administrators need to **support** leadership as it takes place at the bedside. If the administrative leadership is broken at any level—especially at the top—everything else is broken within an organization, and the organization will lose *a lot* of money. Fish rots from the head. But money is only a minor problem compared with patient suffering or death, and poor patient outcomes. Patients are in jeopardy if the administrative and staff leadership is inadequate.

The placement of this chapter is deliberate because we need to pay attention to our administrative leadership before we can expect improved patient outcomes and better reimbursement! If the administrative leadership is ineffective at any level in the organization, other financial problems will follow. But this isn't enough. Staff and patients need to be empowered to be leaders every day in the care given and received.

The third chapter is concerned with organizational strategies. Organizations are complex, as is the healthcare environment. As they become more complex they become bureaucracies. Complexity breeds problems and errors. To deal with this effectively, we need to simplify organizational processes, do only what the patient values, and, as decisions are made, do what is best so that patients can achieve what they value. Thus, the patients, supported by staff at the point of care, make decisions about their care.

Most of the day-to-day decisions need to be made at the bedside. It is important that staff leaders at the point of care make 90% of the decisions about their work. Interdisciplinary shared governance, collaboration, and teamwork promoting healthy collaborative cultures are all part of our administrative work as we design the organization. To stay in touch with what is happening at the point of care all in the organization need to do regular rounds, talking and listening to patients and staff about what is happening. Rounds need to replace some of the meetings so that everyone has a more realistic assessment of the organization.

As we deal with needed changes, we must avoid "quick fixes" that worsen problems rather than repair them. Instead, we need to make small incremental changes that simplify the bureaucracy.

These first three chapters set the stage as the basis of effective financial management. This is supported by the American Hospital Association's 10 "must do" strategies for financial success in this new value-based environment. Financial viability follows when this foundation is in place. It never should be top priority, or the bottom line—as well as the patients—will suffer.

An Open Letter to Nurse Leaders: If We Do What Is Right for Patients, Financial Well-Being Will Follow

Catherine B. Leary, MSN, RN, CNAA

OBJECTIVES

- To understand the importance of developing a personal mission statement.
- To identify resonance between your personal mission statement and the organization's mission statement.
- To accept that it is possible for a nursing leader to create an environment in which both fiscal responsibility and exceptional patient care can coexist.
- To recognize the importance of communication and celebration.
- To embrace the concept of considering what is right for the patient in all thoughts and actions.
- To feel joyful and excited about the opportunity to be a nurse leader who strives daily to connect hearts and minds to the noble calling of patient care.

It is not easy to be a nurse leader/manager. I applaud you for your endeavors and encourage you to bring your best efforts to this very important role. Excellent nurse leaders are the key not only to exceptional patient care, but also to financial health.

Healthcare costs are out of control in this country. Program after program is launched to control the runaway costs of health care and to increase fiscal accountability for the use of the healthcare dollar. This scenario can create a difficult environment for nurses. Our healthcare organizations have reacted to diminishing fiscal resources by downsizing and reengineering. Doing more with less has become a route to survival. In this time of crisis, nurses have come close to the edge—the edge of losing control of our values and our ability to make a difference.

Nurses are good people, compliant with the rules. Nurses want to do the right thing and to be team players. In these years of declining reimbursement, however, there has been an alarming trend to make our decisions on behalf of dollars instead of patients. Nurses have come close to becoming followers instead of leaders.

This letter is a call to leadership to believe in yourself and the nurses you lead. As the gospel hymn says, "We are the people we've been waiting for."

Your calling in life is to do what is right for your patients. It has been my experience (and that of many others) that doing what is right for the patient leads to a positive bottom line. It is important to believe that if you *make decisions on behalf of patients, the dollars will follow.* "A good outcome leads to a good income," as one of my friends declares.

All nurses know this is true. You have seen it with your own eyes. The relative value of nursing care is huge. Evidence supports this. There is no substitute, and there are no shortcuts. It is up to you and other nursing leaders in your organization to carry this message to all corners of your realm of influence—to the community in which you work, to the board that directs your organization, to the physicians, to the patients, and to the nurses whom you lead.

Now is the time. You are fortunate to live in an era in which there is awareness of the need for a values-based workplace. People are seeking a connection between their personal values and their work. It is recognized that there is a need for the practical application of principles and values to breathe spirit and meaning into what people do with their lives. This belief is a natural fit for nurses because it is what true nurses have always believed.

It is easy to catch the wave of "doing the right thing" but difficult to stay on top of it. It takes courage, persistence, and a lot of hard work. It requires that you align your daily work with the dictates of your heart. Having blind faith without looking back helps a lot when you champion a cause. Always remember that you and your nurses embody the standard of care. Know, too, that a high standard of care leads the organization to a profitable position. *Reflect on what is right for the patient in everything you say and do.* It is a winning formula. I guarantee it. Say it out loud a lot. People want to hear it. And best of all, it is catching. Soon you will hear people around you saying it and acting it out.

Another current trend that supports the nursing cause is patient safety—the prevention of errors. The research literature, as well as the popular media, concludes that patients must come first. Errors not only harm patients, but they also cost more. Doing what is right for the patient saves money. Staffing with an adequate number and mix of registered nurses (RNs) prevents errors. Nurses have always known this in their guts. Now there is evidence to prove it. There are many ways to prepare yourself for this crusade on behalf of the patients. Know your business. Be credible. Be smart. And, most of all, communicate and develop relationships. Health care (as with most things in life) is about relationships. Let me explain what I mean.

Mission

To be successful, know (and feel) the relationship between the organization's mission and your personal objectives. **Exhibit 1–1** illustrates this idea.

The first step is to know yourself. What are your personal objectives? What is important to you? What values do you hold dear? What do you mean when you say, "I want to be true to myself"? What is your mission? It is a good idea to develop and write down your personal *mission statement*. This exercise takes time and thought. It is a document you will reflect on and revise throughout life. To get started it is helpful to list your values. Enter *Personal Values Checklist* into your search engine. Many lists are available to get you started on developing your own mission statement. Knowing yourself better will be of great help to you with the many difficult decisions and situations that a nurse leader must address. It will make you a better leader.

Spend some time thinking about this, reflecting on it, and discussing it with others in your workplace. It is important to personally embrace the alignment between your mission and the mission of the organization, and to understand how what you do supports the mission. To feel a resonance between your spirit and the cause of the organization is very powerful. If you believe in what you are doing, work becomes a joyful thing. Your role as a nurse leader is to develop a unit-based mission that supports the organization's mission and strategy. The most effective approach is to engage your team in this effort. Personal involvement for each nurse inevitably leads to buy-in and success. It takes a lot of time up front, but there is a huge return on this investment because when you do this exercise each heart connects personally to the mission. **Exhibit 1–2** shows the basic components of a *balanced scorecard*.

You can see how this concept can be carried to the unit level and connected to personal values. Regular and timely reporting on progress toward goals helps to keep nurses and other caregivers engaged in the process. Pride and teamwork grow with the realization that every individual brings value to the patients and the organization.

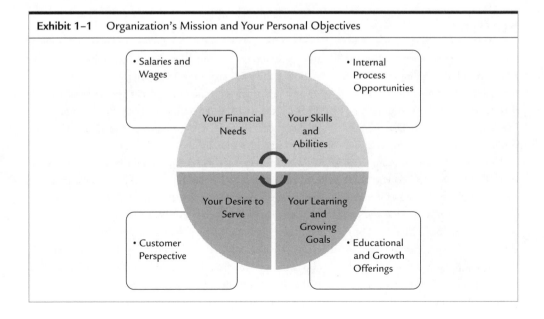

Exhibit 1–1   Organization's Mission and Your Personal Objectives

- Salaries and Wages

- Internal Process Opportunities

Your Financial Needs

Your Skills and Abilities

Your Desire to Serve

Your Learning and Growing Goals

- Customer Perspective

- Educational and Growth Offerings

Exhibit 1–2   Basics of a Balanced Scorecard

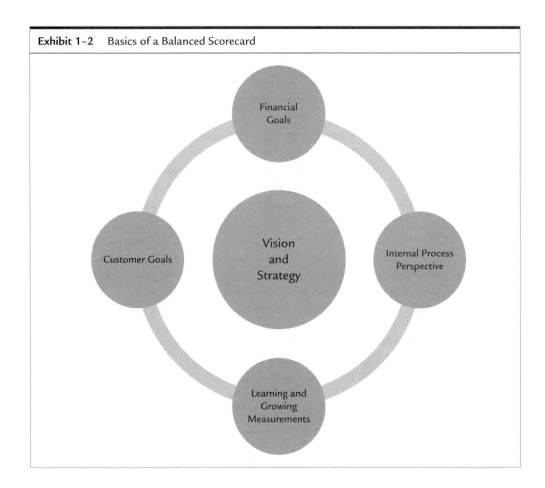

Staffing

One of the biggest expenses of any healthcare organization is personnel cost. Therefore, you must become an expert in knowing how much nurses cost, how many you need, and why. An important key to success is to thoroughly know and understand how your nurses deliver patient care. What are the needs of each patient population that your unit serves? What are the needs of the unit as a whole? Exactly how many full-time equivalents (FTEs) are needed to deliver cost-effective high-quality care? Ask all the questions you need to develop a comprehensive construct of staffing requirements.

Next, sort this out in terms of skill mix. What delivery of care method should you use? Try several ideas. How many RNs do you need? Be reasonable. There really is a shortage of labor and revenue. Be able to justify your request for high-priced personnel to senior management. Know the *hours per patient day* (*HPPD*) or *relative value units* (*RVUs*) that are required to deliver excellent patient care. Turn to the evidence for support. Know this by day, by shift, and by hour. Know exactly what skill mix you need. Be able to visualize who will do what on each shift. What exactly is the role of the RN, and what exactly is the role of everyone else? And, finally, how do these roles mesh to deliver safe, seamless care that satisfies the customer(s)? This exercise, of course, is the first part of the budgeting process. To do it as a group project with your staff is the most effective method. Everyone can then understand where the budget (the staffing) comes from and how important it is to work as a team to care for patients. When they are involved in the process, nurses start to feel more like participants and owners of the process and less like victims of it.

It is essential for you to develop or use quality measures to justify staffing budgets. Be able to show evidence that your requests are necessary to provide patients with safety and high-quality outcomes. It is helpful to develop a balanced scorecard for your unit that measures the same indicators that the overall organization uses to measure its progress toward goals. Enter *Nursing Balanced Scorecards* into your search engine for some examples.

Budgeting Process

Often, the annual budget is developed without much input from managers. Historical performance is used in the forecast, and some adjustments are made based on economic predictions. If this is the case for you, you still have opportunities for influence.

To be effective you need to know the steps of the budgeting process for your organization. Find out who develops the wage and salary budget. It may be a management engineer or someone in the human resources or finance department. The best way to find out is to ask the chief financial officer (CFO). CFOs are usually delighted that someone is interested in learning more about the budgeting process. It is likely that he or she will candidly and eagerly answer all of your questions.

Developing a partnering relationship with the CFO is key. You need each other to be successful. The CFO is often the pivotal contact between the board and the organization. Even if most board members have little healthcare experience, they usually have a lot of expertise with financial reports. Therefore, they scrutinize expenditures and want explanations. The budget for nursing is often one of the biggest, and the CFO must be prepared to defend it. With input from the chief nursing officer (CNO), the CFO is well equipped to defend the nursing budget and to explain the direct link between nurse staffing and excellent patient outcomes.

Get involved in forecasting the budget at the very beginning. If your organization's fiscal year coincides with the calendar year, this may be as early as the middle of the second quarter. Make recommendations to the appropriate person for the staffing your unit needs. Be detailed—include full-time equivalents, skill mix per shift, allocation to each shift, and so on. Be sure to include a line item for education and development. It is a good idea, too, to compare your staffing tables with *benchmarks* recognized as respectable in the industry. These are available online. Comparing to benchmarks helps you verify your work to yourself, your nurses, the CFO, other senior management leaders, and the board. You may not find exact comparisons, but you will be able to find scenarios close enough to your own to be helpful. If you can get both staffing numbers and information about patient outcomes from the benchmark, you are well on the way to building the case for putting patients first.

Most organizations expect managers to review the first draft of the budget before it is finalized. This is an opportunity for you to give valuable input. However, you may need to negotiate with your peers at this late point in the allocation process. In other words, the size of the pie has been determined. All that remains to be decided is the size of the slice for each department. Be fair. There may have to be some give and take. Before you go to budget meetings be clear on what can and what cannot be changed in the budget you are proposing.

As the year progresses you will be asked to talk about your financial performance. You will be expected to monitor and be knowledgeable of revenue and expenses per unit of service. It is important to know what percentage labor is of total expense and the relationship of *productive time* and *nonproductive time* to your unit's overall productivity and labor expenses. There may be the need to calculate *return on investment (ROI)* for capital equipment expenditures.

Take note of what financial indicators are on the organization's balanced scorecard and be able to report on these same indicators at the unit level. It is likely that your organization has an agreement with insurers or payers called *pay for performance*. It used to be that care providers were paid by a system called *fee for service*. The emerging trend is for organizations to be financially rewarded (receive better reimbursement) for delivery of healthcare services that meet preestablished targets. Keep your staff informed of what these targets are and on the progress toward these goals. Providing this information increases buy-in and group synergy.

Nursing Team

You are running a business. You are responsible for influencing a team to walk the fine line between fiscal responsibility and excellent patient outcomes. Your challenge is to find that sweet spot where these goals align. The bad news is that this is difficult. The good news is that you are not alone. Everyone in the organization is trying to do the same thing. It helps to approach your work in the knowledge that you are part of a team. Be collaborative with your colleagues as well as with your direct and indirect reports. Be there for each other.

There is significant power in having a strong nursing leadership team. Know your strengths. Know your plan. Stand as one. In unity there is strength. Be the world's best champion for front-line nurses and for patients. Be quite clear on whom your customers are and how to delight them. Meet frequently as a team and share your progress toward goals. Celebrate. Have fun. Incredible synergy and creativity will emerge. Get worked up. Be excited. Your work is very meaningful. It is a cause worthy of your best effort. Nursing is the noblest calling—serving humankind. What could be more important? Be positive and optimistic. People want to follow a leader who strongly believes that the goals can be met. Praise is a powerful motivator for everyone. People want to be part of a winning team. A strong visionary team can master any challenge.

Group Think

A potentially powerful attribute of having a strong leadership team is the ability to make good decisions. When resources are scarce, every decision about their use must be a careful one. A team that recognizes the strengths of each member and is open and trusting is a vehicle to success. Listen to the stories your colleagues tell about what works in terms of motivating staff and reaching goals. Accentuate the positive. Be open to communication, especially listening. In an environment of open communication, barriers to success can be explored from different perspectives. Divergent opinions and disagreements can stimulate spirited dialogue and new ideas will emerge. Concurrence and convergence on a plan of action result in an even stronger team. Every decision should be tested for its possible short-term and long-term consequences. For example, a short-term plan of conservative staffing to save money may result in a long-term result of poor staff retention and less-than-excellent patient outcomes. It may cost more money in the long run. The more good minds you bring to bear on a problem, the better your decisions will be, as long as you are nimble and quick in getting to the plan of action.

Other Relationships

Depending on your perspective, just about everyone is your partner and/or your customer. The personal relationships you develop with each and all are an important part of your base of power. Nursing leaders usually have excellent interpersonal skills. Building relationships is easy for nurses. Capitalize on this skill. Use every opportunity to communicate and educate. You are the nursing expert. You, better than anyone, can explain why nursing is the backbone of the organization—the key to impeccable patient care and financial health.

Following is a list of leaders in your organization who can be pivotal to a nurse manager's success:

- **Chief Administrator (CEO, COO, CAO):** This person wants to be credible in the eyes of the board and the physicians. His or her goal is to ensure that high-quality health care is provided in a fiscally responsible manner. Your goal is to be seen in the eyes of this person as a key component to the organization in meeting its targets.
- **Chief Nursing Officer (CNO):** The same thoughts apply here. If you report to the CNO, always know what goals the CNO is working toward and mesh into those. Be an asset and not a liability. Suggest solutions to barriers to success. Remember to keep your conversations focused on what is best for the patient(s).
- **Human Resources Director:** This person is responsible for many functions of the organization that are key to your success—recruiting the best people, establishing competitive wages, offering benefits that retain and satisfy employees, developing feedback methods that reinforce goal-oriented performance, gathering information about employee satisfaction, and helping in the process of severing from the organization employees who do not share the values and the goals of the organization.
- **Staff Educators:** The role of these professionals is essential to your success. Collaboration with you and other nursing leaders will help the organization and, therefore, you and them achieve goals. The nurses of the organization are one of its most valuable assets. It is important to make a significant investment in the education of nurses. Start with a stellar orientation—a little extra time and effort up front will pay off handsomely. Offer education abundantly. Nurses like to keep learning. They also like to teach. Pay them a stipend when they mentor new employees. Excellent experienced nurses are the standard of care. Reward them for passing on their knowledge.
- **Chief Information Officer (CIO):** Let the CIO know you are a proponent of the organization's information systems. The electronic health record (EHR) is here to stay. Nurses must embrace it. Timesaving and error-preventing information, monitoring, and documentation systems are an absolute necessity. The learning curve may be steep, but the EHR ultimately eases the paper burden on our nurses and increases patient safety.
- **Chief Financial Officer (CFO):** The importance of this relationship has already been discussed. However, here are some encouraging words from a healthcare CFO. When asked what he expects from nurse managers he states the following: knowledge of the fundamentals of labor management, charge capture, employee satisfaction, patient satisfaction, physician satisfaction, and positive clinical outcomes. In addition, he looks to nurse leaders to maintain an open mind and positive attitude toward their financial responsibilities and to think of their work as shepherding a valuable community asset. He feels it is of prime importance for nurse managers to create a positive experience for themselves and their coworkers, including the finance people like him. He emphasizes his belief that a positive attitude goes a long way in building a collaborative culture that best serves the patient.

- **Physicians:** When nurses consistently provide excellent patient care, their greatest allies are physicians. A culture of teamwork develops. Exceptional patient care becomes the norm. Nursing alone cannot be successful. Everyone needs to embrace the thought that patients come first. Your job is to get all departments to support the work of the nurses. This is not easy to do if you appear superior or demanding. Express your appreciation. Celebrate successes. Share progress toward goals as a mutual endeavor and accomplishment.

- **Governing Board:** The governing board is your ultimate partner and customer. The Joint Commission on Accreditation of Healthcare Organizations (JCAHO) requires that the voice of nurses be heard at the board level. Ideally, the CNO attends all board meetings. At the least, the CNO should report regularly to the board. Use this forum wisely. Report progress on established goals. Emphasize improved performance. Using objective data, make your needs known, e.g., staffing requirements and competitive wages. No whining allowed. Never undercut the CEO. Rehearse your presentations. Remember that you are equal. Do not be intimidated. Communicate that *the board's goals are your goals*. Study after study shows that nurses are the most respected of all professionals. Let your presence reinforce that well-deserved stature.

Keep Your Promises

Strive tirelessly to meet and exceed the goals you establish. This is sometimes the hardest part—especially if you have set "stretch" goals (and you should). In linking mission to strategy to goals, you can develop a dashboard of indicators that helps you steer your course. These indicators include patient outcomes that reflect excellent patient care, clinical and safety outcomes, adherence to evidence-based practice, and so forth. Monitor indications of the well-being of your nurses, such as retention rate, employee satisfaction, and hours of nurse education. And, of course, monitor adherence to your staffing plan, including hours per patient day, skill mix, agency hours, and overtime hours. Review your progress frequently. It is essential that you share timely information with your staff. Celebrate successes. Develop action plans with staff input when you get off track. A good rule of thumb is that three data points are a trend. If you have three data points off track, it is time to act. Think of negative trends as opportunities for improvement instead of problems. Remember also that flexibility is important. That is not to say that you should ever lower the standard of care. Impeccable patient care is sacred. However, health care is changing so fast these days that a goal established 6 months ago might no longer be applicable. Change your plan if the plan no longer fits.

Though objective measurable goals are essential in securing the resources you need and in measuring your success, subjective feedback is also very valuable. Listen carefully to what your customers are saying—patients, families, nurses, other caregivers, and physicians. You will hear compliments and complaints. Pass the compliments on to those who have earned them. Consider the complaints as gifts. This is often free advice on how to make things better. There is a grain of truth in every complaint. Do not let complaints get you down. Remember this: When people bring their concerns to you, they believe in you. They know that you have the power to make a difference. I believe that, too. Godspeed.

There is one question, one answer, one passion: **What is right for the patient?**

Discussion Questions

1. "Make decisions on behalf of patients, the dollars will follow." What does this statement mean to you as you approach your management responsibilities to provide patient care?
2. Based on your experience or understanding, what would you say is the winning formula for achieving good patient care outcomes?

3. Some would say that you can catch more flies with honey. As a nurse administrator, how would you implement this approach?
4. What are the critical statistics that you should have on the tip of your tongue when you are justifying your needs to provide safe, quality care for your patients?
5. As the nurse manager of your unit, give examples of which elements are important for you to provide to achieve an appropriate budget. How will you use your influence as a manager to present your budget to administration to achieve the best possible outcome for your unit?
6. Communication with your nursing team is crucial. Remembering that your front-line nurses are most important for your success and excellent patient care, who are other critical partners essential to ensure exceptional patient care outcomes?

Glossary of Terms

Balanced Scorecard—a strategic management system based on measuring key performance indicators across all aspects of an organization.

Benchmarks—a standard, best practice or point of reference against which outcomes can be compared or assessed.

Evidence-Based Practice—clinical approaches supported by research findings that have proven effective at improving outcomes.

Fee for Service—a payer model in which providers are paid for each patient service regardless of outcomes.

Hours Per Patient Day—the amount of direct and indirect care that is required to provide care to a patient in a 24-hour period.

Mission Statement—a formal summary of the aims and values of a company, organization, or individual.

Nonproductive Time—the amount of employee time spent on vacation, sick days, holidays, and education.

Pay for Performance—a payer model in which providers are given financial rewards for achieving or exceeding specified quality benchmarks, and taken away when certain benchmarks are not achieved.

Productive Time—the amount of employee time spent in providing direct and indirect care to patients.

Relative Value Units or Units of Service—a financial or quantitative method of measuring patient care based on personnel time, level of skill, acuity, and resources required.

Return on Investment (ROI)—the profit made or loss sustained as a result of expenditure.

Relevant Websites

Appreciative Inquiry: http://appreciativeinquiry.case.edu

Balanced Scorecards: www.ache.org

Baldrige Performance Excellence Program: www.nist.gov/baldrige/index.cfm

Evidence-Based Practice: www.ahrq.gov/qual

Healthcare Mission Statement (example): www.nahealth.com/AboutNAH/MissionStatement

The Joint Commission: www.jointcommission.org

Nursing Mission Statement (example): www.ijhn.jhmi.edu

Personal Mission Statement (example): http://allnurses.com/post-graduate-nursing/personal-mission-statement-483464.html

Personal Values Checklist (example): www.lifecoachvictoria.com

Public Opinion, Nurses: www.nurseweek.com/features/99-7

Quantum Leadership: Love One Another

Janne Dunham-Taylor, PhD, RN

OBJECTIVES

- Define quantum leadership.
- Describe the leadership journey.
- Replace leadership fallacies.
- Become a more effective leader.
- Reach for personal mastery.
- Recognize the interconnectedness with others.

The context of leadership has changed. ***Leadership occurs in the space between individuals***. Leadership emerges from relationships, patterns of relationships, and interactions with others. *Any* person can be a leader. Leadership results from how people choose to interact with each other. The more people engage together to accomplish work in an organization, the more leadership is happening between people. Leadership emerges from the relationships taking place as work is being completed. Leadership is needed at all levels in an organization—from the patient or housekeeper to the board chairperson. Using this perspective, *everyone is a leader* as we progress through life. *Please reread this paragraph because this is the new definition of leadership.*

A significant issue in this definition is that staff nurses—what's more, aides and secretaries—do not recognize that they are leaders and that they are participating in leadership activities as they interact with everyone in the environment. Part of our responsibility as administrators is to teach staff about this, refer to it all the time, and make it a regular topic of conversation as everyone interacts together. *Everyone is a leader.* For example, the wonderful aides who provide the backbone of day-to-day care do not describe themselves as leaders, yet they (or the housekeepers) are often the people who are significant to an inpatient or resident. *Patients are leaders too:* they must make decisions about what they receive as they come to us for help. *An important role of the nurse administrator is to promote patient leadership and to develop leadership capabilities of all nursing staff so that they can more effectively perform their work.*

Quantum leadership is a dynamic, integrated process that takes place in relationships. Each of us comes to the relationship in a different leadership stage and has different perspectives. Each of us makes decisions about how we will respond at each decision point in our lives. (When we choose not to be a leader that is a decision too.) This creates a very complex environment (discussed in greater detail elsewhere in the text).

It is important to note here that the American Hospital Association (AHA) supports this concept as being important in order to move successfully from volume-based reimbursement to value-based reimbursement; (AHA calls this the *Second Curve*). As discussed in Chapter 4, reimbursement is lost when "never" events happen, or when protocols are not met as specified. Thus, reimbursement is shifting to include quality patient outcomes, not just volume. AHA (2011) lists ten strategies (given in Chapter 3) for hospitals to implement to be successful in this new climate. Strategy 6 will be shared here because it supports each employee being a leader:

> **Strategy 6: Educating and engaging employees and physicians to create leaders.** Several of the interviewees relayed that the power and success of their organization is completely based on the culture, desire, and dedication of their employees. To thrive in a second-curve market, every clinical and administrative employee must be involved in initiatives to control expenses, improve efficiency, increase quality, and understand the new accountability that hospitals have to overall population health. Interviewees emphasized that change is going to happen, and that their respective organizations must train a new breed of administrative and clinical leadership to manage that change effectively. This can be accomplished with a variety of educational and involvement strategies. Organizations noted that even small engagement in employee health and wellness programs positively impacted turnover rates. As physicians continue to become better aligned with the interests of acute-care facilities, it is a necessity to provide leadership training to clinicians who may be able to guide the integration process. (AHA, 2011, p. 18)

Love One Another

The core essence of effective leadership is *Love One Another*. Such a simple concept. Yet it is something that we may work at for a lifetime and still be able to do better! This is what soul leadership is all about, for love needs to permeate everything we do. Love dissolves conflicts. We feel better when we are loved and when we are loving. Victor Frankl (1984) discusses this in his book *Man's Search for Meaning*, written as he experienced a concentration camp during World War II: "Then I grasped the meaning of the greatest secret that human poetry and human thought and belief have to impart: The salvation of man is through love and in love" (p. 57). It is such a simple statement yet so complex to implement every moment of our lives.

The word *love* has different meanings for different people and is easily misunderstood. Some people would define love as a physical union of two bodies and the pleasure derived from that physical union. That is not the meaning we refer to here. Neither is love merely a sentimental feeling. The definition here is about a more mature love, which grows stronger as we progress through life. It is a love that abides regardless of circumstances or popularity. It is whatever feels right at the "gut level" and is in harmony with the universe. Love gives respect to each person. When love is present, it is possible to achieve very difficult goals.

Love starts *internally* because one must love and respect oneself before one is able to truly love another. Love is not always pleasant and wonderful. Love can be selfless. It can demand giving up personal comfort, where one chooses to *make sacrifices* for another, but one still loves and respects oneself in the process. Think of a mother protecting her child. To achieve this, the mother has to give up certain things.

When one is in an administrative role, it is important that the *intention* behind every thought, word, and action is love. A leader's actions always mirror the intention. (Actions speak louder than words.) People sense the intention rather than the words. Teamwork is strengthened by this mature love.

> Lead with passion, determination, sense of discovery, and commitment to self- discipline. Passion is a necessary driver to establish definiteness of purpose, knowledge of the destination, a burning desire to achieve the destination, and the perseverance to stay focused to reach the destination. A leader with passion can energize others to achieve results that others might not even dream possible. Being a passionate leader requires a great deal of energy and thus entails an equal commitment to personal renewal. Accordingly, leaders must take care of themselves before they can take care of others. (Shirey, 2007, p. 170)

Part of the passion in nurse leaders comes from *caring* for our patients (Pross, Hilton, Boykin, & Thomas, 2011). Many of those we serve are vulnerable, so it is important to serve them to the best of our ability and protect them from harm, helping them to remain true to themselves. When one has empathy and a genuine concern for others, this (love) gains support and loyalty from others. This is why some administrators are so effective.

Love is *honest* and straightforward. Information is shared. Honesty can be difficult at times, especially when it involves sharing unpleasant realities or the need for change. This requires a maturity on the part of a leader to know what is best to share and how to share it. The truth can be painful yet may be necessary to achieve a higher goal. It involves *transparency* (discussed in Chapter 3).

One very important component of administrative competence is generating *trust*. We achieve this by exhibiting consistent behaviors. *Every action the administrator takes, every word out of the administrator's mouth, needs to display honesty and integrity.* Administrators may believe that all they have to do is give lip service to the values. Instead, staff will look at the leader's actions and quickly see whether or not the administrator actually means and lives by the values. And, if the administrator does not have integrity, this has a negative, downward-spiral effect organizationally. When trust is lost, it is very hard to regain it.

When one is in harmony with the universe, this unswerving love actually *protects* an individual. Compare this with someone out of harmony with the universe who draws negativity back from the universe. What we put out there is what comes back. So, it is important to remain positive and loving, regardless of the negativity that others may choose to express. Love and compassion protect one from harm and, in addition, are contagious (Shirey, 2012). We all function best when we can be in a loving environment.

Leadership: A Journey

Welcome to the leadership journey! Every one of us is on this road because we all are in relationships as we pass through life. These principles are true for anyone in any role. However, this chapter is designed to help *nurse administrators* achieve more personal mastery in leadership. No matter where we are in this process, there is always more to learn and change. All the best on your journey!

> Leadership is a journey. It is not a trip, with an identifiable destination and triptiks to keep you on the right road. A journey unfolds gradually. It meanders. You stop and start, take side roads, get bogged down. You meet travel companions and sometimes stay with friends for a while. A journey is not predictable, even though there may be an end goal. On a journey, the process of getting there is part of the overall goal. . . .
>
> Our leadership journeys are only at *midpoint* when we have achieved a position of power.
>
> The second half of the leadership journey comes once we admit our first feelings of dissatisfaction with our leadership, for it is then that we have the opportunity to lead from our souls. . . . Soul leadership begins to emerge when we find our existing leadership style less rewarding, less satisfying than it was; when we must either shift to the inner leadership journey or recycle to an earlier leadership style which is more comfortable and predictable.
>
> The leadership journey is a matter of the soul and that is where the energy and the focus have to be. . . . This is more about inner courage and peace than it is about strategic planning. It is not about skill development, it is about facing fear, letting go of control, gaining self-worth and inner strength, finding inner freedom and moral passion—the things you learn only after you think you know it all. This journey takes you to your core, including your dark core (shame, fear of abandonment, rage), wherein lies the raw power of transformation. It is not an easy journey, and the goal is not to be successful in the traditional sense; it is to be faithful to the journey itself. The only requirement is courage. (Hagberg, 2003, pp. 273–274)

Why Is Leadership in a Financial Book?

Why have a chapter on leadership in a financial book? Because organizations put administrators in charge, and the administrators set the tone for the kind of leadership that will occur. Ineffective administration at any management level of the organization loses money—and it can be *millions* of dollars. "A fish starts to rot from the head." The effects of poor administration result in less reimbursement, more patient complications and legal issues, more unsafe issues, and decreased satisfaction levels from patients and their families, staff, physicians, and other interdisciplinary team members. And as stated in Chapter 1, the patient is the first priority, with the bottom line coming in second.

Ineffective administrative leadership *dramatically* affects the bottom line. Thus, it is very important to pay attention to the quality of administrator leadership in an organization. It is so important that this is the topic of Chapter 2, because if the administration is broken, everything else is. Likewise, effective leadership results in positive outcomes.

Starting Points

All the results of good nursing may be spoiled or utterly negated by one defect—petty management—or, in other words, by not knowing how to manage so that what you do when you are there is done when you are not.

—Florence Nightingale, 1869

The emphasis in this chapter is on the administrative leadership role. As administrators, it is important that we develop our leadership capabilities as much as possible, as well as empower staff to do the same. This achieves better outcomes.

Before we start to discuss this journey, it is important to define terms. The three terms—leadership, management, and administration—mean different things to different people. The Council on Graduate Education for Administration in Nursing (CGEAN) defines them as follows:

Leadership is the process of influencing others toward the attainment of one or more goals. Leadership comprises two types: formal and informal. Formal leadership occurs through official titular designations within an organization or society. Informal leadership occurs when the perceptions and actions of others are influenced by individuals without such official organizational or societal designations. Leadership is not limited to the accomplishment of organizational goals.

Management is the process of aligning resources with needs to attain specific goals. Management includes planning, organizing, motivating, monitoring, and evaluating human and material resources. Although management usually refers to a midlevel formal leadership function within an organization, it is also the process used at any level to align and allocate resources.

Administration comprises working with and through others to achieve the mission, values, and vision of an organization. Administration is an executive function within an organization and has ultimate accountability for defining and achieving the organization's strategic plan. Administration designates responsibility for implementing organizational goals.

Scope and Standards for Nurse Administrators

The American Nurses Association (ANA) *Nursing Administration: Scope and Standards of Practice* (2009) defines nurse administrator standards of practice. It is important for every nurse administrator to have a copy of this and to understand the standards of practice and the standards of professional performance. These are "authoritative statements by which nurses practicing within the role, population, and specialty [are] governed by this document. [This] describes the duties that [nurse administrators] are expected to competently perform" (p. vii). Credentialing in this role at the manager and nurse executive levels can be obtained through the American Nurses Credentialing Center (www.nursecredentialing.org/NurseSpecialties/NurseExecutive.aspx) and the American Organization for Nurse Executives (AONE) (www.aone.org/membership/certification/examprep.shtml).

AONE has defined nurse executive competencies as follows (www.aone.org/):

1. Communication and relationship building
   - Effective communication
   - Relationship management
   - Influence of behaviors
   - Ability to work with diversity
   - Shared decision making
   - Community involvement
   - Medical staff relationships
   - Academic relationships
2. A knowledge of the healthcare environment
   - Clinical practice knowledge
   - Patient care delivery models and work design knowledge
   - Healthcare economics knowledge
   - Healthcare policy knowledge
   - Understanding of governance
   - Understanding of evidence-based practice
   - Outcome measurement
   - Knowledge of and dedication to patient safety
   - Understanding of utilization/case management
   - Knowledge of quality improvement and metrics
   - Knowledge of risk management
3. Leadership
   - Foundational thinking skills
   - Personal journey disciplines
   - Ability to use systems thinking
   - Succession planning
   - Change management
4. Professionalism
   - Personal and professional accountability
   - Career planning
   - Ethics
   - Evidence-based clinical and management practice
   - Advocacy for the clinical enterprise and for nursing practice
   - Active membership in professional organizations
5. Business skills
   - Understanding of healthcare financing
   - Human resource management and development
   - Strategic management
   - Marketing
   - Information management and technology

Sherman and associates (2007) interviewed 120 nurse managers. Six nurse manager competency categories emerged: personal mastery; interpersonal effectiveness; human resource management; financial management; caring for self, staff, and patients; and systems thinking. The researchers list specific activities for each of these competencies. This is an excellent article and one worth having to refer to as a nurse manager orients to the role. Respondents stressed the importance of *personal mastery*. *Interpersonal effectiveness* "includes the ability not only to communicate, listen, and facilitate conflict but also to 'be a visible presence for staff.'" *Human resource management* included retention issues accompanied by "a sound selection and orientation process," understanding generational differences, "identifying what motivates and keeps staff," and keeping "an open mind about scheduling, developing, and rewarding staff" (pp. 90–93).

"Nurse staffing presented the greatest challenge." They identified *financial management* as their weakest area yet a very important one because they constantly needed to justify staffing budgets. They needed more help being able to quantify their needs financially. "The managers we interviewed were most passionate about the need to demonstrate that as a leader, you care—maintaining a connectedness to staff." *Caring for staff, patients, and self* included making rounds on patients but most—except the "very seasoned" nurse managers—needed help with better ways to care for self. "The ability to remain optimistic and resilient during times of turbulence and change" was important (Sherman et al., 2007, pp. 90–93).

Systems thinking involved recognizing the interconnections, that one cannot be isolated. They tried to develop a good organizational assessment so they could be a "big picture thinker" and "respect the perspective of other disciplines." They are "proactive in looking at new initiatives, such as changes in reimbursement, and in assessing what their impact will be on their work teams." They saw the importance of educating staff about these changes (Sherman et al., 2007, pp. 90–93).

Baker and colleagues (2012) found that nurse managers with less than 5 years of experience "spent more time mentoring charge nurses, providing indirect patient care, rounding on the unit, talking to patients and families, and spent time meeting with senior executives and nursing leaders" (p. 27). They also spent more time with their bosses. Nurse managers with more than 5 years of experience "spent the majority of their time preparing and delivering disciplinary action and spent less than half the amount of time of less experienced managers on mentoring charge nurses, rounding and meeting with senior executives and nursing leadership, reviewing resumes, and participating in recruiting activities" (p. 27). These managers also had "more proficiency with unit supplies and medications, attending and facilitating unit meetings, addressing compliance with regulatory agency standards, disseminating urgent mandatory communications, reviewing new equipment, products, and technology; participation in hospital-wide committee or task force meetings; and performing general office/clerical duties" (p. 27).

Chase (2012) discussed a Nurse Manager Competency Instrument (NMCI) and compared it with the AONE Leadership Alliance Framework.

Leadership Theories

There are various theoretical descriptions of leadership. Each captures important components of leadership. **Quantum leadership** is the emergent leadership theory espoused in this chapter.

> According to quantum leadership theory, organizational leadership emerges from the combined active engagement of all members of the organization. Thus as the engagement of individuals in the work of the organization increases, the leadership also increases. In this view, leadership is not attached to individuals but rather occurs in the space between individuals. It is not something done by one person (the leader) to many others (the followers), and it is not a role reserved for the people at the top of the organization. . . . Treating leadership as emergent fits well with the belief that individuals are intrinsically motivated, creative, and capable. (Porter-O'Grady & Malloch, 2011, p. 323)

Quantum leadership fits best with emerging quantum theory, which views change and disruption as always happening. ***Quantum leadership is necessary for survival and growth in an ever changing environment.***

In the past industrial age we had a very different view of leadership, organizations, and the world. At that time we believed the world was fixed and linear, and power was finite. A person's power was measured by how many people reported to that person. Leadership was viewed as a skill people were born with. It was believed that a leader was the person who was the boss, and the boss was the one who needed to learn how to be a better leader; everyone else was a follower. We need to replace this outmoded definition of leadership.

Past leadership theories used the leader/follower dyadic model (Roussel, 2013). These theories

> tend to be equilibrium seeking and structure preserving, taking certainty and stability as important goals. . . . Leadership is treated as a solution to particular organizational problems, specifically problems of performance. . . . [According to these theories] high levels of performance occur only when a leader of superior capability defines and directs the work to be done. (Porter-O'Grady & Malloch, 2011, p. 323)

Can you see the problem with this perspective? Leaders are not just the people in administrative roles. Instead, leaders are each of us as we participate in relationships.

Present evidence shows that we are interconnected and interdependent, that the world is constantly changing, complex, and chaotic. Communication is messy because of these interconnections. Because we are interdependent we have to rely on others to accomplish work. So, it is important for us to learn how to work together more effectively.

Therefore, the leadership theories that called for achieving equilibrium in this environment were not realistic because stasis eventually brings death (since the environment is constantly changing and chaotic). A certain amount of stasis is needed in the work environment, but it cannot be our goal, or the organization will not survive.

Another problem that occurs regularly with healthcare administrators is that many do not understand the service side of the healthcare business—what patients experience. Unfortunately, that is why at the executive level it is often only the chief nursing officer (CNO) who understands the patient perspective. When administrators are clinical professionals, they have an added patient care dimension that makes them more effective in healthcare administration. They understand the care side of our business. Healthcare administrators who lack this dimension can have an eye-opening shock when they experience a life-threatening illness and suddenly see the service side from the patient perspective. They often become more effective administrators after having had this experience. (Actually, this is sometimes the case for nurses and physicians as well!)

Coming back to leadership theories, it is no longer a question of *who* is leader (referring to the boss). Present evidence shows that we all need to be leaders. A better question is, *what* is leadership?

It is certainly important that an administrator possesses excellent leadership capabilities. However, this is not enough. In addition it is necessary for the administrator to empower and encourage all staff to be effective leaders as they do their work. The evidence supports this. Effective administrative leadership is a key factor, but it cannot stand alone. Everyone needs to be an effective leader.

Past leadership theories contribute to our current definition of leadership (Anderson, O'Connor, Manno, & Gallagher, 2010). Therefore, this text describes only a few. For instance, authentic leadership, originally based on the leader/follower dyad, can be applied to everyone's leadership capabilities, not just the leader's. These theories help administrators understand better ways to perform their administrative roles yet should be taken in the context of everyone being a leader, not just the administrator.

Authentic leadership consists of 4 components: *self-awareness* (understanding of and trust in one's motives, feelings, desires, strengths, and weaknesses), *relational transparency* (appropriate expression of one's genuine self through open sharing with followers), *internalized moral perspective* (self-regulation guided by internal moral standards rather than external pressures from groups, organizations, or society), and *balanced information processing* (willingness to objectively analyze data and solicit others' opinions before decision making). . . . Leaders who display these qualities garner the respect and trust of followers by acting in a manner consistent with their values, while facilitating an open and collaborative environment. Authentic leaders assist people to build optimism, confidence, and trust in others and encourage transparent relationships that foster commitment and promote inclusive ethical work climates. (Laschinger & Smith, 2013, p. 25)

Nurse executives identified two important characteristics of the authentic leader—having values (doing what is best for patients) and having the moral courage to do the right thing (Murphy, 2012).

Servant leadership (Neill & Saunders, 2008) is similar. The name was an attempt to get current administrators to change their view of being the authoritarian leader. Servant leadership advocates 10 principles for leaders: listening, empathy, healing, awareness, persuasion, conceptualization, foresight, stewardship, commitment to the growth of people, and community building.

Transformational leadership was first identified by Burns (1978) and Bennis and Nanus (1985). Bass (1998) developed a model that described leaders as having both transformational (charismatic, inspirational motivation, intellectual stimulation, and individualized consideration) and transactional (contingent reward, management by exception—active and passive) leadership characteristics. In his model, laissez-faire leadership also could occur where the leader does nothing. This is a leader/follower model. A number of studies were done with nurse executives using this model. McGuire and Kennerly (2006) examined nurse managers and found that "nurse managers rated themselves as more transformational than their staff perceived, but that staff nurses who perceived their manager as more transformational also demonstrated a higher organizational commitment" (p. 179). The researchers found that many of the nurse manager performance standards required transactional processes (budgets, productivity, and quality monitoring), yet the nurse manager is required to coach, mentor, and lead (transformational characteristics). These are challenging requirements.

Dunham-Taylor (1995) found that nurse executives who were rated as *most highly transformational* by staff actually rated themselves *lower* on transformational leadership scores (staff scores were higher) but higher on transactional scores than staff perceived. These CNOs were highly motivated, optimistic, energetic, and balanced. They were constantly striving to improve, were comfortable with themselves, and possessed humility and integrity. They intuitively knew when to make decisions. They coached others and had a humanistic approach in their interpersonal relationships. They inspired and motivated others and were visionaries, "stressing the importance of establishing close working relationships with people at all levels" (pp. 25–26).

Casida and Pinto-Zipp (2008) suggested that nurse manager transformational leadership

is likely to create or shape an effective nursing unit organizational culture characterized by high levels of cultural traits (mission, adaptability, involvement, and consistency). The transactional contingent reward leadership of the nurse manager is likely to create or shape certain culture traits (for example, consistency and involvement) essential for the internal operations of the nursing unit. (p. 13)

This was supported by Bally (2007).

Bodin (2012) discussed the positive effects of transformational leadership with employee satisfaction, staff retention, resilience, and productivity along with patient safety. Failla and Stichler (2008) and Moneke and Umeh (2013) showed higher levels of job satisfaction when a manager is a transformational leader.

The Magnet Recognition Program advocates transformation leadership (Clavelle, 2012; Drenkard, 2013; Luzinski, 2011; Smith, 2011; Wolf, 2012). Clavelle and colleagues (2012) reported that in magnet organizations, nurse executives' top two practices were enabling others to act and modeling the way. They need to be risk takers and innovators (Crenshaw & Yoder-Wise, 2013). Johnson and associates (2012) discussed transformational leadership and shared governance, both advocated by the Magnet program.

Houston and Wolf (2011) found that successful nurse managers possessed the following transformational leadership skills:

Inspire a Shared Vision
- Engage next level of leadership in spreading the vision
- Discuss with staff the potential barriers to change and solicit their ideas for improvement
- Spend time with staff explaining the "whys" behind proposed organizational changes
- Demonstrate the value to any change and present it with genuine enthusiasm and a positive attitude
- Engage front-line staff in leading practice changes and encourage them to become the experts
- When going through a major change, such as electronic health record or Magnet hospital designation, lead the changes by participating in the classes or becoming certified
- Communicate regularly at staff meetings proposed organizational strategic plans so that changes are not as shocking

Model the Way
- Set professional communication standards and live up to them personally on a daily basis
- Make one-on-one interactions with staff focused and meaningful
- Demonstrate a positive attitude
- Respond to staff questions quickly; demonstrate excellent follow-up in closing the loop on all matters
- Engage staff in unit-based decisions so they can then become the leaders of change
- Take a personal interest in staff and ask them what they need from you
- Assist staff as needed by role modeling behaviors that are expected of all, such as answering call lights, picking up trash, and emulating calming conversations with patients and peers

Challenge the Process
- When possible, allow staff to try out new ideas, even when skeptical, and allow them to learn from their mistakes
- When there is an adverse event, use this as an opportunity to share the story with the staff to effectuate change
- When instituting an important patient care initiative, empower the nursing staff to own the process and to engage with persons of authority
- Engage positive staff and unit-based council members in communications early in any change process so that they can assist leading change initiatives
- Listen to new staff and outsiders to get fresh ideas on current processes
- Involve staff and next-level leadership in the root cause analysis process and share the results with the staff

Enable Others to Act
- See yourself as working for the staff in your role as a nurse manager
- Be able to identify and nurture talented staff nurses to progress along a career advancement path
- Assist the staff to be part of the solution for the unit-based issues

- Be sure that you are approachable and open to staff coming to you with clinical issues—staff need to be able to trust their nurse manager
- Give staff the tools to act, but do not do all the work for them—it is important to coach and mentor, especially with tasks they have never done

Encourage the Heart

- Show the importance of individual recognition by using personalized rewards for a job well done—know when to be public and private with recognition
- Allow staff to get to know their nurse manager personally
- Encourage staff to utilize interdisciplinary rounds as a means to tell stories about their patients and learn from other disciplines
- Conduct staff meetings with a positive attitude
- Taking a personal interest in staff such as knowing their children's names, demonstrating you care about them personally (p. 249).

"Widely touted theories of transformational leadership are based on the belief that administrators have the power needed to transform a low-performing organization into a high-performing organization" (Porter-O'Grady & Malloch, 2011, p. 375). This is good but not enough. The problem with this definition is that *everyone* in the organization needs to transform the environment, not just the administrator; plus, drastic changes are constantly needed within an organization—not just making it high performing at one point in time. The organization needs to constantly change (see Chapter 3) to something better than what it is in the present reality. We are guided by doing what patients value.

There are examples where grassroots administration has produced very effective, more efficient, higher quality companies (Kerfoot, 2011):

> Ruimin, in China, reorganized his business so it could meet the demands of the retail customer faster than any other company. Employees at all levels were assigned to the units with the expectation they would work directly with customers and make necessary decisions. Managers were responsible for ensuring units were provided with key resources, but they were *not in charge* because they were not in direct contact with customers. *If the employees didn't like the way the manager was performing, they could vote that person out.* Employees were informed of productivity and quality numbers daily, allowing for quick corrections if needed. Ruimin's leadership style created the culture where new ideas and expectations can flourish because employees were driven by the quest for quality for their customers. When that is accomplished, everything else, including profitability, falls into place. (p. 290)

Kerfoot goes on to cite how a new CEO and COO came into an inner-city hospital with "a history of dysfunction and mismanagement . . . told managers and staff to solve the problems and had a remarkable turnaround" (p. 290). This is a model of *obliquity leadership* (from making oblique decisions), where staff can take a management plan and adapt it to fit their customers, each time they are with customers. All people need is a big picture of where to go, and then be empowered to get there each day as they work directly with patients. This leadership best fits the complexity issues in our current environment.

For example, medical technology continues to become less invasive and enables us to keep people alive longer. Yet in the midst of all of this we are not giving patients basic nursing care. When we involve all staff taking care of the patient (including the aides) with taking leadership responsibility and understanding the importance of giving the patient what is valued, basic nursing care becomes more valuable. Achieving it becomes a thing of pride, not something to slough off to someone else.

Many RNs do not value this aspect of nursing and expect aides to do it. Often, RN delegation skills are not well developed and teamwork is not effective. They have not learned how to be leaders for the patient, and to give each patient what the patient values. This is a wonderful example for effective shared governance councils (discussed in Chapter 3) to hammer out how to improve this deficit. Perhaps nursing care will improve because reimbursement partially depends on giving good nursing care. Good, effective administrators are a key factor in getting this process started and supporting it. But staff (including aide) leadership is even more important because each person needs to lead as he or she cares for patients. When all of this happens, everyone benefits and the organization makes money. When this does not happen everyone suffers, including the patient, the staff, and the bottom line. Most organizations do not have practice councils. Organizing these councils transforms the organization, but this does not come about just because administrators order it to be so. It takes a lot of effort and commitment across the organization.

We will be discussing *leadership* in this chapter, and ***ways that nurse administrators can enhance the leadership emerging from relationships***. We can understand this better by turning to present evidence. Understanding this information will enhance bringing love to relationships.

The Nurse Manager Role: Challenges and Opportunities

Throughout this text, nurse executive and nurse manager leadership and their effects are discussed, although the main emphasis is on nurse managers. Evidence shows that when nurse managers are effective leaders, patient outcomes are better, nurses and physicians are more satisfied, retention is better, the culture is positive, and the bottom line improves.

The nurse manager role is complicated and accompanied by many stressors. Sherman and colleagues (2007) found that workload and time management were major stressors along with the fact that a lot of the nurse manager's time was taken up with staffing and budgeting. "*Being all things to all people* was cited as a major stressor in the nurse manager role. Staying within budget and dealing with increasing numbers of regulatory issues" were other sources of stress, as were "communicating with patients, physicians, and staff, and managing conflict." Safety and quality concerns were also stressors. "Frustrations expressed about the role included lack of clerical support, staff attitudes, the disengagement of professional nurses from participation on unit issues, union activity, ongoing justification of budget variances, and disciplinary problems" (p. 89). There are many potential sources of stress in this role.

Sherman and colleagues (2007) found that new managers as opposed to more experienced managers were more likely to still be providing direct patient care:

> Experienced nurse managers reported that finding competent staff, dealing with the rising patient acuity levels, and generational issues in the workforce were all challenges they confronted. Medical-surgical nurse managers expressed concern about their ability to recruit new graduates as more nurses now begin their careers in specialty areas. (p. 89)

Zori and Morrison (2009) examined critical thinking in nurse managers.

Cathcart and Greenspan (2012) found that nurse managers need more than just knowledge about the various aspects of the role. They

> engage in demanding relational work, which is at the core of this key leadership practice. Expert managers are able to see the complexity and interrelatedness of all aspects of a situation and know how to work with nurses to support their development. Because the skill of involvement is mastered through experiential learning, relational work was often experienced as a painful challenge for new managers.

Preserving the ethical demand of the practice was, for these nurse managers, a moral source that guided their practice. Ethical demand refers to the trust that the nurse will do for the particular patient and family what needs to be done in ways that respect their concerns. . . . It was their ability to think, perceive, and act ethically as a nurse that determined what leadership actions they took, how they strategized and executed these actions, and whether their interventions were successful. (p. 558)

In addition, *self-care* and *balance* (discussed later in this chapter) were major issues for nurse managers.

Personal wellness and self-care are major challenges for the nurse managers, particularly new managers. Many of the new nurse managers reported that they had completely shut down their private lives and worked long hours. The most seasoned nurse managers discussed the ability to draw the line on how long they stayed at work as being a key survival skill. Few of the nurse managers from either group exercised on a regular basis, but most wished for better work-life balance. (Sherman et al., 2007, p. 89)

Nurse manager turnover occurs for several reasons: being overwhelmed with the responsibilities, not getting positive support/mentoring from bosses, and generational issues. Many current nurse managers are baby boomers with a wealth of experience. As they retire, it may be more difficult to fill their roles. Since the U.S. economic downturn, many baby boomers are taking later retirements. Wendler and colleagues (2009) estimated that 75% of current nurse administrators could leave the role by 2020.

This is compounded by another factor. Bulmer (2013) found that only 12–16% of nurses aspire to administrative roles. Most aspire to administrative roles during the first couple years after they have become a nurse, and the numbers decline as nurses' years in the profession increase. Nurse leadership aspiration scores were higher in nurses with higher educational degrees and lowest in nurses with associate's degrees. So, encouraging more nurses to achieve higher degrees is helpful in increasing the number of nurses who aspire to administrative roles.

A third issue contributes to this possible shortage of nurse managers. As baby boomer nurse managers retire, the newer generations are not as willing to take on all the many nurse manager responsibilities. Both Generation X and Generation Y nurses saw their parents lose positions in organizations after years of loyalty, so they want a more balanced life and are not willing to give as much to organizations. Generation Xers (the "me" generation) do not want all the responsibilities that the baby boomers assumed in manager roles. Actually, Generation Y nurses may be more likely to pursue a nurse manager role. These new nurse managers need good orientation and mentoring programs with more experienced nurse managers, reconfiguration of the role so that they have more direct time with supervisors, more recognition, and more possibilities for achieving career goals. It is likely that they will experience some pushback from older staff nurses as they assume manager roles (Sherman, 2013).

It is important to have a competent charge nurse for each shift. Some facilities have implemented a co-manager role or assistant nurse manager role where two people share manager responsibilities (Creedle, Walton, & McCann, 2012). This way, one can be there each day, Monday through Friday, to attend meetings and do other 24/7 shifts.

The charge nurse role has changed. These nurses are like air traffic controllers. They must possess good communication skills and have good collaborative skills as well as be clinically competent. They are key in meeting reimbursement requirements such as preventing readmissions, bed sores, and never events. Sherman and colleagues (2013) found that charge nurses identified five leadership domains in the role: manages communication, acts as the team coach, seen as approachable, works like an air traffic controller, and viewed as a professional (p. 36). Charge nurses need good organizational skills and need to "effectively manage their time and control their stress levels" (p. 35).

Charge nurses identified *satisfiers* in their role: developing staff, keeping patients happy, leading the team, making a difference, managing unit flow, becoming a leader, and maintaining quality (Sherman et al., 2007, p. 37). Challenges in the role in order of importance include managing conflict on the team, keeping patients and families satisfied, staying current with changes in policies and procedures, delegating care to others, ensuring good communication with team members, meeting regulatory requirements, maintaining a safe patient care environment, making staffing decisions, supervising the work of others, coaching and giving feedback, facilitating education and orientation, communicating with physicians and consulting physicians, making patient care assignments, acting as preceptor for new staff, and arranging patient transfers (p. 38).

Because the nurse manager role is so complicated and time consuming, ***changes are needed in the way responsibilities are organized or in the expectations of the role***.

Administrative Principles: Being in the Actual and Potential Realities

Chaos and complexity apply to everything going on around us. (This is explained further later in the chapter in the section titled "Choice Points: Staying Positively Interconnected.") In the administrative role, we need to be aware of chaos and complexity, as well as helping other employees understand more about them as well. Part of our administrative role is to empower each worker to be a more effective leader in his or her work. Another part of our administrative role is to be aware of both actual reality and the potential reality. As administrators, we need to help everyone make decisions that support a better potential reality, taking into account actual reality. Staff can help with this as they identify potential changes that are occurring and think of potential realities that will more effectively work with these changes. In organizations a constant dialogue about changes/potential realities needs to occur.

As an administrator it is important to always be aware of the bigger picture as well as the smaller units within the organization. Information and decisions need to be made taking both into account. "Leaders must maintain a panoramic view of the world to discern the direction their clients should take. Their ability to see intersections, relationships, and themes is what ensures that the organization will undertake the activities it needs to thrive" (Porter-O'Grady & Malloch, 2011, p. 20).

The problem with potential reality is that it *is constantly changing too*, so we cannot get stuck in one potential, not seeing other clues that are happening that don't agree with our present picture of potential reality.

Porter-O'Grady and Malloch (2011) identify 10 principles for administrators to live by that take into account complexity issues (**Exhibit 2–1**). These are *administrative competencies*:

Principle 1. The whole is actually "a web of simple and discrete networks that cannot survive or function without some intersection and interaction with each other. Complexity is the sum of simplicity" (p. 29). Thus, the whole and parts are not to be viewed in a linear sense. Instead, all are interactive and interconnected. After all, 90% of the decisions need to be made by workers as they do the work. It is like a dance with the dancers (staff) being what the audience (patients) sees, but the choreographers (administrators) are present in the background, viewing the whole and devising ways to make the dance more inspiring (by paying attention to the potential reality). All are involved in the effort, creating, little by little, a wonderful dance for patients. Thus, our work groups (the dancers) cross disciplines and departments to accomplish work (giving patients what they value). The outcome (giving patients what they value) makes the work meaningful. The choreography is played out so that the dance can achieve this outcome in the best way possible.

Exhibit 2–1   Ten Principles for Leaders

Principle 1.	Wholes are made up of smaller units that are always interacting with each other to sustain the whole.
Principle 2.	All health care is local. The integration and effectiveness of health services depend on local relationships, not centralized authorities.
Principle 3.	Anything that adds value to any part of a system adds value to the whole system.
Principle 4.	Simple systems combine with other simple systems to form more complex systems. Complexity grows incrementally through the interconnecting of smaller, simpler systems (called "chunking").
Principle 5.	Diversity is a necessity for life. Only where diversity is present can the ability to thrive be ensured. Diversity makes chaos visible, as it pushes systems to forever adapt to changes in their environment.
Principle 6.	Error is essential to creation. Both random error and conscious error are essential to the process of creation. In fact, error underpins all change. Error contributes to adaptation and thriving.
Principle 7.	Systems thrive when all their functions intersect and interact in a continual dance of relationship and transformation.
Principle 8.	There is a constant and permanent tension between equilibrium (stabilizers) and disequilibrium (challenges). This tension is essential to life and reflects the fact that disequilibrium is the universe's natural state.
Principle 9.	Change moves from the center of a system to all other parts, influencing everything else in the system. Because every system is part of a larger system, there is an ever-evolving dance of interchange between the activities inside the system and between the system and the larger system it is part of.
Principle 10.	Revolution (hyper-evolution) occurs when the many local changes are aggregated to inexorably alter the prevailing reality (called the "paradigmatic moment"). A revolution is a dramatic, almost instantaneous, change in conditions, and it presents living creatures with the challenge of adjusting quickly enough. In a revolution, many events converge to create a situation in which life can no longer be lived in the same way.

Source: Adapted from Porter-O'Grady, T., & Malloch, K. *Quantum Leadership: Advancing Innovation, Transforming Health Care,* 3rd ed. Sudbury, MA: Jones and Bartlett, p. 167.

Principle 2. Health care is accomplished locally. The most important level is where the patient is receiving care. In a linear view, the centralized, top-down model is outmoded and does not achieve the best patient outcomes. Instead, as Tom Peters observed in the past, the patient should actually be at the top of the organizational chart. Administrators serve and guide workers at this point of care to best achieve what patients value and work to improve elements in the organization that impede the workers. This is a very different perspective than the old, obsolete authoritarian system model, which has been shown to be ineffective, yet many of us cling to remnants of the linear model. In the field of organizational models, a *matrix model* is where people at any level on the organizational chart are involved in committee work together. However, in this complexity model, everyone involved at each point of care freely moves around, working together to better achieve what patients value. This happens hour by hour while giving care, during rounds, during committee meetings, and so forth.

Principle 3. We always need to ask ourselves if what we are doing adds value to the care. This is a way to evaluate meetings and processes, whether they are necessary, and whether they are accomplishing what is intended. This is why evidence-based practice is so important at all levels in an organization. "Everyone in a system is obligated to add value to the system. Everyone is doing something, even if it is negative. If someone is not adding value, he or she is taking away value" (p. 53). This is why effective teamwork is so important. If someone is good with patients, yet does not support the team, this aberrant behavior lessens the value. In administration, one sees many of the connections within the whole, and if a connection is not working effectively, this aspect of the organization must be fixed so that it can add value to the system.

Principle 4. "To understand the complexity in an organization, one needs to look for the simplicity that lies at its center" (p. 55). One starts by looking at each individual work group. For instance, a nurse aide teamed with an RN is caring for a group of patients. If the aide and RN are used to working with each other, each can help the other as events happen and still get the work accomplished. But if this dyad is not effective, not accustomed to working together, or is taking care of too many patients, this affects the teamwork and the efficiency of getting the work done. In this case, patients do not get the best care. Next, by looking at the dyads, the administrator can put them all together and assess the effectiveness of the group on the day shift for that particular day. As one does rounds, one can evaluate whether staffing is sufficient for the patient needs and whether the dyads are best organized to meet the patient needs, and so forth. Are they effective in giving patients what is valued? Starting with the smaller groups helps to understand the whole. "Each component system abides by the same rules as the larger system. The component system must have fluidity, fit, and integrity, and its parts must intersect and operate in a way that advances its contribution and value" (p. 55). This maintains the integrity of the whole.

Principle 5. "Diversity is essential for life. Only where diversity is present can the ability to thrive be ensured. Diversity makes chaos visible, as it pushes systems to forever adapt to changes in their environment" (p. 57). Differences (conflict) are a very positive force. They represent different points of view. If we listen to the different points of view, we can arrive at better decisions and be closer to the potential reality. Recognizing the importance of diversity brings new ideas and viewpoints. A system is healthy when this is valued, when people can speak up without being sanctioned to agree with the group. Group think—when everyone has to do the same thing—actually creates stasis and death (Shirey, 2012). When different opinions can be aired and valued, all benefit. This is diversity. This is a must in a complex environment.

Principle 6. "Both random error and conscious error are essential to the process of creation. In fact, error underpins all change. . . . Error is present everywhere in the universe" (p. 59). We think of errors (such as in medication administration) as being something we must eradicate. Yet errors happen even when we have done everything we should have done. This is why it is so important to do sentinel events around errors that teach us about other needed changes. And, if we do this process appropriately, it leads us to take different actions that improve the environment. In a linear system, error is viewed as something for which people are penalized. Instead, we must accept the present reality: Errors are going to happen. We will never achieve a perfect organization. Errors are valuable clues about what needs to be changed.

Principle 7.

> Systems science has taught us that the universe operates as a set of interacting forces and interdependent relationships. There is nothing in the universe that is not in some way acting on or interacting with something else. Because interdependence is an essential characteristic of systems, the leadership role in a system is critically different from the leadership role in [bureaucracies]. (p. 61)

In the linear model we do not see the interdependency existing among everything. This creates an ineffective administration. Instead, we need to see how everything is interconnected and how one action on our part has a ripple effect across the rest of the organization. Recognizing interdependencies also changes how we view workers. We want workers to be knowledgeable, make use of the evidence, and change their care as appropriate for each patient. And all workers, in all departments, are interconnected in providing the best care to the patient. Working together effectively is valued. No one is better than anyone else. All are a team in a relationship dance that transforms care for the patient.

Principle 8. Change is a constant. This creates disequilibrium. However, we need a certain degree of stability to be able to function because if things are constantly chaotic, we cannot be effective in our work. Thus, there is ebb and flow, back and forth between disequilibrium (bringing about our next change) and equilibrium (helping us to function). This always creates tension. The tension forces us to accept change. This is why, for instance, even though we have a strategic plan, something always happens midcourse that changes the direction of where we will go. Having a strategic plan is important, but it must be adaptable and flexible as changes occur. We need to be open to new realities and figure out how to change as we go along day by day, worker to worker, patient to patient. As administrators, we need to be open to change, to recognize it as it happens, and to adjust our course accordingly.

Principle 9. Guess where the center is? It is at the point of service. It includes everyone who is involved in giving patients what they value.

> The delivery of services themselves creates the system's reputation, and thus the people who deliver the services are critical to the ability of the system to thrive. They are, in fact, much more critical to the system than any other single role or factor. . . . No service system can be sustained if the point of service does not deliver. . . . The more the focus of a service system is drawn away from the point of service, the more expensive the structure of service becomes. Consistent with Taguchi's rule, the farther a decision is made from the point of service, the higher the cost, the greater the risk, and the lower the sustainability of the outcome. (pp. 68–69)

(This is Senge's 2nd second law discussed in Chapter 3.) So, we keep coming back to the organization's purpose—to give value to patients at the point of service.

Principle 10. Most changes are evolutionary, taking place gradually over time. However, sometimes a revolution happens—"a dramatic, almost instantaneous, change in conditions" (p. 71). Generally, this occurs when many events converge and make a large enough demand that a big change is needed. Because of all the complexity identified at the beginning of this chapter, healthcare organizations are being forced to make revolutionary changes in the way care is delivered. Our administrative role involves ensuring that others also realize these dynamics so that everyone can make necessary changes to remain viable.

Even though these 10 principles are not part of defined administrative roles discussed earlier in this chapter, **these 10 principles are key components for success in the leader role**. In addition, administrators are most effective if they live by these principles.

Know Thyself

Effective leadership starts from within. Although we never know ourselves completely, we must be able to accurately assess our strengths and weaknesses, know how we respond in certain situations, and be aware of our internal states and resources, our emotional awareness, our spiritual beliefs, our preferences, our biases, and our intuitive capabilities. If we do not realize what our weaknesses are, our judgment could be faulty, our interpersonal relationships may suffer, and we will not achieve our life purpose as well, or at all. Our strengths are related to our life's purpose.

We change as we begin to know ourselves better. (Of course, it is our decision whether or not to change.) This internal process is called *personal mastery*. Personal mastery does not occur immediately in life but follows a great deal of personal work. Even then it can be improved. This continual work can occur as we work internally to improve ourselves or can occur as we experience various difficulties we encounter in our environment. Sometimes hard environmental lessons or personal crises bring about a change within us even though we did not plan to change.

Difficulties we face help us grow and lead us in creative directions we never would have considered otherwise. Shirey (2012) reported studies about *resilience*.

> Employment longevity is important because the longer an individual stays in a challenging work environment, the more resilience they develop. Adequate support from colleagues and individual emotional toughening also lead to the develop of resilience. . . . Individuals with resilience possess protective factors [hardiness, self-efficacy, optimism, patience, tolerance, adaptability, and a sense of humor] that assist them to recover from and thrive despite adversity. (p. 552)

Once we understand our life purpose, it becomes a powerful motivator as we proceed through life. When activated, our imagination lights up, releases creative energy, and new ideas result. We become passionate about it. We achieve fulfillment by maximizing our potential and realizing and using our gifts. Our actualized gifts contribute to our society.

When one is doing one's life work, it is amazing how *what one needs at any point in time suddenly emerges when one needs it.* There is a synchronicity to it all.

The same is true on a larger scale. If each of us explores and develops our special gifts, everything fits together beautifully. Each person's gifts make a contribution because no one else is meeting that particular need. Thus, if we all can stay in tune with our gifts, it all fits together so that we have all we need to live full, productive lives.

Continual learning is part of personal mastery. No matter how competent we are, there is *always more to learn.* Every moment in our lives provides the teaching most needed. It gives us the opportunity to constantly grow and learn. Our choice is to trust the process and allow the lesson to seep in, or we can choose to fight it or ignore it. Learning is dynamic. Our learning changes too. What may interest us at one point in our lives may not later. Then we can learn about something new or different, or we can appreciate certain nuances that we were unaware of before. As we learn, we acquire more wisdom, accomplish our work more effectively, and become more proficient in life. There can be joy in learning new things—exploring new vistas—especially when our explorations match our gifts and interests.

In interviews with "excellent" nurse executives one said, "No matter how much things improve, there always is more that could be achieved." This did not produce frustration, but provided an ongoing commitment. These executives were highly satisfied personally and professionally—yet they balanced this with more to be accomplished (Dunham-Taylor, 1995, p. 25).

As we help others in the work group to achieve better leadership in their work roles, they need opportunities for learning, just as we do. Research has found that people like to have something different to do in their work or they get bored.

We learn in many ways. Learning is more than just passively being a sponge. It involves listening, asking questions, processing information, identifying patterns of similarity, and reflecting on events, processes, issues, or other things that have presented themselves to us. It is actually trying things, changing our behavior when warranted, and learning from the experience.

As we talk about continual learning, we need to consider our mind and its potential. According to various research studies, we use only 5% to 10% of our brains. Think of this untapped resource within each of us. We have so much more potential that could be used as we live our lives! Our minds are capable of things such as superlearning where one listens to certain music (i.e., the Mozart effect), and in this relaxed state, one has the potential to learn more effectively.

Additional personal feedback can be gained by taking work style inventories, such as the Myers-Briggs[1] or the Life-Styles Inventory[2] from Human Synergistics. These inventories can be used to identify what styles one uses when approaching life or work. Then one can determine how this differs from other styles, and how people with this style interact with people who have different styles. The Life-Styles Inventory can also be used by staff directly reporting to a manager. Here, staff members rate their perception of their manager's leadership. This provides a "360 evaluation." This view can help supervisors who may not perceive leadership problems and provide the manager with ways to improve effectiveness.

We can examine left brain/masculine/yang and right brain/feminine/yin at www.mathpower.com/brain.htm. This is a subtle process in which we need to choose the appropriate characteristic for each moment. Each trait is wonderful when used at the right time and is inappropriate when used at the wrong time. This supposes that we have the capability to access both sides of the brain at all times.

Have you noticed how certain people seem to be dominant on one side or the other? This is not balanced because these people are not using a good part of the energy within themselves. These traits are not determined by our biological sex. The attributes are all present in each of us. It is up to each of us to use them. The knowledge of which attribute to use at what time is deep within ourselves if we choose to tune in to it.

Mentors and coaches are helpful. Many excellent webinars, seminars, and educational programs add to our personal mastery. Going back for additional university degrees is also recommended by both the Magnet Recognition Program and the Institute of Medicine report, *The Future of Nursing: Leading Change, Advancing Health* (Institute of Medicine, 2010). Books such as Bolman and Deal's (2001) *Leading with Soul: An Uncommon Journey of Spirit* (a story) further explores administrator issues as one grapples with oneself in becoming more effective. There are infinite ways to develop personal mastery.

Once we possess self-awareness and expand our positive capabilities, our self-confidence and self-worth increase. We begin to be able to regulate our internal states, our impulses, and our internal resources. We have more self-control, keeping disruptive emotions and impulses in check. We strive to improve. We handle change better because we are more adaptable and flexible. We can become more comfortable with new information, different approaches, or novel ideas that help us to be more innovative. We can experience optimism—that "can do" attitude. A growing awareness of our gifts and our life purpose develops. We then can start to manifest these gifts. We can become more persistent in pursuing our goals even when obstacles cross our path or when we experience setbacks. This knowledge increases our ability to relate to the world at large.

All of this is an individual choice; it is like a spiral. The spiral can move upward toward personal mastery and fulfillment or downward in a more negative direction where we become more rigid and entrenched in our beliefs, lose integrity, and become a dictator. Pessimism and depression result. However, at any point we have a choice and can change the direction of the spiral.

From Novice to Expert Administrator

Shirey (2007) discusses administrative competencies using Benner's novice to expert model. The *novice*, in Benner's definition, is at the beginning level of proficiency:

> A novice is someone who has no background in a particular competency related to a specific role or its associated situations. The rule-governed behavior of the novice guides performance; however, this mode of leadership is limited and inflexible and requires further professional growth and development. (pp. 167–168)

The second level, *advanced beginner,*

> is usually a nurse leader who may have dealt with a variety of nursing leadership situations yet may need the frequent guidance of a mentor. They may complete the tasks required of the role, but may or may not have the peripheral vision to absorb an entire context and the implications beyond the focused task or the observable situation. (p. 168)

They learn from failures and from wise mentors.

The third level is a *competent* administrator. When an administrator has been in the role for a period of time (length of time varies), the person acquires skill. This "involves considerable conscious, abstract, and analytic contemplation of problems and issues. The competent leader may demonstrate a sense of mastery and the ability to cope with contingencies of the role. However, they may lack complex multitasking talents and flexibility" (p. 168).

In the fourth level, the *proficient* administrator possesses a holistic understanding of situations and focuses on more accurate and targeted actions in decision making.

> In complex situations, [this person can] assess an overall picture and extract the most salient aspects. This person "uses maxims (tried and tested leadership principles), abstract reasoning, and inductive processes to guide practice. [This person] is most frequently able to recognize the implications of a situation and see potential warning signals before these become apparent. (p. 168)

The *expert* administrator "has an extensive background and repertoire of experiences; is able to zero-in quickly on problems, issues or situations. [This person] has an intuitive grasp from a deep understanding of the total situation and from a sense of knowing what is right" (pp. 168–169). MacMillan-Finlayson (2010) compared seasoned nurse executives with novice nurse executives using Shirey's novice to expert model.

Dunham-Taylor's (1995) research with nurse executives identified four stages of leadership. A nurses in the *first* stage "influences others on a situational basis, is action oriented, is still learning, experiences emotional discomfort, and is working on personal change" (p. 31). *This would be like Shirey's beginner stage.* At the *second* stage, the nurse executives "used common sense; were not afraid to fail and admit mistakes; lacked a leadership definition; thought leaders were born, not made; had difficulty with balance; were aware of strengths and weaknesses; and were inconsistent" (p. 30). *This would be like the advanced beginner stage Shirey identified.*

In the *third* stage, which is highly transformational, executives

> enjoy "cleaning up" difficulties; underestimate their own abilities; are not maintenance people [meaning that they will not stay in the same position for years]; hire the best staff possible; work to develop staff; have people skills; are visionary; have perseverance; enjoy analyzing problems with staff, discussing alternatives, and then have staff decide what to do; want staff to let them know when something goes wrong; are not as balanced; personalize issues; and can become easily frustrated if standards are not met. (pp. 26–27)

This is equivalent to Shirey's competent or proficient stage.

In the *fourth*, or highest, stage, executives

> achieved more balance, were always striving for higher quality—both organizationally and personally—possessed humility, had a dynamic leadership definition and style, were deadly serious about their work, felt that their work mattered, were comfortable with change, had integrity, identified values, experienced intuitive decision making, were a coach and mentor to others, were humanistic, had humor, had charisma, were visionary, and were aware of their own humanity. (p. 29)

They often were in executive positions for years and always believed that there was more that needed to be accomplished. *This is the expert level.*

Kuhnert and Lewis (1987) identified several developmental levels of leadership in business organizations. At the *first* level, leaders are concerned only with their "personal goals and agendas" (p. 652). This approach is a selfish one. The *second* developmental level occurs when the leader is able to see that joining a group and having mutual goals and partnerships are more advantageous than the selfish goals of the first stage. The problem with the second stage is that sooner or later the leader is torn between two groups. For example, a nurse manager might realize that staff want something that is the antithesis of what the higher-level administrative group advocates. The *third* stage of leadership resolves this dilemma. At the third stage, the leader has developed end values—*doing what is best for the patient*—that "transcend" the leader's own goals and agendas. Even though the staff and the higher-level administrative groups do not agree on a goal, the leader makes a decision based on the end value of what is best for the patient.

Developing Leaders

In their nurse manager study, Sherman and colleagues (2007) identified needs of developing leaders: "The lack of career planning to become a nurse manager, a need for formal orientation and mentorship early in the transition to the role, self-care strategies to promote retention, and a need for succession planning for the nurse manager role" (p. 93).

Nurse manager orientation/mentoring programs are important (Cohen, 2013; O'Neil, Hirschkorn, Morjikian, West, & Cherner, 2008). Poor leadership on the part of managers can cause increased turn-over, negative cultures, poorer patient outcomes, and less reimbursement. Fennimore and Wolf (2011) described a leadership development program for new nurse managers, and Cadmus and Johansen (2012) described a nurse manager residency program.

Because the role is so complicated, it is important to have an experienced nurse manager mentor a new manager. Structured mentoring has been linked to nurse manager engagement. In one case, this was accompanied with 360-degree feedback as a baseline for the mentoring (Pedaline, Wolf, Dudjak, Lorenz, McLaughlin, & Ren, 2012). However, because the nurse manager role is so time consuming, the experienced nurse manager mentor may not have enough time to spend with a new nurse manager. One magnet facility hired an experienced nurse executive to coach new nurse managers for the first 4 months in the role (DeCampli, Kirby, & Baldwin, 2010).

Although this book is for nurse managers, we cannot ignore that this role produces potential directors and CNOs. The *CNO* role is also fraught with challenges and turnover issues. The nurse executive being able to influence others (for example, using the Adams Influence Model) has also been explored (Adams, 2012; Adams & Erickson, 2011; Keys, 2011) along with nurse executive turnover.

Executive coaches have been effective when working with new *nurse executives* (Ponte, Galante, Gross, & Glazer, 2006). Thompson, Wolf, and Sabatine (2012) used mentoring and coaching to develop present managers for the nurse executive role. Batcheller (2011) described an in-depth on-boarding experience for nurse executives that included a 360-degree process completed after the nurse executive had been in the role for at least a year. O'Neil and associates (2008) described content needed in leadership development programs.

Along with nurse managers and CNOs having an effective orientation/mentoring program, *charge nurses* often are not oriented to the role. It is important to develop orientation/mentoring programs for them (Homer & Ryan, 2013; Malcolm, 2013; Patrician et al., 2012; Sherman, Schwarzkopf, & Kiger, 2013). They become an excellent resource to become potential nurse managers and CNOs in the future, although Sherman and associates discovered that only 34% of charge nurses indicated they definitely would consider a nurse manager role; 21% would not consider the role; and the remaining 46% would possibly consider the nurse manager role (p. 36). Interestingly, "some charge nurses reported that they currently make more than their managers with overtime and shift differentials. Many also felt they had more job security in their current roles and worked fewer hours" (p. 36).

Succession planning is important (Benjamin, Riskus, & Skalla, 2011; Beyers, 2006; Blouin, Neistadt, McDonagh, & Helfnad, 2006; Bonczek & Woodard, 2006; Cadmus, 2006; Carriere, Cummings, Muise, & Newburn-Cook, 2009; Coughlin & Hogan, 2008; Goudreau & Hardy, 2006; Kim, 2012; Pedaline et al., 2012; Redman, 2006; Sverdlik, 2012; Swan & Moye, 2009). One possible strategy is to develop nurse management internships that allow staff to explore and be mentored in the manager role (Wendler et al., 2009). Benjamin and associates (2011) suggested a 5-day curriculum for leadership development. Wolf, Bradle, and Greenhouse (2006) described a three-level leadership development program. This way there are people ready to assume manager roles as the positions become vacant. However, most organizations do not have a succession plan and need to implement one.

processes: mentoring and coaching others in their learning and development, fostering staff creativity, encouraging growth, determining and trying out new solutions, enhancing and recognizing staff successes, protecting staff from unnecessary work, and respecting and valuing staff contributions.

Because each staff member has different gifts, this process varies with each person. Empowerment also occurs in times of trouble. Giving staff support and help when they are overwhelmed or experiencing a problem, discussing possible alternatives in a difficult situation, or even recognizing mistakes but making sure that someone is not devastated by what they have done are all examples of empowerment. "Employees represent an organization's most valuable asset. Creating an environment that supports coaching and life-long learning nurtures the growth and development of individuals, enhances the value of organizations, and raises the bar for performance" (Shirey, 2007, p. 169).

A difficulty for Fours is their mismatch with the Stage Three environment and the lack of trust among people that that engenders as a result. The people at Stage Three wonder what Fours' agenda is because they are not used to Stage Four behavior. This is not a fault of the Fours but a by-product of them being different from the norm. People who manage Fours soon realize that Fours are not motivated by the same things that Threes are. They cannot be persuaded to do things with the suggestion of rewards such as money or promotions. Because their motives are not traditional, they are sometimes viewed suspiciously (Hagberg, 2003, pp. 114–115).

In Stage Four, there are two traps—both coming from the ego. The first is just struggling with the ego. The second is that Fours have not "experienced a need for a meaningful, other-oriented life purpose" (p. 123). Before a person can move into Stage Five, he or she reaches **The Wall**. Here, the person comes face to face with the ego. At this stage, the only way to overcome the ego is to go within. The individual needs to discover a meaningful life purpose. This process is different for everyone. There is no cookie-cutter approach or one-size-fits-all. The answer is found within.

Stage Five is Power by Purpose:

> Stage Five is unlike all of the preceding stages. Its uniqueness lies in the strength of the inner person relative to the strength of the organizational hold on that person. The guide for behavior in Fives is the inner intuitive voice. They trust it more than they trust the rules. Stage Fives are different internally and externally now. They are more congruent because they no longer have to live two separate lives as Stage Fours do. And it is even harder to spot Fives because they don't care if they're ever spotted. In fact, they may even hide a bit. Fives have a life "calling" that extends beyond them. (p. 145)

Here is where the infinite power definition comes in. "Power is like love: You can't have it truly until you give it away or let it go, and the more of it you give unselfishly, the more it multiplies" (p. 146) and comes back to you in different ways. Fives let others lead. They believe that power is based on values—not on organizational norms or positions—and make decisions accordingly. "They do not attempt to gain or accumulate power because they find the other forms in which it reappears, like caring, appreciation, and friendship, more rewarding" (p. 146). They are humble and possess inner vision. They concentrate on the things that give meaning—both to themselves and to others. Their ultimate objective is to empower others. They do not need to be in charge, preferring to work behind the scenes. It is their faith and their willingness to give up everything that is important to them, that moves them on to Stage Six.

People at *Stage Six, Power by Wisdom*, possess inner vision.

> Stage Six people are very involved with life yet detached from their involvement. They see from a different eye, hear with an unusual ear, and feel with a new heart. They are a paradox, even yet, at the same time, they are deeply moved by the pain and stress in themselves and in the rest of the world. (p. 177)

Sixes are willing to sacrifice themselves for a cause. They often spend a lot of time alone and gain strength from higher sources. They possess an inner calm and have quiet strength. These individuals often go unrecognized because they choose not to take prominent positions. Instead, they prefer to be alone, tuning into higher sources.

Using Hagberg's definitions of power, it becomes more obvious how to define effective leadership. ***"People can be leaders at any stage of personal power, but they cannot be TRUE leaders until they reach Stage Four—Power by Reflection"*** (p. 201).

True leaders:

> Follow a calling, a purpose, an ideal
> Allow for win-win, not just win-lose
> Embrace their own shadows
> Empower others, not themselves
> Have balance in life, between work, community, and family
> Can be vulnerable and reflective
> Treat women, men, and people of color as equals
> Ask why, not how
> Have a spiritual connection to a power within and beyond themselves
> See the bottom line as a means to a larger organizational purpose, not an end in itself
> Live with integrity as their hallmark (p. 205)

In **Exhibit 2–3**, Hagberg portrays how a person at each stage leads. Looking at this, one can see that the authoritarian leader is actually at Stage One. However, leaders at Stage Two are not much of an improvement because they are playing by the rules. At Stage Three, though they still see power as external, leaders use personal persuasion to influence others. Many times this is seen as charisma. Personal persuasion can be confused with getting people to do what one wants. A better approach is to involve, listen to, and empower all stakeholders in deciding upon the change.

No matter where we currently are, we can learn, grow, and change. As we do, this will be reflected in our leadership, which will become more mature.

Exhibit 2–3 Hagberg's Summary of Leadership and Power at Each Stage of Power			
Stage	**They lead by**	**They inspire**	**They require**
Stage 1	Domination, force	Fear of being hurt	Blind obedience
Stage 2	Sticking to the rules	Dependence	Followers to need them
Stage 3	Charisma, personal persuasion	A winning attitude	Loyalty
Stage 4	Modeling integrity, generating trust	Hope for self and organization	Consistency, honesty
Stage 5	Empowering others, service to others	Love and service	Self-acceptance, calling
Stage 6	Wisdom, a way of being	Inner peace	Anything/everything/nothing

Source: Copyright © 2003 by Janet O. Hagberg. Used with permission of author.

Integrity

Leaders at Stage Four lead by modeling integrity. The bedrock of quantum leadership is integrity—remaining true to oneself. It is where one's actions support one's words; where one can look in the mirror in the morning and feel at peace with oneself. When we live it, we are strong and balanced. We are *tuned in to that inner core* that lets us know what is right in a situation. There is a oneness within ourselves. As we work toward this wholeness, every situation we encounter helps us to better understand and reach toward this wholeness.

> Character and values come first. Staying true to one's values and leading in a way consistent with values set the tone for any organization. Leaders who do the right things for people and organizations usually see positive results from their efforts. The true testament of the leader's core values will come from those who observe the leader's character and ultimately equate actions with enhanced credibility. (Shirey, 2007, p. 169)

Integrity becomes our choice each moment in our lives. It is a series of choices, each adding to the other. It is incremental. It spirals. In a previous leadership study with "excellent" nurse executives, they stressed the importance of having very high professional, moral, and ethical standards—and of not compromising those standards. In other words, they stressed the importance of integrity (Dunham-Taylor, 1995).

Simons's (2002) research, which examined managers' behavioral integrity in business settings, found that ***managers that had integrity actually made more money***:

> The ripple effect we saw was stunning. Hotels where employees strongly believed their managers followed through on promises and demonstrated the values they preached, were substantially more profitable than those whose managers scored average or lower. So strong was the link, in fact, that . . . a profit increase of more than $250,000 per year [was noted]. No other single aspect of manager behavior that we measured had as large an impact on profits. (p. 18)

When we have integrity we are *authentic* and appreciate authenticity in others. We are able to accept, and even delight in, others' differences and successes. We put people first and often get recharged by people. This calls for honesty and sensitivity—accuracy in interpreting social cues, recognition of all the interconnections between us, treating everyone with dignity, and knowing that we need to build links among individuals, groups, the community, and society.

Empowerment Based on Gifts and Abilities

> By allowing others to shine, that light will end up somehow reflecting back to you.
>
> —*Nurse executive*[3]

Many definitions of *empowerment* exist. Two people using this term may mean very different things. Some administrators will say, "I empower staff. I let them do the work," meaning "I delegate the work but make sure you do it my way." In actuality, empowerment has a very different definition in quantum leadership. Instead Hagberg (2003) describes "empowering others to be more fully human and more fully satisfied" (p. 215).

Empowerment does not begin to occur until Stage Four when a person begins to realize that power comes from internal sources; Stage Five leads by empowerment. An administrator is not an effective leader until one is able to empower others. Effective leadership involves empowering staff to do work that is a match with their gifts. That is why "Maxwel hypothesized that being immensely secure in yourself is at the heart of serving people" (Kowalski & Yoder-Wise, 2003, p. 30).

Administrators in quantum organizations work to empower employees and ensure they have the freedom to make suggestions, grow and mature, and become sensitized to themselves and others . . . Instead of the chief executive and managers thinking for everyone, all individuals in the organization think (Porter-O'Grady & Malloch, 2011, p. 381).

After all, leadership is not the people in administrative positions; it is the *result of interactions* of all employees with each other and with patients and significant others.

Also, empowerment is necessary because often a worker is better qualified to make decisions about the work than the supervisor is. A worker should make 90% of the decisions about his or her work. This is especially true now, in the Information Age, when information is more technical and complex. When we empower, we trust. Our message is that we know employees can accomplish the work successfully. Actually, **it is best if people's abilities are stretched in an empowering environment**.

In transformational leadership, this kind of empowerment is called *individualized consideration*. Individualized consideration is needed because people have different abilities and gifts. A leader delegates differently to different individuals. Leaders empower by giving as much responsibility to staff and patients at all levels to make the most of whatever talents and experience they have. When empowerment occurs, magic happens!

Laschinger and Smith (2013) reported that "empowering leadership practices and work conditions promote collegial relationships among healthcare team members. Furthermore, authentic leadership, a relational leadership style that employs open interactions between leaders and followers, has been linked to stronger feelings of empowerment" (p. 25).

In an integrated review, Rao (2012) discussed how this achieves decreased burnout, decreased job strain, increased trust in the workplace, increased job satisfaction, improved patient outcomes, increased motivation, risk taking, an achievement orientation, and high career aspirations. In addition, nurses identified having informal power to change things and were engaged in their work. A lack of empowerment results in feelings of failure and frustration among nurses, as well as poorer patient outcomes.

When empowerment is in place, all the positives can happen (Rao, 2012; Shirey, 2012). However, if empowerment does not occur, it spirals negatively.

Pygmalion Effect

Empowerment is linked to the Pygmalion effect that shows in a powerful way how we, in administrative roles, influence others in either positive or negative ways. This concept is discussed in detail in a classic *Harvard Business Review* article, "Pygmalion in Management" (Livingston, 2003). Research has shown, and continues to show, that a **supervisor's beliefs about the person being supervised become a self-fulfilling prophecy**—even when the person may believe the opposite. In other words, if a nurse executive believes that a nurse manager is doing a poor job, even a high-achieving nurse manager will eventually do poor work. And the opposite is true. If the nurse manager believes that a staff member is a wonderful employee, this belief becomes a self-fulfilling prophecy. Conversely, as in the movie *My Fair Lady*, even when the staff member believes he or she cannot do the job, **as long as the supervisor believes the staff member can do the job, the staff member will successfully accomplish the work**. This is why it is important for nurse managers to have good chemistry with their supervisors as well as with those who report to them. When this occurs, anyone can succeed.

This is a powerful message for administrators. *We first need to examine our own beliefs about the people who report to us.* Ask yourself, "Do I believe this person is doing well or is capable of doing well on the job?" Self-examination of one's own likes and dislikes, as well as acknowledging personal biases, is the first step one must take in a supervisory role. An administrator **must** be positive about each employee's capabilities.

The *Harvard Business Review* article makes another important point. Effective leaders provide "high performance expectations that [staff members] fulfill," whereas ineffective leaders "fail to develop similar expectations, and as a consequence, the productivity of their [staff] suffers" (Livingston, 2003, p. 122). *Do we administrators set high performance expectations for staff—and expect that staff will accomplish these?* When we care for the caregiver, the caregiver will then care for the patients.

Supporting the importance of ***having good chemistry with one's boss,*** Laschinger, Purdy, and Almost (2007) reported "higher quality relationships with the nurse manager's immediate supervisor were associated with greater manager structural and psychological empowerment and, consequently, greater job satisfaction" (p. 221). Obviously, this needs to happen from the top down in an organization. "Keep in mind two critical findings from the literature: direct care nurses tend to leave an organization because of their managers, and managers who feel supported by their organizations reciprocate this support with their staffs" (Baker et al., 2012, p. 25). It is best that everyone be empowered to go ahead with their work in ways that support the core value, such as *what is best for the patient.* After all, all have something unique to offer based on their gifts, but our ultimate goal still needs to be the patient.

Empowering is effective because people want to make a difference. We want our lives to have meaning. Each of us comes to this world to accomplish something special that no one else will do. This serves a larger purpose, making this a better world. We reach our highest potential when we pursue and use our gifts. Identification of our personal gifts starts us on the road to achieving our life purpose.

At times people are in jobs that are not a match with their gifts. They may not be performing well because they are not engaged in the work; the work does not tie in with their life purpose and their gifts. They are probably unhappy and are in the wrong job. As a leader, you may need to talk to a person when you perceive a mismatch between his or her work and gifts. A change in jobs might be best.

Humility

By the time people have reached the fifth and sixth power stages, they have humility.

> Eisenhower never fell into the trap, . . . believing the rules no longer applied to him or that he was better than anyone else. . . . He was never arrogant or condescending, and he was thoroughly honest. . . . Humility like Ike's, who conveys absolute assurance but at the same time acknowledges a leader's equality with followers, can be truly inspiring. (Gergen, 2003, p. 21)

Humility comes from being aware of our vulnerabilities and weaknesses. We are aware there is still so much more to learn and improve about ourselves. We are harder on ourselves than others will be. We are brutally honest about our motivations. We are committed to our life purpose. At the same time we begin to see in the scheme of things how insignificant we are. It is being aware of one's limitations, and emotional self-awareness, where one accurately knows one's positive and negative biases (Snow, 2001). As this awareness grows, we become more humble. "It means to act according to one's conscious conviction, but still always having the humility to keep the door open and be proved wrong" (von Franz, 1980, p. 145).

> A leader's most important character traits are humility, the ability to listen to others, and the willingness to give up power. In sharing power, greater influence is achieved for purposes of generating greater good for the organization and the communities served. (Shirey, 2007, p. 170)

Wisdom

Wisdom is the result of learning from our experiences. When things are clouded, then it is not yet time to understand. Once we understand, we have a choice: Do we follow what our inner core tells us, or do we ignore it? If and when we do follow that inner guidance, the world becomes clearer, and more opportunities, including challenges, occur to improve our achievement of our life's purpose.

Wisdom is often enhanced by such events as encountering a crucible experience or achieving a quietness within that help us lose our sense of self (as contained in *self-ish*), gain our sense of selflessness, and realize our interdependence with the world.

One bonus of a quest for personal mastery is that it leads to wisdom. Interestingly, as we become wise and possess wisdom in some areas, chances are we are beginning learners in other areas. After all, there are so many things to explore in this world. Have you ever heard the statement, *the more you know, the more you know you don't know*? Wisdom is enhanced when we develop a broad knowledge base and possess practical knowledge based on life experience yet have insights about situations or people and can perceive the motivations of others. It is a road that spirals ever upward if we are paying attention to what is within.

Choice Points: Staying Positively Interconnected

Administrators need to understand the present reality because we need to help others understand what is happening around us. Many do not realize that change is a constant. Evidence from quantum physics shows that change is a dynamic activity. *Dynamic* means always changing. This dynamic permeates everything except love: Love is the strongest of the constants, and can bring about change. In the next chapter we discuss complexity and chaos. They are also dynamic constants we have no 'control' over these occurring. *Our only choice is how we respond to them.*

However, the good news is that all of this change, chaos, and complexity is self-organizing. Porter-O'Grady and Malloch (2011) observed:

- Everything in the universe is self-organizing. The patterns, webs, and intersections of life create a mosaic of intense goodness of fit that reveals the ultimate connection between all the elements of the universe.
- People, too, are part of the universal network of relationships and are co-creators in the ever-constant unfolding and self-organizing activity.
- Organizations (systems), as smaller reflections of the universe, are self-organizing, complex, and adaptive entities in which people purposefully express their creativity, energy, and meaning together. (p. 467)

For our leadership (and administrative role) to be effective, we need to work to understand current changes so that we can more effectively deal with them. At the same time, we need to help others do the same.

> The science of quantum physics has demonstrated that our world actually occurs in very short, rapid bursts of light. What we believe we see as the swing of a baseball batter on home plate, for example, in quantum terms is actually a series of individual events that happen very fast and very close together. Similar to the many still images that make up a moving film, these events are actually tiny pulses of light called *quanta*. . . . Quantum physics is the study of these minute units of radiating waves, *nonphysical* forces whose movements create our *physical* world. (Braden, 2000, p. 96)

So, it appears that the world and our life force are actually energy—nonphysical forces that move. As an event happens, there are *many possibilities* (*potentialities*) of what could happen because each little force of movement can change direction at any point in time. This fact gives us hope because, although we cannot change how other people choose to respond to events, we ***can*** choose how *we respond to events happening around us.* "The existence of many outcomes for a given event has been predicted by quantum physicists for [ninety] years" (p. 97). These ***choice points*** "make it possible to begin one path and change course to experience the outcome of a new path" (p. 100).

As administrators, we can enhance our leadership capability by realizing that we can choose how we respond at each choice point. Each choice point becomes an opportunity to make situations better.

> Sustainability in organizations comes not from maintaining the status quo, but rather from recognizing change as a constant and supporting a trail blazing spirit. In understanding that excellence is a journey and not a destination, the leader creates possibilities and restores hope in the future. (Shirey, 2007, p. 169)

To better understand choice points, we need to understand another constant—*duality*. In this world there will always be duality—having two parts, a dichotomy: positive and negative, good and evil, male and female, yin and yang. We cannot "control" duality either; it exists. It complicates the situations we face each day. *Our only choice is in how we respond to it.*

Most of us, deep down inside, want harmony and usually make positive choices toward that end. "Happy, well rested, and inspired people will perform better work" (Douglas, 2012, pp. 117, 119.). However, duality is present. Thus, some people will delight in, or out of frustration, will cause, chaos and negativity. They have gotten stuck in negativity as the most effective way to respond to the world.

> Energy comes from knowing that you are significant, that your work is important, and that you can work in an environment that fosters and supports your passions. The leader who is engaged and passionate about the work will communicate this to staff who will then feel the contagion and the excitement. Creating an optimistic culture where people feel they have hope and freedom to grow and mature will create that sense of engagement. (Kerfoot, 2007, p. 48)

If we choose to stay positive, our reality is positive. Positive energy—love and compassion—come back to us (Shirey, 2012). If we choose the negative choice, more negativity comes back to us. This concept was captured in *Zapp! Empowerment in Health Care* (Byham, Cox, & Nelson, 1996)—written as a novel—where a nurse manager begins to realize that specific negative interactions sap the energy of the people involved, whereas people become energized by other positive interactions (zapp).

Mackoff and Triolo (2008a) studied nurse manager engagement.

> This study revealed rich data linking individual signature behaviors to nurse manager vitality and longevity. The analysis identified 10 individual signature behaviors that revealed the experiences, capabilities, and attributes of long-term individual nurse managers: mission driven, generativity, ardor, identification with the work of others, boundary clarity (building strong connections with others—without losing the sense of self; not taking things personally), reflection (learning through the experience of doing things wrong), self-regulation (using restraint to keep emotions in check, suspending judgment, and conserving energy), attunement (learning about a reality quite different from my own, recognition of unique strengths of staff), change agility (challenging the process or status quo, welcoming and initiating change, and seeking change through new learning), and affirmative framework (optimistic explanatory style, positive expectations, resilient behaviors). (p. 123)

This study also identified five organizational culture factors that contributed to nurse manager engagement: a learning culture (organizational support of learning and growth), a culture of regard (being valued as a prime driver in the organization accompanied by being empowered in the role), a culture of meaning (their mindfulness of organizational mission and values), generative culture (a commitment to caring for, and contributing to, the next generation), and a culture of excellence ("We go over the top for everything. We are about being better and having high standards and striving. The bar here is high for everything") (Mackoff & Triolo, 2008b, pp. 167, 169).

Encouraging everyone's *humor*—a positive—enhances relationships. Humor can make the world a better place because it relieves tension. When we enjoy our work and those we work with, life is so much more fun. All can enjoy life, work, and the workplace when everyone can express their lighter side. This is why it is important to stay positive.

> Leaders should create organizational cultures of caring, respect, and dignity for all. Having a sense of purpose and belonging enhances sense of community and creates the joy necessary to freely contribute individual talents to benefit the whole. To sustain a positive workplace for all, leaders should personally model a sense of balance between work and play and humor and seriousness. (Shirey, 2007, p. 169)

Negative emotions—anger, hate, jealousy, revenge—come back to us. The biblical story about Job exemplifies this. Because he worried about various calamities (he put emotion behind his worries), they became his reality. Job chose to put energy into the negative. It is better to replace worry (a negative) with a picture of something positive. Dysfunctional behaviors by administrators, such as having bosses who do not believe in those who report to them and "feeling trapped in the middle, but playing along; and keeping their heads down and paying the price," result in *organizational fatigue* (Connaughton & Hasinger, 2007).

To understand how powerful negativity is, Huseman (2009) observed:

1. We tend to remember failures more vividly than success.
2. We tend to react more strongly to negative stimulus than we do positive.
3. We tend to trust negative information more than we do positive.
4. When we experience joy it is short lived and then we start taking what caused the joy for granted. (pp. 60–61)

How do we deal with negativity? The first clue is that negativity is always a choice we make at each choice point. At any point, we can turn it around. Mentoring and counseling can help. When dealing with negativity in the workplace, studies show that people have three strong needs at work: "1) the need to feel connected to and competent in their work; 2) the need to strengthen/develop their capabilities and build their careers; and 3) the need for recognition" (Huseman, 2009, p. 63). Having an engaged supervisor is key. "Having leaders at every level adopt a leadership style using praise and recognition is one of the quickest ways to counteract negativity" (p. 63).

Negative emotions at work affect productivity, performance, and retention. The problem is that negativity also spreads to patients and can affect patient outcomes. For instance, Huseman (2009) cites one study where nurses' general mood on some cardiac care units was depressed, and the death rate was four times higher than on other similar units.

Evidence supports this. In quantum physics, researchers found that *our thoughts create our reality.* "Recent research has documented that our emotions and feelings directly influence the expression of DNA in our bodies" (Braden, 2000, p. 207). This is why prayer can be so powerful.

Knowing this, we need to examine our thoughts (or the contents of our prayers). Are they negative or positive? For example, someone asked Mother Teresa if she would attend an anti-*war* rally. She refused. She said she would be happy to attend a *peace* rally. *She wanted to put her attention only into positives.* This is also true of prayer. Sometimes we have patients who have whole prayer chains going for their benefit. If the prayer chains are for their good health, that is a positive outcome. If the prayer chains are to do away with their cancer (or whatever is wrong with them), it actually puts more energy into what the patient does not want! What reality do we want to choose?

Examining the negative emotions, fear, for example, is something that most of us do. People's fears vary greatly, but one commonality is that many fears are about things that may never happen. Yet we put energy into them because we get emotionally involved with fear. Giving something a lot of energy, especially when there is emotion behind it, makes it more powerful. We have already mentioned how negativity harms our DNA. So, the question is, *do we realize that when we worry, or when we are fearful or angry, we are emotionally putting energy into negative things?*

Taking this a bit further, Louise Hay (1984) in *Heal Your Body* gives positive affirmations for diseases many people experience.

> Both the good in our lives and the dis-ease are the results of mental thought patterns. We all have many thought patterns that produce good, positive experiences, and these we enjoy. It is the negative thought patterns that produce uncomfortable, unrewarding experiences with which we are concerned. It is our desire to change our dis-ease in life into perfect health. We have learned that for every effect in our lives, there is a thought pattern that precedes and maintains it. Our consistent thinking patterns create our experiences. Therefore, by changing our thinking patterns, we can change our experiences. (p. 5)

So, evidence shows that DNA changes are associated with negative thoughts, and vice versa. It is our choice—and a choice of all those around us—whether to be negative or positive. The Hopi say, "When prayer and meditation are used rather than relying on new inventions to create more imbalance, then humanity will also find the true path" (Braden, 2000, p. 233).

Balance/Listening to the Inner Voice

How is life created? Why do miracles happen? Quantum physics discovered that:

> For there to be an end to one pulse of light before the next pulse begins, there must, by definition, be a space in between. Viewing our experience on earth as a small metaphor for the large-scale experience of the cosmos (as above, so below), is the *breath* of the cosmos. . . . It is in the spaces between, in the silence [stillness] between the pulses of creation, that we have the opportunity to "jump" from one possibility to the next. This space is where the miracles occur. (Braden, p. 101)

The space in between choice points is like the "breath of God" in the Bible. In Sanskrit it is called *prana*. "Like electricity in the air, it is omnipresent. It is also omnipotent. In it lies all energy, either latent or dynamic. It only awaits the proper conditions to express itself as dynamic force in one form or another" (Johnson, 1997, p. 399). It is what gives us life. This is the source of love.

We can tune in to this space. Brooks (1966) suggested that through stillness we can find the answers:

> The cultivation of inner quiet, [gives one] a heightened receptivity. . . . As long as the head is still busy, full sensory receptivity is impossible. With increasing stillness in the head, all perception, traveling unimpeded through the organism, automatically becomes sharper and more in context. In this new stage of more awareness and permissiveness the self-directive powers of the organism reveal themselves ever clearer, and we experience on a deeper level the unexpected transformations we can undergo. . . . [When] one reaches a state of relative balance, simultaneous changes happen throughout the whole person. The closer we come to such a state of greater balance in the head, the quieter we become, the more our head "clears," the lighter and more potent we feel. Energy formerly bound is now more and more at our disposal. . . . We find ourselves being more one with the world where we formerly had to cross barriers. Thoughts and ideas "come" in lucidity instead of being produced. We don't have to try to express ourselves . . . but utterances become just part of natural functioning. Experiences can be allowed to be more fully received and to mature in us. As Heinrich Jacoby once remarked: "Through becoming conscious we have been driven out of paradise, through consciousness we can come back to paradise." (pp. 502–503)

In the West, we do not value *contemplation*. However, contemplation can help us keep things in perspective and keep bringing in love. Love is infinite—there is always more available for us. Instead of getting upset when something goes wrong, it can be helpful to think ahead 5 years: How important will this issue be then? Perhaps we will not even remember it. Or perhaps the incident will lead to something unexpected but better. So, *keeping things in perspective* can help us be more effective administrators.

Consider the following:

> Ultimately we have just one moral duty: to reclaim large areas of peace in ourselves, more and more peace, and to reflect it towards others. And the more peace there is in us, the more peace there will also be in our troubled world. (quote from Etty Hillesum, Holocaust victim; in *Real Power: Stages of Personal Power in Organizations*, Hagberg, 2003, p. 273)

In the West, we are more likely to call this spirituality. Research indicates that "spirituality is associated with better physical, psychological, and social health and that culturally diverse populations and individuals at end-of-life often request spiritual care" (Burkhart, Solari-Twadell, & Haas, 2008, p. 33). Earlier we discussed why prayer is so powerful in quantum perspective. This is important because what we believe is more likely to happen, especially when we add emotion to prayer.

Inner quiet is intertwined with *balance*. When balance is achieved, we are calm yet have energy for whatever we believe is important at that moment. We live in the moment, not the past nor the future. Living in the moment means just what it says: giving our attention to what is happening at that moment, leaving other cares or worries elsewhere, not remembering the past—which has already happened and we cannot change—not thinking of the future—which has not happened and is yet to be.

A discussion of balance cannot avoid the issue of what causes *stress*. *Stress varies for different people.* Eustress is a positive form of stress, and distress is an undesirable form of stress. *Stress is useful when it mobilizes us to take action. It is harmful when it buries us in negativity.* Negative stress can affect our immune system and create disease. What causes stress in one person may not in another. Why is that? It depends on our perspective about issues confronting us. For example, a woman suddenly lost her son in a tragic accident. She said, "It's amazing to think about what used to cause me stress. It was little things that I won't even remember tomorrow. Those things are not important in the scheme of life. *Now I realize that only the far more important matters are stressful issues.*"

Various coping mechanisms can help one keep balance. Smith (2013) recommended: (1) accept that self-care isn't selfish; (2) manage time effectively; (3) learn how to say no comfortably and confidently; (4) set limits; (5) live, love, and laugh every day (pp. 31–32). First, it is important to always remain positive: "Everything will work out perfectly," or "I am in perfect health." Coping mechanisms differ for each person, ranging from swimming, walking, or running to meditation and prayer, to sitting on a mountain looking at the view, to regulating breathing. It is best if this can occur on a regular basis. In fact, to decrease stress and encourage health in employees, some companies encourage staff to exercise in facilities provided by the employer, to not take work home in the evening, to engage in counseling made available for employees, to provide massage therapy for employees, and to have better health habits such as eating more nutritious foods, not smoking, and so forth. Specific ways to achieve balance, as well as encouraging others to achieve balance, are infinite.

Shirey and colleagues (2010) found that nurse managers experienced perceived stress

> when dealing with negative people; with organizational politics—lack of transparency, and lack of interdepartmental collaboration; and people and resource issues—patient and family complaints, maintaining physician relationships, procuring individuals to fill position vacancies, and navigating difficult matrix reporting relationships. (p. 84)

This stress can be increased because of

> high levels of responsibility and knowing what the right thing to do was yet lacking the power to get it done; along with not having enough hours in the day to do the work, being torn in multiple directions, having excessive committee meetings, and experiencing numerous daily interruptions. (p. 84)

Two-thirds of nurse managers "cited issues that included organizational red tape, interpersonal conflict, changing regulatory requirements, multiple ongoing hospital initiatives occurring simultaneously, and system inefficiencies as factors that increase stress" (p. 84).

When asked what factors *decreased their stress*, nurse managers identified four categories:

> Focusing on the positives, having support from others, completing work and achieving targets, and incorporating quality downtime. All of the nurse managers discussed factors that decreased stress, yet only 86%, all experienced nurse managers, actively pursued ways to decrease stress. The experienced nurse managers used mind over matter to "psyche themselves" into avoiding negativity. Having support available was important, and the comanagers reported higher levels of support that empowered them in their roles and helped them get the sheer volume of work completed. Achieving targets was important, yet nurse managers reported that, given the multiple interruptions in their daily work, having the ability to complete a project at work without interruptions was a luxury. Most of the nurse managers (except the comanagers) had difficulty saying no to one more thing on their plates. The less experienced nurse managers reported having the most difficulty saying no and negotiating modifications to their workloads. (pp. 86–87)

Emotions associated with stress fell into three categories: pure positive emotions, pure negative emotions, and mixed emotions. Ninety-one percent of nurse managers stated that they liked their jobs, including loving their work; 14%, both novice and experienced, expressed turnover ideation that had to do with emotions associated with the role's infringement upon their work–life balance and perceived lack of support in their role. All nurse managers verbalized (mixed emotions) associated with the difficult situations: loving all the changes that came with the role, yet feeling the scope of the role was too broad. Nurse managers, both novice and experienced (not the comanagers), described frequent feelings of inadequacy and acknowledged a "fear of losing it" at any moment (pp. 87–88).

Kath and associates (2012) found that nurse manager stress lessens with age (not experience in the role):

> Nurse administrators should give nurse managers as much autonomy as possible in meeting the multiple demands of their challenging roles. When possible, predictability of the job should be increased by freely sharing/communicating information that allows nurse managers to make the most of their autonomy and enhancing their participation in decision making, thus making the work more predictable. Finally, social support mechanisms should be in place such that coworkers and supervisors find ways to offer operational and emotional support to nurse managers. (p. 220)

Paradox

As we face issues, sometimes *paradox* is involved. This is where things are *seemingly contradictory*. For instance, negativity happens, yet *it can bring about good changes*. This is a paradox. Let's explain. Negativity can cause tensions that need resolution. It is like the piece of sand in the oyster causing friction that eventually results in a perfect pearl. Right now we cannot see the pearl, but it is there, and as we work through the tensions, the pearl manifests itself. We can choose to remain in our linear world with the pearl never manifesting and feel the continuing frustrations—or build toward a better future by recognizing the negativity and dealing with what is causing it (such as providing better staffing) or dealing with people who are choosing to be negative. Other paradox examples:

- We want things to be simple yet experience complexity.
- We want to change something, be a risk taker, and push beyond the limits of our comfort zone. Yet we continue to need status quo for comfort and stability.
- We want data, yet sometimes intuition leads us in another direction.

However, with paradoxes, the things that seem contradictory may actually be *complementary at a deeper level*. Let's examine a few instances where this is true:

- Creativity and tension (tension leads to creativity and creativity causes tension)
- Difference and similarity (difference seen at a great distance appears as an integrated whole)
- Complexity and simplicity (complexity is simply the visible connection between aligned simplicities)
- Chaos and order (there is order in all chaos and vice versa)
- Conflict and peace (conflict is necessary to peacemaking, containing in it the elements upon which peace must be built) (Porter-O'Grady & Malloch, 2011, p. 27)

So, what is harmony at this instant (this choice point) will change. Things are always changing. Conflict (a normal element in any environment) helps us get to *something better* (a *potential reality*).

> The techniques for finding common ground, for sorting through the various landscapes representing the diversity inherent in each issue, are now required by every leader. [Thus, it is important to] get people to come together around issues, helping them determine appropriate responses within the context of their own roles. This is a challenge that cannot be met by establishing standardized job procedures or rules. (p. 28)

It is precisely these opposing concepts that provide us with grist for the mill. When we think *linearly*, they present sources of conflict for us, and we want to avoid the conflicts. However, *if we can rise above the seeming differences and find ways to combine the opposing forces, we can resolve these conflicts and create a better workplace.*

Interconnections

Quantum science gives us another clue about leadership—we are all interconnected. Each small effort we make is linked with the whole global system. This causes a ripple effect. As each of us effectively leads, the quantum view is that this energy combines with the energy of others around the globe—all contributing to an improvement of the human condition and the earth as a whole.

The ripple effect occurs not only from our actions but from our emotions. (Remember, our emotions cause DNA changes.) Braden (2000) reported studies showing that "it is our DNA that influences the way atoms and molecules of our outer world behave as well!" (p. 207). So, as our DNA changes, this causes a ripple effect outward into the world. (As above, so below.) Can you see why positivity or negativity is catching? It spreads to others.

Margaret Wheatley (2006) described current scientific thought and applied this to leadership and organizations in *Leadership and The New Science*.

> Changes in small places . . . affect the global system . . . because every small system participates in an unbroken wholeness. Activities in one part of the whole create effects that appear in distant places.

Because of these unseen connections, there is potential value in working anywhere in the system. We never know how our small activities will affect others through the invisible fabric of our connectedness. (p. 45)

The Berlin Wall exemplifies one example of this quantum view. It came down even though the powers that be did not want this to occur. Local efforts—and other similar energies around the world—combined until they were finally strong enough to tumble the wall, even though the government officials wanted the wall to remain.

We see evidence that shows the interconnected relationship of nurse manager effectiveness with other positive outcomes, such as better patient outcomes, positive organizational cultures, more engagement/teamwork among staff, better interdisciplinary relationships, higher nurse and physician satisfaction, and better workforce management practices such as self-scheduling. A ripple effect takes place. In fact, evidence shows that as a person takes an action, it causes a much larger ripple effect than we had previously realized.

Intuition

Our interconnectedness affects each of us. It is reflected in energy fields flowing both through us and all around us. Each of us bumps into and merges with others' energy fields. For instance, how is it that a parent who is not present can know that his or her child is in danger? How does a nurse intuitively know when a patient is nearing a crisis or death? The energy fields transmit this knowledge. Intuition (listening to our inner core) is a capability that many nurses possess.

In nursing, we have been more aware of our intuitive capabilities because we are involved with so many people experiencing life-threatening events. Intuition is what helps us deal more effectively with ambiguity, with situations where we do not have all the facts, when there is uncertainty, and when there is complexity. Intuition can also lead us to have better timing in our actions. Our "gut level" tells us what is right, and when it is the right time to do something. This is a wonderful gift. When we are calm, we are more receptive to this gift. Staying in touch with our intuition improves leadership.

Empathy

Quantum leadership is most effective when we can go beyond selfishness and connect with something that is larger than us. This empathy, or compassion, or sensitivity, or connection with others and their predicaments, reflects an altruism that will better others' welfare. "Without feelings of deep sympathy and sorrow for others struck by misfortune, and a genuine desire to alleviate suffering on the part of caregivers, patient care service would be no more than a robotic endeavor" (Porter-O'Grady & Malloch, 2003).

Empathy means that we are able to learn from others' experiences and expertise (Snow, 2001), and that empathy is reflected in our actions. Empathy also reflects the connection between us and a higher power, found in our integrity. It is the "caring" component so important in health care. It is what we give to others with no motivation other than what is best for them.

Empathy occurs when we understand another person's perspective. To achieve this understanding we need to communicate with others. In fact, as we get to know each other, we often can anticipate a person's response to a situation, decision, or action.

Emotional Intelligence

Another important personal mastery issue is *emotional intelligence*. This "is the capacity for recognizing our own feelings and those of others, for motivating ourselves, for managing emotions well in ourselves and in our relationships" (Snow, 2001, p. 441).

Emotional intelligence is composed of a set of competencies. Emotional intelligence skills and cognitive skills are synergistic; top performers have both. The more complex the job, the more emotional intelligence matters. . . . Emotional competencies cluster into groups; . . . each is based on a common underlying emotional intelligence capacity. The underlying emotional intelligence capacities are vital if people are to successfully learn the competencies necessary to succeed in the workplace. (Vitello-Cicciu, 2002, pp. 441–442)

Goleman (1998) outlines the four capacities that are present when one has emotional intelligence: self-awareness, self-management, social awareness, and social skills. The first two involve an awareness of self, while the last two deal with how well we deal socially with others. Then, using this awareness, one needs to translate it into action.

Self-awareness:
- *Self-confidence*: Certain of one's own expertise
- *Accurate self-assessment*: Conscious of one's limitations
- *Emotional self-awareness*: Cognizant of one's positive and negative biases

Self-management:
- *Self-control:* Remaining poised even when under pressure
- *Adaptability:* Welcoming new ideas
- *Trustworthiness:* Displaying honesty/integrity (Snow, 2001, p. 442)

Social awareness:
- *Empathy:* Learning from other people's experiences, expertise
- *Organizational awareness:* Remaining cognizant of organizational life, politics

Social skills:
- *Visionary leadership:* Inspiring and executing effective tactics
- *Communication:* Establishing positive relationships and managing expectations
- *Conflict management:* Developing consensus and mitigating conflicts (Snow, 2001, p. 442)

Vitello-Cicciu explains what happens when there are deficiencies in any of these capacities:

If they are deficient in social skills, they will be inept at persuading or inspiring others, at leading teams, or catalyzing change. If they have little self-awareness, they will be oblivious to their own weaknesses and lack the self confidence that comes from certainty about their strengths. None of us is perfect in using all of the emotional competencies; we inevitably have a profile of strengths and limits. However, the ingredients for outstanding performance require only that we have strengths in a given number of these competencies (at least six or so), and that the strengths are spread across all four areas of emotional intelligence. (Vitello-Cicciu, 2002, pp. 441–442)

Recent neurobehavioral research on the limbic system indicates that emotional intelligence can be learned through motivation, extended practice, and feedback. Goleman (1998) contended that to enhance emotional intelligence, one must break old behavioral habits and establish new ones through an individualized approach. He also stated:

Building one's emotional intelligence will not happen without a sincere desire or concerted effort on the part of an individual. A brief seminar won't help, nor a how-to manual. Learning to internally empathize as a natural response to people is much harder to learn than regression analysis. (Vitello-Cicciu, 2002, p. 207)

McClelland (1973) found that, *"when senior managers had a critical mass of emotional intelligence capabilities their divisions outperformed yearly earnings goals by 20%."* Emotional intelligence research shows a strong link between an organization's success and the emotional intelligence of its leaders. The research also demonstrates that if people take the right approach, they can develop their emotional intelligence. The research supports the idea that leaders are not born but that people can learn how to manage their emotions and how to motivate people they lead. (Snow, 2001, p. 441)

This research has helped to explain how leaders who are very different can be very effective.

Snow (2001) found that emotionally intelligent nurse administrators help their organizations create a competitive advantage because they achieve: (1) improved performance of nursing personnel, leading to more satisfied patients, physicians, and families; (2) improved retention of top talent; (3) improved team-work among nurses; (4) increased motivation by team members; (5) enhanced innovation in the nursing group; (6) enhanced use of time and resources, and (7) restored trust between nurses and (administrators) (p. 443). Akerjordet and Severinsson (2010) completed an integrated review and found unsubstantiated predictive value, yet Foltin and Keller (2012) found that emotional intelligence was the most important factor in successfully implementing a large change project.

Organizationally, emotional intelligence was one of the characteristics *Fortune* identified in a "Most Admired Companies" survey. These companies:

- Are far more satisfied with the quality and breadth of leadership at both their executive and senior management levels
- Are less tolerant of inappropriate leadership behavior to meet their numbers
- Place more value on leadership development and put more emphasis on ongoing development efforts that are linked closely to strategic business goals and supported by formal rewards programs
- More frequently use competency models and various developmental programs in selecting and advancing their leaders
- Have leaders who are perceived as demonstrating more emotional intelligence (Stein, 2000)

Emotional intelligence research suggests that effective leadership starts with work we accomplish within ourselves. No matter how effective we become, we can always improve.

Diversity/Conflict

As one experiences relationships, it is inevitable that people will not agree with each other and conflicts occur. Porter-O'Grady and Malloch (2011) spend a whole chapter on conflict, and it is an excellent resource for this topic. **Exhibit 2–4** shows sources of conflict. Fisher, Ury, and Patton (1991) is another excellent resource.

Many choose to avoid conflict, and, in fact, many leadership theories discuss processes that can be used to minimize conflict. However, this is dangerous. A certain amount of stasis is good, but if we ignore the conflicts, we are ignoring clues about the potential reality that will help us accomplish changes needed to survive and thrive. "Diversity makes chaos visible, as it pushes systems to forever adapt to changes in their environment" (Porter-O'Grady & Malloch, 2011, p. 57).

Actually, *differences in opinion are a natural occurrence*, and they afford us many *rich opportunities* for different ideas, perspectives, and change. All of us are flawed people, working together to provide care for others. These differences provide a rich resource of possibilities and improve decisions, processes, and relationships.

Thank goodness there is diversity in this world! Wouldn't it be a dull place if everyone were exactly alike? Diversity means differences in our views of the world. For instance, cultural differences can become a strong source of conflict just because we do not understand someone's viewpoint. Such differences exist within work groups. Here is where empathy is put to the test. How well do we understand another

---

Exhibit 2–4   Sources of Conflict

Environmental Sources	Individual Sources
• Ego	• Culture
• Personality	• Nationality
• Identity	• Religion
• Intimate relationships	• Class
• Beliefs	• Economics
• Perceptions	• Politics
• Perspectives	• Society
• Education	• Resources
• Position and role	• Race

Source: Porter-O'Grady, T., & Malloch, K. *Quantum Leadership: Advancing Innovation, Transforming Health Care,* 3rd ed. Sudbury, MA: Jones and Bartlett, p. 167.

---

person's perspective of the world? Are we comfortable enough to let them tell us about it, or are we so uncomfortable that we do not give them a chance to air their beliefs?

Healthy disagreements and honesty provide different perspectives. By paying attention to, and valuing, different points of view, we can make better decisions. Thus, conflict can be very helpful and, when handled appropriately, can help us determine better alternatives. Dialogue and disagreements allow us to consider other ramifications that could occur before choosing the action we will take. Thus, instead of reacting, we can more thoughtfully consider the situation.

When conflict occurs it does not mean that we have been ineffective leaders. Instead, we want to encourage a wide range of views and opinions to accomplish what patients value. It keeps coming back to having basic values and creating/supporting a positive environment. Within a positive environment people will start to be more creative. They will individualize their care in ways that better serve our patients. When conflict occurs in this environment it is energizing and healthy.

Conflicts occur in negative environments as well. The conflicts create ways that the system attempts to adapt to become better. Constant change occurs everywhere, even in negative environments. However, as already discussed, negative environments are toxic and can affect us in negative ways. If a nurse manager takes over a negative environment, with the support of upper-level administration and the boss, the nurse manager can turn this around. It helps to have an assistant or charge nurses who support creating a more positive environment because it requires a lot of consistent work on all shifts. But, little by little, the environment can change to become more positive.

So, differences are good. In our leadership roles (remember everyone is a leader), we encourage others to express their thoughts and opinions, even when we do not agree with them. We need to listen carefully to better understand their perspective. There is a valuable kernel there that will help everyone else to change. We respect others' opinions and encourage open dialogue about issues. We experiment with ideas. Some work and some do not.

Sometimes we *cause* conflicts, for instance, in supporting a needed change to improve care or when implementing technology.

We cannot respond to every conflict that exists. That is not humanly possible. Timing is important. It is important to know which situations to respond to immediately and which can wait. Some decisions are best made after input and dialogue have occurred between a number of people. Other times, when conflict is left unresolved, the situation escalates and interferes with the work getting completed effectively. This is when immediate intervention is needed. A leader needs to know when it is important to get involved in a conflict, what the various viewpoints are in the conflict, and how to negotiate and resolve disagreements.

Negotiating skills can be helpful in conflict resolution. Many times we cannot make decisions alone but must negotiate with others.

"*The secret of good conflict management is simple, but the process is not. The secret is to get the parties in conflict to discern the root issues and mutually agree on actions to be taken*" (Porter-O'Grady & Malloch, 2011, p. 166). As one tries to get at the root issues, it is important to start with the basic value(s), such as *what is best for the patient*. This can help one more effectively deal with disagreements because it lifts the disagreement from being a personal issue to something both people, hopefully, value.

All of this is aided by an environment that welcomes diversity. Here we know that we won't always agree, but that is okay. That is why one person is better with a certain patient. Diversity means that each of us has certain gifts that, when taken all together, create environments that better serve our patients. Effective leaders create an environment where people respect each other and can openly discuss their differences, ideas, and perceptions. It is important that each person has integrity, is trustworthy, and is honest.

We want to create an environment where positive relationships and bonds form a team that is enthusiastic and caring—a team that supports each other to get the work done every day. A team that supports each other's differences.

Within this positive environment, conflicts occur. It is important for the *persons in conflict to directly discuss and resolve the issue*. It is hard because in our society we are not taught to honestly and respectfully discuss disagreements *directly* with the other person involved. Instead, we talk behind their backs about the people we disagree with, don't help them, get passive-aggressive, or even avoid them. When this happens, nothing gets resolved. In fact, the problem can magnify. Too much of this in the workplace creates a toxic, dysfunctional work environment. People may leave. New staff will be eaten alive. It is an environment that we do not want to create or support. As managers, we may need to help staff deal directly with each other as problems occur.

We are all *interconnected*. With this in mind, we need to change the way we have defined conflict. There is no "us" and "them" in quantum physics. Instead there is "we." Because of this it is not appropriate "to impose our will and ideas of change upon the lives of others. . . . As we choose to honor life in our everyday world, we witness the power of our choices to end war and render aggression obsolete" (Braden, 2000, p. 241).

It helps to realize that when a problem occurs, there are usually many different perceptions of it. Hearing different points of view helps to create a solution that is not any one person's idea but that represents a blending of ideas. We take *a risk when we expose our thoughts and feelings*, but this sharing leads to achieving better decisions and more effective teamwork. Thus, when conflicts occur, the leader needs to encourage appropriate expression of conflict as a way to achieve better decision making. No one is wrong or right; there just needs to be dialogue with each person sharing his or her perceptions and ideas about how to resolve issues. It is not a shouting match but rather a dialogue carried out while staying in the adult perspective (explained later).

Many times conflicts are caused by *expectations*. Think about this: If I have an expectation that you will (or should) respond a certain way, when you respond differently there is a conflict. This conflict could have been avoided if I had not had an expectation of how you should respond. This is why *dialogue* is so important—it gives us a chance to check out the other person's perceptions. The most effective leaders *let go of expectations of others*. After all, how a person responds is beyond our control.

We cannot respond to every conflict that exists. That is not humanly possible. Timing is important. It is important to know which situations to respond to immediately and which can wait. Some decisions are best made after input and dialogue have occurred between a number of people. Other times, when conflict is left unresolved, the situation escalates and interferes with the work getting completed effectively.

This is when immediate intervention is needed. An administrator needs to know when it is important to get involved in a conflict, what the various viewpoints are in the conflict, and how to negotiate and resolve disagreements. Negotiating skills can be helpful in conflict resolution. Many times we cannot make decisions alone but must negotiate with others.

The actual conflict can lead us to determine *who* is the most appropriate person(s) to deal with resolving the conflict. Sometimes it is best for one person to make a decision, resolving the conflict, whereas at other times it is best for a group to agree about how best to handle a situation.

Sometimes we can either experience conflict or choose another response. For example, we encourage everyone to find meaning in his or her life and work—even when this may cause us difficulties as leaders. People may not agree with us and speak up about that in team meetings. Or they may make a choice that we do not agree with. Sometimes this can mean that it is best to encourage a valuable staff member to take another job more suited to his or her gifts and life purpose, even when this means we will have to replace that person within the team.

The location of conflict resolution to take place is very important. Usually, it is best if dialogue can take place in a private setting where all involved can be relaxed, feel secure, and not be in the middle of many tasks.

In empowering environments, the work group can resolve many issues *without* any intervention needed by the administrator. It is best when people at any level in an organization can make 90% of the decisions about their work. This is why having practice councils are so important. Effective leaders know when to get involved and when it is more appropriate to have others deal with the issue.

At some point, certain people or behaviors really can hit our hot button. Learning is possible here too because these people or issues probably are a little too close to some problems that exist *within ourselves* that we have not yet resolved. Therefore, an important competency includes encouraging people to discuss issues when they do not agree—and it starts with us. Who is pushing our hot button, and why? What do we need to face within ourselves? How is our problem affecting others? Are we willing to work on this issue, talk about it with others, and ask their help to deal with it?

When our emotions get involved, it makes what we think that much more powerful. If our thinking is positive, it helps to create a better environment for those we serve. When we are negative, one of the emotional intelligence competencies, *self-control*, is important. This is further defined as remaining poised even under pressure (Snow, 2001). Sometimes it helps to ask oneself, "Will I remember this five years from now?" If one is getting emotional and it is not an emergency, it may be time simply to exit the situation, regain balance, and then return to deal with the situation. This is where coming back to the *adult* helps. Let's explain.

Staying in the Adult

In **Exhibit 2–5**, the *P* stands for the *parent* part of us. This side has many aspects. It can be nurturing and helpful; it can be judgmental and full of "should" statements. The *C* stands for the *child* part of us. Children can be playful or angry; they can be loving and responsive. To grow, children often need direction and attention from parents. Finally, the *A* stands for the *adult* part of us. This is the reasoning part. It is more like a computer in that emotion is not attached to it, whereas emotion is attached to the parent and child parts.

Now let's use this exhibit to examine interactions between two people. If Person A comes from the parent when communicating with Person B, Person B will probably respond from the child. If the parental communication is nurturing, the child response is loving and uses the information to learn more about the

---

Exhibit 2–5   Parental Approach

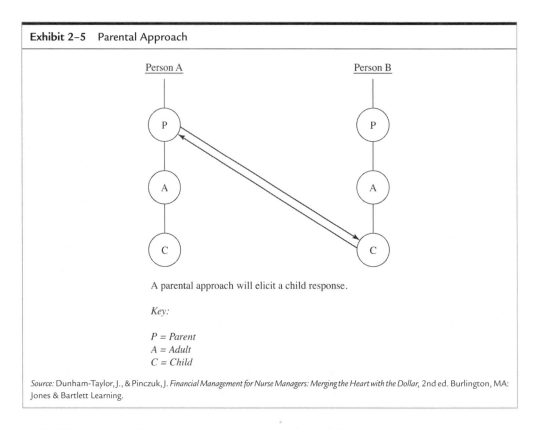

A parental approach will elicit a child response.

Key:

P = Parent
A = Adult
C = Child

Source: Dunham-Taylor, J., & Pinczuk, J. *Financial Management for Nurse Managers: Merging the Heart with the Dollar,* 2nd ed. Burlington, MA: Jones & Bartlett Learning.

---

world. When the parental approach is judgmental, the child may feel ashamed or angry and respond based on those emotions. Emotion is involved in the conversation. The same thing happens if the supervisor comes from the parent when interacting with staff.

In **Exhibit 2–6**, Person A is coming from the child when communicating with Person B. The communication from Person A's child hooks into Person B's parent, so Person B responds from the parent. For example, if the child is angry, the parent may become angry. When someone is angry, the person is not as effective in responding to situations. Anger causes more anger. Issues escalate. This is not desirable.

In **Exhibit 2–7**, Person A is in the adult when communicating with Person B. This is most likely to hook into Person B's adult. This is the reasoning, calm part of both individuals. Emotion is not involved. Person B still has a choice as to how to respond. If Person B chooses to stay in the parent or child mode, his or her response may switch to that approach. However, the greatest likelihood is that each person will communicate from the adult. Ideally, the effective administrator uses the adult approach in communicating with others. In fact, *when we feel ourselves responding to someone using emotion, that is a clue that we are either in the parent or child part of ourselves.* This is a time to rethink, "Do I really want to be in the parent or the child?" It may be time to exit to a place where one can become more calm and balanced before continuing with the communication!

It is important to stay in the *adult*, being factual and keeping emotion out of the conversation as much as possible. In fact, sometimes when we discuss a problem with the person or persons involved, we find out reasons we had not considered about the situation being discussed that can give us a better understanding of why the incident occurred.

Aggression comes from the *parent* or the *child*. Emotion is involved—a sign that one is not reacting appropriately to conflict. We have a greater chance for success when we can stop and think before acting— or reacting—to a situation. If we are immediately emotional in a situation, it is generally better to wait or

Exhibit 2–6   Child Approach

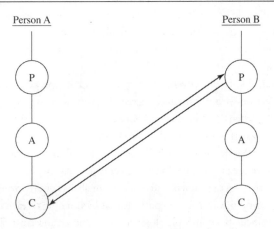

A child approach will elicit a parental response.

Key:

P = Parent
A = Adult
C = Child

Source: Dunham-Taylor, J., & Pinczuk, J. *Financial Management for Nurse Managers: Merging the Heart with the Dollar,* 2nd ed. Burlington, MA: Jones & Bartlett Learning.

Exhibit 2–7   Adult Approach

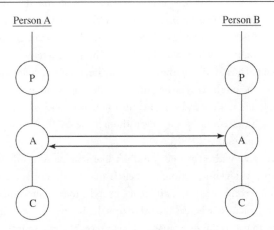

An adult approach will be more likely to elicit an adult response.

Key:

P = Parent
A = Adult
C = Child

Source: Dunham-Taylor, J., & Pinczuk, J. *Financial Management for Nurse Managers: Merging the Heart with the Dollar,* 2nd ed. Burlington, MA: Jones & Bartlett Learning.

step out of a situation until we can get back *into the adult before acting*. Police know this: The best way to live to retirement is to remain calm in the midst of crises.

Many women are in the field of nursing. In the wider society, women have had to learn to be assertive. Similarly, nurses have had to learn how to be assertive while giving care because physicians or administrators have been given more importance than nurses in healthcare organizations, even though nurses spend more time with patients.

Assertiveness, or being able to objectively (staying in the adult), yet respectfully, describe a problem situation directly to the person with whom one disagrees, is a very important skill. Assertion uses "I" statements, such as "I felt _____ when _____ happened," or "I thought _____ was the way we were doing _____." Aggressive statements often start with "You" while expressing disagreement, such as "You did _____," and often are accusing or angry. People can be passive-aggressive in dealing with the situation, too.

Assertiveness is a positive use of dialogue. In a disagreement, it is very possible that once we understand the other person's perspective, we can understand where he or she is coming from and why the other person is doing something a certain way. It is also possible that by listening to each other, we can resolve the conflict easily. Honest dialogue brings people closer together and creates trust. There is also a possibility that both parties may arrive at a better way of doing things than either had thought of in the first place. Also, after dialogue, we may just decide to continue to disagree!

In a safe environment, people feel free to *express disagreement*. This includes the leader having "a willingness to risk exposing thoughts and feelings and to acknowledge how these impact perception and behavior" (Perra, 2000). The more people can be honest about a situation in a calm manner, the better. The goal is to *stay in the adult*: to be "in the storm of conflict and at the same time out of it . . . watching it in serenity" (von Franz, 1980, p. 149).

Even nurturing behaviors can get us in trouble. For instance, a nurse might say, "I will do this myself because I can do it better," and so s/he doesn't delegate tasks to others. This is dangerous because one person cannot possibly take care of everything alone! What the nurse often does not realize is the *child message* this sends to others: "You cannot do this as well as I can." In fact, this attitude is dangerous because then others do not learn. For example, a new nurse is not appropriately mentored about the role, or a patient does not learn how to administer his own insulin or appropriately care for himself. Or, the parental nurse manager expects that all staff will check to see what the manager wants to do before taking action. This is also a trap—what are staff members to do when the manager is absent? Thus, staying in the adult is very important in quantum leadership.

Objectivity, or staying in the adult, is very helpful when dealing with conflict. It enables one to be empathetic with other people and understand why they are doing what they are doing. It is easy for people to see each other as without a redeeming quality, even though the conflict is only caused by a person's behavior or by differences in opinion.

Sometimes when we disagree with someone, we don't like that person. Often, really it is not the *person* we dislike, but the person's words, actions, or beliefs that we do not agree with—not the whole person. In fact, sometimes the conflict is just a difference in style; for instance, one person is very detail oriented, never seeing the big picture, whereas the other sees the big picture and never pays attention to detail. Thus, it is important to get to the *root cause* of the conflict. The *real* source of the conflict may be a person's behavior or way of doing work. One needs to separate the behavior from the person. (This does not mean that we judge others because we have not walked in their shoes.) We understand the person's position and choices—even when we may not agree. Discussing problems and encouraging others not to attach the problem to the entire person are helpful. Staying in the adult, or staying objective, leads to better conflict management and decision making within an entire team. During a conflict, we are compassionate yet want what is best for the patient and to meet standards. This represents justice and fairness.

To a certain extent, our own life experiences cloud our objectivity. But this can be improved. Dialogue helps us to have a dynamic picture of the people involved, take into account all the different viewpoints, and stay in touch with what feels right intuitively.

Our intuition can help us better deal with conflicts. Sometimes we realize that what a person is expressing is not the real issue. This intuitive knowing can help us to be more effective in dealing with conflicting situations. It may be necessary to get to the bottom of the issue, and deal with something else that is actually causing the problem, before the conflict can be resolved.

Our gut level signals us, if we listen to it, and tells us what is right in each life situation. In interviews with nurse executives, some said that they knew they might lose their job at any moment. Yet they identified the importance of following their intuition. For instance, when something happens that is ethically wrong, they face a choice. What should they do? Confront it or overlook it? If one decides to confront it, one may need to go against a powerful physician, or one may not have the support of the CEO, COO, or board. Several executives discussed confronting such situations and leaving their positions because they could not get support to do what was ethically correct. In other situations, both the executive team and physician group rallied around, doing what was right, with the nurse executive continuing to work there. Health care is fraught with such ethical dilemmas.

The bottom line is always, "Can I live with my decision?" Ironically, even when something awful happens to us (like suddenly losing our job or resigning unexpectedly), if we have followed our inner core, it always leads us to something better—something we may never have found if this situation had not happened.

The problem with conflict is that when it is inappropriately expressed, it can result in anger, jealousy, fear, pain, and violence. More often than not, when this happens one of the parties in the conflict has more power, is stronger, or the parties are in some way unequal. This inequality results in one person not being able to express viewpoints in a safe environment. If a change can be made to create more equality, it is important to make the change. For instance, if there is a difficult situation with a physician, having medical staff and administrative support in dealing with the situation is paramount. More about this is included in Chapter 3. It helps if everyone is working toward a common value, such as *what is best for the patient*. It is best when physicians value and respect team members. Research shows that patient outcomes are better on units where this is true.

More conflicts go *unresolved* in unhealthy workplaces. This causes higher staff turnover, and staff play more games, such as being passive-aggressive, talking behind others' backs, and complaining, and nothing is done about poor performance. Most often, problems start with the leader. If the current leader is trying to resolve issues a past leader caused, the new leader first needs to deal with the ineffective administrative leader and then start cleaning up other staff issues.

Conflicts can be caused by *systems problems*, which create barriers to getting the work accomplished. System problems can create unnecessary hassles that, when they occur day after day, prompt staff finally to leave. Staff grumble about these issues. If administrators do regular rounds, these types of problems quickly become apparent. Usually an intraorganizational group that represents different departments or professions must deal with systems problems. Changes that all stakeholders think would work are implemented. And as changes are implemented, additional problems probably will occur that result in further change before the systems problem can be fixed. It is often best to make smaller incremental changes.

Another source of conflict is when our day does not go as planned. We come to work expecting to accomplish certain things, but then an emergency happens, or someone is distressed about something and needs to talk to us, or someone takes an action that adversely affects a patient. Sometimes the whole day passes and the planned activities are not accomplished. This can be upsetting. However, if we think back: We really did what was best at each moment in the day. Perhaps it was *not the right time* to do the planned activities. After all, there is a right time for everything—it just may not be today! We can either experience a great deal of conflict internally—everything kept interfering with the goals we had set—or we can actually have a rewarding day because we know that we responded effectively to more important issues.

As a nurse administrator, we want to create a safe environment for appropriate expression of differences of opinions or viewpoints. The environment is strongest when there is support at higher levels of the organization as well as from other departments for this kind of climate to occur. (If someone is more linear and does not appreciate this climate, it is much harder to have a positive environment.) Dialogue is encouraged, team members feel *valued and respected* and value and respect each other, and better decisions result because all are listening to each other and then deciding what is best.

This is much easier for leaders who are at Hagberg's Stage Four or higher. At Stage Four, empowering others happens. One encourages others to make decisions and be proactive. One also realizes the value in differences of opinion and that differences in opinion are okay. (A person at a lower stage does not understand this.)

An effective leader knows that it is all right *for staff to disagree with the leader.* This concept is hard to understand until one achieves Hagberg's Stage Four. After all, why would we want people to disagree with us? If we listen, we can learn about our misperceptions or about issues we need to resolve. A result is that staff will have more respect for the leader. If someone does not allow others to disagree with them, chances are they are at one of the first three stages.

A participative system is best for this climate. Here people are not in power struggles but instead are part of a team, helping each other as needed, and are proud of their team (and they may even express something like "We are the best unit," or "We do excellent work caring for *any* patient."). They can more comfortably discuss differences together. This does not mean that tension and chaos never occur. But discussion happens and is healthy. The result is better patient care and a happier work environment because people are heard.

In reality, though, other units, or other disciplines, or people at higher levels might not value this climate, and this creates a source of conflict. It is still possible for a unit to achieve this healthy climate, even without support of all the other players. It is just more difficult when team members have a conflict with a person who does not value this because the person may not fairly and honestly deal with others.

Conflict is a natural occurrence. Nurse managers must set up the environment to recognize, support, and, as a team, most effectively deal with the many conflicts that will occur. All the best!

Potential Reality: Innovation

Administrators have an additional responsibility concerning the choice points. We need to *be aware of the potential reality.* There is potential for change at each choice point; there is a potential for something better to happen.

At each choice point, there are two realities—the actual reality and a potential reality. The actual reality we have already experienced, but the potential reality is something that is in the future. We just have not experienced it yet.

> It is in this arena of potential reality that leadership takes its form. The leader is differentiated from the follower in that the leader derives the preponderance of his or her role within the scope of *potential reality.* It is the leader's role to engage unfolding reality in advance of others experiencing it; to see it, note its demands and implications, translate it for others, and then guide others into processes that will act in concert with the demands of a reality that is not yet present but inexorably and continuously becoming. (Porter-O'Grady, 2003, p. 59)

In our administrative role, we need to keep abreast with this unfolding potential reality, bringing it out for others to see, hear, and experience, lifting all of us to new levels not yet achieved. Leaders will see this and do the same. This is why rounds are so important at every level of the organization. As administrators, we need to encourage and support staff leaders as they identify potential realities, as well as look out for potential realities ourselves. As we speak with staff, we can encourage them to identify these potential realities and share perceptions about them. Rounds provide another wonderful resource for potential realities. Excellent suggestions emerge from those around us.

> It is said that 2 heads are better than 1. A greater possibility for creative and catalytic ideas results from the contributions of many minds working collaboratively toward a common goal and shared concerns. To build strong alliances, the leader first must focus on building solid relationships that require effective communication skills and investment in people. (Shirey, 2007, p. 169)

For instance, are we giving the patients what they value? Are we encouraging them to be the leaders in choosing their care? Many practices in health care do not encourage patient leadership, such as having to wear hospital gowns, limitations on visiting hours, and placing dietary restrictions on heavy patients at a time when they are experiencing a health crisis and have not decided to lose weight. It is important to think about how our decisions and policies either limit or enhance patient autonomy and, thus, patient leadership. This helps to set up a new, better potential reality.

The evidence is all around us about potential realities. For instance, there are less invasive treatment modalities, new reimbursement changes, better ways to accomplish workforce management, ways to improve the culture or the way we work with other disciplines, new technology, and, most important of all, beings sure to find out and give patients only what they value. Other changes include landmark reports, legislation, and regulations (Cadmus, 2011).

Porter-O'Grady and Malloch (2011) offered starting points for administrators:

- Deconstructing the barriers and structures of the 20th Century
- Alerting staff about the implications of changing what they do
- Establishing safety around taking risks and experimenting
- Embracing new technologies as a way of doing work
- Reading the signposts along the road to the future
- Translating the emerging reality into language the staff can use
- Demonstrating personal engagement with the change effort
- Helping others adapt to the demands of a changing health system
- Creating a safe milieu for the struggles and pain of change
- Enumerating small successes as a basis for supporting staff
- Celebrating the journey and all progress made (p. 19)

Constant discussion needs to occur because *potential reality is constantly changing*. What is each person seeing, and what needs to change? The goal is that each time there is an interaction between individuals, each person identifies and adapts to the changes that are occurring. It is best to make small, incremental changes. However, some large changes, such as introducing documentation technology, are best done in increments with a lot of planning. As always, the changes need to be based on what patients value.

In leadership theories, potential realities become *shared vision*. Leadership theories often espouse that administrators are responsible for this. In fact, everyone must look for, see, and share potential realities with the team. After all, administrators may not always see a potential reality. We will see some, staff leaders will see some, and the amalgamation of this process becomes the next potential reality.

Leaders should identify a clear vision of a desired future and guide leadership practice in a way that supports *from there to here* thinking to engage others and achieve desired organizational outcomes, leaders should incorporate organizational mission into vision and values. (Shirey, 2007, p. 169)

Because each group is different, leadership resulting from the relationships in each group is different. It is constantly changing and evolving to something better. Dynamic administration involves seeing the whole, understanding how we fit within it, and because this reality is constantly changing, our leadership needs to constantly change. The people we serve—and their needs—change; we change, our work group changes (Cadmus & Holmes, 2013); the community changes; and societal expectations change. Our work is fluid and ever changing. *Everyone we come in contact with is a valuable resource, necessitating our need to change to accomplish the best outcomes.*

From the quantum perspective, the organization is a flexible whole, ever changing, both internally and externally. There is always more to do to make things better. Staff, physicians, and patients are equitable and accountable partners with administrators. Others can think of better ways to do things, or have new ideas, that never occurred to the administrator. All *create* leadership together.

Since we know that people tend to keep doing the status quo, the administrator (along with other staff leaders who see the need for the change) must be a *catalyst for change* (MacPhee, 2007). Administrators and staff leaders

routinely challenge the status quo—indeed, seriously challenge it, which means not asking questions out of curiosity but looking carefully at current dogma and raising issues that open the door to substantial improvements. For quantum leaders, examining the work of their organizations is not a meaningless exercise but is intended to guarantee accountability and make certain that all work is value producing. Asking the unaskable questions about structure, principles, and customs requires an ease with vulnerability and an openness to and passion for new realities. (Porter-O'Grady & Malloch, 2011, p. 256)

As we identify potential realities, change is necessary. Or maybe everyone must *reframe* an issue. When we discussed paradoxes earlier, we described some examples of reframing. To help with this concept, we examine first- and second-order change (Watzlawick, Weakland, & Fisch, 1974). In *first-order change*, a method or person changes. Here, when one asks the question "Why?" the solution is based on common sense. Many changes are actually first-order changes. For example, if there is not enough light in a room to read, the question can be asked, "Why isn't there enough light?" A lamp can be added to supply the needed light and the problem is solved.

At times, though, first-order change does not accomplish anything. Asking "why?" does not solve the problem. For instance, during layoffs some employees in an outpatient department were asked to describe an outpatient role they would like to do, to determine what they would charge to do the role, and to give all of these details to the administrator by a certain date. Otherwise, they would be laid off. Being told this, several employees asked, "*Why* are you doing this to us?" They became stuck in first-order change and could not get beyond the question why. Eventually, they were laid off.

However, a few employees realized that asking "why" did not result in their keeping their jobs. They turned to the question of "what": "What do we need to do?" When using the question *what*, they turned to *second-order change* and reframed the situation. Reframing (Watzlawick et al., 1974) demands creativity and thinking out of the box—thinking about the issue in a different way. For instance, if we look into a house through one window and get one perspective; then we look in another window we get a different perspective. The employees who turned to second-order change began to imagine their work roles in a different way, a way that they had not imagined before. They began to devise the role, develop costs for their services, and gave it in writing to the administrator. The employees choosing to use second-order change still had jobs and were not laid off.

Thinking of options beyond those that seem obvious is something that we are not always taught to do. Actually, thinking is a skill and can be improved. One place to start is with a classic—*de Bono's Thinking Course* (de Bono, 1994). Many people do not actually go through this process as they examine possible decisions. He advocated thinking about a potential decision from three perspectives: (1) P, *Plus*, looking at the good points; (2) M, *Minus*, looking at the bad points; and 3) I, *Interesting*, looking at the interesting points. The I perspective includes points that are neither positive nor negative, things that are both positive and negative, and points of interest about the idea or what it leads to that may move one to think of a different decision or other factors not considered. This helps to train the mind

> to react to the interest inherent in an idea and not just to make judgments about the idea. A thinker should be able to say: "I do not like your idea, but there are these interesting aspects to it. . . ." It is a common enough experience that this sort of reaction is highly unusual. (p. 17)

This helps us to actually improve our thinking.

Another example of reframing (second-order change) occurred in World War II during the Nazi occupation of Denmark. The Nazis told King Christian to issue a decree that all his countrymen should wear the Star of David armband if they were Jewish. King Christian did not want to do this, yet the Nazis in occupation would enforce the decree even if he refused—a dilemma. King Christian used second-order change by very effectively reframing the issue. He issued a decree that all countrymen would wear the Star of David armband. The Nazis soon rescinded the order.

Viewing potential realities involves either first- or second-order change. The best way to determine which to use is to ask the question *Why?*, and if that gets nowhere, ask *What?*

Risk Taking

Mistakes are the portals of discovery.

—*James Joyce*

As we identify potential realities, make changes, meet standards, and do what patients value, both successes and mistakes occur. Nothing ventured, nothing gained. It is a choice. We need to try taking risks and innovating to successfully deal with the changes continually happening around us. Changes and innovations may entail a different way of thinking about a problem, a different solution to address a problem, or an incremental modification to correct an issue.

Even though we do not know what will happen next, we make decisions in each interaction *that we think are best at the time*. This is key. Some decisions make things better, and some bomb. At that point, it is important to recognize the mistake, stop doing it, and take corrective action. If implemented incrementally, when something does not work it is easier to stop whatever is causing the glitch and make a different incremental change to correct the situation.

Any decision and any action are risky. What is pertinent is the *value* of the issue. An effective leader needs to take risks, especially on important issues. If the issue is significant, the risk is probably greater but will result in greater beneficial results.

When we choose not to take risks glitches and errors still occur and will continue to worsen because growth has not happened. The situation goes into decline.

A few issues hamper nurses from taking risks: All the information nurses need to process can be overwhelming and time consuming, and lack of empowerment. Other reasons that nurses do not practice risk taking is that changes and innovations cause *disruption*: The outcome is uncertain and complete informa-tion is not available. "Even though more health care organizations have adopted the idea of a blame-free environment, that concept has not been applied widely and has not been focused on support for risk-taking and innovation" (Crenshaw & Yoder-Wise, 2013, pp. 25–26). "In order to embrace innovation, at least within the profession, nurse leaders must embrace the competency of considered risk taking" (p. 25). Nurses need to implement more innovations and take more risks.

Innovation, or risk taking, is a critical competency of administrators. This means that administrators need to be current on the evidence, guidelines, and policies but also "be willing to sacrifice security by moving out of their comfort zone. 'Risk-taking is the tolerance of uncertainty and ambiguity.' Often attributed to Mark Twain is the quote, 'Why not go out on a limb? That's where the fruit is.'" (Crenshaw & Yoder-Wise, 2013, p. 26). Part of the issue is that the outcome is uncertain, and that complete information is not available.

> Taking risks has personal and organizational benefits. We believe that personal benefits include enhanced self-awareness, self-empowerment, self-confidence, job satisfaction, and professional development. Orga-nizational benefits include moving from the routine to the cutting edge of health care delivery. Consid-ered risk taking can lead to improvements in patient safety, health care quality, fiscal health, healthy work environments, and employee and patient satisfaction. (Crenshaw & Yoder-Wise, 2013, p. 26)

When everyone in the organization is empowered to be a risk taker, positives spiral to bring about bet-ter positives. "As Sinek stated so eloquently in his *Notes to Inspire*, 'New ideas need audiences like flowers need bees. No matter how bright and colorful, they will die unless others work to spread them'" (Crenshaw & Yoder-Wise, 2013, p. 26).

It is important to celebrate the successes—even the small ones that occur daily—with everyone involved. Give credit where credit is due. If a staff member did something wonderful, give him or her credit for the success.

Making Mistakes

Because we are human, mistakes happen. Everyone makes mistakes. When we know we have not been effective in a situation or when a situation really bombs, it can be easy to get bogged down in negativity. However, beating ourselves up about it can actually keep us from being effective in the next situation. Instead, we can admit that we made a mistake, work to repair the damage if needed, and move on, learn-ing from our mistakes. If someone else made the mistake, talk with that person to find out why she did what she did and what she would do differently next time. Mistakes provide fodder for further learning.

Healthcare organizations are emerging from the old Industrial Age authoritarian, blaming way of interacting. Becoming blame free is just the first step. We have learned from sentinel events that one person does not simply make a mistake, but that a whole series of events happens that contribute to the person's mistake. Processes need to be examined and changes are needed to ensure the mistake does not happen again.

When a positive environment exists, everyone is expected to have integrity and identify mistakes to the appropriate people. This assumes that the administration and medical staff have, and continue to, support an environment where it is safe to report errors. "No blame" is a start, but creating a safe environment goes way beyond this. We all know that we make errors and are human. No one is perfect. Instead of punishing a person who has made a mistake (this is getting into the *parent role*), it is best to stay in the *adult* and fac-tually find out what happened, listen to different perspectives, and try to help the person undo the damage that has been done. The same process can be used for ourselves. Beating ourselves up for making a mistake does not help the situation, but it does provide learning for us. It is important to go back and own up to the mistake, and then go on from there, undoing the damage as much as we can.

A mature leader admits to making mistakes. Others see this and have more respect for us because we are able to do this. This also helps to bring about humility. Kerfoot (2009b) explained the neuropsychology of making mistakes. Erickson (2012) leads us through what to do when a serious reportable event happens.

We want to create an environment where everyone can admit their mistakes. Then everyone can begin to investigate what went wrong and what needs to be fixed.

Making Apologies

Many times it is best to apologize. Just saying "I'm sorry" *sincerely* can really help a situation. Some excellent references address apologizing to patients and disclosing what happened. Lazare (2006), a physician, recommended a structure for the apology:

> The first part of any apology is the acknowledgement of the offense, which includes the identity of the offender(s), appropriate details of the offense, and validation that the behavior was unacceptable. The second part of an apology is the explanation for committing the offense. . . . Explanations may mitigate the offense . . . although sometimes saying, "There is just no excuse for what happened" or "We are still trying to find out what happened" can be the most honest and dignified explanation. The third part of an apology is the expression of remorse, shame, forbearance, and humility . . . (arrogance will undo most apologies). The fourth part of an apology is reparation. (p. 1402)

Lazare (2006) goes on to discuss the healing process that occurs when apologies are appropriately given. These include restoration of self-respect and dignity; feeling cared for; restoration of power; lessening of suffering in the offender; validation that the offense occurred; designation of fault; assurance of shared values; entering into a dialogue with the offender; reparations; and a promise for the future. Gallagher and colleagues (2007) and Van Dusen and Spies (2003), pharmacists, concur that apologies are important.

Decision Making: The Importance of Having High Standards

Effective decision making is an art. It involves finding and selecting the best alternative and having the most appropriate person (or people) make and implement the decision at the right time. As one nurse executive said, "It is sifting out the new rules and building for an unknown tomorrow." Decisions are influenced by time constraints, culture, upper-level managerial support, and workforce management issues. Chinn's (2013) Peace and Power model is the best way to reach decisions.

An effective leader possesses the abilities to analyze difficult concepts, listen to and understand different perspectives, get facts needed to make an appropriate decision, see the smaller picture and how it fits with the overall big picture, and make a decision even when unknowns remain. Administrators and staff leaders need these capabilities. Staff leaders need to be making 90% of the decisions about their work. Do you see the importance of staff orientation and mentoring? This is also important for nurse managers. The manager role is very complicated, accompanied by many expectations, as previously discussed.

At the beginning of the chapter *obliquity leadership* was discussed where, once staff know what the overall plan is, they can go ahead and implement it daily as they work with patients. Kerfoot (2011) advocated that this *oblique decision-making* model is most effective in achieving organizational goals. It is a better way to deal with environmental complexity.

Some decision support tools can be helpful in preventing nurse managers and staff from skipping steps necessary to make a decision on action(s) to be taken. Effken and colleagues (2010) recommended a DyNADS tool as one effective way to help managers make decisions. They found that often nurse managers would skip a step (take shortcuts) in decision making that saved time initially, "but if the results are suboptimal, the time saved may be lost later on" (p. 195).

In a complex, messy environment (speaking from a quantum perspective), everyone needs to be making decisions constantly. These decisions are important because patients can suffer if we make erroneous decisions. To do this, we must have the right people in the right positions. Consider the following:

> Hire the right people. Leaders must understand their own strengths and weaknesses. To build an effective team, leaders must hire and retain the best and the brightest. This approach requires leaders to integrate into their teams those individuals who have talents that the leader does not. Once hired, leaders need to believe in the goodness of their people and allow them to do their jobs to the best of their abilities. In doing so, leaders will gain commitment and build on strength while simultaneously cultivating the talents of the next generation of leaders. (Shirey, 2007, p. 170)

"*What we permit, we promote*" (Kerfoot, 2009c, p. 245). Administrators need to set expectations for everyone to give their best. In an organization, it is important for administrators and staff to agree on standards and uniformly promote best practices. Transparency is needed in this process.

> Unfortunately, people become accustomed to working in cultures where low expectations and mediocrity are the norm. They learn to tolerate bad things happening because "it's always been that way." Patients and their families suffer irreparable harm and even death when they are cared for in the culture of low expectations. (Kerfoot, 2009a, p. 54)

When an administrator does not deal with this more errors occur and patients suffer unnecessarily. Mediocrity is not acceptable. It must be stopped. This is an example of poor leadership and takes place in a negative culture. The culture must be changed.

It is important to stress the importance of values and high standards from the beginning of employment. "The leader must be vigilant and have a system in place that will quickly inform people about deviations from the values and standards" (Kerfoot, 2009c, p. 245). Discuss the importance of this in team meetings. Expect that everyone is striving for excellence, and evaluate whether this has been met in performance evaluations.

"Most nurse managers simply don't spend enough time setting expectations, tracking performance, correcting failure, and rewarding success" (Tulgan, 2007, p. 18). He identified eight issues that cause this. First, too often we just leave staff alone instead of making sure they understand and adhere to the expectations. Second, we think that to be fair we need to treat everyone the same way. This is a misinterpretation of the term because some people need more attention and some need less. Third, we want to be a "nice" person. Instead, we need to adhere to the expectations. Fourth, we avoid difficult conversations instead of speaking with staff about expectations not being met, finding out what is going on, and making sure staff are correcting issues. Fifth, we let the red tape stop us instead of learning how to work within and around it. Sixth, we think that we are nurses, not natural leaders. We may need mentoring on how to deal with staff not meeting expectations. Seventh, we say we don't have time. "When you spend time managing, you engage the productive capacity of those you manage and improve the quality and output of their work. . . . That's a good return on investment" (p. 22).

Tulgan (2007) recommended we get back to basics: (1) get in the habit of managing every day—start with doing an hour each day; (2) learn to talk like a performance coach (the most effective managers have a way of talking that's both demanding and supportive, disciplined and patient); (3) take it one person at a time; (4) make accountability a real process; (5) clarify what to do and how to do it; (6) follow performance every step of the way (keep a written record—pay attention to the details); (7) solve small problems before they turn into big problems; and (8) do more for some people and less for others; (8) do more for some people and less for others.

The best way for a nurse manager to work with staff and to understand what is happening is to work on all shifts at some time each month. Also, when staffing is not adequate, the nurse manager can pitch in and help.

Transparency is always the best policy. When all know what is being measured and how well it is actually being achieved, then all can work to improve. Consider the following observation by Cathy Leary:

> Caregivers need to be told what is being measured, how internal processes support this (and are based on best practice), and how the organization is doing, as related to its goals, and as compared with benchmark organizations/practices. Caregivers need to be praised for meeting goals and not punished for not meeting goals. Failure to meet goals should be addressed as an opportunity to learn and to grow, as a failure of systems and processes, not as a failure of individuals or a professional group, such as nurses.
>
> Sounds simple, but my experience shows me that we are still a long way from this. Administrators and organizations tend to focus on short term financial goals and rarely see the long term benefit of building trust, professionalism, and, ultimately, loyalty and high quality by investing time or money in appreciative inquiry approaches to problem solving, or even in adequate orientation and ongoing staff education.
>
> I do think things are better than they were 10 years ago, but change is way too slow. We definitely need more nurses in upper administration and on healthcare organization boards. (personal communication, July 14, 2012)

Many times a leader does not know what to do. Some advocate that a leader bluff at such times, pretending to know the answer. Do not do this. Once people see through this (and they will), they lose trust in the leader. It is much more effective to *admit we do not know what to do, ask for others' ideas, and say that we need time to think about the situation.* If something must be done right away, it is important we listen to our gut after hearing other ideas and take the action we intuitively choose. We arrive at better decisions when we stay in touch with what feels right intuitively and encourage others to follow their intuition.

A number of factors can be helpful to determine the best way to handle a situation. Although many situations have similar themes, individual differences occur that can change the way something should be handled. These processes can aid in making the most appropriate decision. First, go back to the core value of *what is best for the patient.* Decisions are best when the core value is supported. Second, allow others to make the decisions they are best qualified to make. Decision making is tricky for another reason: Sometimes it is best to leave the decision making to others who are fully capable of making better decisions on the matter than we would make. For instance, in the work setting each staff member has the best understanding of his or her work. We do not know the nuances of their work; they are the experts. Each person is a capable adult who must make many decisions to do the needed work appropriately. This is also true for patients—patients need to make the decisions that they determine are best.

Some decisions take *courage.* Connaughton and Hassinger (2007) defined courage as "the ability to take bold action to support the common good, to stay the course in the face of adversity without arrogance or bravado" (p. 468). When the decision is important, we need to stand by it, unless a better way emerges.

Another issue is *prioritizing.* One cannot do it all. In this Information Age, there is so much paper and information we cannot know it all. Instead, we need to listen to our gut and concentrate our time and decisions on important issues. As previously discussed, this can be difficult for some because we need to delegate appropriately and then prioritize what we need to do. Certain things are very important, whereas other things can wait until tomorrow.

Letting others make the decisions—actually encouraging staff to do this—can be difficult. Many nurses and nurse managers do not delegate enough. They say, "I can do it better." In this case, they have not allowed others to make decisions. They have not treated others (including patients and families, as well as other staff, physicians, and administrators) as capable people deserving respect. After all, if one person has to do it all because no one else can do it right, how does all the work get done? It is physically impossible for one person to do everything right. Meanwhile, patients suffer, staff members are unhappy and leave, physicians complain about staff, and so forth.

Instead, the workplace is most effective when everyone delegates effectively. This involves knowing, or learning about, others' capabilities, sharing information, and teaching others if they do not know how to do something. Then it is letting the appropriate people do it at the most advantageous time. This means that others may go about accomplishing something very differently from how we would. Unless this harms someone, let that person do it his or her way. Others' generally know more about themselves, or about doing their job, than we do.

Along with all of this, *timing* is an issue. Knowing when to make the decision is another part of leadership effectiveness. Once again, it is important to stay in touch with one's intuition as well as with others in the environment. At times we must make the decision, but many times others need to make the decision. Knowing when to make the decision and when to leave the situation alone takes experience as well as being in touch with one's intuitive capabilities. Does it feel right to make the decision? If inexperienced, a good mentor can be very helpful in this area. Sometimes it is important to have the courage to make a difficult or unpopular decision, even though others may disagree with it.

Another aspect of decision making is *tenacity*. When something is important yet not easily achieved, it is key to have persistence. We are like a river that flows along, and when there is an obstruction the water finds a way past it, flowing under, over, or around the obstacle in a meandering course. If we are obstructed in pursuing our life purpose, we need persistence to flow around or overcome the obstacle. Sometimes we find that we have created the obstruction within ourselves. In this case, persistence means working through our own blockage. Occasionally, an obstacle is large enough that we cannot find a way around it. Then we must accept what is and move on. It does not make sense to continue to knock our heads against the obstruction. However, when something is really important, we must be tenacious to achieve the objective.

Persistence is needed in any change project. Simply reviewing the change one time with everyone involved does not mean that the change will be made or that anyone will implement it. Tenacity is important in its achievement along with a lot of other potential incremental changes. Hopefully, the end result better serves our patients.

Accountability

With decision making comes accountability for outcomes. As we lead, responsibilities follow. "The buck stops here."

> Leaders are responsible for achieving the organization's desired outcomes and for making things happen. Accountability for one's leadership is a true example of good stewardship in practice. While getting results, however, accountability also involves the generosity to reward and recognize those who contribute toward achieving the expected outcomes. In ensuring accountability, it is important for leaders to have a sense for when to intervene and for when to let go. (Shirey, 2007, p. 170)

We are responsible for our decisions, as well as for the actions of staff who report to us. Were the outcomes what we expected? Was there an unexpected outcome? Should we have made the decision(s) or should others have been more involved? How could we have done it better? How can we fix something that happened as a result of our decisions or our staff's decisions? An effective leader does not blame herself or others when a mistake is made. Instead, effective leaders ask, "How can this mistake be rectified? What will we do differently next time? Did we learn from our mistake?"

Leadership Fallacies

Certain leadership fallacies can negatively affect leadership effectiveness. Fallacies, as shown in **Exhibit 2–8**, are traps that derail us or cause us to be less effective leaders. Once understood, we can overcome leadership fallacies and our leadership will improve.

Perhaps it is best to start by examining our language, which can enhance or detract from our leadership effectiveness. Several words in business do not support quantum leadership. For example, the terms *subordinate* and *superior* indicate that one person is better than another. *Never* use such terms. Each person has gifts and abilities that benefit everyone else. The housekeeper is just as important as the CEO. After all, if the wastebaskets are not emptied and the bathrooms are not cleaned properly, we all suffer and leadership has not occurred. Other terms, such as *staff* and *supervisor, administrator,* or *boss,* can be substituted for *subordinate* and *superior.*

Another example of problematic language is to call everyone *my* staff or *girls/boys/kids.* In the first case, although we all might be in the same work group, no one belongs to anyone else. In the second case, it is demeaning to infantilize people by referring to them as children and indicates that we do not believe they are capable adults. We demonstrate this concept in the nursing profession when we use such expressions as *girls,* implying that staff are children, have not yet grown up, and need parenting. Leadership is the result of interactions where everyone is valued equally.

Another word commonly used in business literature is *control,* such as the *span of control* of a manager—a management term. In fact, control is a myth. We suggest not using this term. After all, controlling ourselves is hard enough! Think of our inability to turn down a wonderful dessert or a bag of chips. How well do we *really* control *ourselves*? It is a fallacy to believe that we control others. Dictators have tried—and continue to try—but no one has been successful. After all, a controlling manager is an ineffective one. We suggest using *responsibilities* as a better word for control. We could list a manager's *responsibilities* rather than talk about her *span of control.*

Another problematic term used in health care is *noncompliance.* Most often we say that patients are noncompliant, meaning that they did not follow our treatment regimen. According to whom? What about the patient's values? This smacks of the attitude, "Do this my way." What about the patient's point of view? Was there interaction between the healthcare professional and the patient to determine the actions needed?

A misconception in the business literature is the implication that administrators are leaders, and all others are followers. We have mentioned already that everyone is at times a leader.

Some question whether leadership can be learned. They say that leaders have inborn qualities that cannot be taught to others. However, *leadership can be learned,* and we can always improve our relationships with others and the leadership that results. This learning happens serendipitously, in infinite ways as we experience life.

Another issue is that leadership is more important than managing day-to-day activities. Both are important. The work needs to be done in a way that the people involved determine is best.

Similarly, a fallacy is that the administrator has all the answers. The first problem here is that leadership is the result of interactions; no one person has all the answers. The answers keep changing and are determined at the time of each interaction. New and different twists in situations must be taken into account. Many times the best answer comes from an interaction or event that triggers us to think about the problem differently. It is okay for an administrator not to know what to do. It is okay to say, "I do not know. Do you have any suggestions or solutions to this problem?" This is all part of the *interaction* that *produces more effective solutions* to problems.

It is a fallacy to assume that when everyone in the work group is empowered, the result is peace and harmony. Instead, many times, there is conflict. Establish a dialogue with each other about the conflicts. *Disagreement and healthy argument on issues provide different perspectives and help a group move to better outcomes* that would not have arisen without the disagreement. Thus, continuous improvement is achieved.

Exhibit 2-8   Leadership Fallacies

Leadership Fallacies	Replace by
Subordinate and superior are appropriate labels for people within organizations, as are my staff and girls, boys, kids.	Instead, use the words staff; supervisor or administrator; and women or men.
Control is a component of effective leadership.	Control of others is impossible. Staff are equitable and accountable partners in the work.
Patients are described as being noncompliant.	What about the patient's point of view?
The administrators are the leaders while other staff are followers.	Everyone is a leader.
Leaders have inborn qualities. Leadership cannot be learned.	Leadership can be learned by anyone. It has more to do with our gifts and life purpose.
Leadership is better than management.	Actually we need a combination to effectively accomplish work. The problem occurs when someone is predominantly management, not taking into account others' perceptions, ideas, knowledge, and relationships.
The administrator, or CEO, has all the answers.	The answers come from everyone.
When everyone is empowered and there is effective leadership, the result is peace and harmony.	Actually the result is that not everyone agrees. Conflicts occur necessitating dialogue to work through issues. Better solutions result.
There is one right way to do the work.	There are many ways that are effective.
What works well in one group will work well in another.	People are different and thus groups of people differ as well. What could work effectively with one group might not work with another.
Administrators strive to have everyone like them.	This is not possible. A better goal is that everyone respects the administrator because the administrator consistently supports the core value.
Effective administrators always use a participative leadership style, involving staff in every decision.	There are times, such as in an emergency, when being participative is not an effective method. In this case someone must make a decision quickly.
A leader must always win.	This is not humanly possible.
Claim another person's idea or work as one's own.	Integrity is important. Give credit where credit is due.
Threatened by more competent people/Do not want staff to outshine oneself.	Competent staff increase a leader's effectiveness, and make the work group more effective.
Leaders do not fear anything.	It is important to recognize our fears and deal with them.
Charisma is an essential aspect of leadership.	Love one another is the essential part of leadership.
Our leadership is perfect; the problems are caused by every else's behaviors.	Our actions may be causing the problem. Thus we always need to examine whether we are contributing to the problem.
We have always done it this way.	The only constant is change.
We think we are better than others because of our administrative title or our degree.	Everyone is equally important.
Pursue one's own selfish agendas.	Think about how each action affects others.
Gender or race bias issues an contribute to erroneous decisions.	It is better to base our assessment of others based on their gifts and contributions.

Leadership Fallacies	Replace by
Successful managers/people are promoted before effective managers/people.	Effective managers do a better job.
A manager who politicks regularly with the supervisor is effective.	The supervisor needs to always do regular rounds to determine manager effectiveness.

Source: Dunham-Taylor, J., & Pinczuk, J. *Financial Management for Nurse Managers: Merging the Heart with the Dollar,* 2nd ed. Burlington, MA: Jones & Bartlett Learning.

An erroneous leadership expectation is that there is one right way to do the work. Expecting others to "do it *my way*" does not necessarily achieve the best possible result. People differ. Work groups are never the same. Change happens. What was right yesterday is outdated today.

It is a mistake for an administrator to think that what works well with one group will work equally well with another. What might work effectively with one collection of people could bomb with another. It is important to know how group members work together. Then, the administrator can better anticipate methods that might work effectively with that group.

Some administrators want everyone to like them. This can be dangerous because, realistically, everyone will not. Their dislike may be as simple as we resemble their Aunt Alice or Grandpa Mike, who treated them badly in the past. When administrators want everyone to like them, they may change decisions depending on the current individual's or group's wants. This causes a lack of consistency in the administrators' actions. People notice this and interactions will be ineffective. This is a trap. A better option is for administrators to have staff *respect* them and to make decisions that support the core value: *what is best for the patient*. Sometimes staff disagree with an administrator's decisions. Interactions may not have been positive. However, even though they may disagree, if staff respect the administrator, that is the most important factor.

Some people think that effective administrators *always* use a participative leadership style, involving staff in every decision. If an administrator never makes a decision without having staff discussion, this is not effective leadership. There are times, such as emergency situations, when the administrator, or whoever is present, needs to make decisions and proceed with action based on current data. The key here is that the administrator knows when it is best to just make a decision, when it is best to have dialogue about a situation, and when it is best to have staff decide what to do.

Another trap is the belief that one must always win. First, when we lose, it can teach us a lot—humility or not to do something a certain way again. Second, maybe we were wrong and made a mistake, and maybe it is a good thing that we lost. Third, how do we know that we have the best solution? Maybe someone else has a better one. If staff interpret the leader's comments as saying that their idea really isn't very good, people will not be as committed to the idea as they were at the beginning of the conversation. Fourth, as people share ideas with us it may be better to encourage them to try their own ideas—and not add how we might do it. Fifth, how important is the incident? Is it something that we will even remember 10 years from now?

Invariably, conflicts arise in the workplace. It is not humanly possible to resolve every conflict. If some issue is really important, such as in a life-or-death situation, it is important that a decision be made. However, if it is a trivial issue, it may be best to just overlook the situation.

An ethical issue is when a manager takes another person's idea or work and claims the success as her or his own. This selfish action does not demonstrate integrity. Generally, word gets out, the manager is "found out," and others lose respect for the manager. When we do not give others credit for their work, we are not effective as leaders. Integrity, discussed earlier in this chapter, is important. We must always give credit where credit is due.

Some administrators do not want staff to shine or to look better than they do. Usually, this happens when someone who seems very competent threatens the administrator's ego. The administrator is ruled by fear because the competent person looks better than the administrator does or might even upstage the administrator. In such cases, the administrator is drawn to and hires incompetent people so as not to confront this issue. Is it any wonder that such a work group usually has problems, being mediocre at best? This administrator may need to be replaced or must do a lot of work to change such behavior. Instead, administrators must realize that when staff shine, it makes us look good.

Another fallacy is that the administrator does not fear anything. Fear is a human trait. We are human. However, fear of any kind interferes with our leadership effectiveness. When we feel fear, we must stop and catch ourselves. Fear causes a downward spiral in our choices of actions and only worsens the situation. The best way to deal with fear is to recognize the feeling and then find a way to deal with it. For instance, in the Judeo-Christian tradition, one comforting place to turn is Psalm 91, which describes the Lord as our protector.

Some identify *charisma* as important in effective leadership, and a lot of research has been done to measure charisma. Some confuse charisma with the ability to convince others to do what we want them to do. Instead, we need to ask, "How do we know that what we want to do is best? What harmful side effects might be caused by this? What will people do when we are not around?" In actuality, many researchers have concluded that being charismatic is not an essential part of effective leadership and can, in fact, be detrimental (Collins & Porras, 1994; Khurana, 2002). The important factors in effective leadership are the administrator's commitment to the mission and values and that the administrator lives the values consistently and humbly. This then inspires and motivates others.

We must never consider our leadership to be perfect or assume problems are caused by everyone else's behaviors. Sometimes, administrators do not realize that they operate under this fallacy, which can be very dangerous. As discussed previously, we must first examine how we might have contributed to the problem. We all have an Achilles' heel. Our own actions may actually be causing the problem. Others may do those things better or think of better ways to handle situations. This is why 360 evaluations are so important. They give us clues as to what we need to improve personally. The people around us every day—staff, colleagues, family members—can give us the best feedback on our issues for improvement. If there is trust, and we invite people to disagree with us, we can have a healthier view of ourselves, and the environment will be more positive for everyone.

We should avoid the fallacy that because something has always been done a certain way, that way is best. Status quo is death. Although it is important to know the history behind certain actions, the world is constantly changing, and so must our practices. Better to know the evidence and use it to make decisions that are best for the current situation.

A misleading notion is to give importance to titles, such as vice president or manager, or academic degrees, such as a doctorate, and believe that we are better than others because of them. Everyone is equally important, regardless of title or degree. Along this line, it can be tempting to pursue our own selfish agenda, not thinking of how it may affect others. People do not thrive under dictators unless they support the dictator's views. And even then, they must be careful not to say or do something unacceptable to the dictator.

Another erroneous belief revolves around gender and race issues. Some people do not believe women or people of a certain race can lead effectively. Some people feel more comfortable dealing with others who are like them. For example, in nursing some among us discriminate against male nurses. On the other hand, female applicants for an administrative position may not be considered because preference is given to male applicants. Evidence shows that when resumes are reviewed, both male and female reviewers rate female applicants lower than males when the applicant's sex is known. Unfortunately, this is also true with race. Biases still exist in our society. To change them, the place to start is within ourselves: It is a better policy to treat *everyone* with respect and to give *everyone* equal treatment based on each person's gifts, abilities, and experiences.

In some cases, the evidence does point to differences in leadership style based on gender. For instance, in business research, studies consistently show that women are more transformational than men (Sharpe, 2000). However, in studies examining nurse executive leadership specifically, the results consistently show that sex and race have no impact on effective leadership. In these nursing studies both men and women are equally transformational in their leadership style. Perhaps this is based on the value of caring—an important philosophy of our profession.

In an observational study, Luthans (1988) discovered a distinct difference between what he labeled *successful* and *effective* managers. Some managers were able to exhibit both traits, but often managers exhibited one trait predominantly:

> Successful managers give relatively more attention to networking (socializing, politicking, and interacting with outsiders) . . . and give relatively little attention to human resource management activities (motivating/reinforcing, managing conflict, staffing, and training/development). (p. 127)

Yet effective managers have a very different work style:

> Effective managers give by far the most relative attention and effort to communicating (exchanging information and processing paperwork) and human resource management activities and the least to networking. (p. 127)

According to this study, a *successful* manager is promoted relatively quickly, whereas the *effective* manager may not be promoted quickly but has "satisfied and committed" staff who achieve higher quantity and quality in their work performance. So, if there is a leadership problem, the manager may be more like the *successful* manager.

Supervisors face another pitfall. A successful manager, by politicking with the supervisor, may be perceived to be a better nurse manager than is actually the case. This is why it is so important for administrators at all levels regularly to do rounds, talking with everyone. In effective rounding, leadership problems are readily apparent, whereas one might not recognize such problems if only interacting with the manager.

By understanding leadership fallacies, we can avoid possible traps that make us less effective leaders. Next, we turn to leadership excellence.

So, What Is Effective Leadership?

Effective leadership is a continuous learning process. It is a path of discovery.

> In this chaotic world, we need leaders. But we don't need bosses. We need leaders to help us develop the clear identity that lights the dark moments of confusion. We need leaders to support us as we learn how to live by our values. We need leaders to understand that we are best controlled by concepts that invite our participation, not policies and procedures that curtail our contribution. (Wheatley, 2006, p. 131)

Effective leadership, or love one another, will continue to evolve. There is so much more to learn! The giving and receiving of love in whatever form it expresses itself can have a more lasting impact than any other single thing we do. All healing finds its roots in the expression of love.

It can reach far deeper places than any pill can go.

Although it is imperative to give physical bodies the support they need, it is equally imperative to give our spirits the love they need to access tremendous healing power (Joy, 2003, p. 26).

Notes

1. This is widely available. One source is Keirsey and Bates (1984), or go to www.humanmetrics.com/cgi-win/JTypes1.htm.
2. Available from Human Synergistics International, 39819 Plymouth Rd., C-8020, Plymouth, MI 48170, Tel: 800-622-7584 or 734-459-1030, Fax: 734-459-5557, e-mail: info@humansynergistics.com, website: www.humansynergistics.com
3. This quote is from a nurse executive interview. Confidentiality was promised, so the person cannot be named here.

Discussion Questions

1. Give an example where poor leadership affects the bottom line. Describe the ineffective leadership, and place dollar amounts on the losses incurred.
2. Describe someone you have known who is an excellent leader. What was he or she like?
3. After reading this chapter, what kind of a leader do you want to be? How can you improve your leadership?
4. Give an example of poor leadership. Which fallacies apply to leadership in this situation?
5. Are you an effective or a successful manager? Has your experience as a manager been like Luthans describes?
6. In your management role, how much are you able to lead versus managing? Do you want to change this ratio? If so, what actions will you take to change it?
7. Think of an example where you have effectively used first-order change. Then, give an example where you have used second-order change (reframing). Were the situations appropriate for the level of change you used?
8. Go through each of the emotional intelligence components and rate your current level of leadership. What are your gifts? What do you want to improve? How will you improve them?
9. Describe an example where effective leadership has saved the organization money. If you had to describe this to a finance person, how would you most effectively present this information? Then, if you had to describe this to a nurse, how would you do so?
10. Nurse managers are caught in a squeeze between delivering quality care to patients, keeping patient satisfaction scores up, and meeting bottom-line requirements. What advice would you give to a new nurse manager to help this person avoid some pitfalls that you have encountered because of this squeeze?
11. How do you achieve balance in your life?
12. What is wisdom? Humility? Integrity? Empathy? How can you tell if people possess these qualities?
13. Have you participated in any assessments of your leadership style? If so, what did the assessment(s) show?
14. Have you experienced intuition in your management role? In your nursing career? Describe it.
15. How does the Pygmalion effect apply to effective leadership?
16. Give an example of staying in the adult when in the midst of conflict.
17. Describe a conflict your work team has experienced. How did you all resolve it? Or, was it not resolved? If it was not resolved, what would you do differently to more effectively deal with this situation if you were the nurse manager?
18. Have you experienced empowerment? Have you empowered others?
19. What is your usual stage of power, as Hagberg describes it, when at work?
20. What are some differences between having a supervisor who empowers others, and one who does not?
21. What are your gifts? Have you identified what gifts each member of the work team has?
22. Describe a situation where it is best for the work group to make a decision about their work. Then, describe a situation where it is best for the nurse manager to make a decision.
23. Have you thought about what your life purpose might be? What is it?
24. Have you experienced a crucible event that changed your approach to life?
25. Have you experienced something significant, such as a sentinel event, where an apology helped to heal?

Glossary of Terms

Administration—the CGEAN definition: *Administration* comprises working with and through others to achieve the mission, values, and vision of an organization. Administration is an executive function within an organization and has ultimate accountability for defining and achieving the organization's strategic plan. Administration designates responsibility for implementing organizational goals.

Authentic Leadership—consists of 4 components: *self-awareness* (understanding of and trust in one's motives, feelings, desires, strengths, and weaknesses), *relational transparency* (appropriate expression of one's genuine self through open sharing with followers), *internalized moral perspective* (self-regulation guided by internal moral standards rather than external pressures from groups, organizations, or society), and *balanced information processing* (willingness to objectively analyze data and solicit others' opinions before decision making).

Laissez-Faire Leadership—is where the leader does nothing.

Leadership—occurs in the space between two individuals. The formal CGEAN definition: *Leadership* is the process of influencing others toward the attainment of one or more goals. Leadership comprises two types: formal and informal. Formal leadership occurs through official titular designations within an organization or society. Informal leadership occurs when the perceptions and actions of others are influenced by individuals without such official organizational or societal designations. Leadership is not limited to the accomplishment of organizational goals.

Management—the CGEAN definition: *Management* is the process of aligning resources with needs to attain specific goals. Management includes planning, organizing, motivating, monitoring, and evaluating human and material resources. Although management usually refers to a mid-level formal leadership function within an organization, it is also the process used at any level to align and allocate resources.

Obliquity Leadership—is where staff can take a management plan and adapt it to fit their customers, each time they are with customers. The name comes from their ability to make oblique decisions.

Pygmalion Effect—is where a supervisor's beliefs about the person being supervised become a self-fulfilling prophecy.

Quantum Leadership—a dynamic, integrated process that takes place in relationships.

Servant Leadership—advocates 10 principles for leaders: listening, empathy, healing, awareness, persuasion, conceptualization, foresight, stewardship, commitment to the growth of people, and community building.

Transformational Leadership—is where leaders are charismatic, providing inspirational motivation, intellectual stimulation, and individualized consideration.

Transactional Leadership—is when leaders use contingent reward, and management by exception—active and passive. It includes more of the management functions.

References

Adams, J. (2012). Exploring influential nurse executive leadership: An interview with Maria Weston. *Journal of Nursing Administration*, *42*(1), 12–14.

Adams, J., & Erickson, J. (2011). Applying the Adams influence model in nurse executive practice. *Journal of Nursing Administration*, *41*(4), 186–192.

Akerjordet, K., & Severinsson, E. (2010). The state of the science of emotional intelligence related to nursing leadership: An integrative review. *Journal of Nursing Management*, *18*, 363–382.

American Hospital Association. (2011, September). *Hospitals and care systems of the future*. Retrieved from http://www.aha.org/about/org/hospitals-care-systems-future.shtml

American Nurses Association. (2009). *Nursing administration: Scope and standards of practice*. Washington, DC: American Nurses Association.

Anderson, B., O'Connor, P., Manno, M., & Gallagher, E. (2010). Listening to nursing leaders: Using national database of nursing quality indicators data to study excellence in nursing leadership. *Journal of Nursing Administration*, *40*(4), 182–187.

Arbinger Institute. (2002). *Leadership and self-deception: Getting out of the box*. San Francisco, CA: Berrett-Kohler.

Baker, S., Marshburn, D., Crickmore, K., Rose, S., Dutton, K., & Hudson, P. (2012). What do you do? Perceptions of nurse manager responsibilities. *Nursing Management*, *43*(12), 25–30.

Bally, J. (2007). The role of nursing leadership in creating a mentoring culture in acute care environments. *Nursing Economic$*, *25*(3), 143–148.

Bass, B. (1998). *Transformational leadership: Industry, military, and educational impact*. Mahwah, NJ: Erlbaum.

Batcheller, J. (2011). On-boarding and enculturation of new chief nursing officers. *Journal of Nursing Administration*, *41*(5), 235–239.

Benjamin, K., Riskus, R., & Skalla, A. (2011). The emerging leader: Leadership development based on the Magnet model. *Journal of Nursing Administration*, *41*(4), 156–158.

Benner, P. (1984). *From novice to expert: Excellence and power in clinical nursing practice.* Menlo Park, CA: Addison-Wesley.

Bennis, W., & Nanus, B. (1985). *Leaders: The strategies for taking charge.* New York, NY: Harper & Row.

Bennis, W., & Thomas, R. (2002, September). Crucibles of leadership. *Harvard Business Review*, *80*(9), 39–45.

Beyers, M. (2006). Nurse executives' perspectives on succession planning. *Journal of Nursing Administration*, *36*(6), 304–312.

Blouin, A., Neistadt, A., McDonagh, K., & Helfnad, B. (2006). Leading tomorrow's healthcare organizations: Strategies and tactics for effective succession planning. *Journal of Nursing Administration*, *36*(6), 325–330.

Bodin, S. (2012). A critical look at critical thinking: What are RN perceptions of leadership skills? *Nursing Management*, *42*(8), 43–46.

Bolman, L., & Deal, T. (2001). *Leading with soul: An uncommon journey of spirit.* San Francisco, CA: Jossey-Bass.

Bonczek, M., & Woodard, E. (2006). Who'll replace you when you're gone? *Nursing Management*, *35*(8), 31–35.

Braden, G. (2000). *The Isaiah effect: Decoding the lost science of prayer and prophecy.* New York, NY: Three Rivers Press.

Brooks, C. (1966). Report on work in sensory awareness and total functioning. In H. A. Otto (Ed.), *Explorations in human potentialities* (pp. 487–505). Springfield, IL: Charles C. Thomas.

Bulmer, J. (2013). Leadership aspirations of registered nurses: Who wants to follow us? *Journal of Nursing Administration*, *43*(3), 130–134.

Burkhart, L., Solari-Twadell, A., & Haas, S. (2008). Addressing spiritual leadership: An organizational model. *Journal of Nursing Administration*, *38*(1), 33–39.

Burns, J. (1978). *Leadership.* New York, NY: Harper.

Byham, W., Cox, J., & Nelson, G. (1996). *Zapp! Empowerment in health care.* New York, NY: Fawcett Columbine.

Cadmus, E. (2006). Succession planning: Multilevel organizational strategies for the new workforce. *Journal of Nursing Administration*, *36*(6), 298–303.

Cadmus, E. (2011). Your role in redesigning health care. *Nursing Management*, *43*(10), 32–42.

Cadmus, E., & Holmes, A. (2013). Leadership's "triple chance": Design, evaluate, implement. *Nursing Management*, *44*(2), 44–48.

Cadmus, E., & Johansen, M. (2012). The time is now: Developing a nurse manager residency program. *Nursing Management*, *43*(11), 18–24.

Carriere, B., Cummings, G., Muise, M., & Newburn-Cook, C. (2009). Healthcare succession planning: An integrative review. *Journal of Nursing Administration*, *39*(12), 548–555.

Casida, J., & Pinto-Zipp, G. (2008). Leadership-organizational culture relationship in nursing units of acute care hospitals. *Nursing Economic$*, *26*(1), 7–16.

Cathcart, E., & Greenspan, M. (2012). A new window into nurse manager development: teaching for the practice. *Journal of Nursing Administration*, *42*(12), 557–561.

Chase, L. (2012). Are you confidently competent? *Nursing Management*, *43*(5), 50–53.

Chinn, P. (2013). *Peace and power: New directions for building community* (8th ed.). Burlington, MA: Jones & Bartlett Learning.

Clavelle, J. (2012). Transformational leadership: Visibility, accessibility, and communication. *Journal of Nursing Administration*, *42*(7/8), 345–346.

Clavelle, J., Tullai-McGuinness, S., Drenkard, K., & Fitzpatrick, J. (2012). Transformational leadership practices of chief nursing officers in magnet organizations. *Journal of Nursing Administration*, *42*(4), 195–201.

Cohen, S. (2013). Transitioning new leaders: Seven steps for success. *Nursing Management*, *44*(2), 9–11.

Collins, J., & Porras, J. (1994). *Built to last.* New York, NY: HarperBusiness.

Connaughton, M., & Hassinger, J. (2007). Leadership character: Antidote to organizational fatigue. *Journal of Nursing Administration*, *37*(10), 464–470.

Coughlin, C., & Hogan, P. (2008). Succession planning: After you, then who?: Mentor up-and-coming nurse leaders to fill your shoes. *Nursing Management*, *38*(11), 40–46.

Creedle, C., Walton, A., & McCann, M. (2012). A better balance: Sharing the nurse manager role. *Nurse Leader*, *19*(6), 30–32.

Crenshaw, J., & Yoder-Wise, P. (2013). Creating an environment for innovation: The risk-taking leadership competency. *Nurse Leader, 11*(1), 24–27.

de Bono, E. (1994). *De Bono's thinking course* (Rev. ed.) New York, NY: Facts on File.

DeCampli, P., Kirby, K., & Baldwin, C. (2010). Beyond the classroom to coaching: Preparing new nurse managers. *Critical Care Nursing Quarterly, 33*(2), 133–138.

Douglas, K. (2012). The return of the smiley face. *Nursing Economic$, 30*(2), 117, 119.

Drenkard, K. (2013). Transformational leadership: Unleashing the potential. *Journal of Nursing Administration, 43*(2), 57–58.

Dunham-Taylor, J. (1995). Identifying the best in nurse executive leadership: Part 2, interview results. *Journal of Nursing Administration, 25*(7/8), 24–31.

Effken, J., Logue, M., Verran, J., & Hsu, Y. (2010). Nurse manager's decisions: Fast and favoring remediation. *Journal of Nursing Administration, 40*(4), 188–195.

Erickson, J. (2012). Leading a highly visible hospital through a serious reportable event. *Journal of Nursing Administration, 42*(3), 131–133.

Failla, K., & Stichler, J. (2008). Manager and staff perceptions of the manager's leadership style. *Journal of Nursing Administration, 38*(11), 480–487.

Fennimore, L., & Wolf, G. (2011). Nurse manager leadership development: Leveraging the evidence and system-level support. *Journal of Nursing Administration, 41*(5), 204–210.

Fisher, R., Ury, W., & Patton, B. (1991). *Getting to yes: Negotiating agreement without giving in.* New York, NY: Houghton Mifflin.

Foltin, A., & Keller, R. (2012). Leading change with emotional intelligence. *Nursing Management, 43*(11), 20–25.

Frankl, V. (1984). *Man's search for meaning.* New York, NY: Washington Square Press.

Gallagher, T., Studdert, D., & Levinson, W. (2007). Disclosing harmful medical errors to patients. *New England Journal of Medicine, 336*(26), 2713–2719.

Gergen, D. (2003, January). How presidents persuade. *Harvard Business Review, 81*(1), 20–21.

Goleman, D. (1998). *Working with emotional intelligence.* New York, NY: Bantam Books.

Goudreau, K., & Hardy, J. (2006). Succession planning and individual development. *Journal of Nursing Administration, 36*(6), 313–318.

Hagberg, J. (2003). *Real power: Stages of personal power in organizations* (3rd ed.). Salem, WI: Sheffield.

Hay, L. (1984). *Heal Your Body.* Carson, CA: Hay House.

Homer, R., & Ryan, L. (2013, March). Making the grade: Charge nurse education improves job performance. *Nursing Management, 44*(3), 38–44.

Houston, M., & Wolf, G. (2011). Transformational leadership skills of successful nurse managers. *Journal of Nursing Administration, 41*(6), 248–251.

Huseman, R. (2009). The importance of positive culture in hospitals. *Journal of Nursing Administration, 39*(2), 60–63.

Institute of Medicine. (2010). *The future of nursing: Leading change, advancing health.* Washington, DC: National Academies Press.

Johnson, J. (1997). *The path of the masters.* New Delhi, India: Baba Barkha Nath Printers.

Johnson, K., Johnson, C., Nicholson, D., Potts, C., Raiford, H., & Shelton, A. (2012). Make an impact with transformational leadership and shared governance. *Nursing Management, 43*(10), 12–14.

Joy, S. (2003, March/April). Is there enough room in my job for love? *Nurse Leader,* 24–27.

Kath, L., Stichler, J., & Ehrhart, M. (2012). Moderators of the negative outcomes of nurse manager stress. *Journal of Nursing Administration, 42*(4), 215–221.

Kerfoot, K. (2007). Staff engagement: It starts with the leader. *Nursing Economic$, 25*(1), 47–48.

Kerfoot, K. (2009a). Good is not good enough: The culture of low expectations and the leader's challenge. *Nursing Economic$, 27*(2), 54–55.

Kerfoot, K. (2009b). The neuropsychology of good leaders making dumb mistakes. *Nursing Economic$, 27*(2), 134–135.

Kerfoot, K. (2009c). What you permit, you promote. *Nursing Economic$, 27*(4), 245–246, 250.

Kerfoot, K. (2011). Direct decision making vs. oblique decision making: Which is right? *Nursing Economic$, 29*(5), 290–291.

Keys, Y. (2011). Perspectives on executive relationships: Influence. *Journal of Nursing Administration, 41*(9), 347–349.

Khurana, R. (2002, September). The curse of the superstar CEO. *Harvard Business Review,* 60–66.

Kim, T. (2012). Succession planning in hospitals and the association with organizational performance. *Nursing Economic$, 30*(1), 14–20.

Kowalski, K., & Yoder-Wise, P. (2003). Five C's of leadership. *Nurse Leader, 5*(1), 26–31.

Kuhnert, K., & Lewis, P. (1987). Transactional and transformational leadership: A constructive/developmental analysis. *Academy of Management Review, 12*(4), 648–657.

Laschinger, H., Purdy, N., & Almost, J. (2007). The impact of leader-member exchange quality, empowerment, and core self-evaluation on nurse manager's job satisfaction. *Journal of Nursing Administration, 37*(3), 221–229.

Laschinger, H., & Smith, L. (2013). The influence of authentic leadership and empowerment on new-graduate nurses' perceptions of interprofessional collaboration. *Journal of Nursing Administration, 43*(1), 24–29.

Lazare, A. (2006). Apology in medical practice: An emerging clinical skill. *Journal of the American Medical Association, 296*(11), 1401–1404.

Livingston, J. (2003, January). Pygmalion in management. *Harvard Business Review,* 121–130.

Luthans, F. (1988). Successful vs. effective real managers. *Academy of Management Executive, 11*(2), 127–132.

Luzinski, C. (2011). Transformational leadership. *Journal of Nursing Administration, 41*(12), 501–507.

Mackoff, B., & Triolo, P. (2008a). Why do nurse managers stay? Building a model of engagement: Part 1, dimensions of engagement. *Journal of Nursing Administration, 38*(3), 118–124.

Mackoff, B., & Triolo, P. (2008b). Why do nurse managers stay? Building a model of engagement: Part 2, cultures of engagement. *Journal of Nursing Administration, 38*(4), 166–171.

MacMillan-Finlayson, S. (2010). Competency development for nurse executives: Meeting the challenge. *Journal of Nursing Administration, 40*(6), 254–257.

MacPhee, M. (2007). Strategies and tools for managing change. *Journal of Nursing Administration, 37*(9), 405–413.

Malcolm, H. (2013, January). Charge nurse university: Preparing future nurse leaders. *American Nurse Today, 8*(1), 38–40.

McClelland, D. (1973). Testing for competence rather than intelligence. *American Psychologist, 46,* 56–62.

McGuire, E., & Kennerly, S. (2006). Nurse managers as transformational and transactional leaders. *Nursing Economic$, 24*(4), 179–186.

Moneke, N., & Umeh, O. (2013). How leadership behaviors impact critical care nurse job satisfaction. *Nursing Management, 44*(1), 53–56.

Morris, T. (1994). *True success: A new philosophy of excellence.* New York, NY: Berkley Books.

Murphy, L. (2012). Authentic leadership: Becoming and remaining an authentic nurse leader. *Journal of Nursing Administration, 32*(11), 507–512.

Nauright, L. (2003, January/February). Educating the nurse leader for today and tomorrow. *Nurse Leader,* 25–27.

Neill, M., & Saunders, N. (2008). Servant leadership: Enhancing quality of care and staff satisfaction. *Journal of Nursing Administration, 38*(9), 395–400.

Nightingale, F. (1869). *Notes on nursing.* New York, NY: Dover.

O'Neil, E., Hirschkorn, C., Morjikian, R., West, T., & Cherner, E. (2008). Developing nursing leaders: An overview of trends and programs. *Journal of Nursing Administration, 38*(4), 178–183.

Patrician, P., Dawson, M., Oliver, D., Ladner, K., & Miltner, R. (2012, October). Nurturing charge nurses for future leadership roles. *JONA, 42*(10), 461–466.

Pedaline, S., Wolf, G., Dudjak, L., Lorenz, H., McLaughlin, M., & Ren, D. (2012). Preparing exceptional leaders. *Nursing Management, 43*(9), 38–44.

Perra, B. (2000). Leadership: The key to quality outcomes. *Nursing Administration Quarterly, 24*(2), 56.

Ponte, P., Galante, A., Gross, A., & Glazer, G. (2006). Using an executive coach to increase leadership effectiveness. *Journal of Nursing Administration, 36*(6), 319–324.

Porter-O'Grady, T. (2003, March–April). Of hubris and hope: Transforming nursing for a new age. *Nursing Economic$,* 59–64.

Porter-O'Grady, T., & Malloch, K. (2003). *Quantum leadership: A textbook of new leadership.* Sudbury, MA: Jones and Bartlett.

Porter-O'Grady, T., & Malloch, K. (2011). *Quantum Leadership: Advancing innovations, transforming health care.* Burlington, MA: Jones & Bartlett Learning.

Pross, E., Hilton, N., Boykin, A., & Thomas, C. (2011). The dance of caring persons: Transform your organization through caring values. *Nursing Management, 42*(10), 25–30.

Rao, A. (2012). The contemporary construction of nurse empowerment. *Journal of Nursing Scholarship, 44*(4), 396–402.

Redman, R. (2006). Leadership succession planning: An evidence-based approach for managing the future. *Journal of Nursing Administration, 36*(6), 292–297.

Roussel, L. (2013). *Management and leadership for nurse administrators* (6th ed.). Burlington, MA: Jones & Bartlett Learning.

Sharpe, R. (2000, November 20). As leaders, women rule. *Business Week*, 75–84.

Sherman, R. (2013). Too young to be a nurse leader? *American Nurse Today, 8*(1), 34–37.

Sherman, R., Bishop, M., Eggenberger, T., & Karden, R. (2007). Development of a leadership competency model. *Journal of Nursing Administration, 37*(2), 85–94.

Sherman, R., Schwarzkopf, R., & Kiger, A. (2013). What we learned from our charge nurses. *Nurse Leader, 11*(2), 34–39.

Shirey, M. (2007). Competencies and tips for effective leadership: From novice to expert. *Journal of Nursing Administration, 37*(4), 167–170.

Shirey, M. (2012). How resilient are your team members? *Journal of Nursing Administration, 42*(12), 551–553.

Shirey, M., Fisher, M., McDaniel, A., Doebbeling, B., & Ebright, P. (2010). Understanding nurse manager stress and work complexity: Factors that make a difference. *Journal of Nursing Administration, 40*(2), 82–91.

Simons, T. (2002, September). The high cost of lost trust. *Harvard Business Review*, 18–19.

Smith, M. (2011). Are you a transformational leader? *Nursing Management, 42*(9), 44–50.

Smith, Y. (2013). How to love and care for yourself unconditionally. *American Nurse Today, 8*(1), 30–33.

Snow, J. (2001, September). Looking beyond nursing for clues to effective leadership. *Journal of Nursing Administration, 31*(9), 440–443.

Stein, N. (2000, October 2). The world's most admired companies. *Fortune*, 183–196.

Sverdlik, B. (2012). Who will be our nursing leaders in the future? The role of succession planning. *Journal of Nursing Administration, 42*(7/8), 383–385.

Swan, B., & Moye, J. (2009). Growing ambulatory care nurse leaders: Building talent from the primed pipeline. *Nursing Economic$, 27*(4), 251–254.

Thompson, R., Wolf, D., & Sabatine, J. (2012). Mentoring and coaching: A model guiding professional nurses to executive success. *Journal of Nursing Administration, 42*(11), 536–541.

Tulgan, B. (2007). It's okay to be the boss—be a great one!: Embrace leadership by saying no to "undermanagement." *Nursing Management, 38*(9), 18–24.

Van Dusen, V., & Spies, A. (2003). Professional apology: Dilemma or opportunity? *American Journal of Pharmaceutical Education, 67*(4), Article 114, 1–6.

Vitello-Cicciu, J. (2002). Exploring emotional intelligence: Implications for nursing leaders. *Journal of Nursing Administration, 32*(4), 203–210.

von Franz, M. (1980). *Alchemy: An introduction to the symbolism and the psychology*. Toronto, Ontario: Inner City Books.

Watzlawick, P., Weakland, J., & Fisch, R. (1974). *Change: Principles of problem formation and problem resolution*. New York, NY: Norton.

Wendler, M., Olson-Sitki, K., & Prater, M. (2009). Succession planning for RNs: Implementing a nurse management internship. *Journal of Nursing Administration, 39*(7/8), 326–333.

Wheatley, M. (2006). *Leadership and the new science: Discovering order in a chaotic world* (3rd ed.). San Francisco, CA: Berrett-Koehler.

Wolf, G. (2012). Transformational leadership: The art of advocacy and influence. *Journal of Nursing Administration, 42*(6), 309–310.

Wolf, G., Bradle, J., & Greenhouse, P. (2006). Investment in the future: A 3-level approach for developing the health-care leaders of tomorrow. *Journal of Nursing Administration, 36*(6), 331–336.

Zori, S., & Morrison, B. (2009). Critical thinking in nurse managers. *Nursing Economic$, 27*(2), 75–80.

Organizations: Surviving Within a Chaotic, Complex, Value-Based Environment

Janne Dunham-Taylor, PhD, RN

OBJECTIVES

- Describe how communication, collaboration, and autonomy impact the organization.
- Understand how chaos and complexity affect organizations.
- Identify ways that nursing can impact the value-based environment (the second curve).
- Describe organizational competence.
- Identify evidence that impacts organizations.
- Understand the soul and spirit in an organization.
- Assess the healthcare organization.

Organizational Evidence

The United States has the highest health care costs in the world, *with third world outcomes.*

— J. Storfjell, O. Omoike, and S. Ohlson, *The Balancing Act:*
Patient Care Time Versus Cost

The real voyage of discovery is not in seeking new landscapes but in having new eyes.

—M. Proust

Healthcare organizations are in the midst of a major change in design. In this past century, we were in a volume-based, tertiary system. However, that perspective will no longer survive. In this new century, a value-based thrust in health care has emerged. *To meet that value-based perspective, healthcare organizations must change drastically to survive.* Consider the following evidence and observations:

Hospitals and health systems in the U.S. face unparalleled pressures to change in the future. Industry experts have projected that multiple intersecting environmental forces will drive the transformation of health care delivery and financing from volume-based to value-based payments over the next decade. These influences include everything from the aging population to the unsustainable rise in health care spending as a percentage of national gross domestic product.

Economic futurist Ian Morrison believes that as the payment incentives shift, health care providers will go through a classic modification in their core models for business and service delivery. He refers to the volume-based environment hospitals currently face as the *first curve* and the future value-based marker dynamic as the *second curve.* Progressing from the *first curve* to the *second curve* is a vital transition for hospitals. This is analogous to having one foot on the dock and one foot on the boat—at the right point, the management of that shift is essential to future success. (American Hospital Association 2011 Committee on Performance Improvement [AHA], 2011)

Half the decisions in organizations fail. Studies of 356 decisions in medium to large organizations in the U.S. and Canada reveal that these failures can be traced to managers who impose solutions, limit the search for alternatives, and use power to implement their plans. Managers who make the need for action clear at the outset, set objectives, carry out an unrestricted search for solutions, and get key people to participate are more apt to be successful. Tactics prone to fail were used in two of every three decisions that were studied. (Nutt, 1999, p. 75)

Even the best concepts or strategies tend to develop incrementally. They rarely ever work the first time out or unfold just as they were planned. (Pearson, 2002, p. 122)

In Honda plants, . . . even relatively routine . . . problems are solved by rapidly created, temporary teams assembled when needed from people who come from throughout the [facility]—not just from the specific area where the problem was first observed. The roots of even seemingly straightforward problems can be far-flung and thus require a surprisingly broad range of institutional knowledge to be resolved. (Watts, 2003, p. 17)

Evidence is all around us. We have been using evidence to identify best practices for the last decade. But best practice goes beyond patient care. It also applies to management practices and organizational improvement. The American Organization of Nurse Executives (AONE)

has taken the strongest possible position on the importance of using best evidence in leadership and management practices. Leadership's use of best evidence in making organizational decisions has potential to impact patient care to a greater extent than does a single clinician using best practices at the bedside. (Marshall, 2008, p. 205)

What we thought worked before (such as the importance of transparency) now often has empirical evidence to support it. It is so important for nurse administrators to keep up-to-date on management and organizational evidence.

The Second Curve of Health Care

One important major shift in health care, supported by the evidence, is the change from a *volume-based environment* (the *first curve*) to a *value-based environment* (the *second curve*). The American Hospital Association (AHA) published two special reports on the major change (AHA, 2011, 2013). In the past century (Industrial Age—first curve), reimbursement was based on volume of insured patients, patriarchal systems and authoritarian leadership abounded, the bottom line was often first priority, and patients were told what to do. Now evidence shows that a major shift has occurred as we enter this new century (Information Age—second curve) that has eroded the old Industrial Age practices.

A number of changes have occurred together (*complexity*), necessitating that we change course in health care. Currently, more information than any one person can possibly know is available. This results in evidence-based care, in evidence that the old patriarchal and authoritarian systems are ineffective and lose money, in research that shows that a bottom-line orientation loses money, and in proof that reimbursement is related to quality and the continuum of care, not just volume (value-based reimbursement). We are realizing that we need to pay attention to what the patient wants and values. This is in the midst of appalling reports that show how many patients are injured or killed because of our poor healthcare practices. Patients have access to a lot of information. Physicians (and nurses) need to listen to patients and work more closely with them so they can make decisions about their care. (*Note:* Although the term *health care* is used throughout this book, in reality *tertiary illness care* is primarily being discussed. This is because historically tertiary illness care was given most of the "healthcare" dollars.)

A review of leadership development—for both staff and patients—at the point of care highlights its importance. The AHA 2011 report agrees with this assessment.

> Several of the interviewees relayed that the power and success of their organization is completely based on the culture, desire, and dedication of their employees. To thrive in a second-curve market, every clinical and administrative employee must be involved in initiatives to control expenses, improve efficiency, increase quality, and understand the new accountability that hospitals have to overall population health. Interviewees emphasized that change is going to happen, and that their respective organizations must train a new breed of administrative and clinical leadership to manage that change effectively. This can be accomplished with a variety of educational and involvement strategies. Organizations noted that even small engagement in employee health and wellness programs positively impacted turnover rates. As physicians continue to become better aligned with the interests of acute-care facilities, it is a necessity to provide leadership training to clinicians who may be able to guide the integration process. (AHA, 2011, p. 18, in reference to Strategy 6 discussed later)

To survive in this new value-based environment, the AHA (2013) recommends 10 *must-do strategies* for hospitals:

1. Aligning hospitals, physicians, and other providers across the continuum of care (p. 3)
2. Utilizing evidence-based practices to improve quality and patient safety (pp. 5–6)
- Effective measurement and management of care transitions
  Fully implemented clinical integration strategy across the entire continuum of care to ensure seamless transitions and clear handoffs

In Strategy 7 in the list of must-do strategies, the AHA Committee on Performance Improvement (AHA, 2011) states:

> Hospitals must prepare for tightening margins. The future of decreased reimbursement and a more severe case-mix commands today's organizations to find the means to cut costs and improve their operating margin without sacrificing any quality in the care provided. Simultaneously, technologies are being designed that significantly improve outcomes but are also a huge financial investment for the majority of institutions. Interviewees commented that without maintaining or improving current operating margins, they would not have the financial resources to perform any of the other must-do strategies such as focusing on quality and patient safety, creating strategic alliances with physicians and other providers, or engaging employees. To achieve the financial status desired for future innovation, organizations will have to fix their current service offerings, capital, and management structure to meet the needs of their population and reduce fixed costs throughout their budget. (p. 19)

In this text, written by a nurse administrator and CFO, we have stressed the importance of nursing and finance working together. People from both areas must understand the issues inherent in this relationship, such as speaking different languages (*linear* versus *relationship* perspectives), not understanding the other's worldview (financial people not understanding the care side; nursing not understanding the financial side), and possible male–female differences. To work together more effectively we need to develop a broader perspective in both professions because it is critical in this environment that frequent communication occurs.

Also, because we anticipate fewer dollars for care, this necessitates an interdisciplinary focus in dealing with this problem. If the administrative leadership is ineffective or stuck in the old authoritarian model, the organization will decline and, if not corrected, eventually fail. Achieving success in this arena depends on having second-curve administrative leadership in place. This chapter focuses on organizations. Evidence shows that a positive organizational culture makes money; achieves patient, staff, and physician satisfaction; allows fewer errors; and provides better quality care. To achieve a positive culture, it is important for everyone in the organization to support the mission and core values in their every action.

In this chapter, first we explore complexity issues that have brought about the need for second-wave organizations. Then, we examine components of a second-wave organization to help ensure that we leave behind first-wave mentality and make the necessary changes to move deeper into a second-wave organization. We define *organizational competence* and discuss how to assess organizations, including the importance of everyone doing regular rounds, to have a better idea of how to best make continuous second-wave changes.

Change Is All Around Us

Presently, we are at an interesting juncture in time because healthcare organizations are changing very significantly.

> Leaders must develop affection for risk and for the edges of agreement and understanding. They must be able to [meander like the river] so that the mental models people bring to the resolution of concerns or the determination of strategies and actions are shifted or even fundamentally altered. There is nothing worse in deliberation than using a mental model or frame of reference that does not fit the circumstances. As we move inexorably into the new age, we must try to understand its characteristics within the context of its becoming rather than of the past. Peter Drucker said it best when he suggested that we must all close the door on the Industrial Age and simply turn around. (Porter-O'Grady & Malloch, 2011, p. 28)

The old model was either based on who had authority (physicians or the executive group) or the location of the service (nursing, laboratory, radiology). As this old model crumbles (including many of the buildings), healthcare leaders are being called into the *chaos* of creativity to produce a good fit between the new framework demanded and the infrastructure that needs to be constructed to support it.[1]

> Changes in technology, service structure, clinical models, consumer demand, and healthcare economics are conspiring to create a need for healthcare organizations that possess the same fluidity and nimbleness required of [other] businesses. The chaos currently being experienced in the system arises from the conflict between the requirement for a radical shift in design and service and the continuing infrastructure. The myriad stakeholders—nurses, doctors, hospitals, pharmacists, etc.—are struggling to hold onto their piece of the healthcare pie without realizing the pie is now being sliced in an entirely different way. (Porter-O'Grady & Malloch, 2011, pp. 33–34)

As we examine organizations, it is important that we understand what is going on around us. A chaotic, complex process has been occurring, not only on the earth (just look at the weather), but within healthcare organizations. *To survive, it is important to be constantly aware of possibilities and find vastly different ways to better serve clients—most of the service will not be in hospitals.*

Consider the following:

- Time is becoming more compressed.
- Change is happening more frequently.
- The unexpected will happen.
- Medical practices continue to become less invasive.
- Eastern and Western medicine are merging.
- Healthcare (a misnomer because it has focused on illness care) is shifting from medical care to genomics integrated with other alternative options.
- Information (including general health information) is instantly available to everyone.
- The hospital bed has ceased to be the main point of service and services will increasingly move out of the hospital. During the next two decades, the number of hospital beds will decline by about 50%. By the end of this decade, more than 70% of the medical services currently provided in hospitals will be provided in clinics and doctors' offices.
- The service structure is more decentralized, more fluid, and more highly mobilized (with service being delivered in small, broadly dispersed units of service).
- Healthcare providers (including physicians and nurses) must be aware of current evidence and change their practices accordingly.
- Core practices of the health professions are being substantially altered.
- Insurers base payment on patient outcomes rather than delivered services.
- The middle class continues to be eroded so fewer people can afford health insurance.
- The Affordable Care Act of 2010 brings healthcare services to many who cannot afford it, and/or who may not want to purchase it. It brings increased taxes for everyone to pay for this, and yet this may not be enough money to provide this service.
- People who can afford it and who value it, are reaching outside the traditional medical focus for alternative, holistic care.
- The locus of control continues to shift from the provider to the user—emphasis has changed from simply rendering services the patient may not want or services not linked with good patient outcomes to what the patient values/wants.

- Patients need to partner with providers to understand options available to them as they undergo care.
- The numbers of elderly people are increasing, many of whom have multiple chronic illnesses.
- There are not enough long-term care facilities to meet the increased needs of elderly adults.
- Better case management is needed to keep patients out of hospitals and long-term care facilities; most patients prefer to be at home.
- Technology continues to proliferate.
- Social media, when misused, can easily violate Health Insurance Portability and Accountability Act (HIPAA).
- Connection between providers and patients (telemedicine) will increasingly be virtual, with supporting technology making clinical services possible without bringing patients to the provider.

In *The New Health Age*, Houle and Fleece (2011) define three forces driving health care: (1) the flow to global—patients can fly anywhere for needed health care and can find it less expensively outside the United States; (2) the flow to the individual—patients have more information available to them to make better healthcare choices; and (3) accelerated connectedness—we can communicate anywhere, anytime, meaning that we can communicate and share new medical treatments and research from various locations around the world.

Houle and Fleece (2011) identify nine dynamic flows operating in the present healthcare environment:

How we think about health care
- Sickness → Wellness
  Currently, health care is about curing sickness. Our current model does not encourage patients to learn how to stay healthy and prevent disease. Yet incentives are increasing to encourage wellness. For example, Knutson and colleagues (2013) describe one model that includes alternative health options.
- Ignorance → Awareness/Understanding
  There is employer recognition that good employee health is critical for business success as well as decreasing health costs.
- Opposition → Alliance
  Currently, there is opposition among patients, payers, and providers. Yet new models (such as accountable care organizations, or ACOs) are encouraging these groups to work *together* to achieve the highest quality at the lowest costs.
  How we deliver health care
- Treatment → Prevention
  Increased focus on prevention will decrease costs of care over time.
- Reactive → Proactive
  Patients with chronic illnesses are expensive. Better ways of monitoring and controlling their illnesses need to be found that cost less money.
- Episodic → Holistic
  Payment will be for preventing illness, including lifestyle changes, rather than treating every episode of illness.
  The economics of health care
- Procedure → Performance
  Now payment is by procedure, but employers can no longer afford this. New payment models [such as ACOs, which could fail] will not only cover necessary care but will reduce coverage and costs. Employees will have to pay more for care.

- Isolation → Integration

  Today care is delivered in silos (hospitals, doctors' offices) with communication and linkages among silos not always effective. More integration is needed between providers and information systems.

- Passive → Active

  Services and insurance claims need to be linked and at lower costs (Mauck & Breitinger, 2012, pp. 8–9).

This environment is complicated by four *financial issues that affect health care*. First, unlike other industries, our customers generally do *not* save up their money because they *want* our services. Instead, they often are vulnerable when they need our services, are afraid of many of the services we offer, and dread that the illness event might deplete their life savings. However, when they experience an illness crisis, they desperately want our services.

Second, the economy is troubled. The middle class is dwindling. Jobs are not plentiful. Inflation has increased costs so that someone who retired 10 years ago can no longer buy as much today, and children are returning to parents' homes because they cannot afford to live on their own.

Third, even when people do not have money to pay for illness services, they still need care. In a retail store they would be told, "No money. No merchandise." In health care, people have indeed been turned away in greater numbers, yet hospital and long-term care providers are forced by law to treat people who cannot pay as specified by federal regulations in the Affordable Care Act of 2010, and to do so in such a way that all providers work together to achieve better outcomes—keeping people in their homes longer. This means that a hospital can no longer be a stand-alone entity but must now pay attention to the *continuum of care* and *prevention*. To keep patients from being readmitted, hospitals must plan for better home care services for their patients, work more effectively with physician offices, and link more closely with long-term care. Accountable care organizations are an initial attempt to achieve this goal, which really affects the bottom line not only of organizations but of the public, who must pay additional taxes.

Fourth, insurance companies continue to cut percentages given to providers for reimbursement. For example, Medicare, which covers the majority of the U.S. population, continues to cut back payments to pennies on the dollar even when positive outcomes are achieved. With pay for performance, reimbursement is taken away when negative patient outcomes occur. In this case, healthcare organizations are left with the additional financial burden of having to pay for the care patients received. In addition, we are now being asked to achieve better coordination of care. In the midst of this environment, healthcare personnel grapple with how to provide quality service, yet make ends meet financially. It is a complicated dilemma fraught with many challenges.

Environmental Chaos and Complexity

Amid all of these changes, what are we supposed to do? Why can't things stay the same? These are good questions.

This complicated group of changes is too much for the old, linear, authoritarian systems to deal with effectively. In the past, we have used a linear *open systems model* to describe organizations:

> The inputs, throughputs, outputs, and feedback loops in a basic system exist in an environment that is influenced by economic, political, social, and cultural factors.

- The *inputs* include the resources, human and nonhuman (materials, equipment, buildings), that come together to provide the desired service. In health care, inputs might be staff labor hours, number and skill mix of nursing staff, other staff needed for various services, technology, equipment, supplies used, and remodeling or building expense.

- *Throughputs* are the processes or work that people do to achieve the output, the final product, or service. In the healthcare system, throughputs are the patient care services provided to the patient and family. Throughput processes use the available inputs to create work processes.
- *Output* results from the interaction of inputs in the throughput process. The output is the material, goods and/or services, produced. Outputs can be both qualitative and quantitative in health care. Reimbursement in health care is driven by the quantitative outputs or documented services produced by the system, regardless of the quality of the output or errors that might have occurred.
- *Feedback* is derived from both the outputs and throughput processes. Feedback is information about the effectiveness of the system and provides support for system changes. When outputs are positive, the system inputs and throughputs are reinforced and supported to continue. When the outputs are less than desired, modifications based on the feedback from the system are made to the throughputs. Similarly, when outputs are not what was expected, modifications to throughputs are considered. (Kathy Malloch, personal communication, June 25, 2012)

Although this linear open systems model is a useful starting point when discussing organizations, actually organizations are complex systems. The dynamic interactions and activities of the system must be considered. For example, Tortorella and colleagues (2013) give an example of improving *throughput* by starting a bed management system. However, as they describe how they did this and how they arrived at this solution, they accounted for the complexity within the system.

Healthcare organizations must be able to change quickly and be more effective. Healthcare administrators *and* workers must continually invent newer, better, more effective and efficient ways to offer services to clients. This is absolutely imperative for survival. We all have to shift our paradigms about how organizations operate. Some chaos and complexity knowledge can help us better understand what is happening and help guide us to change direction in organizations. This complex model better captures what is actually happening. To start with, consider the following statement by Henry Adams, an American journalist and historian born in the 1830s:

Chaos often breeds life, when order breeds habit.

Think about this statement. Chaos and order are opposites. Both are happening at the same time. Too much of either one creates total disruption and death. Both are natural processes. Life is always a dance between the two. As we deal with chaos and order, we need to work continually to balance them.

The linear view of the world—always viewing it the same way, holding accepted values without questioning them—does not capture the complexity of what is happening around us. We professionals can get stuck grasping at sacred cows—"we have always done it that way"—that are now outdated. Evidence supports a better, different way of doing. The linear view can get us stuck when the world is complex and changing. Quantum science provides evidence *that our world is chaotic and complex and ever changing*.

In the midst of the changes, there are some constants (**Exhibit 3–1**). Knowing these helps us deal more effectively with change.

First, *change is constant*. As our Earth changes, so do we. What is orderly at one time or place is chaotic at another time or place.

Change happens all around us and *more quickly than it did in the past*. Yet we don't always perceive change occurring because it happens incrementally outside our field of vision. Changes have a profound impact on us and affect our administrative role in health care. We need to keep abreast of the pulse of this energy and be open to it even though we don't know what is going to happen next.

Hints of changes are all around us. It is important to be on the lookout for these and to encourage staff to look for them as well. As we communicate with each other, together we can better identify what

---

Exhibit 3–1   Constants in the Midst of Change

- Change is constant, and is happening more quickly.
- Time is compressed and is gaining momentum.
- We are all different and very complex.
- Duality will always be present. Paradoxes reveal that where things seem contradictory, at a deeper level they are complementary.
- Chaos happens but we are attached to stasis. Our choice is how to respond to it.
- There is order within the chaos.
- "Living systems continually seek to renew and reinvent themselves, yet maintain their core integrity" (*autopoiesis*).
- New information enters into a system "in small fluctuations that continually grow in strength, interacting with the system and feeding back upon itself" (*autocatalysis*).
- At times we choose to create chaos—cause disorder (*dissipative structures*).
- In the midst of chaos and change, there are some things we cannot explain (*strange attractor*).
- We are all interconnected.
- We are all interdependent.
- Organizations become increasingly more complex over time.
- Unexpected events occur "that have a significant and disproportionate impact on a system" (Clancy, 2008a, p. 273). These are called *black swans*. The more complex a system is, the more frequently these events occur. The vast majority are positive.
- As above, so below (fractals). Example: The patterns in a leaf have the same form as the tree that contains the leaves. "The smallest level of a single organization and the most complex array of the large aggregated system containing the organization are connected inexorably through the power of fractals."
- "At every level of the organization there exists a self-organizing capacity and this capacity maintains a balance and harmony even in the midst of the most chaotic processes. To the extent the balance and harmony are sustained, the organization's life is advanced. To the extent that they are upset or cannot be articulated, visualized, and acted on at every level of leadership, the organization's actions tend to impede its integrity and effectiveness."
- "No decision, action, or undertaking can occur any place in the organization without ultimately having an impact on every other action, decision, and undertaking."
- Quoted material, except where indicated, from Porter-O'Grady and Malloch, 2011, p. 14.

Source: Porter-O'Grady, T., & Malloch, K. *Quantum Leadership: Advancing Innovation, Transforming Health Care*, 3rd ed. Sudbury, MA: Jones and Bartlett, p. 167.

---

is changing. It is important to be open to the possibilities. Change happens throughout our lives, although here we focus on healthcare organizations.

The fact that everything is complex, ever changing, and seemingly chaotic can lead us to question what we see. So, when we see something that does not make sense, we must be open to it and think about possibilities. A quantum perspective better explains what is happening and what we might expect to happen. Linear ways of thinking do not capture or explain complexity.

As change happens, healthcare organizations need to continue to adapt (change) to this new environment by *de*constructing health services and changing to newer models of service. For instance, Ackman and associates (2012) found that better information was obtained from nurses who used a trial admission assessment and referral sheet than those who used a nursing history. Clavelle (2012) got better patient services in a small rural hospital in Idaho using a collaborative team effort with physicians expanding advanced practice RN privileges.

Change is not just a one-time event; it is a *journey*.

> It is premature to claim victory or arrival. Every arrival point is also a debarking point. There really is no permanent point of respite from change. Since everything in life is a journey, it is important for the nurse leader to keep an honest perspective. The arrival points are merely points of demarcation, of momentary rest. The wise leader carefully balances the moments of rest and celebration with those of effort and action. Depending upon the demand, the timeframe, and the circumstances, leaders choose the moments of marking success carefully so that they can serve to reenergize when necessary, refresh when possible, and challenge when appropriate. (Porter-O'Grady, 2003, p. 64)

Part of the journey involves the death of what we have gotten used to. At first, we mourn this loss. However, something better is replacing it, so there is hope along with the loss. Death is part of the cycle of life. We cannot avoid it. "Not everything in the universe that thrives will continue to do so. When circumstances change radically, some formerly vigorous systems fail" (Porter-O'Grady & Malloch, 2011, p. 35).

So, change is happening all around us.

A second constant is *compressed time*. Since the earth was formed, time has continued to become more compressed. This was not as noticeable 100 years ago, but we feel it today because it is happening more rapidly than in the past and is gaining momentum. Have you noticed how quickly time is passing? Today what had been measured as 24 hours has been compressed into 18 or 19 hours. Scientific evidence supports your thoughts about not having as much time!

A third constant is that *we are all different and very complex*, like snowflakes and organizations. This is why what works in one workplace does not work in another. This is because the people are different, the environments are different, and so forth. Because we are all different it is not right to superimpose our beliefs on others. Each person must decide what is best for himself or herself. It is important to respect every person for his or her differences. In fact, in an effective team, members celebrate their differences, knowing that these differences make the team more effective.

Imagine how boring this world would be if everyone was exactly like us! Our definitions about the world create different pictures. Think of what we view as "perfect." In actuality, when we want things to be perfect, the problem is that (1) nothing is perfect because it is ever changing, and (2) what is considered perfect to one person is not by another.

When we apply this concept to organizations, no organization is perfect, and what is perfect for one organization probably will not be for the next. It also means that as we make changes and choose strategies, *there is no one best way,* even within the same organization, and no one best way to structure organizations (Clancy, 2007a, p. 535).

A fourth constant is that we live in a *world of duality*—positive and negative, good and evil, male and female, and so on. We cannot control this. Duality complicates the situations we face each day. Our only choice is what we do, how we respond to it, and how we treat others around us. We can react positively or negatively. The choice is ours. *The only choice each of us has in this world is to choose how to respond to our environment.*

Most of us, deep down inside, want harmony and usually make positive choices. "Happy, well rested, and inspired people will perform better work" (Douglas, 2012, pp. 117, 119). However, duality is present. Some people delight in it or, out of frustration, cause chaos and negativity. They have gotten stuck in negativity as the most effective way to respond to the world.

How do we deal with this? Negativity needs to be dealt with by mentoring and counseling. But negativity can bring about good changes. Let's explain. Sometimes in duality, *paradox* is involved. This is where things are *seemingly contradictory*. For instance, data and intuition seem to be opposites. Other examples are as follows:

- We want things to be simple. Yet we experience complexity.
- We want to change something, be a risk taker, and push beyond the limits of our comfort zone. Yet we continue to need status quo for comfort and stability.
- We want to be able to change instantly, try things, improvise, experiment. Yet we want order, neatness, and consistency following procedures for patient safety.

However, in paradoxes, the things that seem contradictory may actually be *complementary at a deeper level*. Let's examine a few instances where this is true:

- **Creativity and tension:** Tension leads to creativity, and creativity causes tension.
- **Difference and similarity:** Difference seen from a great distance appears as an integrated whole.
- **Complexity and simplicity:** Complexity is simply the visible connection between aligned simplicities.
- **Chaos and order:** There is order in all chaos and vice versa.
- **Conflict and peace:** Conflict is necessary to peacemaking, containing in it the elements upon which peace must be built. (Porter-O'Grady & Malloch, 2011, p. 27)

What is harmony at this instant will not remain harmonious because of change. Conflict, a normal element in any environment, helps us to get to *something better*, a **potential reality**.

> The techniques for finding common ground, for sorting through the various landscapes representing the diversity inherent in each issue, are now required by every leader. [Thus it is important to] get people to come together around issues helping them determine appropriate responses within the context of their own roles. This is a challenge that cannot be met by establishing standardized job procedures or rules. (Porter-O'Grady & Malloch, 2011, p. 28)

It is precisely these opposing concepts that provide us with grist for the mill. When we think *linearly*, these opposing concepts present sources of conflict. However, if we can realize that our responsibility is to rise above the seeming differences and find ways to combine the opposing forces, we can resolve these conflicts to create a better workplace.

New tensions that need resolution always exist. It is like the piece of sand in the oyster that creates friction that eventually results in a perfect pearl. Right now we cannot see the pearl, but it is there, and as we work through the tensions, the pearl manifests. We can choose to remain in our linear world where the pearl will never manifest and we continue to feel the frustrations—or we can build toward a better future.

The fourth paradox, chaos and order, is another constant: *We are attached to order, but chaos happens.* Our linear beliefs can help us as we move through our daily routines (habits); this is stasis. But our habits also get in our way. Our daily routines gradually need to change. Stasis, over time, leads to death if we choose not to change. Enter chaos.

What is chaos? Generally, it is perceived as something unpredictable or random. Chaos happens whether we want it to happen or not. Chaos helps us change—*even when we do not choose to do so*. Our only positive choice is to see chaos as a positive force that gets us out of our habits and brings about a better reality. Of course, in a world of duality, another choice is to view chaos as a force to be dreaded. Someone who chooses a negative way of dealing with the world may cause chaos to disrupt the environment and achieve negative goals.

We do *not* have a choice about whether chaos will occur. *Our only choice is how we respond to chaos.*

However, take heart. Quantum scientists have found that *there is order in the chaos*. When looking at a situation overall across time, *chaos leads us to a better reality*. "Chaos is a class of system behavior that appears random but has underlying structure and is deterministic" (Clancy, 2007b, p. 436).

> Even at the fundamental levels of life, chaos is hard at work. Creatures as small as one cell are constantly undergoing accidental modifications that give them a better chance of thriving. It is a basic requisite of all life to adapt to changing conditions. The demise of the dinosaur is a good example of what happens when living beings fail to adapt. (Porter-O'Grady & Malloch, 2011, p. 27)

3. *Behavior grows better before it grows worse* talks about systems that may make things look better in the short run, only to return in 2 or 3 years to haunt you.

4. *The easy way out usually leads back in* discusses how we often apply familiar solutions to problems. This idea of sticking to what we know best is comforting, but very often the real solution is not obvious and the answer is hiding somewhere in the darkness, so we create more complexity by keeping with the familiar.

5. *The cure can be worse than the disease* is seen when familiar solutions are not only ineffective but sometimes addictive and dangerous. For instance, many organizations become dependent on consultants, instead of training their own staff and solving problems themselves.

6. *Faster is slower* comes from the old story of the tortoise and the hare. Making a change quickly without involving all the players results in many unanticipated problems that could have been avoided with more dialogue between all the players in the first place, and with making a change more incrementally.

7. *Cause and effect are not closely related in time and space* uses the example where there are sagging profits and unemployment in the nation. The "cause," which happened earlier, is that companies have moved beyond our borders seeking cheaper labor.

8. *Small changes can produce big results—but the areas of highest leverage are often the least obvious.* Large changes often have the least effect. How easy it is for people to go back to the status quo after a large change, especially when they were not involved in planning it. Smaller, incremental changes involving many stakeholders are better.

9. *You can have your cake and eat it too—but not at once.* For instance, organizations can improve on processes and achieve better quality (the cake) that in the long run result in lower costs (eat it too).

10. *Dividing an elephant in half does not produce two small elephants* describes how many organizations can see problems within individual departments but do not realize how they interconnect with the "whole" organization.

11. *There is no blame* indicates that the real problem probably involves a complicated group of processes that occurred.

This list shows how important it is to have dialogue with all those involved in the change before implementation.

Quick fixes can easily occur. Clancy (2010, 2011a) gives two quick-fix examples with preventing medication errors and MRSA. When we experience similar situations, we implement quick fixes that actually make things worse because other factors or stakeholders affecting the process were not identified. The quick fixes add to the complexity instead of decreasing it.

"It is rare that a project unfolds in the precise manner it was planned. . . . *Intensely prescriptive plans have a higher likelihood of leading to unexpected outcomes*" (Clancy, 2011b, p. 340). It is better to use a trial-and-error process that tests new ideas in small increments and to throw away the unsuccessful ones while only keeping the ideas that are successful. This method achieves the best result.

Clancy (2010) suggests a *positive deviance (PD) method* as a better way to deal with making improvements in organizations:

> In most organizations there are individuals and groups whose different (deviant) practices or strategies produce better (positive) outcomes than do colleagues who have access to the same resources. The PD process helps members of the community uncover the positive deviants in their midst and identify their successful practices and then, through widespread engagement, amplify and spread these practices. . . . One of the mantras of PD is: "Who else needs to be here?" (p. 152)

The PD process brings about new connections within the organization as those who did something successfully share what they did with others. As a result of the increased communication and collaboration occurring among diverse individuals in different roles and different places, a new self-organizing process is created that results in better outcomes.

In addition, unexpected events occur "that have a significant and disproportionate impact on a system" (Clancy, 2008a, p. 273). These are called *black swans*. In actuality, most black swans are often *positive* improbable events—when we think, This is a *miracle!* However, negative events can happen too. "The death of a patient from a medication error is a black swan, and *the more complex a system is, the more frequently these events occur*" (p. 273). *Black swans occur even when the procedures have been followed to the letter.* It is *so* important to treat the information discovered from a sentinel event (or any outlier) as *valuable* information. We need to pay attention to these outcomes and immediately implement changes based on the results. Usually, several systems processes have caused the error. So, instead of doing a quick fix that increases complexity, we can take actions that decrease complexity. The main issue is to recognize black swans, be adaptable, and make changes accordingly.

As chaos happens we often do not appreciate the complexity involved. Yet there is another concept or constant that helps us understand. Consider the saying, *As above, so below.* For instance, the veining patterns in a leaf have the same format as the tree that contains the leaves. We can look at any leaf on the tree and see the same pattern. Same with holograms. This is the nature of *fractals.* "The smallest level of a single organization and the most complex array of the large aggregated system containing the organization are connected inexorably through the power of fractals" (Porter-O'Grady & Malloch, 2011, p. 13). Fractals occur within our own bodies, within organizations, and throughout the world.

> Fractals have tremendous implications for organizations. From the smallest structural elements to the very complex patterns of behavior existing throughout an organization, the same patterns appear and are played out in precise detail. This fact implies that *at every level of the organization there exists a self-organizing capacity and that this capacity maintains a balance and harmony even in the midst of the most chaotic processes.* To the extent that the balance and harmony are sustained, the organization's life is advanced. To the extent that they are upset or cannot be articulated, visualized, and acted on at every level of leadership, the organization's actions tend to impede its integrity and effectiveness. It is important, therefore, that the leaders of the organization be aware of the continuous and dynamic action of fractals in all organizational behavior and structure so that they can advance the consonance and value of the employees' activities and enhance the organization's ability to fulfill its mission.
>
> *Perhaps it is even more important for leaders to recognize that, within the context of the fractals' dynamic action, their own actions have cascading and rippling implications in every other part of the organization. In fact, they should understand that no decision, action, or undertaking can occur any place in the organization without ultimately having an impact on every other action, decision, and undertaking. In addition, once they are cognizant of the web of interaction and interdependence that exists in the organization, the leaders will approach deliberation and decision making only with extreme care, caution, and thoroughness.* (Porter-O'Grady & Malloch, 2011, p. 14)

This concept is so important. Please reread the quote. We must understand how this concept is critical to being an effective administrator and why, if things are broken, it takes time to fix them. The entire contents of this text are interrelated—just as all contents within an organization are interrelated.

Some excellent resources on chaos and complexity include *Resilience: Why Things Bounce Back* (Zolli & Healy, 2012), *On the Edge: Nursing in the Age of Complexity* (Lindberg, Nash, & Lindberg, 2008), *Edgeware: Lessons from Complexity Science for Health Care Leaders* (Zimmerman, Lindberg, & Plsek, 2008), and *Inviting Everyone: Healing Health Care Through Positive Deviance* (Singhai, Buscell, & Lindberg, 2010). Many of these are sponsored by Plexus Institute (www.plexusinstitute.org). In addition, *Nursing Economic$* has a regular column on managing organizational complexity.

Organizations—Living Ever-Changing Systems

Our concept of organizations is moving away from the mechanistic creations that flourished in the age of bureaucracy. We now speak in earnest of more fluid, organic structures, of boundaryless and seamless organizations. We are beginning to recognize organizations as whole systems, construing them as "learning organizations" or as "organic" and noticing that people exhibit self-organizing capacity. These are our first journeys that signal a growing appreciation for the changes required in today's organizations. . . . We can forgo the despair created by such common organizational events as change, chaos, information overload, and entrenched behaviors if we recognize that *organizations are living systems, possessing the same capacity to adapt and grow that is common to all life.*

What is it that [rivers] can teach me about organizations? . . . The stream has an impressive ability to adapt, to change the configurations, to let the power shift, to create new structures. But behind this adaptability, making it all happen, is the water's need to flow. Water answers to gravity, to downhill, to the call of ocean. The forms change, but the mission remains clear. Structures emerge, but only as temporary solutions that facilitate rather than interfere. There is none of the rigid reliance . . . in organizations on single forms, on true answers, on past practices. [Rivers] have more than one response to rocks; otherwise, there'd be no Grand Canyon. Or Grand Canyons everywhere. The Colorado River realized there were many ways to find ocean other than by staying broad and expansive. . . .

Organizations lack this kind of faith, faith that they can accomplish their purposes in varied ways and that they do best when they focus on intent and vision, letting forms emerge and disappear. We seem hypnotized by structures, and we build them strong and complex because they must, we believe, hold back the dark forces that threaten to destroy us. . . . [Rivers] have a different relationship with natural forces. With sparkling confidence, they know that their intense yearning for ocean will be fulfilled, that nature creates not only the call, but the answer. (Wheatley, 1999, pp. 15, 17–18)

Where Are We Headed? Determining Purpose

What is a healthcare organization's ocean? Where are we headed? And, the greater question is, How do we get to that ocean? It is important to understand this organizational perspective to survive in the value-based (second-curve) environment.

The ocean is the organization's primary purpose. *Purpose* remains unchanged for years. It needs to be aimed at achieving what patients' value. It may be similar to the purpose of other healthcare organizations. Purpose is similar to quality, where one is always working toward achieving it, but it is never totally accomplished. The purpose statements *do not* give a specific description of the various services (products). Nor do they specifically define the customer.

Purpose helps to give clarity and direction to all in an organization.

When leaders make their strategic intent abundantly clear—as Wal-Mart's management has in proclaiming its strategy of "low prices, every day"—employees know what to do without requiring myriad further instructions. Achieving that clarity, however, is often far more difficult than managers appreciate. (Useem, 2001, p. 57)

We are mistaken if we believe that our ocean, our primary purpose, is making money. Many healthcare organizations are run by administrators who believe that the bottom line runs the organization, the antithesis to the mission statement above their entrance that defines various values. When we make the bottom line first, finances plummet, whereas *when purpose is the first priority, with the bottom line in second place, finances are sustained or improved.*

This is not to say that revenue is unimportant. We still need money to operate. The money simply must remain *secondary* to the primary goal. Money is part of the meandering that the stream does while looking for the ocean. If revenues are unavailable from one source or service, they might be available elsewhere. *The primary issue is, Which services does the patient want or need?* Then, we go from there to determine what we do. The research shows this to be true:

> Profitability is a necessary condition for existence and a means to more important ends, but it is not the end in itself. . . . Profit is like oxygen, food, water, and blood for the body; they are not the point of life, but without them, there is no life. (Collins & Porras, 1994, p. 55)

If the CFO, and perhaps most of the executive team, really believes that the bottom line is the ocean, conflict and frustration occur for others in the organization who believe the patient comes first. What is important to workers, *what makes the work worth doing,* are the outcomes achieved—not the bottom line. (Just like being paid is important but not the most important aspect of the work.)

Stewardship

We discussed *as above, so below.* The organization must be considered within its larger community. It is important to consider the facility's obligations to and interactions with the community.

Walter Gast rightly claimed that to be successful in the long term:

> A business has to follow six laws: 1) provide a just return on capital; 2) produce a useful commodity or service; 3) increase the wealth or quality of society; 4) provide productive employment opportunities; 5) help employees find satisfying work; and 6) pay fair wages. (O'Hallaron, 2002, p. 125)

If the community flounders, the organization could be at risk, or vice versa. Just as all departments need to be integrated and working together within an organization, all organizations are better off if they are integrated and working effectively with others in the community, helping the community to better serve its citizens. This is called *stewardship.*

The concept of stewardship is discussed in Magnet Force 10: Community and the Healthcare Organization: "Relationships are established within and among all types of health care organizations and other community organizations, to develop strong partnerships that support improved client outcomes and the health of the communities they serve" (American Nurses Credentialing Center [ANCC], 2013b).

In a discussion of second-wave strategies, the AHA's (2013) first must-do strategy supports community involvement: "Aligning hospitals, physicians, and other providers across the continuum of care" (p. 3). Within the community all need to work together to improve prevention as well as provide a seamless continuum of care.

The Soul and Spirit of the Organization

For organizations, two energies are necessary to navigate the meandering river to the ocean successfully: *soul* and *spirit.* Understanding and believing in the ocean (giving patients what they value—the purpose) is the soul. Spirit comes from doing meaningful work. We feel it very deeply. Spirit is the energy that fuels getting to the ocean. Our relationships with each other reflect soul and spirit. We need to understand and feel these to be successful in the value-based (second-curve) environment. If relationships are not good, chances are we have lost touch with the soul part of our business and the spirit is not strong.

If relationships are collaborative and positive, chances are the soul and spirit are present, alive, and well. Remember this Chinese proverb:

> If there is light in the soul, there will be beauty in the person.
> If there is beauty in the person, there will be harmony in the house.
> If there is harmony in the house, there will be order in the nation.
> If there is order in the nation, there will be peace in the world.

Let's start with defining the importance of the *soul* part—understanding and believing in the purpose. This is where the spirit gets its energy. Collins and Porras (1994) reported an enormous research project that lasted 50 to 100 years with premier companies that are known for excellence and yet have experienced multiple leaders and different product lines through the years. They report:

> A visionary company almost religiously preserves its core ideology—changing it seldom, if ever. Core values in a visionary company form a rock-solid foundation and do not drift with the trends and fashions of the day; in some cases, the core values have remained intact for well over one hundred years. And the basic purpose of a visionary company—its reason for being—can serve as a guiding beacon for centuries, like an enduring star on the horizon. Yet, while keeping their core ideologies tightly fixed, visionary companies display a powerful drive for progress that enables them to change and adapt without compromising their cherished core ideals.
>
> There is no "right" set of core values. . . . Indeed, two companies can have radically different ideologies, yet both be visionary. . . . The crucial variable is not the content of a company's ideology, but how deeply it believes its ideology and how consistently it lives, breathes, and expresses it in all that it does. Visionary companies do not ask, "What should we value?" They ask, "What do we actually value deep down to our toes?" (pp. 8–9)

The *core value,* or belief, is described in a sentence or two that capture the general guiding principle of the organization. It can provide a common cause for people who work in the organization. (It can be useful for nurse managers to identify core values with staff for a unit or department as well.) When sound, *these beliefs provide the backbone of every policy or action people within the organization take.* The core values come first, before goals, policies, or procedures. If a goal, policy, or procedure violates a core value, then it must be changed. Generally, one core value will remain unchanged for many years. An example of a core value is *To treat the patient the way we would want a family member to be treated.*

Examples of core values from other businesses are as follows:

- **Sam Walton's value for Wal-Mart:** "[We put] the customer ahead of everything else. . . . If you're not serving the customer, or supporting the folks who do, then we don't need you."
- **John Young's core value for Hewlett-Packard:** "The HP Way basically means respect and concern for the individual; it says 'Do unto others as you would have them do unto you.' That's really what it's all about." (quoted material p. 74)

The core value must be authentically identified by people in the organization, not copied from some other organization (even though it is possible that a core value for one company is the same as for another). The core value does not have to be unique, but it is imperative that all within an organization support it with words, actions, and goals.

Core values are extremely important. In premier companies, as described in *Built to Last,* **one becomes an outcast if one does not support the values**:

> A visionary company creates a total environment that envelops employees, bombarding them with a set of signals so consistent and mutually reinforcing that it's virtually impossible to misunderstand the company's ideology and ambitions. . . . Because the visionary companies have such clarity about

who they are, what they're all about, and what they're trying to achieve, they tend to not have much room for people unwilling or unsuited to their demanding standards, both in terms of performance and congruence. (Collins & Porras, 1994, p. 121)

These companies promote from within, encouraging managers to immerse themselves in the company ideology for several years to make sure they understand what is expected from them, before being promoted.

We are most successful in defining our core values when they go *deeper* than just surface direction. Consider how people accomplish the impossible for a cause.

> Shared values are the primary vehicle through which people experience the highest form of trust in one another and their leader. A clear vision and mission can unify the values of external and internal stakeholders. In a study of 418 project teams, a clearly stated vision and mission was the only factor that predicted collaborative teamwork and success.
>
> The vision and mission can also be a springboard for personal values examination and a means to build a stronger organizational culture with shared values and a collective identity. (MacPhee, 2007, p. 408)

Several authors discuss the importance of core values in rallying staff but stress the difficulties of really living by the core values. For instance, Lencioni (2002a) observes:

> Coming up with strong values—and sticking to them—requires real guts. Indeed, an organization considering a values initiative must first come to terms with the fact that, when properly practiced, values inflict pain. They make some employees feel like outcasts. They limit an organization's strategic and operational freedom and constrain the behavior of its people. They leave executives open to heavy criticism for even minor violations. And they demand constant vigilance. (p. 114)

When the bottom line has the greatest importance, facilities lose the *soul* of the organization. Morale and job satisfaction of staff plunge. As budget cuts occur, workers feel depersonalized and suffer from battle fatigue and survivor guilt (Tuazon, 2008). The problem is that staff do not feel valued, and they will turn around and not treat patients well. Problems spiral because clients coming for care sense that they are not important, that staff do not care. Any organization using this approach cannot survive in the long run.

Shared vision arises from the core values. There continue to be new ways to operationalize the core values in the changing environment.

> With a quantum sensibility, there are new possibilities for how to create order. Organizational behavior is influenced by the invisible. If we attend to the fields we create, if we help them shine clear with coherence, then we can clean up some of the waste of organizational life. . . . In a field view of organizations, we attend first to clarity. We must say what we mean and seek for a much deeper level of integrity in our words and acts than ever before. And then we must make certain that everyone has access to this field, that the information is available everywhere. Vision statements move off the walls and into the corridors, seeking out every employee, every recess in the organization. . . . We need to imagine ourselves as beacon towers of information, standing tall in the integrity of what we say, pulsing out congruent messages everywhere. We need all of us out there, stating, clarifying, reflecting, modeling, filling all of space with the messages we care about. If we do that, a powerful field develops—and with it, the wondrous capacity to organize into coherent, capable form. Let us remember that space is never empty. If it is filled with harmonious voices, a song arises that is strong and potent. If it is filled with conflict, the dissonance drives us away and we don't want to be there. When we pretend that it doesn't matter whether there is harmony, when we believe we don't have to "walk our talk," we lose far more than personal integrity. We lose the partnership of a field-rich space that can help bring order to our lives. (Wheatley, 2006, pp. 56–57)

The *spirit* is the energy that fuels getting to the ocean. Spirit comes from our belief that we are doing meaningful work. It is the "radical loving care" that is given (Chapman, 2004). Work becomes meaningful when we strongly believe in, and are committed to giving, what our patients value. It is the synergy that exists between team members, physicians, suppliers, patients, families, and the community as what the patient values is realized. Spirit is the energy that works to achieve getting to the ocean.

Spirit is enhanced by Magnet Model Component II: Exemplary Professional Practice:

> The true essence of a Magnet organization stems from exemplary professional practice within nursing. This entails a comprehensive understanding of the role of nursing; the application of that role with patients, families, communities, and the interdisciplinary team; and the application of new knowledge and evidence. The goal of this Component is more than the establishment of strong professional practice; it is what that professional practice can achieve. (ANCC, 2013c)

Magnet Force 5 further defines professional models of care:

> There are models of care that give nurses responsibility and authority for the provision of direct patient care. Nurses are accountable for their own practice as well as the coordination of care. The models of care (i.e., primary nursing, case management, family-centered, district, and wholistic) provide for the continuity of care across the continuum. The models take into consideration patients' unique needs and provide skilled nurses and adequate resources to accomplish desired outcomes. (ANCC, 2013b)

Spirit is so important. Evidence supports this:

> As nurses became more involved in testing and implementing changes in care on their units, vitality increased. . . . It is also supported by previous research on magnet hospitals that have demonstrated a relationship between the level of nurse job satisfaction and access to empowering factors in the workplace and the ability to exercise judgment and implement changes related to their work environment. (Upenieks, Needleman, & Soban, 2008, p. 393)

Nurse engagement (spirit) is linked with patient satisfaction (Bacon & Mark, 2009).

Throughout this discussion of spirit, money is not mentioned. A theme we pursue is that *if we do what the patient values, the money will follow*. This discussion follows on that theme. This intrinsic motivator is more important than pay to nurses. First, nurses have to find their work meaningful. Research shows this. Still, we continue to get tripped up believing that paying bonuses, or some other payment scheme, will achieve success with employees. Just like the bottom line, the pay helps but is not the most important factor.

Magnet Force 4: Personnel Policies and Programs states that "salaries and benefits are competitive," but mostly support professional nursing practice:

> Creative and flexible staffing models that support a safe and healthy work environment are used. Personnel policies are created with direct care nurse involvement. Significant opportunities for professional growth exist in administrative and clinical tracks. Personnel policies and programs support professional nursing practice, work/life balance, and the delivery of quality care. (ANCC, 2013b)

Spirit, or motivation, comes from within. There is not a magic wand we can wave to achieve a motivated workforce. Instead, in the right environment, under the right conditions, the opportunity is there for personnel to be motivated about their work. But remember, duality is present, so whether someone is motivated remains that person's choice. Motivation is an intrinsic factor that comes from within.

Trust is an important factor that relates to our spirit. It is important for all in an organization to trust each other. This contributes to more effective teamwork, and getting what the patient values delivered. Trust is important between nurse administrators and finance people who know that the nurse administrator is being honest about financial issues, and vice versa. Employees trust administrators when administrators have integrity, believe in and live by the core values. Any achievement is possible in a trusting environment. Trust is something to value very highly because it is not lightly given and, once lost, can probably never be regained.

When an organization derails and administrators want to fix the problems, it is important they start with the core values. Can administrators live by the core values and support the core values in all their actions? (Or, if core values have not been identified, can administrators and staff dialogue about—and agree on—core values?) Next, administrators must talk about the core values with all employees. Can everyone support them? If all believe and live by the core values, *their beliefs will provide the energy, or spirit, to achieve success*. If an administrator cannot support the core values in his or her words and actions, that person may need to be dismissed. It takes time and commitment to recover from this change because the trust has been lost. Trust must be earned again, or new administrators will have to prove they can be trusted, before the situation can be turned around.

The *soul* provides meaning for the *spirit* to remain alive and well. It permeates our feelings of belonging and engagement. It is the heart of teamwork and connectedness within an organization. "Courage comes from the French word which means heart. Once our heart is engaged, we operate with passion, and not power, and we can find ways to transform our world together" (Kerfoot, 2002, p. 298).

When soul is there but the spirit is missing, we need to question within ourselves whether we are doing something to cause this problem. Curran (2000) reports that the Gallup organization, after doing 25 years of research on 400 companies with 80,000 managers, concluded that one could measure the strength of the workplace using 12 simple questions. *Spirit* is more likely to be energized when these 12 aspects are present in the workplace:

1. Do I know what is expected of me at work?
2. Do I have the materials and equipment I need to do my work right?
3. At work, do I have the opportunity to do what I do best every day?
4. In the last 7 days, have I received recognition or praise for doing good work?
5. Does my supervisor, or someone at work, care about me as a person?
6. Is there someone at work who encourages my development?
7. At work, do my opinions seem to count?
8. Does the mission/purpose of my company make me feel my job is important?
9. Are my co-workers committed to doing quality work?
10. Do I have a best friend at work?
11. In the last 6 months, has someone talked to me about my progress?
12. This last year, have I had opportunities at work to learn and grow?

> Buckingham and Coffman . . . demonstrated that these 12 questions separate great organizations from average ones. . . . Individuals may join organizations, but it is their immediate manager who directly influences how long they stay and how productive they are. Employees do not leave organizations, they leave managers. (Curran, 2000, p. 277)

This is really what patient satisfaction is all about. In "Serving Up Uncommon Service," Doucette (2003) points out the difference between quality, the "measurement of outcomes," and service, "a measure of perception of what matters to the patient." "Quality outcomes are a baseline. The one feature that units demonstrating consistently high-ranking customer satisfaction scores share is satisfied employees. The conclusion seems clear: To improve patient satisfaction, improve staff satisfaction" (Doucette, 2003, pp. 26–27).

It is easy to diagnose whether spirit is present. It is reflected in productivity—or the lack of it. You can also see spirit in workers' eyes: Their eyes shine. Or, if lacking, they look overwhelmed and discouraged, even depressed. Employees want to be a part of important work that is accomplished through collective effort. *Soul* and *spirit* are not management techniques. They are available to us through personal commitment to values. They are intangible things surrounding us when we have a healthy workplace. They energize us.

The Nursing Organizations Alliance™ believes that a healthful practice/work environment is supported by the presence of the following elements:

1. ***Collaborative Practice Culture***
   Respectful collegial communication and behavior
   Team orientation
   Presence of trust
   Respect for diversity
2. ***Communication Rich Culture***
   Clear and respectful
   Open and trusting
3. ***A Culture of Accountability***
   Role expectations are clearly defined
   Everyone is accountable
4. ***The Presence of Adequate Numbers of Qualified Nurses***
   Ability to provide quality care to meet client/patient's needs
   Work/home life balance
5. ***The Presence of Expert, Competent, Credible, Visible Leadership***
   Serve as an advocate for nursing practice
   Support shared decision-making
   Allocate resources to support nursing
6. ***Shared Decision-Making at All Levels***
   Nurses participate in system, organizational, and process decisions
   Formal structure exists to support shared decision-making
   Nurses have control over their practice
7. ***The Encouragement of Professional Practice and Continued Growth/Development***
   Continuing education/certification is supported/encouraged
   Participation in professional associations encouraged
   An information-rich environment is supported
8. ***Recognition of the Value of Nursing's Contribution***
   Reward and pay for performance
   Career mobility and expansion
9. ***Recognition by Nurses for Their Meaningful Contribution to Practice***
   These nine elements will be fostered and promoted, as best fits, into the work of individual member organizations of the Alliance

Source: Copyright 2005 by the Nursing Organizations Alliance. All rights reserved.

Nobre (2001) suggests that "*Soul + Spirit + Resources + Leadership = Results.* The fruits of spirit are enthusiasm, motivation, and performance" (pp. 287–288).

The key to an effective organization is that *the goals, organizational strategies, policies, and administrators—along with staff—support the purpose and core values.* This gives life to the soul and spirit and helps us to know how to meander along as we head toward the ocean. It varies from organization to organization, from one healthcare worker/administrator to another, and from patient to patient because we are all different.

We provide some possible strategies, processes, or landmarks throughout this chapter, but because each organization is different and serves a different community, there will be differences in the strategies used as well as outcomes achieved. Just as no river is the same, no organization is the same. *There are an infinite number of possibilities of how to more effectively reach our ocean and how to keep the spirit energized. There is no one best way to achieve any of this.*

The Power of Meaningful Work

When we discuss spirit, we need to better define *meaningful work.* Work is meaningful when we give our patients what they value. This is why most of us became nurses. This is the goal in a second-wave healthcare organization.

However, sometimes people get confused about the importance of the work outcome versus the organizational processes. The processes can be in place, yet patient outcomes can be negative. The processes are not the most important thing. Processes only become important, or have value, when they are directed toward specific outcomes. *Outcomes give processes their value.*

This concept can also be applied to work. The work itself is not valuable. It is the *outcome* of the work that makes the work fulfilling. When burnout occurs, it is not the work itself, but the outcomes of the work that have not occurred. Nurses can become burned out when their workplace is understaffed and patient outcomes suffer. *Outcomes not occurring causes burnout, not the work itself.*

This is currently an issue in healthcare organizations. We become focused on the processes, forgetting that the most important issue is a good patient outcome. If our processes do not achieve the outcome, we need to change the processes—*always focusing on the outcome we want to achieve.*

To improve patient outcomes sometimes it is necessary to change care delivery models. These changes can be major and critical to achieving better patient-centered care, better patient and staff outcomes, physician satisfaction, lower costs, and better reimbursement (Cropley, 2012; DiGioia, Bertoty, Lorenz, Rocks, & Greenhouse, 2010; Mellott, Richards, Tonry, Bularzik, & Palmer, 2012; Morjikian, Kimball, & Joynt, 2007; Novak, Dooley, & Clark, 2008; Reineck, 2007; Storey, Linden, & Fisher, 2008; Thompson et al., 2011; Tonges & Ray, 2011).

Vestal (2012) gives one example when she suggests ways to make a quick turnaround. First, it is important for the nurse executive to get an honest, objective assessment of the issues by obtaining *feedback* from a number of sources. Then, based on that feedback, the nurse manager develops a plan to improve along with a timeline in 100-day increments, making sure that key managers, educators, clinical leaders, and mentors all agree with the issues and the plan.

> The plan should be detailed, have timeframes, and establish outcome measurement points and goals. Share the plan widely to make it clear what will be expected throughout the process and how the benefits will accrue to everyone. Ensure the necessary resources are committed. (p. 11)

The nurse executive should be sure that key staff are involved. For instance, if there has been staff turnover, it may be necessary to replace and orient staff as the first part of the plan. Or an expert may be brought in to ensure proper care is given to meet different patient population needs. "Lead the process with quality and safety as the first focus" (Vestal, 2012, p. 11). Sometimes that is all that is needed. For instance, if staff learn how to better care for a new patient population, their confidence and capability will increase. "Post and constantly review progress and results" (p. 11). It is important, when implementing a change, not to lose interest in it partway through.

> Additionally, it was noted that organizational culture is an essential foundation to the success of the strategy execution. A culture of performance improvement, accountability, and high-performance focus is critical to enhancing the organization's ability to implement strategies successfully. The right culture will enable the transformation to the hospital and care system of the future. (AHA, 2011)

Each person must tweak the processes as he or she perceives the individual nuances in what patients value and need. It is important to keep the outcome in mind and then determine the next action that will best achieve this outcome. This is supported by evidence that stresses the importance of nurse engagement and identifies factors that decrease engagement, such as having too many patients and not enough support services/equipment—these diminish the possibility of nurses achieving the outcome.

In this text, we keep coming back to what the patient values. As we consider care delivery models, it is important to first get the *patient perspective*. DiGioia and associates (2010) suggest shadowing and care flow mapping to be sure we understand in detail what patients and families are actually experiencing. To accomplish this, we can select a care experience and define the beginning and end points. Then, we establish a care experience guiding council. Council members can be anyone who touches patients' care experiences, such as nurses, physicians, therapists, technicians, dietitians, appointment schedulers, parking attendants, and janitors, as well as hospital leaders, purchase and supply chain employees, and financial representatives whom patients may never see. Next, a tool kit that includes patient shadowing, care flow mapping, patient storytelling, and patient surveys is used. This is followed by developing a work group that creates a shared vision of the ideal patient and family care experience. Last, we can identify improvement projects and project teams and implement the changes. In a surgical experience, the authors thought their ideal experience seemed impossible in 2007, and by 2010 they had realized the goal. Viewing a care experience through the eyes of the patient and family resulted in excellent outcomes.

When asked how they make sure best practices are used at the bedside, *staff nurses*

> emphasized the need to begin with building clear understandings as to how best practice actually resonates at the bedside. Moreover, nurses need to clearly establish and make visible a lived philosophy of care that embraces a priority for best practices. (Novak et al., 2008, p. 452)

They suggested the following strategies to achieve this:

1. Develop a clear grassroots understanding of the current state of affairs and degree of readiness for practice changes.
2. Start the dialogue by gauging the degree of staff commitment and soliciting ideas about how to make it happen.
3. Appraise to what extent nurses take ownership and responsibility for continuously updating clinical practices.
4. Solicit focused unit-based ideas for examining care efficiencies and/or effectiveness.
5. Establish performance review recognition and systemwide reward mechanisms for organizing and implementing clinical best practices.
6. Allocate budgetary resources to directly support the development of best practices through equipment and/or clinical nurse leader positions. (Novak et al., 2008, p. 452)

Clinical shift leader influence is important when making practice changes. Clinical shift leaders need to support the practice changes with each staff member and on each shift (Storey et al., 2008).

As new care delivery models are implemented, the *CNO role* is critical. "Executive leadership selects the [larger] change initiatives for the organization. Success is promoted by crafting change initiatives that are realistic, valued, manageable, and locally applicable to employees" (MacPhee, 2007, p. 405). Morjikian and colleagues (2007) completed interviews with CNOs who had successfully implemented changed delivery models. They identified four challenges:

1. The first challenge was the importance of completing a rigorous, formal business planning process for the implementation of the new care delivery model that includes formulation and analysis of key assumptions; strategy; operating plan and tactics; resource requirements; financial plan/ analysis identifying costs and benefits as well as revenues and expenses; evaluation/measurement plan (including measurable benefits such as fewer readmissions, lower rates of complications and mortality, lower inpatient costs, patient and physician satisfaction, staff retention); and contingency plans.
2. The second challenge was communication effectiveness, internally (in an interactive way with the care team, the nursing department, physicians, senior executives, and board members) and externally (with other hospitals, the broader nursing profession, relevant professional associations, policy makers, consumers, and other community leaders). This included providing information people needed to know to do their jobs, and providing information in a timely manner so that individuals could make accurate decisions. CNP approachability was important—they could be easily approached, built rapport, put others at ease, and listen. This meant having the patience to hear people out and being able to accurately restate the opinions of others even when the CNP did not agree. They identified a set of core values that were the basis for the change.
3. Resistance to change was the greatest obstacle. Communicating the need for the change and persuading experienced nurses to accept the change were critical. Dealing with this early is important.
4. Communicating expectations around the change process, that it is a journey. (pp. 400-401)

When implementing the change Morjikian and colleagues (2007) found that: (1) Using patient care facilitators was a cornerstone because the new model would change how all clinicians worked together to provide the care. (2) It was important that physicians recognized and valued the facilitators as well as the change. (3) It was important that other stakeholders were involved in the change, such as the executive group as well as other disciplines. (4) Having at least one nursing champion who had credibility and respect across the organization was critical. This person could energize the group (pp. 402–403).

Change fatigue is an issue to be reckoned with when implementing any new procedures and can derail a change. Reineck (2007) identifies six signs of change fatigue:

1. The value and objectives of the change effort are increasingly questioned.
2. Resources become diverted to other strategic initiatives.
3. Impatience with the duration of the change effort.
4. Data and results of the change are shared with hesitation.
5. Key leaders no longer attend status updates about the change project.
6. Change leaders become stressed and often leave. (p. 389)

"Traditional models of change are often linear and, unfortunately, do not account for the circular, chaotic change experienced today" (p. 389). Reineck recommends using six change strategies that are more successful in complex environments.

1. Change through Power—empowering others to build the change
2. Change through Reason—appealing to logic and rationale
3. Change through Reeducation—providing information, knowledge, and skills
4. Structural Approach—altering structures or processes
5. Behavioral Approach—developing new communication and collaboration patterns
6. Technological Approach—harnessing the power of computers and automation (p. 389)

Promoting Clinical Autonomy

Work is meaningful when staff autonomy is promoted. This is a must in a second-wave environment. Ditomassi (2012) identified organizational characteristics that are highly correlated with RN work satisfaction: autonomy, control over practice, and internal work motivation. The ANCC Forces of Magnetism Force 9 is Autonomy:

> Autonomous nursing care is the ability of a nurse to assess and provide nursing actions as appropriate for patient care based on competence, professional expertise and knowledge. The nurse is expected to practice autonomously, consistent with professional standards. Independent judgment is expected within the context of interdisciplinary and multidisciplinary approaches to patient/resident/client care. (ANCC, 2013b)

For nurses to have autonomy they need to be valued. Joseph (2007) recommends specific measurements that can be identified within an organization that portray the impact of nurses on patient and organizational outcomes.

One seminal research study by Kramer and associates (2007) examines "structures, practices, elements in the environment, and interventions that nurses, nurse managers, and physicians identify as promoting staff nurse clinical autonomy" (p. 41).

The first issue they identified revolves around *renegotiation of scope of practice.*

> Doing something that the patient needs right now without an order is not buried under a bushel basket or whispered about in the dark. We openly talk about it and what is the best way to handle the situation and whether that activity should be added to our scope of practice. (p. 44)

It is helpful to discuss this regular meeting of physicians and nurses (some places have designated rapid response teams for this function) (Gibson, 2011). As treatment evidence changes, these groups renegotiate and evaluate, or create, critical pathways or protocols based on best practice evidence. (Note that this can actually impede nurse autonomy when it reflects physician preferences instead of best practices.) "Renegotiating scope of practice enables autonomy by lessening feelings of risk and providing sanctioned power and authority for staff nurses to make decisions in the best interests of patients" (Kramer et al., 2007, p. 44).

The second issue identified in the study was *administrative/departmental sanction,* which was important to both nurses and physicians.

> [Each] hospital had a council structure designed to foster organizational autonomy, that is, formulation, regulation, and standardization of policies and practice across clinical services; guidance and development of educational, recruitment, and retention activities; and design of mechanisms to evaluate practice. Councils vary in goals, but all have one in common that is related to autonomy, that is, the promotion, regulation, and implementation of research and EBP initiatives. (Kramer et al., 2007, p. 44)

This was sanctioned in shared governance councils (discussed later in this chapter), department documents (such as scope of practice, definitions of nursing, or models of professional practice), performance appraisals, and career ladders documents.

A third element the study identified was the importance of a *cohesive, supportive peer group*. Effectiveness of teams and a culture of "helping one another without having to ask" were important to nurses. They trusted each other and worked well together.

A fourth element was *physician trust, respect, and support*. This mutual trust and respect create a synergistic, interdependent alliance based on recognition of each other's competencies. "Trust and support are based on meeting mutual expectations: the nurse will do what needs to be done for the patient; the physician will provide feedback and will cover with an order" (Kramer et al., 2007, p. 45). This is supported by the third point in the Institute of Medicine report *The Future of Nursing: Leading Change, Advancing Health*: "Nurses should be full partners with physicians and others in redesigning U.S. healthcare" (Cadmus, 2011, p. 34).

A fifth element supporting nurse autonomy was *specialization, focus, and mission*. The specialized, focused body of knowledge helped to create autonomy among nurses and physicians. "Focus or mission also promotes a distinct and constant group of nurses and physicians working together where . . . trust earned by some group members is extended to others who are new to the team" (Kramer et al., 2007, p. 46). The unit culture also promotes this.

Not surprisingly, *nurse manager support* was another factor. In the Magnet precepts, control over nursing practice is essential. Nurse managers supported positive clinical autonomy, promoted staff cohesiveness, supported a positive unit culture, and wanted "staff to function autonomously in scheduling, assignments, organizing tasks, and direct patient care" (Kramer et al., 2007, p. 46). The group worked together "to select equipment, review policies/practices, and manage scheduling" (p. 47). In this study, unit culture was identified as being more important than organizational culture. A cultural premise was being dedicated to the patient. Nurse manager support was particularly important with new employees.

Physicians and nurses identified combined, interdisciplinary evidence-based practice activities that promoted autonomy and teamwork. Various educational programs were cited as essential, including certification review sessions.

Lastly, in this study two nurse attributes were important: (1) "that the nurse is experienced, knowledgeable, and smart [learns from experience, and even applies for certification]; and (2) nurses must want, desire, and enjoy autonomous practice and have confidence in their ability to make decisions" (Kramer et al., 2007, p. 48).

Culture

Culture reflects the way people work together, the spirit that moves the organization forward. Weiss (2001) defines an organization's culture as "shared values, beliefs, norms, expectations, and assumptions that bind people and systems" (p. 348). Culture is a pattern of assumptions or behaviors, often implied and not formally recognized, that are indirectly taught to new members as they enter an organization. A strong culture (such as the expectation that all will give 200% effort, or that each staff member helps other staff complete the work when help is needed) has great impact on team members and results in effective teams, goal fulfillment, innovations, and a strategic capacity (Gordon, 2002). In the most effective cultures, self-management can flourish. In this environment, nurses can make critical decisions with minimal supervision. "Nurses are actually self-managing themselves" just as chaos and complexity are self-managing. "Although implicit, each nurse follows a set of social rules or norms that stress the importance

Some additional domains may need to be examined for further insights:

Learning/mentoring: Is learning from one another encouraged, and are new staff mentored?

Patient-centered involvement: Are patients and their families treated as part of the care team? Are the risks and benefits of care fully disclosed to patients? Are the decisions about care by an informed patient respected and supported?

Resources/staffing: Patient deaths are associated with fewer nurses. [It is also important] that nurses *perceive* that staffing is adequate. Education and skill level of resources are also factors.

Mindfulness: Is situational awareness always paramount, and is deference given to expertise depending on environment and circumstance?

Job design: Are pains taken to support the needs of caregivers who work in a highly fragmented environment fraught with latent conditions that can undermine [what patients value/safety]?

Change: Are management and staff open to incorporating [best practices]? (p. 50)

The authors suggest that other ways to measure culture include "recent hire and exit interviews, executive rounding, focus groups, staff satisfaction and turnover rate, performance evaluations, and testing of [best practice] knowledge" (Smetzer & Navarra, 2007, p. 51).

An example of an organizational culture in which nursing practice is valued is when nurses have the option to close units to new patients—and physicians and administrators *cannot override this decision*. The most important thing to remember is to model the behavior that one wants to promote. Actions speak louder than words.

> Two factors contribute to a deeply satisfying work culture. The quality of worker engagement at the point of service, the first factor, is similar to the caring concept of presence with the patient, which nurses find deeply satisfying. The second factor is the ability of front-line leaders to move out of supervision to focus on motivating and enabling workers to do their work effectively. These factors are challenged by emphases on efficiency and economics, such that employees often feel depersonalized as an expense item. (Sherwood, 2003, p. 37)

Nurse manager leadership is a key factor in achieving a strong culture. Laschinger and colleagues (2009) cite the importance of unit leadership in creating empowering work environments that increase nurses' commitment to the organization. Thompson and associates (2011) found nurse managers who were higher on leader–member exchange had higher supervisor safety expectations, were more committed to organizational learning and continuous improvement, had better total communication, gave more feedback and communication about errors, and had a nonpunitive response to errors. Warshawski and colleagues (2012) found that interpersonal relationships with the people nurse managers reported to were most predictive of nurse managers' work engagement:

> [Evidence shows that] the driving force behind top performance is an engaged workforce. Engaged employees are energized, dedicated, and motivated to persevere and complete their work. Managers are critical for creating environments fostering employee engagement. Managers must be engaged in their own work to create these stimulating work environments. (p. 423)

In a study with 323 nurse managers, Warshawski and colleagues (2012) found that nurse managers were highly engaged in their work. They felt their work was meaningful. They had access to sufficient job and personal resources to mitigate job demands. These findings support the importance of both supervisor and coworker relationships as key in building work engagement.

The organizational culture is enhanced when nurse executives support and communicate the importance of collaborative interpersonal relationships and mentor nurse managers to achieve this on their units.

Organizational designs, such as reduced spans of control for nurse managers, promote the development of quality interpersonal relationships with staff nurses by having time to coach and build connections.

Organizational designs may also improve nurse manager relationships with physicians. For example, employing physicians as hospitalists encourages physicians to align their goals with the organization. By creating partnerships of nurse managers and physicians, responsibility for achieving quality patient outcomes can be shared. (Warshawski et al., 2012, pp. 423–424)

The authors suggest that staff, physicians, and nurse administrators are all involved in interviewing potential nurse managers. This achieves support of the new candidate by all involved in the interviews and sends the message to staff and physicians that interdisciplinary teamwork is valued.

"Recognition and rewards need to be based on team performance and achievement of shared goals. . . . Shared rewards for exemplary team performance reinforce team behaviors" (Warshawski et al., 2012, p. 424).

The evidence shows that culture is influenced from the top down. When nurse managers are supported by their supervisors, they become more engaged. Then, the nurse managers can support staff on the unit to become more engaged.

Now let's turn to *negative cultures*. "Culture can kill the best strategic plan" (Curran, 2002, p. 257). Evidence shows negativity is most often caused by

> (1) an excessive workload; (2) concerns about management's ability to lead the company forward successfully; (3) anxiety about the future, particularly longer-term jobs, income, and retirement security; (4) lack of challenge in their work, with boredom intensifying existing frustration about workload; and (5) insufficient recognition for the level of contribution and effort provided, and concerns that pay isn't commensurate with performance. (Huseman, 2009, p. 61)

Bohn (2000, p. 84) warns that if at least three of the following symptoms are present, the organization is in trouble, productivity will suffer, and everyone will burn out rushing from crisis to crisis:

1. There isn't enough time to solve all the problems. (Not enough nurses are present for the current number of patients.)
2. Solutions are incomplete. (As nurses try to deal with everything, they patch the present problem but do not fix it.)
3. Problems recur and cascade. (The same problems come up again or are even worse because they were not dealt with properly in the first place.)
4. Urgency supersedes importance. (There is never any time to examine processes or work on improvements because of all the crises the nurses are dealing with.)
5. Many problems become crises. (Smaller problems flare up to larger ones that may require heroic efforts on the part of the nurses.)
6. Performance drops.

To understand how powerful negativity is, Huseman (2009) observes:

1. We tend to remember failures more vividly than success.
2. We tend to react more strongly to negative stimuli than we do positive.
3. We tend to trust negative information more than we do positive.
4. When we experience joy it is short lived and then we start taking what caused the joy for granted. (pp. 60–61)

In the workplace:

> Negativity is contagious and spreads quickly [like a virus], especially within an organizational culture. . . .[one large study] found that, on average, more than half of workers' current emotion is negative at work and a third is intensely negative. (Huseman, 2009, p. 61)

Negative emotions at work affect productivity, performance, and retention. The problem is that it also spreads to patients and can affect patient outcomes. For instance, Huseman (2009) cites a study where nurses' general mood on certain cardiac care units was "depressed," and the death rate was four times higher than on other similar units.

How can we make the workplace more positive? Studies show that satisfying three strong needs of nurses brings about a positive culture; the needs are as follows: "(1) the need to feel connected to and competent in their work; (2) the need to strengthen/develop their capabilities and build their careers; and (3) the need for recognition" (Huseman, 2009, p. 63). The immediate engaged supervisor is key here. "Having leaders at every level of a hospital adopt a leadership style using praise and recognition is one of the quickest ways to counteract negativity" (p. 63).

Once the causes of negativity are identified, they need to be fixed. For instance, if staffing is inadequate, problems will continue until the administration increases staffing. The nurse administrator may need to emphasize that evidence shows that negative cultures result in higher nurse turnover, more patient safety issues, more potential lawsuits, and less reimbursement. If administrators are using linear thinking, the nurse administrator can supply numbers for all of these points.

Sometimes the issue can be the nurse manager (or higher levels of administrators). Is this person effective in the role? If not, this must be dealt with. The person may need mentoring, or perhaps the person does not like the administrative role and would prefer to do something else. The person may need to be counseled and, if changes do not occur, may need to be terminated or asked to step down from the role. Leadership issues must be fixed before the culture can change.

Once any leadership issues are fixed, correcting the issues on a unit (or in the organization) takes time and consistent, positive leadership by administrators. Often the culture gets worse as the manager begins work to change it because the behaviors are static and employees do not want to change—even though many hate the culture! Having support from the top down and having support of informal leaders really help the nurse manager turn this around.

Within a positive, empowering culture, some individuals do not fit. Sometimes this results from a style difference or is an example of the Pygmalion effect. Moving to another work area with a different supervisor may better suit these individuals. It may be necessary for certain people to leave, if they decide not to support the changes.

If an individual has a negative effect on the culture and needs to be counseled, the best way to counsel is to recognize that it is an individual's personal responsibility to change negative behaviors. Campbell, Fleming, and Grote (1985) published a classic on disciplinary action that *involves the employee in solving the problem*. This includes the use of reminders rather than warnings and actually gives the employee a paid leave day to decide whether (1) to change, specifying how behaviors will change, or (2) to quit and submit his or her resignation. This method of disciplinary action is preferable to action where the supervisor *tells* the employee what to do.

Bates (2003, p. 38) gives five tips for building a credible culture:

- Reward people who communicate openly and build trust in the workplace; counsel those who don't.
- Talk about the values of your organization from the top down and encourage conversation about issues.
- Build your own credibility bank by practicing open communication; if you make a mistake, you will get the benefit of the doubt.

- Encourage questions. Trust thrives on open lines of communication. The people who work for you know it's okay to question a decision or priority.
- Don't assume people know what is expected; be clear about the kind of behavior and communication you expect and find acceptable.

Organizational Design: Shifting to Complexity

Now let's turn to organizational design because it is needed for best outcomes in this value-based environment (the second curve). As we examine design, it is important to shift our linear views to *relational and whole systems thinking* that incorporates complexity and chaos. As previously discussed, the mission and core values are important underpinnings—as long as they support what patients value.

> Organizations are like icebergs. They float above the water with characteristics that are easily visible. Characteristics and events tell the story. Often we make the mistake of reacting to events without considering what is lying below the water line: patterns behind those events and system structures that support those patterns. Patterns tell you what has been happening over time and allow you to predict or anticipate what is likely to occur in the future. Structures, both tangible and intangible, drive those patterns and support those events. Tangible system structures include organizational structures, policies, and procedures. Intangible structures include culture, beliefs, and mental models. (Wolf, 2012, p. 309)

For an organization to be viable, everyone must be flexible and adapt in ways that better achieve patient outcomes. As problems occur, each person must figure out how to change to better achieve what patients value. *Administrators and staff need to work together to achieve this.*

Organizationally, the design needs to be the best way to accomplish this goal. At this point, some terms need clarification. *Structure* in linear language refers to the way an organization delineates jobs and reporting relationships. The arrangement of roles within an organization is portrayed in the organizational chart. Structure is needed to provide a starting place to organize the work, yet it must be ever changing. It is a linear picture that does not capture all the complexity of relationships within the organization as people (regardless of placement on the chart) interact to achieve what the patient values. It also does not capture group effectiveness. Porter-O'Grady and Malloch (2011) warn:

> When any system has too much structure, it begins to support the structure rather than accomplishing its objectives. Unnecessary structure draws resources away from the system's services and interferes with its ability to do its work. Structure drains the energy and creativity out of a system and obstructs relationships and interactions necessary for the system's function. The same holds true for unnecessary management. (pp. 25, 69)

The *design* of an organization describes the process of "setting up" or the "appearance" of the organization. Though the terms *structure* and *design* are closely related, there is a lack of consistency and clarity in the use of these words. Many times these terms are used interchangeably. *Design* goes beyond structure to include the identified work units and how they are interconnected internally and externally. Design reflects the relationships and processes used (the complexity) within an organization.

> The design that best coordinates resources to achieve [patient outcomes] should be contingent on the evolving environment. For example, an organization competing in an externally complex environment must match that complexity internally to remain viable. A complex environment means that there are multiple states the overall system could evolve to. (Clancy, 2007a, p. 535)

Earlier we discussed, *As above, so below*. This also applies to design. Organizational design must match the complexity in the greater community, and individuals in the organization need to match the complexity found in the overall organization. Each worker in an organization must own his/her work processes and take part in bringing about the necessary changes because chaos happens in incremental bits. It takes each person in the organization doing his/her best to give patients what they value and support others to give their best.

> By focusing on different descriptors in portraying how human dynamic systems work and how processes get sustained, we have created a new framework for considering design and function within the workplace and within the entire human community—and for considering what is and is not effective in the workplace and in relationships between people, as well as for looking at issues of accountability, productivity, and value.
>
> For example, no longer is it enough for leaders to assess the functional proficiency of individual workers as a way of determining whether a work process is fully effective and sustainable. Instead, they must also examine whether each worker's competence fits with the competence of the other workers. "*Goodness of fit*," not the individual proficiency of any single participant, leads to effectiveness and sustainability. (Porter-O'Grady & Malloch, 2011, pp. 14–15)

In organizational design, Senge (2006) suggests we create a *learning organization*. He refers to five disciplines that build the learning organization:

1. **Building shared vision:** The practice of unearthing shared "pictures of the future" that foster genuine commitment
2. **Personal mastery:** The skill of continually clarifying and deepening our personal vision
3. **Mental models:** The ability to unearth our internal pictures of the world, to scrutinize them, and to make them open to the influence of others
   Mental models are the beliefs and assumptions that we have about almost everything—the lens through which we view the world. They are usually unconscious and yet have a very powerful effect on our behavior. Often they act as a filter, limiting the information we are able to absorb. . . . The culture of an organization has a strong impact on the mental models of employees. (Wolf, 2012, p. 310)
4. **Team learning:** The capacity to "think together" that is gained by mastering the practice of dialogue and discussion
5. **Systems thinking:** The discipline that integrates the others, fusing them into a coherent body of theory and practice

Senge coined the term *systems thinking*, describing it as a framework for seeing interrelationships. Systems thinking "lies in a shift of mind: seeing interrelationships rather than linear cause and effect and seeing processes of change rather than snapshots" (p. 73). As thinkers we often see things in straight lines, whereas reality is actually made up of circles.[2]

By using systems thinking, we can picture the entire organization and how it functions, not just our own department. It is dynamic (ever changing). How will people across the organization, and even in the community, respond to a change? What outcomes might result if a decision is implemented?

When decisions are made using systems thinking, the decisions are carefully crafted to include dialogue by all who would be affected by a change and incorporate issues they identify. This achieves the best result and avoids possible pitfalls that could actually worsen the situation. Without using systems thinking, it is easy to implement quick-fix solutions that actually generate more problems and result in other unanticipated effects because they did not account for the entire system response to the change. In today's complex organizations, *systems thinking is a necessary administrative competency*.

Understanding systems thinking begins with understanding the concept of feedback. The word *feedback* can be used in many different ways. When we ask for feedback, we are often asking for someone's opinion, encouraging both positive and negative remarks. Systems thinkers use feedback as a broader concept. Senge (2006) describes feedback as any "reciprocal flow of influence," an "axiom that every influence is both cause and effect," and that "nothing is influenced in just one direction" (p. 75). Ongoing dialogue helps us better understand what is going on by providing feedback in this circular process.

In systems thinking, we need to understand feedback issues. According to Senge (2006), there are two types of feedback: reinforcing and balancing. *Reinforcement feedback* (the "engine of growth") occurs in many ways throughout the organization, such as when leaders or team members praise those who have done well (positive) or when low performers are ignored (negative). When feedback is negative, reinforcing processes may become vicious cycles. For example, if a person is interfering with other team members' work and this behavior is allowed to continue, another more positive team member may leave for a healthier work environment.

The second type of feedback in systems thinking is *balancing feedback* (or goal-oriented behavior). This occurs as we encounter limits or boundaries. A classic example is when managers, under budgetary constraints, cut team members to help meet or decrease the budget. In turn, the remaining team members become overworked, and the budget does not improve because of an increase in turnover and required overtime. If the managers had used systems thinking, they would have anticipated this result and would have met the budget constraints in other ways.

Balancing feedback is often difficult to manage because the goals are implicit and go unrecognized. No one realizes that they even exist. One example that Senge uses is the leader who tries relentlessly to decrease burnout among professionals by decreasing work hours and locking offices so that people stop working late. This backfires when professionals start taking work home because the offices are locked. Balancing processes are more difficult to handle than reinforcing processes; we often do not see change occurring because of an actual balancing process.

The issue of responsibility often complicates the concept of feedback. Linear thinkers always search for someone or something to blame, for instance, in regard to patient safety issues. When we become accomplished systems thinkers, we renounce the idea that one individual is responsible and begin to realize that responsibility is shared; it is interconnected.

Everyone in an organization needs to use systems thinking. Work teams are more effective when the entire team can view the organization as a whole. Unfortunately, team members' confidence and responsibility can be undermined by the complexity of a situation. How often do we hear team members and front-line leaders comment, "You can't change the system?" Systems thinking can drastically help to change this helpless feeling.

Senge (2006) lists several qualities that are apparent in most successful change initiatives:

- They are connected with real work goals and processes.
- They are connected with improving performance.
- They involve people who have the power to take action regarding these goals.
- They seek to balance action and reflection, connecting inquiry and experimentation.
- They afford people an increased amount of "white space," opportunities for people to think and reflect without pressure to make decisions.
- They are intended to increase people's capacity, individually and collectively.
- They focus on learning about learning in settings that matter. (p. 43)

Formal Organization

Two forms of organizational structure and design are usually described: formal and informal. The *formal* organization, or "official" structure, is described by the organizational chart. The organizational chart displays the chain of command, or the relationship of authority. The solid lines that connect the boxes show the formal channels of communication and reporting relationships; the dotted lines show an informal reporting relationship. Doesn't this sound linear?

Most often the *organizational chart* has the board and the CEO, or president, at the top of the chart. (Some suggest that this chart should be inverted, with the patient at the top and the president and board at the bottom.) The organizational chart provides clarity and specifies areas of responsibility, which are needed for stability. However, an organizational chart is a very *imperfect* linear picture because it does not capture the relationships (complexity) that exist. Relationships are more important to getting the work accomplished. Therefore, the chart must be taken in context with the actual workings of the organization.

In authoritarian linear structures, the organizational chart is tall, meaning that there are many layers in the hierarchy. This is a centralized model. In this text, we advocate a decentralized organizational model, which works much better because everyone is interconnected and communication occurs throughout the organization. In decentralized models,

> Organizational structures are generally flat, rather than tall, and decentralized decision-making prevails. The organizational structure is dynamic and responsive to change. Strong nursing representation is evident in the organizational committee structure. Executive-level nursing leaders serve at the executive level of the organization. The Chief Nursing Officer typically reports directly to the Chief Executive Officer. The organization has a functioning and productive system of shared decision-making. (ANCC, 2013b)

This is the second Force of Magnetism.

The formal structure also includes the regularly scheduled meetings that take place within the organization. Hopefully, these meetings aid those in the organization to function more effectively. However, there is great divergence in actual meeting effectiveness. Some organizations have so many meetings the administrators cannot get their work done or do not do regular rounds! Often the meetings have a more linear focus. In a complex environment, better information can actually be obtained from rounds (discussed later in this chapter).

In nursing, staff are generally expected to attend and participate in certain meetings. The problem becomes finding a way to relieve staff of patient care responsibilities long enough to attend and participate in meetings. In an authoritarian environment, meetings might not be considered as important, and other issues might easily interfere with staff being able to attend these meetings. Meetings are linear, just giving information.

In a participative, value-based environment, release times for meetings have more importance because administrators realize the complex nature of important functions and the need for transparency. A shared governance model encourages everyone to deal with issues that staff face every day. Meetings, when functioning well, more than pay for the release time needed.

Informal Organization

> In every organization there is a formal structure and process and an informal network. This network is primarily relational and carries most of the information about how people in the organization think or feel and what their sentiments are regarding almost anything in the system. It is as vital and valid a part of the system as any other, and it requires attention because, among other things, it

typically contains essential pieces of the dynamic that have been overlooked or missed as well as the "undiscussables," and opinions that do not reflect the prevailing point of view. Embedded here too are some of the most dynamic notions of what should happen or what should be done.

All elements of the system, whether formal or informal, are a part of the dynamic of change in the organization. Each can be a vehicle for action and even transformation. Leaders need to pay notice to all the informal pathways and networks of communication and relationship, from hallway conversations to lunchtime discussions, from whispered comments to sarcastic asides—each plays a role in the complex web of interactions necessary for sustaining the organization. Taking an opportunity to hear, communicate, or join with the others, contributes to discovering the state of the organization and determining the proper actions to take to strengthen it. (Porter-O'Grady & Malloch, 2011, pp. 28–29)

The informal organization reflects all the interpersonal relationships among people that are not reflected on the organizational chart but that affect operations. For instance, a nurse manager may value the unit secretary's informal leadership, which might really enhance the nurse manager's effectiveness and help the unit to function much more efficiently. If the nurse manager chooses to ignore or suppress this person's leadership capabilities, unnecessary conflicts can result, patient care may suffer, and the dysfunctional situation spirals downward from there.

When there are flaws or inefficiencies in the administrative leadership, such as when a nurse administrator is secretive or does not share information, the informal information network runs rampant. When most information is shared (transparency) and nurses trust administrators, the informal network becomes relatively inactive.

In the informal organizational structure, free-flowing communication is known as "the grapevine." This type of communication reaches every corner and level of the organization, introducing complexity. When team members do not receive credible information from administrators, the grapevine takes over. Generally, information spread through the grapevine is about 75% correct. Leadership can use the grapevine to gauge employee responses by allowing new ideas and policies to be spread through the grapevine. Although it is critical for nurses to learn formal channels of communication, the informal communication networks cannot be ignored.

Increased Communication in a Value-Based Environment

In the past, three common types of communication patterns prevailed in a formal organization: downward, upward, and lateral. Presently, we realize there is another communication pattern that is most effective: It is *circular and messy*—the most appropriate kind of communication in a value-based environment. People at all levels talk with one another. They talk with those within and those who touch the organization. For instance, we have open-door policies that break the rigid barriers of the protected office with a secretary out front to prevent others from reaching the administrator, and we do regular rounds (discussed later in this chapter).

This circular communication pattern is messy because it opens up the realization that we may have misperceptions about a situation (in an authoritarian system we were not aware of this). It *changes our judgmental attitude to one of curiosity*. At the same time, it *creates synergy and belonging*.

This brings about another change in the value-based environment—we need to *increase* the information flow within the organization. Studies in the field of social network theory demonstrate that *by increasing the number of communication links among individuals, an organization can generate more solutions to environmental threats* (Clancy, 2007a, p. 535). Communication among all stakeholders (including physicians and patients) is paramount.

Ideally, there is *transparency*. "Transparency is about being open about what you do and how you do it" (Scalise, 2006, p. 35). This not only takes place within the organization but also in the greater community. For instance, quality, charity care, and/or financial data can be shared openly with others. Many states have passed transparency laws requiring healthcare organizations to report sentinel events, nurse staffing levels, and/or hospital charges/payment rates. Obviously, risks are involved. Sometimes administrators fear that other similar entities will look better, or that competitors will exploit their weaknesses. Physicians may fear that published mortality rates will give them a bad reputation. But secrets have a way of eventually becoming public knowledge. All of this is chaos and complexity at work.

In today's explosion of information technology, communication has become even more complex. Misunderstandings, misreadings, and unclear or selective hearing all play into faulty communication exchanges within an organization.

> The most powerful way to make a significant change is to convene a conversation. But we know that often that is the most difficult thing to do. It is easier to talk about the person than to the person, but no progress is made toward solving a particular problem or learning about new ways to interact to make a real change.
>
> A sign of professional maturity is a person's capacity and appreciation for conversation. Our world and our organization's world would be in a much more peaceful state if the capacity for conversation between the parts were more mature.
>
> The art and science of focused conversation [is] . . . a collaborative dialogue of discovery where you invite others to share differing views and you test your thinking and understanding in the context of this dialogue so you can hear in a different manner . . . trusting the wisdom of the person or group and believing that this is the right person or group to solve the problem. . . . The leader will only succeed if he/she truly believes in the group's wisdom and does not come armed with solutions. . . .
>
> We must be open to seeing the issues in a much more messy context than our little world of making judgments has allowed us. When you open yourself to a conversation among equals, you open yourself to the necessity of questioning your positions and the "truths" from which you operate. The only way to enter a productive conversation is to give yourself permission and willingness to be disturbed. . . . Real conversations change you and the people/groups you are talking to. That is the whole point: to make new relationships and synergies out of old dysfunctional patterns of parts interacting with each other. To have a conversation, you must allow for messiness and for being disturbed and confused as a way to make new growth.
>
> The only way to improve the world is through relationships, and conversations are the prelude to creating that change. (Kerfoot, 2002, pp. 298–299)

Pilette (2006) cites a study where *60% of U.S. hospital deaths each year can be attributed to poor, faulty, or absent communication*. "Participants acknowledged their inability to structure and handle the conversation as the most frequent reason for not addressing faulty behaviors" (p. 26). Honesty is important here, but the first issue is that people may not realize that they are not communicating appropriately. She recommends doing a 360-degree evaluation or having an executive coach. This provides feedback for each administrator.

> Some experts believe that we're frequently defending against fears or concerns about our own significance, competence, and likability. They further distinguish that we're not defending ourselves from other people, but from painful feelings inside us that we don't want to experience. For example, if we feel we're not competent, we may be very critical of others, try to shame them, use sarcasm to berate them, treat them with indifference, or bully them.
>
> Now the good news. With genuine introspection, defensiveness is advantageous as "an early internal warning system," which can be used to consciously shift us out of a conflict-generating posture to

one of relationship building. Knowing our trigger points for defensiveness makes it easier to recognize similarities in another's response, thereby affording us an opportunity to step out of an emotional discussion and rebuild safety into the conversation. (Pilette, 2006, pp. 26–27)

Faulty communication on the part of administrators is only part of the problem.

The communication skills of the physician, nurse, and hospital staff topped the list as the most critical to positive patient satisfaction scores. Physicians are charged with not taking the time to really listen to patients. Meetings with physicians are usually hurried and impersonal. The patient isn't included in the care decisions about his or her health and lacks the knowledge on how to proceed with treatment options and medication regimens. Poor communication with patients can result in dangerous situations, noncompliant patients with prescribed treatment regimens, negative outcomes, and patient dissatisfaction. (Squires, 2012, p. 28)

Ajeigbe and associates (2013) found that when a teamwork intervention was completed with nurses and physicians in EDs, it enhanced autonomy and control over practice for both nurses and physicians. Participants felt it was a more positive work environment.

Nurses can help the faulty communication issue by treating the patient with respect, listening to the patient, paying attention to nonverbal clues, explaining what the physician wants, giving the patient helpful suggestions in discharge information, as well as managing pain and protecting the safety of the patient.

Physicians and nurses communicate with patients differently. Physicians usually speak to patients from a medical point of view using technical terms. . . . Nurses explain how behavior patterns determine health conditions and the importance of taking responsibility to improve health status. (Porter-O'Grady & Malloch, 2011, p. 28)

Physician communication can cause other issues. Physicians sometimes exhibit abusive behavior toward nurses.

Doctors commonly get frustrated when nurses present information differently than they would or provide more detail than they believe necessary. Nurses get frustrated when doctors seem uninterested in information nurses deem essential to their patients' health and well-being. Of course, these differences in communication styles don't justify disruptive outbursts—but understanding them can help nurses and doctors avoid them.

Power dynamics within healthcare organizations may contribute too. Even as nurses are poised to take on a greater role as health care turns to a more team-based care model, physicians still cling to traditional positions and roles. Also, physicians remain central to revenue models, perpetuating traditional hierarchies. And while the problem of nursing shortages waxes and wanes, universal agreement exists that physicians are in short supply and will be for decades to come.

For most nurses, the first step in addressing disruptive physician behavior is internal. It starts with an absolute belief that nobody deserves to be yelled at for making or witnessing a mistake, much less while doing their job correctly and competently. . . .The best approach is to be assertive and confront the physician directly at the time of the occurrence. How this is done marks the difference between a healthy workplace culture and a toxic one. (Gessler, Rosenstein, & Ferron, 2012, p. 9)

When inappropriate physician behavior is not dealt with by administrators and by the medical staff it results in negative patient outcomes, errors, and adverse events. This behavior also causes nurses to leave positions (Squires, 2012). Education can help nurses and administrators better deal with this issue and can help physicians to learn how to deal with conflict more appropriately (Casanova et al., 2007; Crawford, Omery, & Seago, 2012; Rosenthal, 2013; Squires, 2012).

Many issues contribute to this communication problem—variance in knowledge, differing educational perspectives, stereotypes, language/cultural issues, and organizational culture issues (Crawford et al., 2012). Both physicians and nursing professionals work in a stressful environment with frequent interruptions. Physicians value rounding, whereas nurses do not always believe they have the time. Some physicians continue to think that nurses' main function is to follow MD orders. Both types of professionals are pressed for time. When nurses ask for clarification of orders, physicians can perceive this as "undermining their authority." Another challenge is "coordination between multiple patients with multiple physicians" (Casanova et al., 2007, p. 69). Lastly, some are still caught up in the doctor–nurse game involving "passive communication structures and male–female autonomy issues." The rules of this game:

> Nurses are required to be bold, take initiative, and make significant recommendations while appearing to be passive and submissive. Properly done, the recommendations appear physician-initiated. In return, physicians request a recommendation from nurses without appearing to ask for it. The avoidance of open disagreement is a key game feature. Mutual dialogue must be established in order to achieve interdisciplinary collaboration and overcome this cumbersome milieu. (Crawford et al., 2012, p. 549)

In an integrated review of the evidence on nurse–physician communication, Crawford and associates (2012) suggest the following evidence-based recommendations for both physicians and nurses:

- Respectfully greet each other and introduce new staff members to other care providers.
- Establish a nonhierarchical and collaborative communication structure emphasizing respect, openness, active listening, and a free flow of patient-centered information.
- Use a structured tool to focus communication on patient care needs.
- Increase opportunities for sharing about the differences between the work of the nurse and the physician, using that knowledge to create a collaborative common ground meeting patient needs.
- Encourage active participation among the team involving all disciplines in programs such as multidisciplinary rounds or care conferences.
- Nurses should be timely and prepared with accurate and relevant patient information when communicating with physicians and other team members. Succinct communication needs to be refined. This is particularly relevant when communicating condition changes and patient care needs over the phone.
- Establish specific procedures to eliminate unnecessary telephone calls, such as bundling redundant phone calls and the development of clinical algorithms when appropriate.
- Implement effective strategies that support chain-of-command procedures and enforcement of disruptive behavior policies.

Manojlovich and Antonakos (2008) found that "openness, understanding, and accuracy of communication are important communication satisfiers for nurses" (p. 241).

Pilette (2006) suggests that we can help ourselves if we learn to dissect a conversation into *content*, *pattern*, and *relationship*. It is relatively easy to recognize *content*. This is the subject of the conversation (problem, event, person, or idea). *Patterns* reflect "habits, which affect *relationship* predictability. Good habits foster dependability and reliability, while a string of bad habits erode interpersonal trust" (p. 27). To determine if habits are good or need improving, consider the consequences of the conversation. Is that what you really wanted or intended?

If the subject is the issue, Pillette (2006) advocates using a *Ladder of Inference*:

1. Observe "data" (information, evidence, etc.).
2. Select specific data from what you've observed.
3. Add meaning to the data from a personal and cultural perspective.
4. Make assumptions based on the meaning.
5. Draw conclusions based on assumptions.
6. Adopt beliefs based on conclusions.
7. Take action based on conclusions. (p. 27)

Using this model, think about these in the order given. If someone says something that we think is inappropriate or harmful, instead of emotionally reacting to this (because we are drawing conclusions about how bad this is), we can take a breather, if necessary, and then go through the seven steps. We can ask for clarification (What are the assumptions you used to determine this?). Then, we use active listening with the goal of understanding the other person's perspective. The same process can be used with problematic patterns: What are the consequences of the actions? Is this what we intended and really wanted?

Communication is also complex because of gender differences and the ways men and women do work. Rutan (2003) reports that female nurse managers discuss "domestic, family, personal, and social issues before the meetings" and sometimes these issues are interwoven in meeting discussions, whereas male leaders stick to business and work-related subjects. On the other hand, male leaders discussed meeting agenda items before the meeting in various locations, and, in one example, once a meeting started,

> The male [leader] acted as a coach in charge of a team, with the other males helping him carry out the play. Female team members were never part of this "meeting before the meeting." . . . [During the meeting] the male participants communicated more actively, asking more questions, contributing information and data, and making frequent recommendations and suggestions. Males avoided both eye contact and exchanging personal thoughts and feelings. They were interested in getting to the point of issues by being assertive, dominant, competitive, independent, and aggressive. (p. 184)

Females often do not understand this dynamic and, instead, would bring ideas up in the meeting:

> Women see the leader's competence, respect, and fairness as significantly more important to team effectiveness than men do. Women see the team members' knowledge of their jobs as significantly more important to team effectiveness than men do. Women see the team members' liking, trusting, and helping each other as significantly more important to team effectiveness than men do. (p. 184)

A nurse manager is more effective if he or she understands these differences. For women, it is important not only to be attentive to nurturing and socializing roles but to be task oriented with well-developed business and financial skills. For men, it is important to incorporate more of the interpersonal skills and be open to changes occurring during the meeting. Rutan (2003) suggests that the following learning needs to take place:

> Females must understand that males do not share personal experiences primarily because they do not want to appear vulnerable. Nurse leaders should . . . devote time prior to a formal meeting for idea generation, problem solving, and information sharing, just as the . . . male administrators . . . need to concentrate on being more open to new ideas as they are proposed or be prepared to present ideas and work out solutions while team meetings are in session. (p. 185)

Staff development activities that identify gender differences and encourage everyone (regardless of gender) to understand and use the positive aspects of both perspectives go a long way to achieve better teamwork. We recommend the Pat Heim tapes (1996) as a helpful tool to accomplish this goal.

Some organizations have used *scripting*, where people say prescribed words in certain situations. This can be helpful for employees. Be aware that if the underlying emotion is negative, actions speak louder than words, and in such cases, the scripted response is not effective. A second issue is that workers can resent having to use scripting, and the resentment builds.

Collaboration: The Key to the Future

Collaboration is the glue that holds together the relationships, the teamwork, and the communication among everyone involved in the organization. It incrementally increases horizontal, messy communication. It is presented as a separate category here in this chapter, but in reality it is interwoven with teamwork, giving care the patient values, meeting reimbursement requirements, and so forth. The better the glue, the more effective the organization in this value-based environment.

This is magic, dynamic glue. It is not permanently adhesive, but, when needed, it is removable. The bond is strong, yet ever changing. The bond forms between people who know and trust each other. Magic happens within a messy process when people work effectively together. Everyone respects each other, communicates with one another, and works together in ways that will best serve patients. Evidence shows that everyone, including the patients (residents, clients), staff, and physicians, fares better when collaboration is present. Laschinger and Smith (2013) found that as much as *70% of adverse events occur because of a lack of communication and collaboration among healthcare team members.*

> Collaboration focuses on trying to reach agreement among divergent opinions to accomplish mutual goals. Weiss suggests that the conflicts between nurses and physicians are due to the overlapping nature of their domains and the lack of clarification between their roles. Adding to the difficulty of achieving agreement, doctors and nurses use different methods of conflict resolution. When resolving differences, physicians tend to bargain or negotiate while nurses avoid, accommodate, or compete.
>
> Collaboration . . . involves a high level of concern for others (cooperativeness), as well as a high concern for self (assertiveness). . . . Dechairo . . . found that self-confidence was a predictor of nurse case manager satisfaction with nurse/physician collaboration.
>
> The Thomas and Kilman model of conflict resolution is one of problem solving, and it is useful in complex situations where parties have common interests and the stakes are high. Inherent in this model is the assumption that conflict resolution [and mediation tools] can be taught and that effective collaboration will be the outcome. Using this model, willing participants can overcome the handicaps of a history of competition and style of avoidance or dominance. (Dechairo-Marino, Jordan-Marsh, Traiger, & Saulo, 2001, p. 225)

Sometimes collaboration does not happen even though it would have been a better approach. For instance, some use *competition,* thinking it is all important to win, regardless of the cost. Eventually, everyone loses in this situation, even the person who wins. Another approach that is not as effective is *compromise,* where each person gives up something but agrees on the best alternative. Even worse, one could *accommodate,* where one concedes to others, letting them get their way. The most ineffective approach is to *avoid situations* and not take any action.

Collaboration is most effective. When individuals collaborate, they work together to come up with a mutually acceptable solution. Although this takes more time, no one loses. This results in higher nurse satisfaction and better patient outcomes (Houser, Ricker, ErkenBrack, Stroup, & Handberry, 2012).

Collegiality, or collaboration between nurses and physicians, when effective, affects patient outcomes. Kramer and Schmalenberg (2003) cite lower mortality rates in intensive care units when collaboration is achieved. In their research, they came up with a five-category scale describing nurse–physician relationships:

Category 1: Collegial. Described as excellent, the essential ingredient in these relationships is equality based on "different but equal" power and knowledge.

Category 2: Collaborative. In these "good" or "great" relationships, staff work together very well. Nurses describe mutuality but not equality of power.

Category 3: Student–Teacher. Physicians are willing to discuss, explain, and teach. Power is unequal, but outcomes are beneficial. Either nurse or physician acts as the teacher.

Category 4: Neutral. A near absence of feeling marks this relationship. Often, there's only information exchange. But physicians frequently fail to acknowledge receiving the information, which leaves the nurses feeling they aren't contributing much.

Category 5: Negative. Frustration, hostility, and resignation characterize this relationship. Power is unequal and outcomes are negative because of their reactions to power plays. (pp. 36–37)

From this research, they suggest it is important to plant and nurture the "equal but different" seed: Create a culture that values, expects, and rewards collegial nurse–physician relationships and fosters, supports, and encourages education programs of all types (so that all stay clinically competent). This collegiality improves with ongoing relationships over time.

The Magnet approach supports this equal but different seed. Forces of Magnetism Force 13: Interdisciplinary Relationships states:

Collaborative working relationships within and among the disciplines are valued. Mutual respect is based on the premise that all members of the health care team make essential and meaningful contributions in the achievement of clinical outcomes. Conflict management strategies are in place and are used effectively, when indicated. (ANCC, 2013b)

Magnet Force 12: Image of Nursing discusses the importance of respect for nurses:

The services provided by nurses are characterized as essential by other members of the health care team. Nurses are viewed as integral to the health care organization's ability to provide patient care. Nursing effectively influences system-wide processes. (ANCC, 2013b)

Collaboration is a competency (Hill, 2006). When we have a competent organization, collaboration occurs everywhere—millions of times—as work gets done. It is messy. It is something that each person in the organization understands and works to achieve.

Collaboration among disciplines, particularly among medical staff members, is one of the most challenging and often daunting tasks for the nurse leader. In today's pay-for-performance environment, collaboration between disciplines, particularly medicine, nursing, nutrition services, respiratory, radiology, and pharmacy, is essential to produce top-tier performance and, thus, optimal patient outcomes. (Hill, 2006, p. 390).

Collaboration occurs when we realize that we need to be true to ourselves and to others equally. Conflicts arise because we do not recognize that another person's perspective is different from ours. Neither perspective is wrong—each is just different from the other. Fisher and associates (1991) found that it is best to "separate the people from the problem; focus on interests, not positions; generate a variety of possibilities before deciding what to do; and insist that the result be based on some objective standard" (p. 11). It is always best to base this on giving the patient what is valued.

A must-read book, *Peace and Power: New Directions for Building Community,* by Chinn (2013), provides ways to facilitate collaboration.

> When your group uses Peace and Power to its fullest extent, you do not have a structure of elected officers in the same way that many groups do. Instead, leaders emerge based on the needs of the group at any one time, and needs and leaders can shift at any time.
>
> For example, group meetings are led by a convener, and the responsibility to convene a meeting shifts in a rotation that is agreed upon by the group. The more the group values everyone learning to be a leader, the more often they will rotate convening to make sure that every member of the group gains this important skill.
>
> When a task requires specific knowledge, people in the group who have the knowledge or experience to do the task assume responsibility for it initially, but they gradually orient others to the task so that others can learn and assume the responsibility. . . . [This includes finances.]
>
> When your group needs to make a decision, you can take "straw votes" to get a sense of the whole, but your decisions are made using a process of value-based decision making. This is similar to what is commonly understood as "consensus," but differs dramatically in that rather than getting everyone to agree, you make sure that everyone appreciates why one option is better than others. And most important, this process ensures that everyone is able to fully support the decision of the group even if it is not their personal preference. (p. 44)

Chinn's approach to collaboration supports the quantum view of complexity and chaos. We are all interconnected, and we all have responsibility to work together effectively so we can best give the patient what the patient values. This results in, and continues to result in, a positive environment as well as positive outcomes. Conflict happens. Diversity is present. The environment is chaotic and complex. As collaboration transpires, the ultimate value question is, *What does the patient value and need?* Members of the group *may not agree with the patient's decisions,* yet these decisions *are the all-important basis and goal* of interdisciplinary groups involved in the collaborative process.

> Peace and Power decision-building focuses on the quality of the process that you use to get there, and in the end ensures the best possible decision that everyone understands. It also ensures that what you do is the same as what you value.
>
> Peace and Power decision-building combines individual preferences (as in voting), hearing all points of view (as in consensus), and brainstorming all possibilities (as in creative problem solving). In addition, Peace and Power decision-building incorporates processes of values clarification, conflict mediation, and critical thinking.
>
> Peace and Power decision-building is always grounded in your group's purpose [what the patient values], and is built consciously to be consistent with the group's values—your principles of solidarity. At the same time, decision-making processes contribute to clarifying and revising your group's purposes and your principles of solidarity.
>
> A common concern when you first consider Peace and Power decision-building is that the process will be time consuming and inefficient. It sometimes does take more time to reach a decision using Peace and Power decision-building. However, groups that shift to this approach almost never have to retrace their decision, nor do they have to spend time later making sure that everyone is on the same page. It is not possible to determine the time and effort saved when everyone understands and supports the decision while you are making the decision. But to take shortcuts in building a decision is a sure setup for wasted time and frustration later. The overall benefits of cohesiveness, acting in accord rather than at cross-purposes, and mutual understanding more than compensate for the time invested in reaching a decision using Peace and Power. (Chinn, 2013, p. 70)

The Peace and Power approach to making decisions can be found in **Exhibit 3–2**. This may seem very simple, but it captures the complexity and keeps everyone interconnected at the same time. The first step, *Define the Question*, also seems simple. Yet, does everyone truly know what the patient values—not what we *think* the patient values, but what he or she actually wants? This means that we have to involve the patient and the family in this process and get their perspective(s). We have to *listen* and actually hear what is important to them. It often is not what we think but instead is their perspective(s). It can be complicated in that the family may want something different from what the patient wants, so, in such cases, the patient may need some support in dealing with the family.

The second step, *Identify Your Key Principles of Solidarity*, also can seem deceptively simple. The group needs to first identify the basic value(s) they will work by, and support those values. "*Principles of solidarity* express the values and ideals that everyone in the group shares. They form your common ground that you intend to remain constant regardless of whatever happens in the group" (Chinn, 2013, p. 31). After finding what the patient values, it is important to think about resources that will be necessary to supply this. "The group may come to realize that they need to stretch the limits of what might be possible beyond the constraints of the budget as they now see it in order to achieve certain goals that they also value highly" (p. 72). But it always comes back to the basic value(s) identified, and agreed upon, by the group.

The third step, *List the Benefits You Seek*, "describe[s] the benefits that your group envisions for any decision that arises from this process" (Chinn, 2013, p. 72). However, the benefits need to support the underlying value(s).

> In typical decision-making, people who favor a certain decision use benefits that can come from the decision they prefer as a way to convince the group to go along with what they want. When you use Peace and Power, you identify the benefits you want from any decision *in advance* of considering possible options. Then when you know what the options are, you compare how each one measures in bringing the benefits your group seeks. (p. 73)

The fourth step, *Brainstorm the Options*, then follows. Here, everyone thinks of as many options as possible. The sky is the limit. Even when something seems impossible or ludicrous, it is brought to the table and listed as an option.

In the fifth step, *Gather Information You Need and Compare the Options*, the group revisits each option and gathers as much information as possible about it. A group member may have the expertise needed in a specific area, or the group may need to go to someone else for consultation and expertise. Gathering information can involve going into the community to find knowledge.

Exhibit 3–2   Approach to Making Decisions

1. *Define the Question*
2. *Identify Your Key Principles of Solidarity*
3. *List the Benefits You Seek*
4. *Brainstorm the Options*
5. *Gather Information You Need and Compare the Options*
6. *Make Your Decision*

Source: Data from Chinn, P. (2013). *Peace and Power: New Directions for Building Community*, 8th ed. Burlington, MA: Jones & Bartlett Learning.

> If at any time the group wants to know how many people prefer one option over others, pause to take a straw vote that gives everyone information about where people stand on the issue at this point in time. Votes are not taken to decide an issue, but rather to inform the deliberation. After the group votes, take the time to have people speak to why they favor one option over others.
>
> As you reach a point where you have considered many possibilities and you have before you all the information you can gather, begin to weigh the most viable options seriously against the benefits you set forth early in the process. Narrow the possibilities to those options that are most congruent with these benefits. (p. 73)

The last step is *Make Your Decision*. When everyone is in agreement about an option that seems best, the decision is made. But often everyone is not in agreement.

> If this is the case, take a deep breath and decide how urgent this decision is. If it is truly not urgent, or if you can make an interim decision, the group leaves the matter open and places it on the agenda for the next gathering.
>
> If the decision is urgent, then your group must focus on the necessity of reaching a decision that everyone can live with for now, and plan for more discussion of the issues involved. Even in this circumstance, the more that the group is able to identify the values upon which the decision is built and select the option that best expresses your values, the more satisfactory the decision will be in the long run. (Chinn, 2013, pp. 73–74)

This process is so valuable and results in much better patient outcomes and staff satisfaction. Each person and his or her knowledge, experience, and perspectives are given significance. If anyone disagrees, that person is encouraged to express his or her views. Dissenting views are valued, which means that people need to be within an environment where this perspective is encouraged. This decision-making process must be accepted and supported by each person in the group as the best method to use.

In the Information Age, collaboration must happen in different ways. Richards (2001) suggests that "collaborative practice involves a community of electronically connected practitioners providing a richer and more scientific foundation for practice" (p. 6). Chinn's method can also occur using technology. It is best if people can actually see each other as they interact.

Erickson and colleagues (2012) advocate creating a new role: attending registered nurse. This person coordinates the work of the interdisciplinary team in addressing overuse, underuse, and misuse of services.

In the hospital setting, Hill (2006) recommends that it is particularly positive when both a physician and a nurse can provide leadership for the interdisciplinary process on a unit, with the goal of giving patients what they value. Hill discusses how each profession can be more effective with each other and the team by using executive coaches who facilitate discussions between physicians and nurses "to verify the importance of accountability within the organization and to explore the notion of shared and independent domains of practice" (p. 391). Coaching can also help each discipline deal with the politics involved and, in such cases, help them (1) develop a joint strategy before meetings, and (2) deal with issues that come up in large meetings.

One nurse executive stated:

> I have found that the best decisions are supported through the informal communications before and after the meeting, where issues and political landmines can be more informally addressed and where a constituent can influence the outcome of a process or decision before it is presented. (Hill, 2006, p. 391)

It was important for nurse executives to mentor others in their profession so that they can more effectively work together.

This nurse executive recommended the following:

(1) be inclusive in groups; (2) be transparent in your ideas. Often, the best ideas come from an open discussion on the issues. Leaders need to be open to input from multiple perspectives; (3) attainment of doctoral education created a level field for credibility with physicians as peers; (4) participate in a 360-degree evaluation so one is aware of one's own "blind spots"; (5) be explicit about what you want. (Hill, 2006, p. 392)

Collaboration is most effective with different professionals in an organization. We are educated differently from each other. We do not use the same terminology. Plus, we are all learning how to move away from the old frameworks when what the physician wanted was key. Now, we are on a more even playing field, although this is not always recognized. Our challenge is to work out ways to collaborate more effectively with each other, valuing each other's contributions.

Interprofessional collaboration is essential to deliver unified, cohesive, patient care; yet our work in evidence-based practice is often profession-specific, without exchange of theories, models, or tools in a unified approach focusing on a specific patient outcome. Efforts of each individual profession are grounded in specific knowledge, value, and belief systems, with resulting variations in forms of and values for specific types of evidence. Social boundaries result in poor diffusion across professions. This status quo is intolerable if we are to advance the quality of care for patients in all settings. (Newhouse, 2008, p. 414)

Bleich and associates (2009) recommend that we restructure some of the common meetings, such as staff meetings, patient huddles, and rounds, to include other departments and services. We also need to create more feedback loops among staff, patients, families, and other caregivers, examining clinical problems in context.

With these new decision-making models at the point of service, team effectiveness or relationship building is enhanced when *collaboration* occurs. When we collaborate, we are working with others to achieve shared goals. We are proactive; that is, a person does not just complain about problems but thinks of ways to solve them. We cooperate and share knowledge with each other. There is an element of shared meaning within the group. We create group synergy in the pursuit of collective goals. We make sacrifices to achieve the group goals. Group energy is harnessed. Different views are encouraged and it is safe to express these views.

Work Teams

Work teams help us to better achieve what the patient values in a second-curve environment. Work teams are necessary because we are all interconnected and interdependent with one another. Although many times patients are not included in team efforts, the team is most effective when the patient is a valued member. Work teams may include just nursing staff and patients, but it is best when work teams are interdisciplinary to achieve what each patient values.

Very few people work by themselves and achieve results by themselves. . . . Most people work with others and are effective with other people. . . . Managing yourself requires taking responsibility for relationships. This has two parts. The first is to accept the fact that other people are as much individuals as you yourself are. They perversely insist on behaving like human beings. This means that they too have their strengths; they too have their ways of getting things done; they too have their values. To be effective, therefore, you have to know the strengths, the performance modes, and the values of your coworkers. . . . Each [coworker] works his or her way, not your way. And each is entitled to work in his or her way. What matters is whether they perform and what their values are. . . . The first secret of effectiveness is to understand the people you work with and depend on so that you can make use of their strengths, their ways of working, and their values. Working relationships are as much based on the people as they are on the work.

The second part of relationship responsibility is taking responsibility for communication. . . . Personality conflicts . . . arise from the fact that people do not know what other people are doing and how they do their work, or what contribution the other people are concentrating on and what results they expect. And the reason they do not know is that they have not been asked and therefore have not been told. . . . Even people who understand the importance of taking responsibility for relationships often do not communicate sufficiently with their associates. They are afraid of being thought presumptuous or inquisitive or stupid. They are wrong. Whenever someone goes to his or her associates and says, "This is what I am good at. This is how I work. These are my values. This is the contribution I plan to concentrate on and the results I should be expected to deliver," the response is always, "This is most helpful. But why didn't you tell me earlier?" [It is important for the leader to ask,] "What do I need to know about your strengths, how you perform, your values, and your proposed contribution?" . . . Trust . . . means that they understand one another. (Drucker, 1999, pp. 71–72)

Does this sound familiar? It is what we explored in the chaos/complexity section of this chapter. We are all interconnected and interdependent with one another. Yet each person has different perspectives and different ways of going about work that can cause conflict. This conflict, if recognized, can be used to foster a better understanding of each other's perspectives and can help to lead us to make needed changes. It is very valuable information. If we pay attention to this, patients are more likely to receive what they value.

The team involves all stakeholders who communicate with each other and who are committed to solving problems. If possible, it is best if all involved can remain unattached to current paradigms. The ultimate goal is providing what will better achieve what patients value. The team needs to build consensus around goals, realizing that changing one component of a system generally affects another part of the system. All of this needs to be coordinated. This is why making small, incremental changes is a good way to fix a problem. Then, if something that is tried only creates more problems, it can be changed or stopped until another process can facilitate the change successfully.

Systems dynamics is now an important concept for all in an organization to understand. In complexity science, we recognize that a large number of people/objects have many connections in different spaces and at different times. This approach is "used to model processes over time. [It] focuses on the information-feedback characteristics of a process or activity" (Clancy, 2009a, p. 251). The author explains complexity by using a social network example where physician consultation referral patterns are examined as one way to decrease length of stay.

Benham-Hutchins and Clancy (2010) further explain social network analysis.

Social network analysis is a set of methods and analytical concepts that focuses on the structure and pattern of relations in a social network. Social network analysis is beneficial in workflow analysis because it can uncover explanatory factors or variables that influence individual and group behavior. (Clancy, 2009a, p. 251)

"Effective teamwork depends on leadership clarity, role clarity, shared goals, and frequent communication" (MacPhee, 2007, p. 407). "Leadership is a catalyst for teamwork" (Castner, Schwartz, Foltz-Ramos, & Cervolo, 2012, p. 470). The catalyst is not only the nurse manager, but we must include the charge nurse. Leaders "must encourage participation, mobilization, and innovation" (Smith, 2012, p. 46). Evidence shows that ambiguous leadership roles and responsibilities result in low levels of team support for innovation. We do not always discuss the importance of teams with staff, let alone have expectations that each worker is an effective team member. Evidence shows that when team roles and expectations are not clarified, there is more conflict and outcomes/reimbursements plummet.

To gauge how effective a team is, MacPhee (2007, p. 410) recommends the following checklist for assessment:

Communications
1. Is there sufficient vertical (formal) team communication?
2. Is there sufficient horizontal (informal) team communication?

Coordination and mutual support
3. Are individual efforts assimilated into team efforts?
4. Do team members help and support each other to achieve team goals?

Contributions
5. Is each team member maximizing his or her contributions?
6. Is the team taking full advantage of each member's expertise?
7. Is the team acknowledging the contributions of its members in an equitable or balanced fashion?

Cohesion
8. Are there team spirit and a collective identity?
9. Are team members focused and motivated to achieve the team goals?

"An important personality trait of people who enjoy working with others and who are team players is agreeableness, which helps form social cohesion" (MacPhee, 2007, p. 407). Nurse managers can expect and mentor these behaviors, and these behaviors can be specified in performance evaluations.

Each team member brings certain gifts to the team that, when valued, are instrumental in achieving team effectiveness. Gifts can be clinical expertise, or certain people work better with certain kinds of patients. Gifts also include team roles. A few will be innovators.

> Innovators (about 2.5% of a group) are well connected to outside knowledge sources and recognize innovation opportunities, such as cutting-edge technologies and best-practice approaches. Innovators, however, are not always well connected within their organization. Their ideas need to be championed by the "early adopters" or opinion leaders, who comprise about 13.5% of a group. These transformational leaders inspire others to follow the new idea, and they have the power to make things happen. Although they have earned the trust of others, not everybody will immediately follow them. Their immediate audience consists of the "early majority," another 34% of the group. These followers are comfortable taking a new idea, adopting it to their local environment, and conducting small-scale pilots. Their successes pave the way for more innovation diffusion. The "late majority" followers, another 34% of the group, watch and see what happens among the early majority. They change when successful outcomes are more certain. The last 16% consists of "traditionalists." These individuals are rooted in habits and routines; "We've always done it this way." They eventually convert, but not until the innovation has become the new status quo. There needs to be a 15% to 20% critical mass of innovators, adopters, and early majority personalities to tip the scale toward innovative change. (MacPhee, 2007, p. 407)

The best way to achieve *innovation* within a team is to have a diverse team mix. Low-diversity group members are homogenous. They tend to keep on with the status quo. However, if diversity is too high, members often cannot develop shared goals and objectives. "The right mix consists of people with diverse but overlapping knowledge domains and skills" (MacPhee, 2007, p. 407). This is why a group of nurses needs other professionals (physicians, therapists, pharmacists, dietitians, etc.) on the work team and vice versa.

Educational programs can teach about role clarity, the importance of functioning as a team member (both with unit staff and with other disciplines), and teamwork expectations. Providing practice opportunities is important.

Frequent communication is needed because we don't know what each patient values until we talk with that person. If all on the team share what they find, the patient is more likely to receive what he or she values. This process of communication has different nuances for each patient situation.

Communication is complicated by needing to continually improve the care given. Current evidence specifies changes in the way we actually perform care. For instance, Shermont and colleagues (2008) suggest the importance of 10-minute huddles in the middle of a shift, for example, when suddenly several nurses have fallen behind, a patient takes a turn for the worse, another patient needs to be taken for an emergency magnetic resonance imaging scan, and the charge nurse finds out there will be another admission. By calling a huddle, the charge nurse, along with the rest of the nursing staff, can quickly get updated on what is happening and make more effective decisions on who will do what.

The huddle is a good example because, while the team is dealing with the patient situations, they need to be aware of the strategic plan goals and achieve pay-for-performance goals. This is further complicated because change is always occurring. Thus, each member of the team must help identify incremental changes that are necessary to better achieve what patients value. And this needs to be communicated to the rest of the team.

Another issue with teams can involve *delegation*. For instance, when care omissions occur (with ambulation, turning, delayed or missed feedings, patient teaching, discharge planning, emotional support, hygiene, intake and output documentation, and surveillance), evidence showed that nurses inconsistently or inappropriately delegated tasks to nursing assistants (NAs). This is a messy problem because reasons for these occurrences often are intertwined. There is

> inconsistency in the nature of the tasks delegated, a possible knowledge deficit in expectations by the nurse regarding the capability and functioning of NA, tension in the nurse and NA relationship, role confusion between practitioners, poor communication, and insufficient system support. (Bittner, Gravlin, Hansten, & Kalisch, 2011, p. 510)

To fix this problem, nurses and NAs may need to learn better communication techniques. Promoting positive relationships can also be helpful. Positive relationships occur when a team regularly works together and team members develop trust so that when things get busy good teamwork happens and the care continues to be delivered.

The delegation problem is affected by other factors—workload and NA competence. When nurses (and NAs—although this has been reported less frequently) are overwhelmed, even if for only part of a shift, they may not have time to make sure all the necessary care is occurring. Evidence also shows that NAs can become complacent about performing care, and nurses need to be more vigilant in making sure the care is given. This type of situation is often complex with intertwined causes.

Having *continual team dialogue* helps to determine what is happening and how best to deal with these changes. Each member brings small changes he or she is experiencing, and by having continual dialogue with other team members and communicating these changes, the team comes closer to achieving what the patient values. In addition, the workplace is a better environment for employees and physicians. Everyone wins.

We must realize that when team dialogue is working well, it is messy, but the energy is positive. Something is always happening, and something is always changing. It is worth experiencing this messiness because of the outcome achieved with the patient.

Group energy can increase or decrease what is accomplished. When teamwork is excellent, outcomes are very positive. Magic happens. We advocate that self-managed teams be used as much as possible because *90% of the decisions need to be made at the point of service.*

There are several reasons why using the team approach to decision making is advantageous in organizations. First, the knowledge and skills that each individual brings to the group create synergy. Second, an increase in creativity occurs, often as a result of the diversity of multidisciplinary teams and the different worldviews that each team member brings to the group. The whole is greater than the sum of the parts. *Most organizations experience a 20% to 40% increase in productivity when employees are deeply involved in their work* (Porter-O'Grady & Malloch, 2011, p. 341).

Teamwork is not as effective as it can be unless the leaders share power and foster interdependence. To be most effective teams need to have shared goals and, of course, support the core values.

Efforts to improve teamwork have positive effects. Kalisch and associates (2007) used a team enhancement and engagement intervention (that unit staff chose) to achieve a lower patient fall rate and lower turnover and vacancy rates. Staff reported better teamwork. Hall and colleagues (2008) designed a workplace intervention to improve resource availability on patient care units. "After participation in the intervention, nurses in this study reported higher perceptions of their work and work environment" (pp. 43–44).

Sometimes trained group facilitators are needed to help team members achieve better working relationships and more effective teamwork. Once the team functions effectively, the group facilitator may no longer be needed. Further education of team members and facilitation of their work can save countless hours of wasted time and advance the team toward successful completion of the goal.

According to Wellins, Byham, and Wilson (1991), there are six key factors in team development: commitment, trust, purpose, communication, involvement, and process orientation. All of these occur as a team evolves. In the first stage of team development, *getting started*, the purpose, or goal, of the group needs to be clearly defined, and all members need to get acquainted with it.

In the second stage, *going in circles,* team members know who they are and where they are going and need to decide how to get there. They often feel an urge to pull out of the team to work alone or to work in subgroups. Members sort out whom they do and do not trust and those they are unsure of at this point. The team has a better understanding of its purpose but still requires reassurance and guidance. Often, much time is spent on describing how meetings will be conducted, setting agendas, and setting up ground rules with task completion as the goal.

In this stage, conflict begins to arise, especially if certain members attempt to dominate the team. This conflict is disturbing to members who want the team to succeed. It is important for the team to keep returning to the group goal. Power moves tend to decline as more effective group process develops, feedback occurs, and members begin to identify specific gifts each member brings. However, if this does not occur, the team will be stuck and probably not accomplish the original purpose.

The third stage of team development, *getting on course*, is focused on achieving the goal. Team members are more comfortable with each other, more comfortable with their roles in the group, and are committed to getting the job done. The group process is more natural because members understand the team's purpose, are beginning to know and appreciate each other, and can begin to explore solutions different from the status quo.

The final stage, *full speed ahead*, is when teams are more comfortable with the benefits of being empowered. They are committed to both the team and the organization at this stage. Trust is a stable commodity and extended openly. A clear sense of mission and vision is maintained, and the team becomes more flexible. Changes in meeting frequency and communication occur at this level. Members are constantly involved and accept new roles and responsibilities. The team focuses on quality and continuous improvement.

Porter-O'Grady and Malloch (2011) have divided this stage into three substages: competent, proficient, and expert. At the *competent* stage, team members want to hear each other's concerns and ideas and integrate this information into a cohesive group collective. The members have established an effective set of ground rules. They may mentor and coach each other for increased effectiveness. They may find solutions that challenge the status quo.

> Teams at the competent stage can meet the requirements for standard success but find it impossible to become passionately optimistic while recreating the future or to maintain resilience in the face of negative events. They accomplish the assigned work but seldom move beyond the assigned boundaries. (p. 348)

At the *proficient* stage, team members are more likely to have a total organizational assessment, be passionately optimistic, be aware of individual differences, and can arrive at consensus decisions, not just saying that the majority rules. They honestly recognize team member limitations and give emotional support to help the person deal with personal failings. They consider the emotional components of the conflicts and work through them, supporting both the emotions and the actual work that needs to be accomplished. Relationships stay intact and are based on honesty.

At the *expert* stage, all the healthy internal group work occurs, and the group recognizes the organizational issues and culture making sure that the proposed solutions fit within the existing organizational components. The group is proactive and affirmative, recognizing and dealing effectively with each member's emotional needs and undercurrents and arriving at effective solutions for the individuals, the group, and the organization. At times, this could extend to the community as well.

Teams develop over time and progress through the stages of team development at different rates, depending on internal and external influences. In fact, if team membership changes or goals are not well defined or change, the group may revert to a previous stage or may never resolve the ensuing conflicts, thus never achieving the goal.

Team development is not a linear process. Often teams are composed of very diverse members with a variety of values and backgrounds. Some members may be into negative, selfish behaviors. The team will probably fail unless it can reach such individuals and pull them into the team or these individuals are effectively dealt with, asked to leave the team, or asked to leave the organization. Team development takes time, patience, and effort.

In *The Five Dysfunctions of a Team,* Lencioni (2002a) identifies other issues that surface. The book is written as a novel, presents some individual issues that can lead a team astray, and presents how to fix the problems. The five dysfunctions are invulnerability (absence of trust), artificial harmony (fear of conflict), ambiguity (lack of commitment), low standards (avoidance of accountability), and status and ego (inattention to results). These barriers create tremendous costs to the organization. First, there is the cost of everyone's salaries that are wasted, but there are many larger costs: This lack of teamwork will occur in other work areas, unresolved conflicts will resurface, administration will be viewed as ineffective, patient care and patient outcomes/reimbursements will suffer, physicians will prefer to be somewhere else, and legal issues will result. The higher the level of dysfunction, the more it permeates the entire organization.

As conflicts occur, if the team is able to resolve the conflict without decimating members and use the situation as an opportunity for learning, the team is more likely to make good progress with group development. They begin to develop a group identity and a feeling that they are making a difference. The *spirit* increases because of each person's involvement and commitment to the goals of the group. The team can become *self-actualized and believe they can make things happen.*

> Self-actualized teams . . . use the whole potential of each team member to remain incredibly focused on "their" work, and they use skepticism in a healthy and productive way. They are willing to live at the border and do not eliminate ideas, no matter how outrageous. All ideas are reviewed with the typical constraints

of finance, practicality, time, and ethics. More importantly, self-actualized teams effectively deal with members who are congenital victims and continually tell us that this and that will not work now because it didn't work in 1947. Self-actualized teams regulate behavior and focus it toward innovation and away from the troubles of the day. They are able to be in the moment and image the future simultaneously, rearranging existing patterns into new and innovative strategies that will solve problems. (Crow, 2003, p. 35)

The leader is only as effective as the team, and the team only as effective as the leader. Part of leadership effectiveness is recognizing the individual differences in team members:

Some people work best as team members. Others work best alone. Some are exceptionally talented as coaches and mentors; others are simply incompetent as mentors. . . . A great many people perform best as advisers but cannot take the burden and pressure of making the decision. A good many other people, by contrast, need an adviser to force themselves to think; then they can make decisions and act on them with speed, self-confidence, and courage. This is the reason, by the way, that the number two person in an organization often fails when promoted to the number one position. The top spot requires a decision maker. Strong decision makers often put somebody they trust into the number two spot as their adviser—and in that position the person is outstanding. But in the number one spot, the same person fails. He or she knows what the decision should be but cannot accept the responsibility of actually making it. (Drucker, 1999, pp. 68–69)

Magnet Force 8: Consultation and Resources discusses the importance of having experts available for staff. This is a critical component of organizational competence:

The health care organization provides adequate resources, support and opportunities for the utilization of experts, particularly advanced practice nurses. The organization promotes involvement of nurses in professional organizations and among peers in the community.

Shared Governance: A Collaborative Model

Interdisciplinary shared governance is a necessity in the value-based environment. If it does not exist in the organization, it is important to at least start with nursing shared governance. Remember that in the second-curve environment, administrators serve the leaders who are at the point of care, and it is those leaders who need to make 90% of the decisions about their work environment.

Shared governance (**Exhibit 3–3**) is a structural team framework that affords nursing professional autonomy at the point of care (Brody, Ruble, Barnes, & Sakowski, 2012; Church, Baker, & Berry, 2008; Dunbar, Park, Berger-Wesley, & Cameron, 2007; Gokenbach, 2007; Johnson et al., 2012; Kear, Duncan, Fansler, & Hunt, 2012; Moore & Hutchison, 2007; Moore & Wells, 2010; Nolan, Laam, Wary, Hallick, & King, 2011). This is where staff members make decisions about their work. "Shared governance is not a democracy. It is an accountability-based approach to structure in which there is a clear expectation that all members of a system participate in its work" (Porter-O'Grady, 2009, p. 45). Costs and time allotments for staff to participate in shared governance are spelled out by Rundquist and Givens (2013).

Shared governance isn't an end-point but a journey with continual "mile markers." It is based on two expectations: First, previous governance will be redistributed from managers to staff following implementation of shared governance. (So administrators need to release control and transition previous authority roles into educator, advocate, and coach roles.) Second, nurses want to be active participants in decision making. (So staff need to learn how to work out practice issues—not just have gripe sessions—yet still have a relationship with the administrators). (Church et al., 2008, pp. 36–38)

Outcomes are better with shared governance. This includes higher RN satisfaction scores, higher patient satisfaction scores, lower mortality and healthcare-acquired infection rates, and lower RN turnover and vacancy rates (Church et al., 2008).

Exhibit 3–3   Principles of Shared Governance

Partnership
- Role expectations are negotiated.
- Equality exists between the players.
- Relationships are founded upon shared risk.
- Expectations and contributions are clear.
- Solid measure of contribution to outcomes is established.
- Horizontal linkages are well defined.

Equity
- Each player's contribution is understood.
- Payment reflects value of contribution to outcomes.
- Role is based on relationship, not status.
- Team defines service roles, relationships, and outcomes.
- Methodology is defined for team conflict and service issues.
- Evaluation assesses team's outcomes and contributions.

Accountability
- Accountability is internally defined by person in the role.
- Accountability defines roles, not jobs.
- Accountability is based on outcomes, not process.
- Accountability is defined in advance of performance.
- Accountability leads to desired and defined results.
- Performance is validated by the results achieved.
- Processes are generally loud and noisy.

Ownership
- All workers are invested in the enterprise.
- Every role has a stake in the outcome.
- Rewards are directly related to outcomes.
- All members are associated with a team.
- Processes support relationships.
- Opportunity is based on competence.

Source: Porter-O'Grady, T. (2009). *Interdisciplinary shared governance: Integrating practice, transforming health care.* Sudbury, MA: Jones and Bartlett.

Shared governance operates in a true *environment of empowerment*. Empowerment does not even happen until a leader is at least at stage 4 of Hagberg's power model (Hagberg, 2003). With shared governance, staff and leaders are empowered to contribute collectively to the decision-making process related to clinical practice, standards, and procedures. Shared governance also provides the organization with a mechanism to make decisions that improve patient care and the workplace environment. For example, nurses know how processes can be improved, so the nurses who deliver the care can directly make the decisions to do so.

Shared governance benefits an organization because staff members (all staff members, not just nurses) are involved in the design of their work. Authoritarian environments are not effective. If there is an ideal time for shared governance and true empowerment, it is now. This is the only way to achieve positive patient outcomes and better reimbursement and, for that matter, organizational longevity.

Creating an empowering environment is hard work, meaning that *decision making is increased at the point of service*. It takes constant effort. It can be painful. It means staff should be making 90% of the decisions and may choose directions that never occurred to us. Staff need to be involved in the decision making with hiring, budgeting, allocating, discipline, and policy. An empowering environment is time consuming to maintain, but the time taken is well worth the outcomes achieved. As staff become used to working effectively with shared governance, the process becomes more automatic and takes less time.

Not all shared governance efforts are successful. Ballard (2010) discusses factors that lead to success and failure:

> Successful ventures happen when there is successful communication of a vision by senior nursing leaders, along with support of managers. It is helpful if both these groups along with staff nurses plan together, and continue this process as the governance model gets off the ground. One issue is that some managers have difficulty giving up authority patterns, rather than becoming a coach/mentor. Managers need a lot of mentoring before implementation can be successful. Another barrier to success can be staff apathy. It is better to start with staff that really believe in it, and then mentor them for the new role. This may involve their learning how to read and interpret various data reports, how to run meetings, set agendas, "shepherd" discussion, and reach consensus. It is important to be clear on boundaries— what kinds of decisions can be made by the group, other types of decisions will be recommendations to administrators or other departments, and certain organizational boundaries cannot be changed. Gradual transition is helpful using transition teams. Then it is trial and error. As they begin to function they need to learn how to substantiate need for changes, the timing of requests, and how to initiate changes. For first efforts it is probably best to do so with 3 guidelines: 1) must be congruent with hospital policies and procedures; 2) proposed changes must improve patient care/quality outcomes/work environment; and 3) financial outcome must be budget neutral or justified. Staff must have support to attend meetings; also, attendance is an expectation from the administrative team. (pp. 411–415)

Today, many nurse managers feel overwhelmed, especially when they are in environments where they are not empowered and not supported by supervisors. This leads to higher nurse manager (and nurse executive) turnover. So, in this chaotic time, it is time to support each other as we create this new reality.

In a *whole-systems shared governance model*, each member has equal power and responsibilities in the decision-making process, giving first priority to what the patient values. Porter-O'Grady (2009) advocates having an *operations council* (concerned with resources, linkage, planning, market strategy, implementation, and compliance), a *patient care council* (concerned with service delivery, system models, disciplines, service design, roles, quality, and process), and a *governance council* (concerned with mission, strategy, priorities, policy, and integration). Physicians have had a medical staff organization historically, but Porter-O'Grady advocates that

> many of the current separate functions of the medical staff will disappear as they become more integrated within the system. . . . The real struggle for physicians is seeing themselves as partners in the health system rather than the controllers of it. (pp. 264–265)

In this model, a shared governance steering group shares information and integrates decisions among the three councils. It is important that "every key role in the system, staff or management, should be represented in the steering group. The majority of planners, however, should be from the staff, not from management" (Porter-O'Grady, 2009, p. 80). "Integration is evidence of the attempt to configure services around the point of care and to bring providers together in a service partnership. . . . Compartmentalization is the death of integration" (p. 40).

To make all of this work effectively, caregivers who are at the point of service need access to accurate information, need to tune in to what the patient values, need administrative support from the top down to make these decisions, and need to feel accountable for their decisions. Shared governance structure ensures "that the decisions made there are correct, implementable, and do not require broad organizational approval or a long decision making process (which might reduce the efficiency and effectiveness of the clinical delivery system)" (Porter-O'Grady, 2009, pp. 77–78). It is a system based on accountability of staff who want to give their best effort to their work.

Professional Development

Keeping up with the latest clinical, educational, and administrative evidence requires time and commitment. Yet, this is a key necessity in a value-based environment.

Knowledge management "addresses how organizations leverage their knowledge or intellectual assets" (MacPhee, 2007, p. 408). There are three kinds of knowledge: "human knowledge or expertise, social knowledge or collective knowledge that develops as a result of people working together, and structured knowledge or the knowledge embedded in an organization's policies, procedures, and routines." (MacPhee, 2007, p. 408).

All are necessary for organizational competency. Sharing this knowledge is important.

Human knowledge includes the expertise of various employees of different disciplines. For instance, nursing work teams are enhanced when a nurse has expert knowledge as defined by Benner. Educational/orientation/mentoring programs usually exist to expand the expertise of employees. *Social knowledge* is about what happens in the organization as various teams work to provide care for patients, or do their work. Social networks exist, including who goes to lunch with whom. *Structured knowledge* is fairly standardized knowledge, which is shared and can be used repeatedly. Generally, this is codified data that can be stored in and retrieved from computer databases. Organizations tend to favor one of these three types of knowledge. If an organization emphasizes one strategy over the others, it will not be successful.

Often social knowledge is not as fully developed as it needs to be.

> Most healthcare organizations require viable social networks to effectively manage/share expertise and collective wisdom. Berwick describes the importance of "spannable social distance," where each person hears the news from someone socially familiar and credible to them. Networking opportunities among employees require organizational investment, such as meeting spaces and time away from work responsibilities to generate discussion.
>
> What are the outward signs of an organizational culture that supports social networking? Vertical interactions between different lines of authority are known for leaders' approachability and willingness to discuss all kinds of topics, even sensitive ones, openly and honestly. Horizontal interactions among individuals at the same organizational level support seeking out existing expertise versus "reinventing the wheel." High levels of interaction and collaborative problem solving are organizational norms. This is a high-trust organizational culture: Where trust exists among the organization, its leadership, and their followers. (MacPhee, 2007, p. 408)

The goals and objectives of the organization often give clues as to which knowledge strategy is favored. Organizations must learn to balance all three types of knowledge (another change).

The Magnet Recognition Program recognizes the importance of education of employees. Magnet Force 14: Professional Development follows:

> The health care organization values and supports the personal and professional growth and development of staff. In addition to quality orientation and in-service education addressed earlier in Force 11, Nurses as Teachers, emphasis is placed on career development services. Programs that promote formal education, professional certification, and career development are evident. Competency-based clinical and leadership/management development is promoted and adequate human and fiscal resources for all professional development programs are provided. (ANCC, 2013b)

Professional education is an important organizational strategy that enhances staff capabilities to better understand what is coming in the future. It helps everyone to stretch and grow. Every member of the organization—from housekeeping to board members—can benefit from additional learning opportunities. Generally, every staff member should experience learning opportunities both within and outside the organization. Because we learn differently—some by seeing, some by hearing, some by experiencing—we need to provide various opportunities that correspond to a person's learning style. And sometimes we learn best when we have to teach someone else. The sky is the limit here because there is an infinite number of possibilities.

Unfortunately, often the education budget gets cut. This is a major error. In the current environment, which is constantly changing, educational offerings provide effective strategies for remaining viable, as well as meeting generational needs. If no educational opportunities are available, this ignores the fact that we all need to do meaningful work and have opportunities to continue to grow. Scott (2002) makes the following observation:

> When learning and professional development are viewed only in terms of an optional opportunity for improvement—rather than as *a threat to your organization's survival if ignored*—the commitment to sustain successful change will be missing. Thus, look at professional development from two angles: what you and your team will gain if everyone worked differently, and what you and your team will lose by simply maintaining the status quo. Bottom line, will you achieve your strategic goals if you and your staff continue to lead the way you are leading today? (p. 17)

We have discussed the shifts that all of us need to be living in this new Information Age. Scott (2002) names 10:

> From a provider orientation to customer obsession; from silo thinking to an organizational perspective; from directing to coaching; from status quo to courage, risk, and change; from busyness to results; from telling to facilitating dialogue; from protecting turf to building relationships; from a function manager to a business leader; from the employee as expendable to the employee as precious; and from pressure and overwork to perspective and balance. (p. 18)

There are many more examples of needed shifts sprinkled throughout this text. The exciting thing is that there is so much more to learn, which is true of the nurse aide all the way to the board members.

Another educational aspect cannot be forgotten in organizations. By providing organizational learning opportunities for students, we are facilitating future potential or current employees' knowledge base. The magnet program recognizes the importance of providing organizational opportunities for students. Magnet Force 11: Nurses as Teachers states:

> Professional nurses are involved in educational activities within the organization and community. Students from a variety of academic programs are welcomed and supported in the organization; contractual arrangements are mutually beneficial. (ANCC, 2013b)

It is important to have a development and mentoring program for providing staff preceptors for levels of students (students, new graduates, experienced nurses, and so forth. In all positions, staff serve as faculty and preceptors for students from a variety of academic programs. There is a patient education program that meets the diverse needs of patients in all of the care settings of the organization.

Organizational Competence

Now we turn to organizational competence in the (second-curve) value-based environment. In fact, there are *organizational competencies* that are necessary for survival (Gibson, 2011):

> A competent institution is characterized by individual and collective knowledge, skills, and attitudes that enable an organization to operate effectively. In the context of patient safety, a competent organization is one whose structures and processes enable care that is safe, effective, patient centered, timely, efficient, and equitable. Nurses and all health care professionals function best when the systems in which they work are competent and enable them to provide high-quality care. It's time hospitals and other organizations are held accountable for being competent in quality and patient safety, when nurses and other health care professionals are being called upon to do the same. (p. 46)

Part of our administrative responsibility is to build a competent organization. *However, even if achieved, it is only at one point of time, and then, because life is dynamic, it will need to continue to change or become obsolete.* Because the world is ever changing, achieving and keeping organizational competency take constant work. The organization, like us, needs to keep on changing with the times to survive.

What is a competent healthcare organization? First, we need to make sure all are aware of, and support, the purpose and mission or values of the organization. If this is not the case, we need to pay attention because it is important that everyone's actions always support the purpose and values. This is hard but always supplies our direction.

Second, it is important to *stay current with the evidence and with all the changes taking place in our healthcare environment* (external environments). This means that all staff, including staff nurses, physicians, and administrators, stay updated and practice accordingly. Because it is important to stay current with the surrounding environments, make needed incremental changes hourly (to keep re-creating the potential reality) to stay viable. This includes paying attention to

> Providers (healthcare institutions), payers (federal, state, private, and managed care insurers), individuals (patients, physicians, nurses, support staff, and educators), and technology (the Internet, information systems, medical equipment, and pharmaceuticals). Collectively, the interactions of these parts converge and create the emergence of a dynamic, highly complex state space. . . . Eventually, the environment will favor those institutions that are creative, robust, adaptable, and able to solve an ever-changing set of problems. (Clancy, 2007a, p. 535)

Administrators must also update their views of reality. For instance, in school we were taught to pay attention to the competition (note that part of this word is *compete*), which is what we needed to do to stay viable. Business journals discuss the importance of the competition. However, the competition really is not important.

> Capitalism treats competition as fundamentally a personal exercise—a contest between oneself and others for profitability and success. What it does not always recognize is that whether success is achieved has less to do with one's competitors than with one's adaptability, creativity, energy, and commitment to succeed. In other words, the pursuit of success should not be viewed as a contest with others but as a personal effort to give one's best and to thrive in the environment one has chosen to live in. (Porter-O'Grady & Malloch, 2011, p. 31)

The issue is not what the competition is doing; the issue is survival. It is giving it our best effort. All of us need to change, but this starts at home. The key is *survival and adaptability.* This is why it is so important to pay attention to the internal and external environments and look to the evidence for clues as to what we need to do next (new potential realities) to survive. It is not competition but *innovation* that is needed so that we can thrive.

> All living systems seek to thrive. At a fundamental level, they are not concerned with each other's survival unless it is somehow related to their need to thrive. Adaptation is not about competition between the fittest but about survival of the fittest, and the survival of the system is more dependent on its inherent adaptability to its environment than on anything else. To thrive, the system must have beneficial interactions with its environment and must also have the capacity to adjust to the prevailing conditions quickly and effectively. A system is fundamentally in competition with *itself*, not with anyone or anything else. (Porter-O'Grady & Malloch, 2011, p. 32)

The AHA (2011) suggests seven competencies for healthcare organizations:

1. Design and implementation of patient-centered, integrated care
2. Creation of accountable governance and leadership
3. Strategic planning in an unstable environment

4. Internal and external collaboration
5. Financial stewardship and enterprise risk management
6. Engagement of employees' full potential
7. Collection and utilization of electronic data for performance improvement (p. 23)

The AHA accompanies these competencies with competency questions in each category.

For the nursing profession and nurse administrators, perhaps the Magnet/Excellence precepts for internal organizational competencies are the best defined. These precepts continue to evolve. (There is a pattern here: They continue to evolve, too, to keep up with potential reality.) We need to keep *improving our internal environment so that we can best achieve what patients value.*

Magnet/Excellence Precepts

Both the Magnet Recognition Program and the Pathway to Excellence Program provide wonderful resources for nurse administrators, *whether one has applied for Magnet status or not.* Evidence supports this. Ulrich and associates (2007) found in a national sample of 1,783 nurses that *those in magnet organizations and those in organizations in the process of applying for magnet status had significantly better results when asked about characteristics of the work environment and professional relationships. Magnet hospitals enjoy higher percentages of satisfied RNs, lower RN turnover and vacancy, improved clinical outcomes, and improved patient satisfaction.*

In a four-state survey of 26,276 nurses, Kelly, McHigh, and Aiken (2011) reported:

> Magnet hospitals have better work environments and a more highly educated nurse workforce. Outside of California where nurse staffing mandates decrease variation in staffing, Magnet hospitals have significantly better nurse staffing reflected in nurses caring for fewer patients each. Nurses in Magnet hospitals are significantly less likely to experience high burnout or be dissatisfied with their jobs than nurses in non-Magnet hospitals. Our results are consistent with a substantial and growing research base on Magnet hospitals that has accumulated over several decades showing significantly better work environments in Magnet hospitals and better nurse outcomes. (p. 432)

Houston and colleagues (2012) found that decisional involvement is higher among Magnet-designed than non-magnet facilities. Kovner and associates (2009) reported that it is not Magnet status per se, "but rather common characteristics of Magnet hospitals such as autonomy and lower organizational constraints . . . that are related to satisfaction and organizational commitment" (p. 90). Trinkoff and colleagues (2010) found that "nurses who worked in Magnet hospitals were less likely to report having mandatory overtime and on-call as part of their jobs, although 'reported hours worked' did not differ" (p. 313). Kelly and associates (2011) found that magnet hospital nurses were 18% less likely to be dissatisfied with their job and 13% less likely to report high burnout. Vartanian and colleagues (2013) found that nurses' perceptions of their workplace were more positive in magnet environments. Boyle and colleagues (2012) found that magnet recognition is associated with increases in nursing specialty certification rates.

Although most of the evidence is positive, there are some exceptions. Goode and colleagues (2011), in a study of 19 magnet hospitals and 35 non-magnet hospitals, found that the magnet hospitals had fewer total staff and a lower RN skill mix compared with non-magnet hospitals. The non-magnet hospitals had better patient outcomes, except that the magnet hospitals had slightly better outcomes for pressure ulcers.

Higdon and colleagues (2012) advocate magnet designation in small hospitals with fewer than 100 beds, presenting a business plan (cost-benefit analysis, outcome measures, and financial impact data) to support this. Small hospitals can apply for the Pathway to Excellence Program® instead of the larger magnet Recognition Program®.

The Pathway to Excellence program focuses on the quality of the nursing practice environment, whereas the Magnet program focuses not only on the practice environment, but also on research, outcomes, and innovation. According to the ANCC, the Pathway program is appropriate for facilities of all sizes where nurses work, but, in particular, it's viewed as a way for small- and medium-sized facilities (clinics, long-term-care facilities, and critical access hospitals) to demonstrate their commitment to excellent nursing practice environments. (Shaffer, Parker, Kantz, & Havens, 2013, p. 27)

The Pathway to Excellence Program has 12 standards:

1. Nurses control the practice of nursing.
2. The work environment is safe and healthy.
3. Systems are in place to address patient care and practice concerns.
4. Orientation prepares new nurses.
5. The CNO is qualified and participates in all levels of the facility.
6. Professional development is provided and utilized.
7. Competitive wages/salaries are in place.
8. Nurses are recognized for achievements.
9. A balanced lifestyle is encouraged.
10. Collaborative interdisciplinary relationships are valued and supported.
11. Nurse managers are competent and accountable.
12. A quality program and evidence-based practices are utilized.

The Excellence program is intended for small, rural hospitals, which comprise 41% of U.S. community hospitals. Havens and associates (2012) found that rural nurses viewed their work environments as favorable. Newhouse and colleagues (2009) found that 280 nurse executives in small, rural hospitals actually scored lower total Essentials of Magnet scores. "As a smaller system entity, nurse executives may perceive higher system oversight, control, and a lower level of influence" (p. 194). One hospital, working through the Excellence process stated:

After a careful self-assessment, you may be pleasantly surprised to learn that many of the standards are already met in your organization. However, if your assessment reveals that the standards aren't in place, the Pathway program provides a framework to guide development of an excellent nursing practice environment. Involve as many staff members, disciplines, and departments as possible. Assign sections of the application and documentation of standards to staff and leaders from different disciplines. Inclusion of ideas from nonnursing colleagues contributes important perspectives and shows an appreciation for nursing's contribution to patient care across the organization.

Communication is critical throughout the process. . . .

Appreciative inquiry (AI), a method that focuses on increasing what works within an organization and removing what doesn't work, [was used]. (Shaffer et al., 2013, p. 31)

Appreciative inquiry was also used by Havens and colleagues (2006) to improve communication and collaboration, to increase nurse involvement in decision making, and to enhance cultural awareness and sensitivity. Appreciative inquiry is when a group completes the following cycle in this order: (1) discovery—appreciate "what works"; (2) dream—imagine "what might be"; (3) design—determine what "should be"; and (4) delivery/destiny—create "what will be" (p. 464).

Meraviglia and associates (2009) worked with 30 rural or small hospitals, providing consultation visits and ongoing support on strategies to achieve the 12 criteria. There was "significant improvement in nurses' appraisal of their work environment" (p. 70). Reineck (2007) suggests strategies for building capacity for magnetism (Havens et al., 2012, p. 390). In non-magnet rural hospitals, Newhouse and colleagues (2011) found:

> Larger rural hospitals are more likely than small hospitals to have a clinical ladder, more baccalaureate-prepared RNs, greater perceived economic and external influences, lower shared vision among hospital staff, and higher levels of quality and safety engagement. Most nurses employed in rural hospitals are educated at the associate degree level. (p. 129)

The Magnet Recognition Program is a credentialing process that has been awarded to approximately 6.78% of all registered hospitals in the United States. The application process is extensive and fairly expensive. Often, a project director within an organization is designated to work on this (Lavin, 2013). The term *Magnet hospital* is equated with excellence.

Magnet criteria value further education, supporting the Institute of Medicine's *Future of Nursing* report. The second recommendation in the report focuses on increasing the proportion of registered nurses with baccalaureate degrees to 80% by 2020. Although the evidence is mixed on this issue, many studies have linked higher education with better patient outcomes. Blegan and associates (2013) found that "hospitals with a higher percentage of RNs with baccalaureate or higher degrees had lower congestive heart failure mortality, decubitus ulcers, failure to rescue, and postoperative deep vein thrombosis or pulmonary embolism, and shorter length of stay" (p. 89).

The Magnet Recognition Program was started 30 years ago by the American Nurses Credentialing Center (ANCC) for healthcare organizations that provide the services of registered nurses. The ANCC has continued to refine and improve the Magnet program. The program identified 14 common components, or Forces of Magnetism (FOM), in the 1980s, and in the late 1990s expanded this program to include long-term care facilities and international healthcare organizations, as well as hospitals.

The 14 Forces of Magnetism are as follows:

Force 1: Quality of Nursing Leadership
Force 2: Organizational Structure
Force 3: Management Style
Force 4: Personnel Policies and Programs
Force 5: Professional Models of Care
Force 6: Quality of Care
Force 7: Quality Improvement
Force 8: Consultation and Resources
Force 9: Autonomy
Force 10: Community and the Health Care Organization
Force 11: Nurses as Teachers
Force 12: Image of Nursing
Force 13: Interdisciplinary Relationships
Force 14: Professional Development

(These can be found at www.nursecredentialing.org/Magnet/ProgramOverview/HistoryoftheMagnetProgram/ForcesofMagnetism.)

After conducting several studies on the organizational culture of Magnet facilities, Kramer and Schmalenburg (2003) identified eight essentials of magnetism, now called the Nursing Work Index:

1. Working with other nurses who are clinically competent
2. Good nurse–physician relationships and communication
3. Nurse autonomy and accountability

4. Supportive nurse manager–supervisor
5. Control over nursing practice and practice environment
6. Support for education (inservice, continuing education, etc.)
7. Adequate nurse staffing
8. Paramount concern for the patient

As research continued on Magnet facilities, in 2008 a panel of experts examined the evidence from magnet facilities and reconfigured the 14 Forces of Magnetism into 5 model components. These make up the Magnet Model:

- Transformational Leadership
- Structural Empowerment
- Exemplary Professional Practice
- New Knowledge, Innovation, and Improvements
- Empirical Quality Results

The following subsections provide the Magnet definitions of these components and some additional helpful evidence to further explain how organizations can achieve each component.

I. Transformational Leadership

Today's health care environment is experiencing unprecedented, intense reformation. Unlike yesterday's leadership requirement for stabilization and growth, today's leaders are required to transform their organization's values, beliefs, and behaviors. It is relatively easy to lead people where they want to go; the transformational leader must lead people to where they need to be in order to meet the demands of the future.

This requires vision, influence, clinical knowledge, and a strong expertise relating to professional nursing practice. It also acknowledges that transformation may create turbulence and involve atypical approaches to solutions.

The organization's senior leadership team creates the vision for the future, and the systems and environment necessary to achieve that vision. They must enlighten the organization as to why change is necessary, and communicate each department's part in achieving that change. They must listen, challenge, influence, and affirm as the organization makes its way into the future.

Gradually, this transformational way of thinking should take root in the organization and become even stronger as other leaders adapt to this way of thinking.

The intent of this Model Component is no longer just to solve problems, fix broken systems, and empower staff, but to actually transform the organizations to meet the future. Magnet-recognized organizations today strive for stabilization; however, healthcare reformation calls for a type of controlled destabilization that births new ideas and innovations.

Forces of Magnetism Represented

- Quality of Nursing Leadership (Force #1)
- Management Style (Force #3) (ANCC, 2013c)

This component supports the previous material in this chapter. This type of leadership constantly transforms the organization, recognizing the chaos/complexity issues and the potential realities. Throughout the organization, it is important to have organizational advocacy and support for giving patients what they value from housekeeping to board members. This is an important model for all administrators within an organization.

II. Structural Empowerment

Solid structures and processes developed by influential leadership provide an innovative environment where strong professional practice flourishes and where the mission, vision, and values come to life to achieve the outcomes believed to be important for the organization.

Further strengthening practice are the strong relationships and partnerships developed among all types of community organizations to improve patient outcomes and the health of the communities they serve. This is accomplished through the organization's strategic plan, structure, systems, policies, and programs.

Staff need to be developed, directed, and empowered to find the best way to accomplish the organizational goals and achieve desired outcomes. This may be accomplished through a variety of structures and programs; one size does not fit all.

Forces of Magnetism Represented

- Organizational Structure (Force #2)
- Personnel Policies and Programs (Force #4)
- Community and the Healthcare Organization (Force #10)
- Image of Nursing (Force #12)
- Professional Development (Force #14) (ANCC, 2013c)

Elements of structural empowerment are discussed later in this chapter.
This criterion includes Magnet Force 4: Personnel Policies and Programs that states:

Creative and flexible staffing models that support a safe and healthy work environment are used. Personnel policies are created with direct care nurse involvement. Significant opportunities for professional growth exist in administrative and clinical tracks. Personnel policies and programs support professional nursing practice, work/life balance, and the delivery of quality care. (ANCC, 2013b)

III. Exemplary Professional Practice

The true essence of a Magnet organization stems from exemplary professional practice within nursing. This entails a comprehensive understanding of the role of nursing; the application of that role with patients, families, communities, and the interdisciplinary team; and the application of new knowledge and evidence. The goal of this Component is more than the establishment of strong professional practice; it is what that professional practice can achieve.

Forces of Magnetism Represented

- Professional Models of Care (Force #5)
- Consultation and Resources (Force #8)
- Autonomy (Force #9)
- Nurses as Teachers (Force #11)
- Interdisciplinary Relationships (Force #13) (ANCC, 2013c)

Exemplary professional practice is emphasized throughout this text, and autonomy and interdisciplinary relationships are discussed in this chapter.

IV. New Knowledge, Innovation, and Improvements

Strong leadership, empowered professionals, and exemplary practice are essential building blocks for Magnet-recognized organizations, but they are not the final goals. Magnet organizations have an ethical and professional responsibility to contribute to patient care, the organization, and the profession in terms of new knowledge, innovations, and improvements.

Our current systems and practices need to be redesigned and redefined if we are to be successful in the future. This Component includes new models of care, application of existing evidence, new evidence, and visible contributions to the science of nursing.

Forces of Magnetism Represented

• Quality Improvement (Force #7)

This book helps to give readers new knowledge, as well as ideas for innovation and improvements. As Magnet Force 7: Quality Improvement states: "The organization possesses structures and processes for the measurement of quality and programs for improving the quality of care and services within the organization" (ANCC, 2013b).

V. Empirical Quality Results

Today's Magnet recognition process primarily focuses on structure and processes, with an assumption that good outcomes will follow. Currently, outcomes are not specified, and are minimally weighted. There are no quantitative outcome requirements for ANCC Magnet Recognition. Recently lacking were benchmark data that would allow comparisons with best practices. This area is where the greatest changes need to occur. Data of this caliber will spur needed changes.

In the future, having a strong structure and processes are the first steps. In other words, the question for the future is not "What do you do?" or "How do you do it?" but rather, "What difference have you made?" Magnet-recognized organizations are in a unique position to become pioneers of the future and to demonstrate solutions to numerous problems inherent in our healthcare systems today. They may do this in a variety of ways through innovative structure and various processes, and they ought to be recognized, not penalized, for their inventiveness.

Outcomes need to be categorized in terms of clinical outcomes related to nursing; workforce outcomes; patient and consumer outcomes; and organizational outcomes. When possible, outcomes data that the organization already collects should be utilized. Quantitative benchmarks should be established. These outcomes will represent the "report card" of a Magnet-recognized organization, and a simple way of demonstrating excellence.

Forces of Magnetism Represented

• Quality of Care (Force #6) (ANCC, 2013c)

Strategic planning identifies the process needed to move forward into potential reality. Magnet Force 6: Quality of Care states:

Quality is the systematic driving force for nursing and the organization. Nurses serving in leadership positions are responsible for providing an environment that positively influences patient outcomes. There is a pervasive perception among nurses that they provide high quality care to patients. (ANCC, 2013b)

Organizational Assessment: An Administrative Competency

Now we turn to an administrative competency: organizational assessment. Organizational assessment is the ability to have a fairly accurate, dynamic picture of the total organization, such as how various people work together, which departments are more effective, how different departments have different cultures, how clients perceive the organization, and how the organization fits within the community that surrounds it. This picture is dynamic, meaning that it changes constantly as various components, relationships, and people change within and outside the organization.

> Organizational agility exemplifies knowing and understanding how the organization works; knowing how to get things done both through formal channels and informal networks; understanding the origin and reasoning behind key policies, practices, and procedures; and especially critical, understanding the organizational culture. (Morjikian et al., 2007, p. 401)

This organizational assessment capability helps the administrator to know, with fair accuracy, how different individuals and departments might respond to situations. No matter how well we know an organization, we still experience surprises, but this organizational assessment capability is a key factor for effectiveness.

Assessment is a lived experience that takes time and effort. The resulting picture is never totally accurate because there are always hidden factors that we do not know, both about ourselves and about others, and because everyone in the organization is constantly changing.

Porter-O'Grady and Malloch (2009) suggest that it is necessary for the nurse administrator to possess synthesis and contextual capacity.

> *Synthesis*, the ability to "see" flow, movement, connection, and integration, is becoming an essential skill for both leader and innovator. The ability to articulate the product of the creative effort and the value of the innovation process and to know when to move with it has become an important competence for the leader. The ability to distinguish between emergent properties and coalescence is critical to the viability and sustainability of the products of innovation.
>
> *Contextual capacity* is critical if leaders of innovation are to enable the financial, strategic, and process viability of the innovation dynamic: facilitating proposal rendering for innovation, critically appraising innovation and the diffusion processes, assess the evidence-driven constructs underpinning an innovation, enabling successful diffusion and adoption of innovations, and evaluating innovation feasibility and sustainability. The 7 areas of content capacity essential to this approach are concept, evidence, policy, finance, technology, communication, infrastructure, and outcomes. (p. 246)

Organizing the Assessment Data

As part of the organizational assessment process, it is important to discuss the various components of an organization. If we use linear thinking, we can look at each component as a separate entity. *Yet we must remember that all of these components are actually intertwined and interconnected to make the whole.*

An organizational assessment is like describing a person. We cannot take a person apart and look at each separate body system or organ to get a true description of that person. We can only describe how the whole person seems to operate. At each moment, this whole person is changing as events happen and he or she responds. Similarly, although we can describe the components of an organization, we must go beyond linear thinking and see the organization as a *whole, ever-changing, dynamic entity.*

As we assess an organization, we need to define not only our own department but the overall organization, which could be a single facility or a larger corporate healthcare system. Large corporate systems have their own dynamic, as do individual facilities. For instance, the corporate system might have one culture, the individual facility another, and the specific department or unit yet another.

Collins and Porras (1994, pp. 259–260) defined nine organizational categories that are helpful to use when assessing an organization:

- **Category 1: Organizing Arrangements.** "Hard" items, such as organization structure, policies and procedures, systems, rewards and incentives, ownership structure, and general business strategies and activities of the company (e.g., acquisitions, significant changes in strategy, going public).

  When considering *rewards and incentives*, if not carefully thought out, they can produce negative results. For example, one incentive for an executive team might be a bonus if they can keep costs below a certain level for the quarter or for the year (a linear model). But this has significant downsides. First, bonuses are not linked with a quality dimension and so encourage executives to save money even when patient outcomes may worsen as a result of their decisions—in the long run costing more money, not to mention patients' lives. Second, these bonuses reward only executive-level administrators, yet the people doing the everyday work with patients are not rewarded. Bonuses are more effective when given to everyone in the organization.

  Another disincentive for nurses is that they are professionals, yet we make them use time cards to clock in and out. What if their patients need care beyond their shift time? Some organizations have chosen to pay nurses annual salaries rather than hourly rates. (Sometimes salaries have been abused by administrators as a way to avoid paying for overtime. That is not the intent here. Salaries should pay a fair wage.) This can have *positive results when nurses are given the freedom to work when their patients need them.* In inpatient settings, nurses could choose their hours while others cover actual shift times. The main idea is that nurses accomplish meaningful work—satisfying experiences with patients and families that enhance nurse retention and better serve the patients.

  Another disincentive in some organizations is the high amount of money paid for traveler nurses, which ignores our best and loyal workforce already present day after day working for us and costing less money. By hiring traveler nurses, we send the message that this loyal group is not as important as the traveler nurses. Who deserves the higher salary? Surely the loyal workforce!

  It is important to give careful thought to the rewards and incentives provided in an organization because they must support desired behaviors. For instance, employee performance evaluations have no clout if they are not used to determine merit increases. And organizational performance evaluations are worthless if not everyone in the workplace is rewarded for meeting performance standards. When incentives are used to reward certain behaviors, it is important to provide the staff with educational activities that teach them the specific behaviors. For instance, if rewards are given for being patient centered, it is important to supply educational activities to teach everyone what *patient centered* actually means in daily behaviors, including the thinking and decision-making processes to be used. In addition, it is helpful if all, including top-level administrators, model and support the desired behaviors.

  Another important incentive is to pay for staff to attend conferences. During budget meetings, conference monies are often cut—a short-sighted decision—yet sometimes executive travel expenses for national conferences remain fully paid. This sends a message to staff that they are not valued (actions speak louder than words). It is important that all staff, including aides and housekeeping staff, are up-to-date doing meaningful work.

- **Category 2: Social Factors.** "Soft" items, such as the company's cultural practices, atmosphere, norms, rituals, mythology and stories, group dynamics, and management style. (Collins & Porras, 1994, pp. 259–260)
  Social factors are discussed earlier in this chapter.
- **Category 3: Physical Setting.** Significant aspects of the way the company handled physical space, such as plant and office layout or new facilities. This included any significant decisions regarding the geographic location of key parts of the company. (Collins & Porras, 1994, pp. 259–260)
  The physical setting can be a significant factor and can use many budget dollars. For instance, as more elderly people navigate our health systems, it is important for them to have easy access to services (i.e., not having to walk long distances). The physical setting can also affect how well we can accomplish our work. If the environment is always too hot or too cold, or we have only double rooms available, or we have to go to different locations for equipment, supplies, and so forth, we are less effective. Many older work settings are not adequate to handle the newer technology necessary for care. One goal in many healthcare organizations is to have everything the healthcare worker needs present at the point of care. Pati and colleagues (2012) found this reduced total walking time on a 12-hour shift by 67.9%. Fixing physical setting factors can create considerable expense, but these factors are very important.
- **Category 4: Technology.** How the company used technology: information technology, state-of-the-art processes and equipment, advanced job configurations, and related items. (Collins & Porras, 1994, pp. 259–260)
  We are in the Information Age. Technology has exploded across the healthcare landscape. Healthcare organizations, if they are not keeping up with state-of-the-art processes and equipment, are becoming obsolete. Yet technology is a huge expense. Is it worth the cost, not only of the initial purchase but implementation, regular updates, and so forth? This is a big issue that looms larger as reimbursements continue to decline. At the same time, organizations are faced with how to keep confidential information safe (meeting HIPAA laws).
- **Category 5: Leadership.** Leadership of the firm since its inception: the transition between key early shapers of the organization and later generations, leadership tenure, the length of time the leaders were with the organization before becoming CEO (Were they brought in from the outside or grown from within? When did they join?), and leadership selection processes and criteria. (Collins & Porras, 1994, pp. 259–260)
  Leadership can make or break organizational effectiveness. It is so important that when a work group is dysfunctional, the first place to look to resolve the problem is the administrative leadership. Most likely, the administrator is ineffective, which leads to more and more dysfunction in the group.
  Currently, there is a high level of turnover in the nurse manager group. Many experience feelings of overwhelm about their role. They are caught in the middle: expected to "keep staff happy"; do what the administration wants them to do even when administrators do not understand how their decisions affect staff; keep patient satisfaction scores up; maintain quality in a safe environment; keep budgets balanced; and keep up with current technology, not only for patient treatments, administering medications, and documentation but to understand administrative systems and respond to data using these systems. A big issue is that the administrators they report to may need to grow themselves. We are all in this dance together.
- **Category 6: Products and Services.** Significant products and services in the company's history. How did the product or service ideas come about? What guided their selection and development? Did the company have any product failures, and how did it deal with them? Did the company lead with new products or follow in the marketplace? (Collins & Porras, 1994, pp. 259–260)

Products and services, such as oncology or cardiology services, are a key factor to organizational success. As we serve clients, it is important to pay attention to what our healthcare clients value and want. This is what we need to provide rather than what we personally might like if we were the patients. As services are delivered, an organization needs to pay attention to ethical and legal issues as well.

As organizations examine which services to offer, it is important for them to assess the local community to identify what is already available and what is needed. For example, with baby boomers approaching retirement, managing chronic illnesses is a huge issue in health care. As healthcare services are delivered, case management is critically needed for better management of the patient and better reimbursement. More attention needs to be given to develop a seamless continuum of care. The AHA (2013) must-do strategies focus on these issues for survival in a value-based environment.

- **Category 7: Vision: Core Values, Purpose, and Visionary Goals.** Were these variables present? If yes, how did they come into being? Did the organization have them at certain points in its history and not others? What role did they play? If it had strong values and purpose, did they remain intact or become diluted? Why? (Collins & Porras, 1994, pp. 259–260)

  The first part of this chapter is devoted to core values and organizational purpose—these are so important that we started the chapter discussing them. Vision and goals support the must-do strategies the AHA (2013) has identified.

- **Category 8: Financial Analysis.** Ratio and spreadsheet analysis of all income statements and balance sheets for every year going back to the date when the company became public: sales and profit growth, gross margins, return on assets, return on sales, return on equity, debt to equity ratio, cash flow and working capital, liquidity ratios, dividend payout ratio, increase in gross property plant and equipment as a percentage of sales, asset turnover. Also examine stock returns and overall stock performance relative to the market (if applicable). (Collins & Porras, 1994, pp. 259–260)

  Although most of this is the purview of the finance department, it is important for nurse administrators to understand ratio and spreadsheet analysis. Nursing personnel are most concerned with budgets; developing and analyzing budgets and understanding how to compare reimbursements with the costs of services provided—important mandates in the value-based environment.

- **Category 9: Markets/Environment.** Significant aspects of the company's external environment: major market shifts, dramatic national or international events, government regulations, industry structural issues, dramatic technology changes, and related items. (Collins & Porras, 1994, pp. 259–260)

The micro- and macroeconomic environments contribute significantly to our present illness care system.

Moving Toward Decision Making at the Point of Care

As one assesses an organization, Likert's (1973) model (**Exhibit 3–4**) continues to be useful to show how organizational variables interact with one another at different stages.

System 1 represents a very authoritarian system. Here, there is little dialogue, communication occurs only in a downward direction (assuming the CEO is at the top—an authoritarian model), the informal rumor mill is rampant and needed because it is the best source of information for staff, decisions are made at the top, orders are given, no one dares to question the orders, staff often resist the orders covertly, and control is all important. Linear thinking is rampant.

Exhibit 3–4   Likert's Organizational Systems

Organizational Variables	SYSTEM 1	SYSTEM 2	SYSTEM 3	SYSTEM 4
Leadership				
How much confidence and trust is shown in staff?	Virtually none	Some	Substantial amount	Great deal
How free do staff feel to talk to supervisors about job?	Not very free	Somewhat free	Quite free	Very free
How often are staff's ideas sought and used constructively?	Seldom	Sometimes	Often	Very frequently
Motivation				
Is predominant use made of (1) fear, (2) threats, (3) punishment, (4) rewards, and/or (5) involvement?	1, 2, 3, occasionally 4	4, some 3	4, some 3 and 5	5, 4, based on group
Where is responsibility felt for achieving the organization's goals?	Mostly at top	Top and middle	Fairly general	At all levels
How much cooperative teamwork exists?	Very little	Relatively little	Moderate amount	Great deal
Communications				
What is the usual direction of information flow?	Downward	Mostly downward	Down and up	Down, up, and sideways
How is downward communication accepted?	With suspicion	Possibly with suspicion	With caution	With a receptive mind
How accurate is upward communication?	Usually inaccurate	Often inaccurate	Often accurate	Almost always accurate
How well do administrators know the problems faced by staff?	Not very well	Rather well	Quite well	Very well
Decisions				
At what level are decisions made?	Mostly at top	Policy at top, some delegation	Broad policy at top, more delegation	Throughout but well-integrated
Are staff involved in decisions related to their work?	Almost never	Occasionally consulted	Generally consulted	Fully involved
What does the decision-making process contribute to motivation?	Not very much	Relatively little	Some contribution	Substantial contribution
Goals				
How are organizational goals established?	Orders issued	Orders, some comments invited	After discussion, by orders	By group action (except in crisis)
How much covert resistance to goals is present?	Strong resistance	Moderate resistance	Some resistance at times	Little or none

(continues)

Exhibit 3–4 Likert's Organizational Systems (*continued*)				
Organizational Variables	**SYSTEM 1**	**SYSTEM 2**	**SYSTEM 3**	**SYSTEM 4**
Evaluation				
How concentrated are review and evaluation functions?	Very highly at top	Quite highly at top	Moderate delegation to lower levels	Widely shared
Is there an informal organization resisting the formal one?	Yes	Usually	Sometimes	No—same goals as formal
What are cost, productivity, and other evaluation data used for?	Policing, punishment	Reward and punishment	Reward, some self-guidance	Self-guidance, problem solving

Source: Adapted from *The Human Organization: Its Management and Value* by Rensis Likert. Copyright 1967 by McGraw-Hill, Inc.

Compare this to a system 4 model, which is participative, reflecting complexity. Here, matrices exist where communication occurs between and within all levels, communication is open and shared, dialogue occurs, decisions are made at the appropriate level, the organization consists of well-integrated staff, goals are determined by group action except in crisis, there is no need for an informal organization because information is transparent, and productivity is enhanced by each person, with everyone doing their own problem solving. Circular thinking exists here with people understanding the inner connectivity of everyone in the system. Systems 2 and 3 fall between these two extremes, with system 2 being slightly authoritarian whereas system 3 starts to become more participative.

Using Likert's model, we need to assess where our organization currently is and base our actions on this assessment. For instance, if we are a transformational leader who believes in a system 4 yet we are in a system 2, we become very frustrated and staff do not understand our leadership style if we interact with them as though we were in a system 4. Instead, we must respond based on the current system level and gradually move toward the desired system. So, in a staff meeting, when we want to get information from staff on an issue or a piece of equipment and we ask for feedback, we might not get much response. It is easy to wonder what we have done wrong. (This is internalizing the problem. Try not to do this.) Instead, realize that staff are suspicious of us, thinking, "What does she want from me? I'm not going to stick my neck out." Continue forward with transparency; it may take repeated meetings before staff begin to trust enough to start offering suggestions. Even then, it occurs only on issues that are perceived to be safe or not as emotionally laden. When this breakthrough happens, the group starts to move to a more participative model.

When we want to move an organization, department, or floor from a system 2 to a system 3, it takes repeated, consistent efforts for a year or two before we begin to see movement in the desired direction. This cultural change is enormous and particularly hard if administrators at the executive level are still authoritarian. We must not get impatient and must look for small changes. Maybe a staff member starts to give honest feedback in private, even though in meetings this person remains silent. This is an important breakthrough; it means that this staff member is starting to trust and starting to move to the next level.

When we are looking for a job, identifying the organization's system level is an important factor to assess in the interview process. Nurse administrators can assess the system level of the overall organization and the workgroup where he or she will be working.

Movement in the opposite direction is also possible, for example, nurse executives operating at a system 4 level could move to a system 2 organization. This can work but most often presents many problems.

In such cases, it is especially important to know what the nurse executive's boss is like. If the boss functions as a system 2 administrator and likes this system, this boss will not understand the nurse executive's leadership style and might even believe that the nurse executive is incompetent! System 4 characteristics can seem like a foreign language to those who operate in systems 1 or 2. When the new nurse executive asks staff what they think about issues, the system 2 boss might think, "Isn't the new nurse executive able to make his/her own decisions?" In other words, "Doesn't this nurse executive know what to do? Is this person incompetent? Why doesn't this person just tell staff what to do?" The boss operates in a system 2 mode by issuing edicts. Staff members are to follow the edicts, and there is no room for questions or dialogue. This approach can be very frustrating for the system 4 nurse executive unless the executive understands this systems model and deals with the boss on a system 2 level. Unfortunately, in this situation, most often the nurse executive is fired within a year.

This model can also help explain why a successful program in one facility will not work in another. Perhaps the successful strategy worked in a system 3 environment. Is it any wonder that it will not work in a system 2 setting?

Rounds

Another way to assess organizations is by doing *rounds*. In this value-based environment, this is the best way to stay in tune with what is actually happening with patients—the primary purpose of our business. This is important for everyone from board members and executives to floor nurses and nurse aides. It is the best way to discover the small, incremental changes that are around us every day. The focus is the patient and what the patient values. Frequent *administrative rounding* provides valuable information about organizational dynamics. It enables nurse administrators to get to know employees, see how organizational processes are actually working—or not, hear concerns from everyone—at all points of service, note physical environment issues, and more. *It is critical that administrators at all levels of management, as well as nursing staff, do frequent rounds.*

Rounds are times to share information, be open to questions and concerns, eliminate or reduce barriers to care, and have roundtable gatherings around issues. We can get a feel for the total organization, and an additional bonus is that many issues can be resolved on the spot. This also means that when there is full census, or a unit or department needs help, the administrators are empathetic to the situation and pitch in.

Nurse administrators can find out all sorts of helpful information by visiting staff, physicians, patients and families, and other interdisciplinary staff while doing rounds. Rounds allow feedback to be gained from and given to staff without having too many meetings. This is greatly facilitated when all administrators—from board members and the president to the nurse manager—do rounds *daily*, being visible for the sake of more effective communication as well as giving support and living the core values. In a value-based environment, this is a much more productive way to spend administrative time than many of the meetings are.

Rounds provide opportunities for regular dialogue with the people at the point of service about major issues that need to be fixed. During rounds, nurse administrators can identify the appropriate individuals to work on and discern solutions to fix the problem issues, and then continue to involve appropriate people to implement the chosen solution, to tweak it when needed, and to evaluate the effectiveness of what occurred to make sure the desired outcomes were achieved.

In fact, an *administrative competency* is *the ability to sense the atmosphere* in a department or on a unit when coming to round. Sometimes it is quiet or involves the usual hustle and bustle, but sometimes one can sense that something is wrong—or that magic is happening. Duality again. It may be time to celebrate when magic is happening. But it may be necessary to intervene and help if something is wrong. This competency of being aware of the energy (atmosphere) as one rounds is something that develops over time.

Evidence supports the importance of doing rounds. Lee and Manley (2008) and Rondinelli and colleagues (2012) share how nurse director rounds support patient-centered care, and how nurse administrators who value staff rounding support this concept in meetings, staffing decisions, and so forth. Rondinelli and colleagues (2012) and Tonges and Ray (2011) describe nurse manager rounding, which includes whether staff have rounded on patients. Setia and Meade (2009) bundled nurse manager rounding with discharge telephone calls. This significantly raised patient satisfaction. They found that nurse manager rounds identified "many outcomes including identification of service recovery opportunities, setting expectations about the care that the patient will receive, and building confidence in the team of nurses who will care for the patient" (p. 140). Interestingly, they found that when the nurse manager rounds with patients, the patients "feel better about the nurses taking care of them."

There are fewer lawsuits when the patient and family perceive that the caregivers—and administrators—care. A healthcare administrator is always more effective when doing rounds because the real patient issues are more likely to be identified earlier and many can be addressed on the spot.

While doing rounds, it is important for nurse administrators to coach and mentor staff, rather than be too task oriented. We want staff to think, make decisions, and take actions, not depend on someone else, such as the administrator, the physician, or the nurse manager, for all the answers. The goal is to encourage and empower staff as much as possible to deal with issues as they arise.

There are some potential traps to avoid. First, the administrator needs to exhibit certain behaviors. While walking down the hall of an inpatient unit, if the administrator does not pay attention to call lights or patients/families that are having obvious problems, the message the administrator sends is that patient issues are not important. If the administrator does not greet staff but just goes to find the manager, staff get the message they are not valued. They can view the administrator as not caring about them.

Second, it is best not to be Attila the Hun. If one reacts to a situation and heads roll, everyone becomes afraid of the administrator, hides information from the administrator, resents the administrator, and does not actually change behavior—unless the administrator is around. It is more advantageous to converse with staff and to help staff explore more effective options.

A third trap to avoid is micromanaging. When an administrator micromanages, the message is that staff members, or the manager, are not capable of doing the job right. However, the real problem is that the administrator has not learned to delegate effectively.

The most effective way to do rounds is to pay attention to everyone present, talk with people, demonstrate caring, and use rounds as a learning process. All actions support the core values and the purpose. As crises occur, remain calm and decisive and, when necessary, pitch in and help resolve the situation. As problems become evident, talk with those involved to explore how best to handle a situation, or get into a dialogue about what happened and determine what could have been done to more effectively deal with the problem.

Round-the-clock meetings enable everyone, regardless of shift or work schedule, to learn what is important from other perspectives. This way the midnight or weekend personnel do not feel as isolated. Administrators at all levels should hold these meetings regularly.

Roundtable gatherings can be a helpful way to deal with the many issues that staff experience as they do their work. It is best if all attend a gathering based on interest in the topic to be discussed. It is especially helpful if those attending from administration represent various levels, and depending on the topic to be discussed, special invitations should go out to departments that deal with the issue being discussed.

An *open-door policy* means that someone who has an important issue is welcome to share it with any administrator at any level in the organization. An open door does not mean that a secretary intercedes, although, if the secretary is empowered, this person is invaluable to an administrator and actually deals with many issues directly, saving the administrator time.

Multidisciplinary rounds range from daily to biweekly or weekly, often led by a physician and/or nurse (Squires, 2012). Case managers are included. Geary and colleagues (2009) found daily rapid rounds to be most effective and decreased length of stay.

Many advocate hourly *staff nurse rounds* where nurses talk with patients about current issues patients are concerned with and make sure all patients' needs are met (pain medications, repositioning, patient and environmental assessment). Rondinelli and associates (2012) advocate: "A—activity, B—bathroom, C—comfort, D—dietary, and E—environment" (p. 328).

Sherrod and colleagues (2012) and Tonges and Ray (2011) advocate "purposeful" hourly rounding. This allows "nurses to spend more time with their patients addressing care needs. By increasing care quality, patient satisfaction improves, positively affecting the image of a facility for patients and families" (p. 37). Tonges and Ray (2011) advocate staff nurses and nursing assistants round on alternative hours. Both Neville and colleagues (2012) and Bourgault and colleagues (2008) advocate involving patient care technicians (PCTs) in rounding so that when a nurse needs to spend more time with one patient, the PCT can visit the other patients.

Rounds shows patients that someone cares about them. Rounds might be done by the primary nurse or by a nurse/PCT team, and frequently charge nurses assist in rounding (Minnier et al., 2012). Rounds needs to vary in certain areas, for example, in postpartum it may be to help with feeding the baby, and in the OR it may be to talk with relatives waiting during the patient's procedure.

> Routine patient [rounds], once considered a standard of care in the nursing profession, has recently reemerged with a twist. New research shows that hourly patient rounding increases patient satisfaction and decreases patient falls and call-light usage when performed in a standardized and consistent manner. (Bourgault et al., 2008, p. 18)

Berkow and associates (2012) advocate that nurses who are not assigned to certain patients round on similar patients for about 5 minutes. This gives the nurses more of an organizational team experience/picture than just being caught up with their own patients.

There are issues, however. Shepard (2013) discusses barriers to rounds. "Nurses described how complex patients, necessitating additional and prolonged time, frequently altered their rounds protocol, leaving them concerned and frustrated about caring and rounding for other patients" (Neville et al., 2012, p. 87).

> Although the findings support the practice of rounding, thematic analysis revealed that nurses' strong sense of professional autonomy and identification of patient needs through assessment were the most important factors in determining the frequency and duration of time spent with patients. Findings revealed that a mandated [rounds] protocol minimized the sense of professional autonomy and self-directed practice. It was felt that their presence at the bedside was oftentimes far more frequent than every 1 hour. Nurses reported challenges in the provision of rounding due to increased patient acuity levels, time constraints, and the nurses' awareness of their need to be physically present. (Neville et al., 2012, p. 86)

Other issues included documentation of the rounds—another task to do that takes more time; inadequate workloads and skill mix are barriers; and interruptions that interfere with rounds being completed.

Rounds work best when staffing is adequate; when technology is available, such as computerized physician order entry (CPOE), electronic medical records (EMRs), and Vocera; when the staff involved have good communication skills; and when there is a collaborative relationship between staff so that, as one nurse has to spend more time with one patient, someone else helps to cover the rest of the patients.

Education is needed. There is a "need for stronger delegation, [time management,] collaboration, team building, and role clarity between nurses and ancillary personnel" (Neville, et al., 2012, p. 86), as well as a stronger formal orientation to rounds. As rounds are implemented, it can be helpful to have each work group work out how to accomplish it, and then have project leaders/staff be available to share best practices and tools as others start the process. The project leaders can also identify barriers, which can be worked out for each area. During implementation, a collaborative phone call where anyone can call in to discuss the rounds process can be helpful (Rondinelli et al., 2012). Generally, some customized tool is developed to show that rounds are occurring every hour. Flexibility is important in determining the process and changes to this process. Rounds can also be tied in with performance evaluations and can be added to questions asked of patients when assessing their healthcare experience. Patient feedback is also helpful and can provide additional ideas.

Some aspects of physical design may be issues that need to be resolved as well. It is best if all the equipment and supplies needed are located right by the patient room. Charting can be done as nurses see patients in the room. All of this saves valuable nurse time.

The improved outcomes from rounds can also help to get staff and manager buy-in to the rounds concept. Rondinelli and associates (2012) found that outcomes included fewer patient falls, fewer hospital-acquired pressure ulcers, increased patient satisfaction scores, lower number of patient call lights, better pain management, increased number of patient compliments versus complaints, staff satisfaction, less staff turnover, fewer sitters, less restraint use, and fewer patient requests made at the nurses' station. They also identified some unintended positive outcomes: patients' perception of being well cared for, efficient nursing practice, expert nursing practice, and realization of both unit and individual practice culture (p. 330).

Conclusion

This chapter is only the beginning. As we head toward the ocean, we take various paths. Some meander here and there. Some get there successfully despite many obstacles. Many experience temporary setbacks but know that sometimes setbacks lead in a better direction. The charted course is different for each organization. Money can continue to be adequate or, if bottom-line thinking prevails, will be scarce. We continue to evolve, either into better systems that run closer to the mission or as antiquated relics of days gone by, floundering and disappearing midstream. The choice is ours.

Notes

1. A helpful resource on tearing down the old structure and replacing it with something healthier is Lencioni's *Silos, Politics and Turf Wars: A Leadership Fable About Destroying the Barriers That Turn Colleagues into Competitors* (2006).
2. To explore thinking patterns, see de Bono (1976, 1994).

Discussion Questions

1. Identify changes in the healthcare environment that affect you at work.
2. What actions can a healthcare organization take to increase reimbursement?
3. Why is it important for an administrator to understand chaos and complexity?
4. What are some ways that chaos and complexity could be used to achieve change in a healthcare organization?
5. Why do many changes result in more complexity, and not actually fix the problem?
6. Is the purpose in your facility an effective one? Is it followed by everyone in the organization as they work?
7. How can nursing help to achieve the 10 must-do strategies the AHA has identified to be most successful in the value-based (second-curve) environment?
8. From your perspective, what is the most important core value in a healthcare organization? What are the core values at work?
9. As a nurse manager, what actions can you take to facilitate more meaningful work for each staff member?
10. Assess the spirit within your organization. How can this be increased?
11. How much autonomy do staff nurses have in your organization? How could this be improved?
12. Assess the culture where you work. What would you do to make it even better?
13. Describe the design of your organization. Is this the best design to achieve what patients value? To achieve reimbursement?
14. Why is it important for administrators to use systems thinking?
15. What would improve communication in your work setting?
16. How does evidence affect your role as an administrator?
17. How can collaboration be improved within your department and across the organization?
18. What measures can a nurse manager take to increase team effectiveness?
19. How can a nurse manager increase staff decision making at the point of service?
20. Give an example where shared governance could improve the work setting.
21. What professional development changes would you make for your work setting?
22. How could the Magnet/Excellence precepts be useful in your organization?
23. Assess your organization. As you assess it, start with the corporate organization, and then the facility, and then the unit/department where you work.
24. Why is it so important for everyone from the CEO to the nurse aide to do rounds? Give examples of what can be accomplished during rounds.
25. What are five major organizational competence issues that need to be dealt with more effectively in your organization? How would you resolve them?

Glossary of Terms

Appreciative Inquiry—"a method that focuses on increasing what works within an organization and removing what doesn't work (Shaffer et al., 2013, p. 31).

Autocatalysis—"a process in which information enters into a system in small fluctuations continually grow in strength, interacting with the system and feeding back upon itself" (Porter-O'Grady & Malloch, 2011, p. 14).

Autopoiesis—"the process by which living systems continually seek to renew and reinvent themselves, yet maintain their core integrity" (Porter-O'Grady & Malloch, 2011, p. 14).

Black Swans—unexpected events that occur "that have a significant and disproportionate impact on a system" (Clancy, 2008a, p. 273).

Chaos—forces that work to unbundle attachment to whatever is impeding movement. Chaos challenges us to simultaneously let go and to take on. It reminds us that life is a journey of constant creation (Porter-O'Grady & Malloch, 2011, p. 22).

Complexity—dynamic, interactive, nonlinear systems that adapt to changing environments. When many different interconnected agents interact at all levels to affect each other. Has a self-organizing structure that is spontaneous, adapts, and is flexible. Finds order within seemingly random complexities. Recognizes that actions are reciprocal.

Dissipative Structures—"Structures in which disorder is the source of order and vice versa. In this 'dance' between order and disorder, old form ends and new form begins" (Porter-O'Grady & Malloch, 2011, p. 14).

Feedback—is derived from both the output and throughput processes. Feedback is information about the effectiveness of the system and provides support for system changes. When outputs are positive, the system inputs and throughputs are reinforced and supported to continue. When the outputs are less than desired, modifications based on the feedback from the system are made to the throughputs. Similarly, when outputs are not what was expected, modifications to throughputs are considered (Porter-O'Grady & Malloch, 2011).

Fractals—"the smallest level of a single organization and the most complex array of the large aggregated system containing the organization are connected inexorably through the power of fractals" (Porter-O'Grady & Malloch, 2011, p. 13).

Inputs—the resources, human and nonhuman (materials, equipment, buildings), that come together to provide the desired service. In health care, inputs might be staff labor hours, number and skill mix of nursing staff, other staff needed for various services, technology, equipment, supplies used, and remodeling or building expenses (Porter-O'Grady & Malloch, 2011).

Linear—processes based on Newton's theory in which the environment is viewed as mechanistic and events are vertical and linear, compartmental, hierarchical, reductionistic, and controlling.

Outputs—result from the interaction of inputs in the throughput process. The output is the material, goods, and/or services produced. Outputs can be both qualitative and quantitative in health care. Reimbursement in health care is driven by the quantitative outputs or documented services produced by the system, regardless of the quality of the output or errors that might have occurred (Porter-O'Grady & Malloch, 2011).

Positive Deviance Method—a method to bring about improvements in an organization where those having different (deviant) practices/strategies that produce better (positive) outcomes share them with others.

Shared Governance—a structural team framework that affords nursing, and other disciplines, professional autonomy at the point of care.

Strange Attractor—"The activity of a collective chaotic system composed of interactive feedback between and among its various 'parts' and evidencing 'attraction' to its pattern of behavior" (Porter-O'Grady & Malloch, 2011, p. 14).

Throughputs—the processes or work that people do to achieve the output, the final product or service. In the healthcare system, throughputs are the patient care services provided to the patient and family. Throughput processes use the available inputs to create work processes (Malloch, 2011).

Value-Based Environment (second curve)—presently, reimbursement is changing to include organizational performance mandates. When protocols are not met, and when never events occur, insurers do not pay providers for the event or for the hospital stay. Reimbursement is value based.

Volume-Based Environment (first curve)—in the past, when reimbursement was determined by the volume of insured patients. Industrial Age organizational design was used.

References

Ackman, M., Steckel, C., Perry, L., Hill, C., & Wolfard, E. (2012). Changing nursing practice: Letting go of the nursing history on admission. *Journal of Nursing Administration, 42*(9), 435–441.

Ajeigbe, D., Leach, L., McNeese-Smith, D., & Phillips, L. (2013). Nurse–physician teamwork in the emergency department: Impact on perceptions of job environment, autonomy, and control over practice. *Journal of Nursing Administration, 43*(3), 142–148.

American Hospital Association 2011 Committee on Performance Improvement. (2011, September). *Hospitals and care systems of the future.* Chicago, IL: Author.

American Nurses Credentialing Center. (2013a). Announcing a new model for ANCC's Magnet Recognition Program. Retrieved from http://www.nursecredentialing.org/MagnetModel.aspx

American Nurses Credentialing Center. (2013b). Forces of magnetism. Retrieved from http://www.nursecredentialing.org/Magnet/ProgramOverview/HistoryoftheMagnetProgram/ForcesofMagnetism

American Nurses Credentialing Center. (2013c). Magnet Recognition Program model. Retrieved from http://www.nursecredentialing.org/Magnet/ProgramOverview/New-Magnet-Model

American Organization of Nurse Executives. (2004). *Principles and elements of a healthful practice/work environment.* Retrieved from http://www.aone.org/resources/leadership%20tools/PDFs/PrinciplesandElementsHealthfulWorkPractice.pdf

Autrey, P., Howard, J., & Wech, B. (2013). Sources, reactions, and tactics used by RNs to address aggression in an acute care hospital: A qualitative analysis. *Journal of Nursing Administration, 43*(3), 155–159.

Bacon, C., & Mark, B. (2009). Organizational effects on patient satisfaction in hospital medical-surgical units. *Journal of Nursing Administration, 39*(5), 220–227.

Ballard, N. (2010). Factors associated with success and breakdown of shared governance. *Journal of Nursing Administration, 40*(10), 411–416.

Bates, S. (2003, January/February). Creating a credible culture. *Nurse Leader,* 37–38.

Benham-Hutchins, M., & Clancy, T. (2010). Social networks as embedded complex adaptive systems. *Journal of Nursing Administration, 40*(9), 352–356.

Berkow, S., Workman, J., & Aronson, S. (2012). Strengthening frontline nurse investment in organizational goals. *Journal of Nursing Administration, 42*(3), 165–169.

Biron, A., Lavoie-Tremblay, M., & Loiselle, C. (2009). Characteristics of work interruptions during medication administration. *Journal of Nursing Scholarship, 41*(4), 330–336.

Bittner, N., Gravlin, G., Hansten, R., & Kalisch, B. (2011). Unraveling care omissions. *Journal of Nursing Administration, 41*(12), 510–512.

Blegen, M., Vaughn, T., Goode, C., Spetz, J., & Park, S. (2013). Baccalaureate education in nursing and patient outcomes. *Journal of Nursing Administration, 43*(2), 89–94.

Bleich, M., Hatcher, B., Cleary, B., Hewlett, P., Davis, K., & Hill, K. (2009). Mitigating knowledge loss: A strategic imperative for nurse leaders. *Journal of Nursing Administration, 39*(4), 160–164.

Block, P. (1993). *Stewardship.* San Francisco, CA: Berrett-Koehler.

Bohn, R. (2000). Stop fighting fires. *Harvard Business Review, 74*(4), 82–91.

Bourgault, A., King, M., Hart, P., Campbell, M., Swartz, S., & Lou, M. (2008). Circle of excellence: Does regular rounding by nursing associates boost patient satisfaction? *Nursing Management, 39*(11), 18–24.

Boyle, D., Gajewski, B., & Miller, P. (2012). A longitudinal analysis of nursing specialty certification by Magnet status and patient unit type. *Journal of Nursing Administration, 42*(12), 567–573.

Brewer, C., & Frazier, P. (1998). The influence of structure, staff type, and managed-care indicators on registered nurse staffing. *Journal of Nursing Administration, 28*(9), 28–36.

Brody, A., Ruble, C., Barnes, K., & Sakowski, J. (2012). Evidence-based practice councils: Potential path to staff nurse empowerment and leadership growth. *Journal of Nursing Administration, 42*(1), 28–33.

Cadmus, E. (2011). Your role in redesigning health care. *Nursing Management, 42*(10), 32–42.

Campbell, D., Fleming, R., & Grote, R. (1985, July–August). Discipline without punishment—at last. *Harvard Business Review,* 162–178.

Casanova, J., Hendricks, B., Day, K., Theis, L., Dorpat, D., & Wiesman, S. (2007). Nurse–physician work relations and role expectations. *Journal of Nursing Administration, 37*(2), 68–70.

Casida, J. (2008). Linking nursing unit's culture to organizational effectiveness: A measurement tool. *Nursing Economic$, 26*(2), 106–110.

Castner, J., Schwartz, D., Foltz-Ramos, K., & Cervolo, D. (2012). A leadership challenge: Staff nurse perceptions after an organizational team STEPPS initiative. *Journal of Nursing Administration, 42*(10), 467–472.

Chapman, E. (2004). *Radical loving care: Building the healing hospital in America.* Nashville, TN: Baptist Healing Hospital Trust.

Chinn, P. (2013). *Peace and power: New directions for building community* (8th ed.). Burlington, MA: Jones & Bartlett Learning.

Church, J., Baker, P., & Berry, D. (2008, April). Shared governance: A journey with continual mile markets. *Nursing Management,* 34–40.

Clancy, T. (2007a). Organizing: New ways to harness complexity. *Journal of Nursing Administration, 37*(12), 534–536.

Clancy, T. (2007b). Planning: What we can learn from complex systems. *Journal of Nursing Administration, 37*(10), 436–439.

Clancy, T. (2008a). Control: What we can learn from complex systems science. *Journal of Nursing Administration, 38*(6), 272–274.

Clancy, T. (2008b). Fractals: Nature's formula for managing hospital performance metrics. *Journal of Nursing Administration, 38*(12), 510–513.

Clancy, T. (2009a). Putting it altogether: Improving performance in heart failure outcomes. *Journal of Nursing Administration, 39*(6), 249–254.

Clancy, T. (2009b). Self-organization versus self-management: Two sides of the same coin? *Journal of Nursing Administration, 39*(3), 106–109.

Clancy, T. (2010). Positive deviance: An elegant solution to a complex problem. *Journal of Nursing Administration, 40*(4), 150–153.

Clancy, T. (2011a). Hitting your natural stride. *Journal of Nursing Administration, 41*(11), 443–445.

Clancy, T. (2011b). Improving processes through evolutionary optimization. *Journal of Nursing Administration, 41*(9), 340–342.

Clancy, T. (2012). Complexity and change in nurse workflows. *Journal of Nursing Administration, 42*(2), 78–82.

Clavelle, J. (2012). Implementing Institute of Medicine future of nursing recommendations: A model for transforming nurse practitioner privileges. *Journal of Nursing Administration, 42*(9), 404–407.

Collins, J., & Porras, J. (1994). *Built to last: Successful habits of visionary companies.* New York, NY: Harper Business.

Cornell, P., & Riordan, M. (2011). Barriers to critical thinking: Workflow interruptions and task switching among nurses. *Journal of Nursing Administration, 41*(10), 407–414.

Cornell, P., Riordan, M., & Herrin Griffith, D. (2010). Transforming nursing workflow, Parts 1 and 2: The chaotic nature of nurse activities & The impact of technology on nurse activities. *Journal of Nursing Administration, 40*(9,10), 366–373, 432–439.

Crawford, C., Omery, A., & Seago, J. (2012). The challenges of nurse–physician communication: A review of the evidence. *Journal of Nursing Administration, 42*(12), 548–550.

Cropley, S. (2012). The relationship-based care model: Evaluation of the impact on patient satisfaction, length of stay, and readmission rates. *Journal of Nursing Administration, 42*(6), 333–339.

Crow, G. (2003, March/April). Creativity and management in the 21st century. *Nurse Leader,* 32–35.

Curran, C. (2000). Musings on managerial excellence. *Nursing Economic$, 18*(6), 277, 322.

Curran, C. (2002). Culture eats strategy for lunch every time. *Nursing Economic$, 20*(6), 257.

de Bono, E. (1976). *Teaching thinking.* New York, NY: Penguin.

de Bono, E. (1994). *De Bono's thinking course* (Rev. ed.). New York, NY: Facts on File.

Dechairo-Marino, A., Jordan-Marsh, M., Traiger, G., & Saulo, M. (2001). Nurse/physician collaboration: Action research and the lessons learned. *Journal of Nursing Administration, 31*(5), 223–232.

Demir, D., & Rodwell, J. (2012). Psychosocial antecedents and consequences of workplace aggression for hospital nurses. *Journal of Nursing Scholarship, 44*(4), 376–384.

DiGioia, A., Bertoty, D., Lorenz, H., Rocks, S., & Greenhouse, P. (2010). A patient-centered model to improve metrics without cost increase: Viewing all care through the eyes of patients and families. *Journal of Nursing Administration, 40*(12), 540–546.

Ditomassi, M. (2012). A multi-instrument evaluation of the professional practice environment. *Journal of Nursing Administration, 42*(5), 266–272.

Doucette, J. (2003). Serving up uncommon service. *Nursing Management, 34,* 26–29.

Douglas, K. (2012). The return of the smiley face. *Nursing Economic$, 30*(2), 117, 119.

Drucker, P. (1999). Managing oneself. *Harvard Business Review, 77*(2), 65.

Dunbar, B., Park, B., Berger-Wesley, M., & Cameron, T. (2007). Shared governance: Making the transition in practice and perception. *Journal of Nursing Administration, 37*(4), 177–183.

Elganzouri, E., Standish, C., & Androwich, I. (2009). Medication Administration Time Study (MATS): Nursing staff performance of medication administration. *Journal of Nursing Administration, 39*(5), 204–210.

Erickson, J., Ditomassi, M., & Adams, J. (2012). Attending registered nurse: An innovative role to manage between the spaces. *Nursing Economic$, 30*(5), 282–287.

Erickson, J., Hamilton, G., Jones, D., & Ditomassi, M. (2003). The value of collaborative governance/staff empowerment. *Journal of Nursing Administration, 33*(2), 96–104.

Fisher, R., Ury, W., & Patton, B. (1991). *Getting to yes: Negotiating agreement without giving in.* New York, NY: Penguin.

Geary, S., Quinn, B., Cale, D., & Winchell, J. (2009). Daily rapid rounds: Decreasing length of stay and improving professional practice. *Journal of Nursing Administration, 39*(6), 293–298.

Gessler, R., Rosenstein, A., & Ferron, L. (2012). How to handle disruptive physician behaviors: Find out the best way to respond if you're the target. *American Nurse Today, 7*(11), 8–10.

Gibson, R. (2011). Making the trains run safely on time: How competent is the organization where you work? *Nursing Economic$, 29*(1), 46–47.

Gokenbach, V. (2007). Professional nurse councils: A new model to create excitement and improve value and productivity. *Journal of Nursing Administration, 37*(10), 440–443.

Goode, C., Vaughn, T., Blegan, M., Spetz, J., & Park, S. (2011). Comparison of patient outcomes in Magnet and non-Magnet hospitals. *Journal of Nursing Administration, 41*(2), 517–523.

Gordon, J. (2002). *Organizational behavior: A diagnostic approach* (7th ed.). Upper Saddle River, NJ: Prentice Hall.

Gravlin, G., & Bittner, N. (2010). Nurses' and nursing assistants' reports of missed care and delegation. *Journal of Nursing Administration, 40*(7/8), 329–335.

Hagberg, J. (2003). *Real power: Stages of personal power in organizations* (3rd ed.). Salem, WI: Sheffield.

Halbesleben, J., & Rathert, C. (2008). The role of continuous quality improvement and psychological safety in predicting workarounds. *Health Care Management Review, 33,* 134–133.

Halbesleben, J., Rathert, C., & Bennett, S. (2013). Measuring nursing workarounds: Tests of the reliability and validity of a tool. *Journal of Nursing Administration, 43*(1), 50–55.

Hall, L., Doran, D., & Pink, L. (2008). Outcomes of interventions to improve hospital nursing work environments. *Journal of Nursing Administration, 38*(1), 40–46.

Hall, L., Pedersen, L. C., & Fairley, L. (2010). Losing the moment: Understanding interruptions to nurses' work. *Journal of Nursing Administration, 40*(4), 169–176.

Hardin, D. (2012). Strategies for nurse leaders to address aggressive and violent events. *Journal of Nursing Administration, 42*(1), 5–8.

Havens, D., Warshawsky, N., & Vasey, J. (2012). The nursing practice environment in rural hospitals; practice environment scale of the nursing work index assessment. *Journal of Nursing Administration, 42*(11), 519–525.

Havens, D., Wood, S., & Leeman, J. (2006). Improving nursing practice and patient care: Building capacity with appreciative inquiry. *Journal of Nursing Administration, 36*(10), 463–470.

Health Research and Educational Trust. (2013, April). *Metrics for the second curve of health care.* American Hospital Association. Retrieved from http://www.hpoe.org/future-metrics-1to4

Heim, P. (1996). *Gender differences in the workplace series.* Videotapes produced by Cynosure productions, LTD.

Higdon, K., Woody, G., Clickner, D., Shirey, M., & Gray, F. (2012). Business case for Magnet in a small hospital. *Journal of Nursing Administration, 43*(2), 113–118.

Hill, K. (2006). Collaboration is a competency! *Journal of Nursing Administration, 36*(9), 390–392.

Houle, D., & Fleece, J. (2011). *The new health age: The future of health care in America.* New Health Age Publishing.

Houser, J., Ricker, F., ErkenBrack, L., Stroup, L., & Handberry, L. (2012). Involving nurses in decisions: Improving both nurse and patient outcomes. *Journal of Nursing Administration, 42*(7/8), 375–382.

Houston, S., Leveille, M., & Luquire, R. (2012). Decisional involvement in Magnet, Magnet-aspiring, and non-Magnet hospitals. *Journal of Nursing Administration, 42*(12), 586–591.

Huseman, R. (2009). The importance of positive culture in hospitals. *Journal of Nursing Administration, 39*(2), 60–63.

Institute of Medicine. (2011). *The future of nursing: Leading change, advancing health.* Washington, DC: National Academies Press.

Johnson, K., Johnson, C., Nicholson, D., Potts, C., Raiford, H., & Shelton, A. (2012). Make an impact with transformational leadership and shared governance. *Nursing Management, 43*(10), 12–14.

Johnson, S., & Rea, R. (2009). Workplace bullying: Concerns for nurse leaders. *Journal of Nursing Administration, 39*(2), 84–90.

Joseph, A. (2007). The impact of nursing on patient and organizational outcomes. *Nursing Economic$, 25*(1), 30–34.

Kalisch, B., Curley, M., & Stefanov, S. (2007). An intervention to enhance nursing staff teamwork and engagement. *Journal of Nursing Administration, 37*(2), 77–84.

Kalisch, B., & Lee, K. (2012). Congruence of perceptions among nursing leaders and staff regarding missed nursing care and teamwork. *Journal of Nursing Administration, 42*(10), 473–477.

Kalisch, B., & Williams, R. (2009). Development and psychometric testing of a tool to measure missed nursing care. *Journal of Nursing Administration, 39*(5), 211–219.

Kear, M., Duncan, P., Fansler, J., & Hunt, K. (2012). Nursing shared governance: Leading a journey of excellence. *Journal of Nursing Administration, 42*(6), 315–317.

Kelly, L., McHugh, M., & Aiken, L. (2011). Nurse outcomes in Magnet and non-Magnet hospitals. *Journal of Nursing Administration, 41*(10), 428–433.

Kerfoot, K. (2002). Messy conversations and the willingness to be disturbed. *Nursing Economic$, 10*(6), 297–299.

Kerfoot, K. (2006). Reliability between nurse managers: The key to the high-reliability organization. *Nursing Economic$, 24*(5), 274–275.

Kersey-Matusiak, G. (2012). Culturally competent care: Are we there yet? *Nursing Management, 43*(4), 334–339.

King, T., & Byers, J. (2007). A review of organizational culture instruments for nurse executives. *Journal of Nursing Administration, 37*(1), 21–31.

Knutson, L., Sidebottom, A., Johnson, P., & Fyfe-Johnson, A. (2013). Development of a hospital-based integrative healthcare program. *Journal of Nursing Administration, 43*(2), 101–107.

Kovner, C., Greene, W., Brewer, C., & Fairchild, S. (2009). Understanding new registered nurses' intent to stay at their jobs. *Nursing Economic$, 27*(2), 81–98.

Kramer, M., Donohue, M., Maguire, P., Ellsworth, M., Schmalenberg, C., Poduska, D., Andrews, B., Smith, M., Burke, R., Tachibana, C., & Chmielewski, L. (2007). Excellence through evidence: Structures enabling clinical autonomy. *Journal of Nursing Administration, 37*(1), 41–52.

Kramer, M., & Schmalenberg, C. (2003). Securing "good" nurse/physician relationships. *Nursing Management, 34*(7), 34–38.

Lalley, C. (2013). Work-arounds: A matter of perception. *Nurse Leader, 11*(2), 36–40.

Laschinger, H., Finegan, J., Shamian, J., & Almost, J. (2001). Testing Karasek's demands—control model in restructured healthcare settings: Effects of job strain on staff nurses' quality of work life. *Journal of Nursing Administration, 31*(3), 233–243.

Laschinger, H., Finegan, J., & Wilk, P. (2009). Context matters: The impact of unit leadership and empowerment on nurses' organizational commitment. *Journal of Nursing Administration, 39*(5), 228–235.

Laschinger, H., & Smith, L. (2013). The influence of authentic leadership and empowerment on new-graduate nurses' perceptions of interprofessional collaboration. *Journal of Nursing Administration, 43*(1), 24–29.

Lavin, P. (2013). Boots on the ground: The role of the Magnet project director. *Nursing Management, 44*(2), 50–52.

Lee, S., & Manley, B. (2008). Nurse director rounds to ensure service quality. *Journal of Nursing Administration, 38*(10), 435–440.

Lencioni, P. (2002a). *The five dysfunctions of a team.* San Francisco, CA: Jossey-Bass.

Lencioni, P. (2002b). Make your values mean something. *Harvard Business Review*, 113–117.

Lencioni, P. (2006). *Silos, politics and turf wars: A leadership fable about destroying the barriers that turn colleagues into competitors.* San Francisco, CA: Jossey-Bass.

Lindberg, C., Nash, S., & Lindberg, C. (2008). *On the edge: Nursing in the age of complexity.* Washington, DC: Plexus Press.

Longo, J., & Sherman, R. (2007). Leveling horizontal violence. *Nursing Management, 38*(3), 34–37, 50.

MacPhee, M. (2007). Strategies and tools for managing change. *Journal of Nursing Administration, 37*(9), 405–413.

Manojlovich, M., & Antonakos, C. (2008). Satisfaction of intensive care unit nurses with nurse–physician communication. *Journal of Nursing Administration, 38*(5), 237–243.

Marshall, D. (2008). Evidence-based management: The path to best outcomes. *Journal of Nursing Administration, 38*(3), 205–207.

Mauck, J., & Breitinger, A. (2012). Future of health care in America; what nurse leaders need to know about the shifting landscape. *Voice of Nursing Leadership, 11*(2), 8–9.

Mellott, J., Richards, K., Tonry, L., Bularzik, A., & Palmer, M. (2012). Translating caring theory into practice: A relationship-based care experience. *Nurse Leader, 10*(5), 44–45.

Meraviglia, M., Grobe, S., Tabone, S., & Wainwright, M. (2009). Creating a positive work environment; Implementation of the nurse-friendly hospital criteria. *Journal of Nursing Administration, 39*(2), 64–70.

Minnier, T., Brownlee, K., Kosko, R., Kowinsky, A., Martin, S., McLaughlin, M., Shovel, J., & Young, J. (2012). Reliable and variable rounder care delivery model for nursing assistants and patient care technicians. *Nurse Leader, 10*(5), 28–31.

Moore, S., & Hutchison, S. (2007). Developing leaders at every level: Accountability and empowerment actualized through shared governance. *Journal of Nursing Administration, 37*(12), 564–568.

Moore, S., & Wells, N. (2010). Staff nurses lead the way for improvement to shared governance structure. *Journal of Nursing Administration, 40*(11), 477–482.

Morjikian, R., Kimball, B., & Joynt, J. (2007). Leading change: The nurse executive's role in implementing new care delivery models. *Journal of Nursing Administration, 37*(9), 399–404.

Neville, K., Paul, D., Lake, K., Whitmore, K., & LeMunyon, D. (2012). Nurses' perceptions of patient rounding. *Journal of Nursing Administration, 42*(2), 83–88.

Newhouse, R. (2008). Evidence-based behavioral practice: An exemplar of interprofessional collaboration. *Journal of Nursing Administration, 38*(10), 414–416.

Newhouse, R., Colantuoni, E., Morlock, L., Johantgen, M., & Pronovost, P. (2009). Rural hospital nursing: Better environments = shared vision and quality/safety engagement. *Journal of Nursing Administration, 39*(4), 189–195.

Newhouse, R., Pronovost, P., Morlock, L., & Sproat, S. (2011). Rural hospital nursing: Results of a national survey of nurse executives. *Journal of Nursing Administration, 41*(3), 129–137.

Nobre, A. (2001). Soul + spirit + resources + leadership = results. *Journal of Nursing Administration, 31*(6), 287–289.

Nolan, R., Laam, L., Wary, A., Hallick, S., & King, M. (2011). Geisinger's proven care methodology: Driving performance improvement within a shared governance structure. *Journal of Nursing Administration, 41*(5), 226–230.

Novak, D., Dooley, S., & Clark, R. (2008). Best practices: Understanding nurses' perspectives. *Journal of Nursing Administration, 38*(10), 448–453.

Nutt, P. (1999). Surprising but true: Half the decisions in organizations fail. *Academy of Management Review, 13*(4), 75–90.

O'Hallaron, R. (2002, October). Letter to the editor: Corporate values. *Harvard Business Review*, 125.

Pati, D., Harvey, T., & Thurston, T. (2012). Estimating design impact on waste reduction: Examining decentralized nursing. *Journal of Nursing Administration, 42*(11), 513–518.

Pearson, A. E. (2002). Tough-Minded Ways to Get Innovative. *Harvard Business Review 80*(8), 117–124.

Pendry, P. (2007). Moral distress: Recognizing it to retain nurses. *Nursing Economic$, 25*(4), 217–221.

Pilette, P. (2006). Collaborative capital: Conversation for a change. *Nursing Management, 37*(11), 24–28.

Porter-O'Grady, T. (2003). Of hubris and hope: Transforming nursing for a new age. *Nursing Economic$, 21*(2), 59–64.

Porter-O'Grady, T. (2009). *Interdisciplinary shared governance: Integrating practice, transforming health care.* Sudbury, MA: Jones and Bartlett.

Porter-O'Grady, T., & Malloch, K. (2009). Leaders of innovation: Transforming postindustrial healthcare. *Journal of Nursing Administration, 39*(6), 245–248.

Porter-O'Grady, T., & Malloch, K. (2011). *Quantum leadership: Advancing innovations, transforming health care.* Burlington, MA: Jones & Bartlett Learning.

Reineck, C. (2007). Models of change. *Journal of Nursing Administration, 37*(9), 388–391.

Richards, J. (2001). Nursing in a digital age. *Nursing Economic$, 19*(1), 6–11, 34.

Rondinelli, J., Ecker, M., & Crawford, C. (2012). Hourly rounding implementation: A multisite description of structures, processes, and outcomes. *Journal of Nursing Administration, 42*(6), 326–332.

Rosenthal, L. (2013). Enhancing communication between night shift RNs and hospitalists: An opportunity for performance improvement. *Journal of Nursing Administration, 43*(2), 59–61.

Rundquist, J., & Givens, P. (2013). Quantifying the benefits of staff participation in shared governance: Organizations can save money and avoid costs by involving staff in the work of shared governance. *American Nurse Today, 8*(3), 38–42.

Rutan, V. (2003). The best of both worlds: A consideration of gender in team building. *Journal of Nursing Administration, 33*(3), 179–186.

Sayers, P. (2008). It's in the air: Census and weather. *Nursing Management, 39*(9), 29–31.

Scalise, D. (2006, November). The see-through hospital. *Hospital & Health Networks*, 34–40.

Schwartz, D., & Bolton, L. (2012). Leadership imperative: Creating and sustaining healthy workplace environments. *Journal of Nursing Administration, 42*(11), 499–501.

Scott, G. (2002, November/December). Coach, challenge, lead: Developing an indispensable management team. *Healthcare Executive*, 16–20.

Sellers, K., & Millenbach, L. (2012). The degree of horizontal violence in RNs practicing in New York state. *Journal of Nursing Administration, 42*(10), 483–487.

Senge, P. (2006). *The fifth discipline: The art and practice of the learning organization.* New York, NY: Doubleday/Currency.

Setia, N., & Meade, C. (2009). Bundling the value of discharge telephone calls and leader rounding. *Journal of Nursing Administration, 39*(3), 138–141.

Shaffer, D., Parker, K., Kantz, B., & Havens, D. (2013). The road less traveled. *Nursing Management, 44*(2), 26–31.

Shepard, L. (2013). Stop going in circles! Break the barriers to hourly rounding. *Nursing Management, 44*(2), 13–15.

Shermont, H., Mahoney, J., Krepcio, D., Baccari, S., Powers, D., & Yusah, A. (2008). Meeting of the minds: Ten-minute "huddles" offer nurses an opportunity to assess unit workflow and optimize patient care. *Nursing Management, 39*(8), 38–44.

Sherrod, B., Brown, R., Vroom, J., & Sulllivan, D. (2012). Round with purpose. *Nursing Management, 43*(1), 33–38.

Sherwood, G. (2003). Leadership for a healthy work environment: Caring for the human spirit. *Nurse Leader, 1*(5), 36–40.

Shirey, M. (2012a). Group think, organizational strategy, and change. *Journal of Nursing Administration, 42*(2), 67–71.

Shirey, M. (2012b). How resilient are your team members? *Journal of Nursing Administration, 42*(12), 551–553.

Singhai, A., Buscell, P., & Lindberg, C. (2010) *Inviting everyone: Healing health care through positive deviance.* Washington, DC: Plexus Press.

Smetzer, J., & Navarra, M. (2007). Measuring change: A key component of building a culture of safety. *Nursing Economic$, 25*(1), 49–51.

Smith, L. (2012). The recipe for success? Invest in your team: Containing costs while promoting quality care can be complex. Rise to the challenge! *Nursing Management, 43*(9), 46–48.

Squires, S. (2012). Patient satisfaction: How to get it and how to keep it. *Nursing Management, 43*(4), 26–31.

Storey, S., Linden, E., & Fisher, M. (2008). Showcasing leadership exemplars to propel professional practice model implementation. *Journal of Nursing Administration, 38*(3), 138–142.

Storfjell, J., Ohlson, S., Omoike, O., Fitzpatrick, T., & Wetasin, K. (2009). Non-value added time: The million dollar nursing opportunity. *Journal of Nursing Administration, 39*(1), 38–43.

Storfjell, J., Omoike, O., & Ohlson, S. (2008). The balancing act: Patient care time versus cost. *Journal of Nursing Administration, 38*(5), 244–249.

Thompson, D., Wold, G., Hoffman, L., Burns, H., Sereika, S., Minnier, T., Lorenz, H., & Ramanujam, R. (2011). A relational leadership perspective on unit-level safety climate. *Journal of Nursing Administration, 41*(11), 479–487.

Tonges, M., & Ray, J. (2011). Translating caring theory into practice: The Carolina care model. *Journal of Nursing Administration, 41*(9), 374–381.

Tortorella, F., Ray, R., Ukanowicz, D., Triller, M., & Douglas-Ntagha, P. (2013). Improving bed turnover time with a bed management system. *Journal of Nursing Administration, 43*(1), 37–43.

Toussaint, J., & Gerard, R., with Adams, E. (2010). *On the mend: Revolutionizing healthcare to save lives and transform the industry.* Cambridge, MA: Lean Enterprise Institute.

Trbovich, P., Prakash, V., & Stewart, J. (2010). Interruptions during the delivery of high-risk medications. *Journal of Nursing Administration, 40*(5), 211–218.

Trinkoff, P., Johantgen, M., Storr, C., Han, K., Liang, Y., Gurses, A., & Hopkinson, S. (2010). A comparison of working conditions among nurses in Magnet and non-Magnet hospitals. *Journal of Nursing Administration, 40*(7/80), 309–315.

Tuazon, N. (2008). Survivor guilt after downsizing. *Nursing Management, 39*(5), 19–23.

Ulrich, B., Norman, L., Buerhaus, P., Dittus, R., & Donelan, K. (2007). Magnet status and registered nurse views of the work environment and nursing as a career. *Journal of Nursing Administration, 37*(5), 212–220.

Upenieks, V., Needleman, J., & Soban, L. (2008). The relationship between the volume and type of transforming care at the bedside innovations and changes in nurse vitality. *Journal of Nursing Administration, 38*(9), 386–394.

Useem, M. (2001, October). The leadership lessons of Mount Everest. *Harvard Business Review*, 51–58.

Vartanian, H., Bobay, K., & Weiss, M. (2013). Nurses' perceptions of sustainability of Magnet efforts. *Journal of Nursing Administration, 42*(3), 166–171.

Vestal, K. (2012). When is it time for a turnaround? *Nurse Leader, 10*(5), 10–11.

Walrafen, N., Brewer, M., & Mulvenon, C. (2012). Sadly caught up in the moment: An exploration of horizontal violence. *Nursing Economic$, 30*(1), 6–13.

Warshawsky, N., Havens, D., & Knaft, G. (2012). The influence of interpersonal relationships on nurse managers' work engagement and proactive work behavior. *Journal of Nursing Administration, 42*(9), 418–425.

Watts, D. (2003, February). The science behind six degrees. *Harvard Business Review*, 16–17.

Weiss. K. (2001). *Organizational behavior and change* (2nd ed.). Cincinnati, OH: South-Western College Publishing.

Wellins, R., Byham, W., & Wilson, J. (1991). *Empowered teams: Creating self-directed work groups that improve quality, productivity and participation.* San Francisco, CA: Jossey-Bass.

Wheatley, M. (1999). *Leadership and the new science: Discovering order in a chaotic world.* San Francisco, CA: Berrett-Koehler.

Wilson, B., & Diedrich, A. (2011). Bullies at work: The impact of horizontal hostility in the hospital setting and intent to leave. *Journal of Nursing Administration, 41*(11), 453–458.

Wolf, G. (2012). Transformational leadership: The art of advocacy and influence. *Journal of Nursing Administration, 42*(6), 309–310.

Zimmerman, B., Lindberg, C., & Plsek, P. (2008). *Edgeware: Lessons from complexity science for health care leaders.* Irving, TX: VHA, Inc.

Zolli, A., & Healy, A. (2012). *Resilience: Why things bounce back.* New York, NY: Free Press.

Providing Value-Based Service

Now that we have discussed the importance of both effective leadership and achieving change in organizations along with the importance of working as part of a team, we need to get to the basics—the main reason we exist—our patients. *What does each patient value?* Is this what we are providing? This is so important that we devoted a separate section to providing value-based services. As previously noted, this is first priority, not the bottom line.

Chapter 4 is concerned with how to best support patients being the leader in their care. To do this, we need to find out and provide only what patients value within a safe environment. In healthcare settings, we have not always stressed the importance of listening to our patient to find out what he or she wants and needs. Also, we must give our patient information so that he or she can make the best decisions on needed care.

The old patriarchal system where we made decisions for the patient, and many times did not tell our patients what would happen, is outdated. Along with this, we, as nurses, need to get out of the "task" box and become leaders to make sure that patients are receiving only what they really want. So, this new perspective—listening to the patient, providing information, and having the patient make the care decisions—is *so* important. Then, as leaders, we support the patient decisions.

Chapter 4 also includes information on both quality and patient safety. This is more familiar territory for a nurse. Nurses understand more about quality and patient safety than our patients do. This is another aspect of leadership needed at the point of care.

We are still harming too many patients in our healthcare systems. We would never choose an airline with that kind of record! So, why should patients choose our services? In fact, many patient safety issues are caused by a series of events or organizational processes that are broken. It is time to fix these problems and processes and leave blame behind (after all, we are all human, and chances are, one person alone did not cause the problem). Every single one of us needs to do everything in our power to ensure quality service and patient safety.

As we provide care patients value in a safe environment, chances are we *healthcare providers have a knowledge deficit*—it is not possible to keep up with all the current treatments, drugs, and research results that could improve our practice and benefit our patients. There is so much information that no one can keep track of it all. Now that we are in the Information Age, this research evidence is not a big secret anymore. Yet research indicates that caregivers—both physicians and nurses—tend to go on doing what we were taught in school (sacred cows), even though evidence-based best practices have been identified that should change our practices.

Chapter 5 is devoted to evidence-based practice. Here, we are shown how easy it is to access information.

> *Evidence-based practice* is analyzing the research available as critically as possible, placing the findings in the context of your organization, and adding the perspectives and judgment of clinicians and patients. (Russell-Babin, 2009, p. 27)

Many nurses are not very computer literate. Thus, the dedicated librarians in Chapter 5 show us how to find evidence-based information as we need it (using the just-in-time concept). *This is a must-read chapter for all healthcare professionals.*

Chapter 5, however, has a much broader focus than just identifying the best clinical care for our patients. *Evidence-based administrative and educational information is available to help us more effectively manage and lead the healthcare team.* Finding information on the latest administrative/educational evidence can be very helpful as we work on various issues each day. We note here that we have sprinkled administrative evidence throughout this book. However, it is important to continuously find new information on best practices for clinicians, for administrators, and for educators.

Reference

Russell-Babin, K. (2009, November). Seeing through the clouds. *Nursing Management*, *27*(11), 27–33.

Providing Patient Value While Achieving Quality, Safety, and Cost-Effectiveness

Sandy K. Diffenderfer, PhD, MSN, RN, CPHQ, Janne Dunham-Taylor, PhD, RN, Karen W. Snyder, MSN, RN, and, Dru Malcolm, DNP, MSN, RN, NEA-BC, CPHRM

OBJECTIVES

- Articulate the goal of quality patient care.
- Explain the four most important hospital strategies to be implemented to prepare for value-based payments.
- Describe administrative practices that support performance improvement efforts.
- Analyze the nurse administrator's role in patient safety.
- Propose ways that nurse administrators can promote evidence-based practice.
- Synthesize how nurse administrators can promote patient value while achieving quality, safety, and cost-effectiveness.

The most important priority in all healthcare settings is to determine what the patient wants and values; to provide safe, loving, quality care; and to constantly improve care delivery and continuity across the continuum in a cost-effective way. This is true for staff and physicians at the point of care and for administrators in all decisions and actions.

Introduction

This is a demanding goal! Thankfully, at times this is achieved. When this goal is met the patient and caregivers recognize that it was worth the effort. As healthcare payments are transformed from volume-based to value-based reimbursement over the next decade (American Hospital Association 2011 Committee on Performance Improvement [AHA], 2011), this goal *must* be met. A compelling book, *Radical Loving Care: Building the Healing Hospital in America* (Chapman, 2004), provides some answers regarding ways to achieve this goal.

The Malcolm Baldrige Quality Award criteria (National Institute of Standards and Technology [NIST], 2013) recognize that "patients and other customers are the ultimate judges of performance and quality" (p. 37). To date, 12 healthcare organizations have been awarded the Malcolm Baldrige National Quality Award since the gold standard *Criteria for Performance Excellence* was broadened to health care in 1998 (NIST, 2012). This is important because there is a link between top-performing hospitals that use the criteria and successful operations, management practices, and overall performance (NIST, 2012). Although this reference is related to hospitals, the principles apply to long-term care, home care, ambulatory care, and primary care settings. We return to this goal after a discussion of the contemporary healthcare environment and some of the problems that have surfaced.

There are four significant challenges and related goals confronting contemporary health care (**Exhibit 4–1**):

1. **To habitually determine what our patient/client/resident wants and values**. Healthcare workers often miss the goal related to this challenge. Many individuals in health care do not know how to discover what the patient wants and values. Often, workers are focused only on the current care setting rather than continuity across the continuum. Determining what the patient wants and values needs to be assessed by staff at the point of care. In addition, everyone in the organization from board members and the chief executive officer (CEO) to the nurse aide and housekeeper should make regular rounds to speak and interact with patients to determine whether their needs are being met. Often healthcare workers are not good listeners; active listening must begin with those in administrative roles because executive leaders set the tone for the organization.

   Thus far, healthcare leaders have not clearly identified how to determine what the patient wants and values, and the current quantitative outcome measures do not capture whether this goal has been accomplished. Instead, healthcare measures focus on patient satisfaction scores, complications, financial ratios, and/or staffing or turnover metrics—none of which captures whether the patient

---

Exhibit 4–1   Four Significant Challenges in Health Care

1. To habitually determine what our patient/client/resident wants and values
2. To provide the very best quality care, once we know what the patient wants and values
3. To keep our patient/client/resident safe
4. To accomplish the first three challenges in a cost-effective way

got what was wanted or valued. The core principle of patient care quality is to determine what the patient wants and values and to make the patient the leader of his or her care. These are misunderstood principles. Thus, a section of this chapter is devoted to patient values; see the section titled "Our First Priority: Discovering What the Patient Wants and Values" later in this chapter.

2. **To provide the very best quality care, once we know what the patient wants and values**. Care that is provided must take into account what the patient wants and values while collectively using the nurses' professional judgment along with evidence-based care. When discussing the importance of evidence-based care, O'Grady (2009) points out a paradox that must be acknowledged: "The idea is that all of health care can be delivered with an evidence-base, yet we have no metrics on some of the more compelling aspects of nursing, such as therapeutic presence" (p. 337). Thus, nurses in collaboration with patients and the healthcare team need to determine and measure therapeutic presence. What we believe is quality care may be at odds with what the patient wants and values. Quality, as measured by the patient, is the focus of this chapter. Nevertheless, healthcare providers must be cognizant of their patient advocacy and teaching responsibilities because the patient may not be aware of quality and safety standards.

3. **To keep our patient/client/resident safe**. To accomplish this, everyone in health care must constantly consider ways to improve safety. Healthcare organizations and systems are complex. As the complexity of healthcare delivery increased, bureaucracies were formed. The complexity has resulted in increased healthcare errors. Our goal is to simplify our organizational environment by carefully examining what we do to determine whether these activities reflect the organization's mission and values. This means that everyone is a leader, especially the staff nurse and nurse aide, who make 90% of their work decisions at the point of patient care. These leaders continuously make small incremental changes as they interact with each patient and determine the need for change. Thus, it is important that administrators recognize, value, and support leaders at the point of care, and for administrators to be a part of the *patient care team*.

    The 2013–2014 Malcolm Baldrige *Healthcare Criteria for Performance Excellence* (NIST, 2013) emphasizes the

    > "voice of the customer" . . . process for capturing patient- and other customer-related information. . . . Processes are intended to be proactive and continuously innovative so that they capture . . . customers' stated, unstated, and anticipated requirements, expectations, and desires. The goal is customer engagement. (p. 13)

    In order to hear the "voice of the customer" (NIST, 2013, p. 13), administrators and staff must commit to routine patient rounds because these listening opportunities are recognized as the most important way to speak and interact with patients to determine whether their needs are being met. When problems are identified, the issues are recognized as critical opportunities to simplify the patient environment and make it safer. Interdisciplinary shared governance and the accompanying complex communication are essential to hear the "voice of the customer" (NIST, 2013, p. 13) and keep patients safe. Safety is also related to contemporary workforce management practices, such as nurse managers with responsibility for more than 35 to 50 full-time equivalents (FTEs) on open units, inadequate staffing especially during peak times, and 12-hour shifts. These practices have resulted in an increase in errors that result in poorer patient outcomes and reimbursement.

4. **To accomplish the first three challenges in a cost-effective way**. Cost-effectiveness is listed fourth because it should never be given a higher priority than the previous three goals. As stated in other discussions, "If we do what is right for the patients, financial well-being will follow." The bottom

line is never the first priority. To accomplish this goal financial information needs to be transparent across the organization because staff at the point of care must understand costs to complete delivery of care in the most cost-effective way. Because ineffective leadership is linked to poorer outcomes and reimbursement, it is important to nurture a positive interdisciplinary culture throughout the organization (negative cultures also are linked with poorer outcomes and reimbursement). Everyone in the organization needs to make decisions based on the organization's mission and values—what is best for patients—with the bottom line always being second.

We Have a L-O-N-G Way to Go to Fix Our Healthcare System

In the emerging age, a large part of the leadership role will involve facilitating the transition to a new way of living and working. Leaders will increasingly devote their energies to helping others adapt the new rules for thriving in the world of work.

—T. Porter-O'Grady and K. Malloch, *Quantum Leadership: Advancing Innovation, Transforming Health Care*

There are major healthcare problems in the United States. According to the World Health Organization (WHO, 2013), in 2011 the United States spent more per capita ($8,607.88) on health care than any other country. This is compared to the Central African Republic, which spent $30.90 per capita on health care in 2011 (WHO, 2013). Storfjell and associates (2008) state, "The United States has the highest health care costs in the world, *with third world outcomes*" (p. 244). In addition, the Commonwealth Fund (2013) reported that the 2011 *National Scorecard on U.S. Health System Performance,* which assessed health and health care in the United States based on quality, access, efficiency, and equity, assigned the United States a score of 52 out of a possible score of 100. This is far short of what is attainable considering the U.S. per capita expenditure on health care.

Care is often fragmented and depersonalized. Unintentional harm to patients is common. At times, the patient's condition becomes worse rather than better—or the patient dies when he or she comes in contact with healthcare workers. Patients' needs and values are often not considered in the plan of care. This is compounded by the 2011 statistic that 18.2% of the U.S. population was uninsured (Centers for Disease Control and Prevention [CDC], 2013). Over the next several years, as the Patient Protection and Affordable Care Act (PPACA; U.S. Government Printing Office, 2010) is implemented, many of these individuals will have health insurance; nevertheless, some individuals, for example, migrant workers, will remain uninsured. How these newly insured people will afford the cost has not been determined, nor has it been determined how the United States will finance health insurance for individuals who are up to 400% over the poverty level. An increase in our taxes has already occurred. Considering deficits in federal and state budgets, the outcome remains unknown.

Preparing for the future state of health care requires leadership, planning, and change management. In their seminal work *Hospitals and Care Systems of the Future* (AHA, 2011), the authors outlined 10 must-do strategies that hospitals must implement in preparation for the future value-based market dynamic, termed the "second curve" (p. 3). An organizational culture of performance improvement, accountability, and quality is critical to implementation of these strategies (AHA, 2011). The entrenched hierarchal, patriarchal culture that continues to thrive in the U.S. healthcare system will change in organizations that remain viable. Nevertheless, organizational culture develops over time and is resistant to change. What is needed are transformational change agent leaders who understand the complex nature of the healthcare system.

"Understanding complexity is a requisite for understanding relationships. Complexity science teaches us that everything is related at some level" (Porter-O'Grady & Malloch, 2011, p. 43). Complexity change agents refute the traditional assumptions of organization change that envision organizations as machines (Crowell, 2011). The complexity view of the leader/change agent recognizes that change starts with those closest to the work of the organization, efficiency does not come from control, and that prediction is not possible (Crowell, 2011). Leaders who will be successful in navigating the turbulent coming years in healthcare recognize that improvements are emergent, not hierarchical. Examples of emergent patterns include structure, culture, and behavioral norms (Crowell, 2011). According to Porter-O'Grady and Malloch (2011), "We witness emergence any time individuals come together and accomplish more than what was thought possible. The collective wisdom and creativity of individuals seldom disappoint us" (p. 90). Successful leaders/change agents may be at any level of the organization or even outside the organization; nevertheless, they recognize how and when to influence the system toward self-organization. Although incremental improvements are positive and need to continue, the entire healthcare system must change to meet the challenges of the upcoming healthcare reality.

Of the 10 strategies set forth by the AHA (2011), 4 are identified as major priorities. The underpinnings for all four of these strategies are concomitant with quality and value. The first priority addresses the need for seamless patient care across the continuum (AHA, 2011). Whereas all members of the healthcare team are involved in implementation of this priority, it is recognized that nurses play a key role in patient continuity of care, including patient education and communication. As the focus of health care transitions to value across the continuum of care, the role of nurses, nurse practitioners, and case managers will come to the forefront. This priority is also linked to priority 2, second-curve metrics, "Utilizing evidenced-based [*sic*] practice to improve quality and patient safety" (p. 4) because the expectation is measurement and management of care transitions (AHA, 2011).

The second priority set forth by the AHA (2011) proclaims the use of evidence-based practice to improve quality and safety. In addition to measurement and management of care transitions, second-curve metrics related to this priority include the following:

> Management of utilization variation
> Preventable admissions, readmission, ED visits, and mortality
> Reliable patient care processes
> Active patient engagement in design and improvement (AHA, 2011, p. 4)

Most contemporary nurse leaders have experienced the challenge of linear measurement models such as those described earlier (Porter-O'Grady & Malloch, 2011). Nevertheless, successful nurse leaders recognize the potential for integration of complexity principles into such measurement models and are positioned to lead change related to current measurement assumptions to create models that reflect the complex nature of healthcare delivery (Porter-O'Grady & Malloch, 2011). Because leaders are duty bound to ensure regulatory compliance—especially considering value-based purchasing mandates—measurement models must include industry standards and measures that reflect the mission, values, and context of the organization as well as what the patient wants and values.

The third priority identified by the AHA (2011) is improved efficiency. It is well known that unnecessary operational inefficiency is a significant source of healthcare costs. Fortunately, healthcare workers have some control over this dynamic (de Koning, Verver, van den Heuvel, Bisgaard, & Does, 2006). This priority is a familiar one; nevertheless, robust performance improvement work must continue using methods such as such as Lean Thinking and Six Sigma to increase productivity and improve financial management. These methods (discussed later in this chapter) can be combined to provide a framework for systematic improvements in health care (de Koning et al., 2006). A reliable quality-driven organizational framework for obtaining distinction is the Baldrige *Healthcare Criteria for Performance Excellence* because the focus is on a systems perspective to achieve organizational alignment (NIST, 2013). It is important here to point out that there is tension among professionals in regard to the best approach to improving quality, specifically whether an incremental approach or a systems approach is most effective. It is our opinion that both approaches are needed to survive in the ever-changing healthcare environment.

The final top priority for hospitals in preparation for the value-based market is the development of integrated information systems (AHA, 2011). Technological advances contribute significantly to the increasing cost of care. However, it is evident that data must be readily available for analysis and improvement work. Regardless of what happens financially, *health care will change*! At this point, if you need an uplifting experience, read Bargmann's (2002) "The Top Hospital in America: The Heart and Soul of a Great Medical Center."

Patient Safety Issues

The priority for quality improvement work is always to provide a safe environment. The focus is to design quality and safety into our processes. The focus on safety is evident because publications about patient safety are published daily. For example, the Leapfrog Group (2013) published recommended "leaps" that organizations should take that promote quality. The recommendations include: (1) implementing computerized physician order entry (CPOE), (2) having an electronic health record (EHR) (also called electronic medical record [EMR]), (3) implementing intensive care unit staffing with physicians experienced in critical care medicine, and (4) attaining a high Leapfrog Safe Practices score. The safe practices score measures the organization's progress in meeting and implementing the safe practices endorsed by the National Quality Forum that are aimed at reducing the risk of harm in certain processes, systems, or environments of care (Leapfrog Group, 2013). It is estimated that if all hospitals implemented the first three leaps, "over 57,000 lives could be saved, more than 3 million medications errors could be avoided, and up to $12.0 billion could be saved" (para. 3) annually. Again, focusing on prevention of human pain and suffering is the priority.

In a groundbreaking report, the Institute of Medicine (IOM, 1999) estimated that as many as 98,000 hospital deaths per year were the result of avoidable medical errors. The landmark study noted that hospital medical errors were the eighth leading cause of death in the United States. These statistics did not take into account errors that may have occurred in the vast array of other healthcare settings. This report startled the healthcare community and consumers to action, yet authors noted in a 2005 follow-up report that progress toward improved patient safety was slow (Leape & Barwick, 2005). In 2007, the IOM published findings from a workshop, Creating a Business Case for Quality Improvement Research. This report acknowledged a "reluctance to invest in quality improvement" (p. 1) throughout the country. Resources are limited and tend to be spent on "highly visible technology-driven programs" (IOM, 2007, p. 1). Although technology can improve systems, it is not the single answer to a safer healthcare system.

The Eighth Annual HealthGrades Patient Safety in American Hospitals Study (Reed & May, 2011) reported that from 2007 through 2009:

- There were 708,642 identified patient safety events. This is daunting considering that only 13 potential patient safety indicators were evaluated in the study, and thus this number represents only a small portion of total patient safety events.

- Based on the total hospitalized Medicare patients, 1.6% experienced one or more patient safety events.
- Patient safety events cost Medicare nearly $7.3 billion and resulted in 79,670 potentially preventable deaths.
- One in 10 surgical patients died following serious, but treatable complications.
- A total of 52,127 Medicare patients developed a nosocomial acquired bloodstream infection, of these patients, 8,114 died. Nosocomial acquired bloodstream infections cost the federal government approximately $1.2 billion.
- If all hospitals performed at the level of top ranked facilities, approximately 174,358 patient safety events and 20,688 deaths could have been avoided, saving the federal government $1.8 billion.

These authors noted that preventable medical errors are so prevalent and expensive that selected indicators will be part of a hospital's performance score for the value-based incentive plan. The Hospital Value-Based Purchasing Program, which was established by the Patient Protection and Affordable Care Act of 2010 (U.S. Government Printing Office, 2010), represented the first time that U.S. hospitals were paid for inpatient service based on quality rather than quantity. Beginning in fiscal year 2013, Medicare made incentive payments to hospitals based on how well they performed on 12 clinical measures and 8 measures based on patients' experiences or based on improvement of the measures compared to their baseline (CMS, 2011). Although the definitions of several of the indicators in the study were changed from the previous report, it is clear that patient safety events remain a problem in U.S. hospitals (Reed & May, 2011). The *most important issue* is human pain, suffering, and loss and death related to these preventable events. The healthcare system must be fixed.

Additional provisions of the Patient Protection and Affordable Care Act were designed to improve care while decreasing costs. For example, beginning in 2013, hospitals will receive a reduction in payment for excessive 30-day readmissions for myocardial infarctions, heart failure, and pneumonia (Centers for Medicare & Medicaid Services, 2011).

Being proactive, preventing patient safety events is important. However, when mistakes occur, administrators must react from the complexity, "no blame" perspective rather than from the patriarchal Industrial Age view. The traditional approach to patient safety violations was to identify what an individual practitioner did wrong. Serious errors resulted in occurrences being "reported to the board for disciplinary investigation because of an error or breach in the standards of safe practice" (Woods & Doan-Johnson, 2002, p. 45). Many facilities have adopted "no-blame" policies rather than focusing on blame and punishment.

There are two issues here. First, assigning blame encourages individuals to hide or to not report errors. Second, even when one individual made the error, upon critical examination, usually there are underlying process problems. Most often there are multiple factors that caused the error. Administrators must consider the most important issue about errors—what can be done to prevent the error from occurring again?

A more effective solution is to report the error and undertake a root cause analysis to determine what process changes—or patterns or trends—occurred that provide clues for needed changes. Medical errors usually involve more than one individual and require a systems approach to find solutions. Usually, an organizational systems process went wrong or a better process needs to be implemented. Administrators must establish systems to prevent reoccurrence. A systems approach is best.

Establishing a just or blame-free culture is critical if organizations are to focus on process and system improvements rather than assigning blame. Without the occasion for open discussion, many opportunities for improvement are hidden or go unreported because team members are fearful of losing their jobs or getting into trouble. To this end, the problem will reoccur.

Creating a just culture begins with executive leaders and must be reinforced each time an incident occurs. Administrators must be informed. Being informed starts with personal continuing education. The Institute for Healthcare Improvement (IHI, 2011c) toolkit Strategies for Leadership: Hospital Executives and Their Role in Patient Safety provides a checklist of actions that executives and leaders should use to establish a just culture. Once informed, it is important that administrators role model expected behaviors, speak publicly about safety, set expectations, establish policy, and personally participate in significant event root cause analyses.

Another important source for patient safety opportunities is the organization's incident reports or variance reports. Healthcare risk managers have used these tools for years; nevertheless, the information provided in these reports needs to be used more effectively. Incident or variance reports are traditionally used to alert risk managers of potential litigation. The risk manager's role has historically been to identify, manage, and reduce risk to support the delivery of safe health care while reducing organizational legal risks. Most risk management activities occur after an incident; thus, these functions are not the best way to achieve safe care. Nevertheless, administrators need to pay particular attention to these resources because these reports provide valuable information regarding organizational issues that need to be resolved to ensure patient safety.

An emerging role in health care is the patient safety officer. This position promotes safety through education; examination of issues to determine better, safer organizational processes; discovering the root cause; creating system changes to prevent future incidents of the same kind; and involvement in implementing programs designed to foster safety. The IHI (2011a) recommends that this role be part of the executive team in the organization and be solely dedicated to patient safety with no overlapping duties. The patient safety officer works closely with risk management personnel to discover the root cause of patient safety events and create system changes to facilitate a safer environment.

Medication Errors

The IOM released a report in 2006 on prevention of medication errors. The research discovered that "a hospital patient can expect on average to be subjected to more than one medication error each day" (p. 1). This is a frightening statistic. Errors occurred in every step of the medication process, but more occurred during prescribing and administration. Experts estimate that error rates are actually higher than the numbers reported. One of the studies cited in the report documented an additional cost of $8,750 per hospital stay for each adverse drug event. IOM (2004a) reported in an earlier study that "two hospitals over a 6-month period found that nurses were responsible for intercepting 86 percent of all medication errors made by physicians, pharmacists, and others involved in providing medications for patients before the error reached the patient" (p. 3). The IOM (2006) asserts that most of the errors and the additional costs were preventable.

The risks of adverse drug events are higher for nursing home patients. Garcia (2006) predicted that nearly "two thirds of nursing facility residents will experience an adverse drug event over a 4-year period of time, with 1 in 7 of these residents requiring hospitalization" (p. 306). Simonson and Feinberg (2005), in extensive work reviewing the medication issues in elderly adults, identified that one-half of adverse drug events in nursing home facilities are preventable.

Caution is advised related to computerized provider order entry (CPOE). Although electronic health records, which include CPOE and clinical decision support (CDS), have improved some aspects of patient safety (Agency for Healthcare Research and Quality [AHRQ], n.d.), Wetterneck and associates (2011) reported an increase in duplicate medication order errors following implementation of CPOE and CDS. These researchers identified improved communication, teamwork, and CPOE usability and functionality as approaches to reducing such errors. This is important because electronic health records are expensive and technology is often viewed as a fail-safe way to prevent medication errors. Medication administration is a complicated process; most errors are system errors rather than user errors. Healthcare leaders need to monitor and analyze medication errors carefully because identified problems may warrant the time and expense of a performance improvement (PI) team.

Healthcare-Associated Nosocomial Infections

Healthcare-associated nosocomial infections continue to be an issue in organizations across the country. Healthcare-associated infections that occurred in U.S. hospitals were estimated at 1.7 million and were associated with approximately 99,000 deaths (Klevens et al., 2007). Scott (2009) estimates the range of overall annual direct medical costs of hospital-associated infections as between $28.4 billion and $33.8 billion. Scott estimated the range for the cost benefits of prevention as $5.7 billion to $6.8 billion (low) to $25.0 billion to $31.5 billion (high). Reed and May (2011) reported that hospital-acquired bloodstream infections among hospitalized Medicare patients for the period of 2007 to 2009 were serious and costly. According to the researchers' report, hospitalized Medicare patients acquired 52,127 bloodstream infections, 8,114 patients died, and the cost to the federal government was an estimated $1.22 billion. Again, the *most important issue* is human pain, suffering, and loss and death, related to these preventable events. The healthcare system must be fixed. *Methicillin-resistant Staphylococcus aureus*, or MRSA, has reached endemic levels in hospitals and long-term care facilities, and rates continue to rise. The increasing numbers of patients with healthcare-associated infections provide evidence that *healthcare workers are not following the basic preventive measures—good hand hygiene.*

Nevertheless, complexity theory provides an underpinning for approaching such dearth. Crowell (2011) describes complexity science as "nonlinear, dynamic, often uncertain, and very much relationship-based" (p. 3). The focus needs to be bottom-up rather than top-down management. Lindberg and Clancy (2010) propose that within organizations some individuals or groups have different "deviant" practices that produce better "positive" (p. 152) outcomes. *Positive deviance* holds that staff at the point of care are best equipped to solve the problem. The job is to discover positive deviant practices, and then through widespread engagement spread these best practices throughout the organization and system. Positive deviance is a potentially dramatic breakthrough related to the culture of change for hospitals. An increasing number of hospitals are using this philosophy to solve the problem of MRSA (AHC Media, 2008).

Falls

Falls among older adults (age 65 and older) continue to be a safety issue. Falls are the leading cause of death among older adults, and the death rate from falls for this group has increased over the past ten years. In 2009, 20,400 people 65 and older died from injuries from unintentional falls. In 2010, 2.3 million people 65 and older were treated in emergency departments (EDs) for nonfatal injuries from falls and more than 662,000 of these patients were hospitalized (CDC, 2012). In the report of their study, Stevens, Corso, Finkelstein, and Miller (2006) estimated the direct costs of falls was $19.2 billion per year, while the CDC (2012) estimated that the direct medical costs of falls in 2010 alone was $30.0 billion. These figures to do include subsequent long-term care costs or loss of quality of life.

The Institute for Healthcare Improvement (IHI, 2013a) reported that patient falls are the most prevalent adverse events in hospitals. Of upmost concern is that " . . . injuries from falls are often associated with morbidity and mortality" (IHI, 2013a, para 1). Research suggests an increasing risk of falls with lower nurse staffing levels (Whitman, Kim, Davidson, Wolf, & Wang, 2002).

Missed Care

Missed care is distressing to nurses, but most important these omissions can result in patient morbidity and mortality. The omission of simple, yet missed vital care tasks such as turning, ambulating, feeding, mouthcare, and toileting can lead to patient complications, for example, decubitus ulcers and pneumonia. Although the patient is always the priority, pay-for-performance/value-based purchasing, described later in this chapter, emphasizes the significant reimbursement ramifications of these two complications alone. It is important to acknowledge that nurses must be accountable for the patient care they provide.

Accountability includes an advocacy role for the nursing team and patients. It is unacceptable to complain about poor staffing or other problems in the care environment and do nothing to improve the situation. For example, despite years of efforts to improve healthcare quality including Lean (discussed later in this chapter) and Transforming Care at the Bedside (IHI, 2013b) (which was launched as a way to improve care of medical/surgical units), the literature does not support a direct relationship between these quality practices—touted to transform ineffective processes and standardize work—and *the time nurses spend at the bedside* (Brackett, Comer, & Whichello, 2013). To the contrary, the focus on quality efforts and using fewer resources has resulted in nurses spending more time *away* from patients (Brackett et al., 2013). This is a distressing report and certainly nurses are not to blame.

Nevertheless, nurses cannot abandon efforts to improve quality and safety; however, leaders can use complexity theory to adapt to the natural aspects of life within the healthcare system. Missed care may be related to poor professional nurses' delegation skills or failure to properly supervise assigned care. When opportunities to improve are identified, real-time corrections must be made. Or, if the issue is more complex, follow-through is needed to determine next steps; improve and sustain the gains; and never give in to complacency because "that is just the way it is." Regardless of the method used to improve quality, the complex nature of health care mandates a culture change in which all healthcare workers make safety the priority focus every day and in all settings.

Non-Value-Added Time

The report of Storfjell and colleagues (2008) of excessive amounts of nursing time being spent on support activities and the resultant waste of $1 million in annual nurse salaries per unit (Storfjell, Ohlson, Omoike, Fitzpatrick, & Wetasin, 2009) reflects the need for PI work. Cookson and associates (2011) described the seven Lean wastes as waiting, overproduction, rework/defects, motion, (over) processing, inventory, and transportation, all of which were reported by Storfjell and colleagues (2008).

Healthcare leaders have embraced *Lean thinking*, which originated with Toyota Motor Corporation in the 1950s, as a way to improve processes by removing non-value-added steps or waste (Radnor, Holweg, & Waring, 2012). It is an effective method for identifying and eliminating non-value-added time. In fact, the aims of Toyota's production system are to reduce *non-value-adding work*, overburden (which applies here to nurses), and unevenness of flow (Cookson et al., 2011).

Radnor and associates (2012) describe Lean improvement activities such as rapid improvement events (RIEs) or "kaizen blitz" (p. 365)—held over 3 to 5 days—in which staff evaluate, develop, and redesign identified processes followed by monitoring to measure whether the gains are sustained. These RIEs tend to produce small-scale localized gains rather than systemwide approaches, which are seen in manufacturing (Radnor, Holweg, and Waring, 2012). Lean is discussed in more detail later in this chapter.

Interruptions

Interruptions in the work environment are frequently occurring safety issues. When the work of nurses is interrupted, errors occur and efficiency is decreased (Biron, Lavoie-Tremblay, & Loiselle, 2009; Trbovich, Prakash, & Stewart, 2010). An example of process improvement that decreased the frequency of inter-ruptions during medication administration involved the use of red aprons (Relihan, O'Brien, O'Hara, & Silke, 2010) or sashes (Pape, 2008) worn by the medication nurse which identified that the nurse was not to be disturbed (AHRQ, 2008; Relihan et al., 2010). This improvement example demonstrated Lean thinking related to unevenness of flow (Cooksen et al., 2011). *Value-stream mapping* is the primary analyti-cal tool in Lean activities and can be used effectively to identify interruptions to make improvements in work flow. This tool is an extended process flowchart that focuses on speed, continuity of flow, and work in progress to identify non-value-added steps and bottlenecks (de Koning et al., 2006).

These are a few of the safety issues facing today's healthcare system. Administrators must find ways to create a culture of safety that does not tolerate continuation of these problems. Ethical principles and standards of care mandate a focus on patient safety.

Workforce Management Issues

We examine what happens when RNs or nursing budgets are cut. Presently, nurses are dissatisfied with their work. Studies have shown that the dissatisfaction rate is four times greater for hospital nurses than all other U.S. workers (Aiken, Clarke, Sloane, Sochalski, & Silber, 2002). Dissatisfaction is often related to high patient-to-nurse ratios. A poll of RNs by the ANA (American Nurses Association, 2008) revealed that close to half of the respondents are considering leaving their job because of inadequate staffing. Data from respondents were reported as follows:

- 73% of nurses asked don't believe the staffing on their unit or shift is sufficient.
- 59.8% of those asked said they knew of someone who left direct care nursing because of concerns about safe staffing.
- Of the 51.9% of respondents who are considering leaving their current position, 46% cite inad-equate staffing as the reason.
- 51.7% of respondents said they thought the quality of nursing care on their unit has declined in the last year.
- 48.2% would not feel confident having someone close to them receiving care in the facility where they work. (para. 2)

Research supports the gravity of inadequate staffing. Aiken and associates (2002) reported that nurse staffing ratios are linked to quality of care and patient outcomes. Adding one additional patient to the nurse assignment increases the likelihood of patient death by 7% within 30 days of hospital admission. On a positive note, ANA (2013b) cited that "*each additional patient care RN employed (at 7.8 hours per patient day) will generate over $60,000 annually in reduced medical costs and improved national* **productivity**" (para. 5). Evidence shows that improving the work environment for nurses can lead to improved job satisfaction and increased patient satisfaction and safety (Dunton, Gajewski, Klaus, & Pierson, 2007;

Vanhey, Aiken, Sloane, Clarke, & Vargas, 2004). Likewise, Boev (2012) found preliminary support for the relationship between nurses' and patients' satisfaction in adult critical care.

Researchers analyzed data from the National Database of Nursing Quality Indicators (NDNQI) regarding the nursing environment in relation to patient outcomes. These researchers concluded that multiple factors, including nurse staffing, percentage of RN staff, and RN years of experience, affect patient safety and nurse-sensitive outcomes. For example, the incidence of hospital-acquired pressure ulcers decreased with a more experienced staff along with having a higher percentage of RNs caring for the patient (Dunton et al., 2007).

The IOM (2004b) supported the following in their report *Keeping Patients Safe: Transforming the Work Environment of Nurses* (IOM, 2004b):

> Leaner nurse staffing is associated with increased length of stay, nosocomial infection (urinary tract infection, postoperative infection, and pneumonia), and pressure ulcers. . . . These studies . . . taken together, provide substantial evidence that richer nurse staffing is associated with better patient outcomes. . . . Greater numbers of patient deaths are associated with fewer nurses to provide care . . . and less nursing time provided to patients is associated with higher rates of infection, gastrointestinal bleeding, pneumonia, cardiac arrest, and death from these and other causes. . . . In caring for us all, nurses are indispensable to our safety (p. 3).

Additional researchers have reported similar outcomes. A recommended reading is a meta-analysis by the Agency for Healthcare Research and Quality (Kane, Shamliyan, Mueller, Duvai, & Witt, 2007) that found strong evidence that higher RN hours per patient day related to lower complication rates and lower mortality.

Based on these data, the ANA (n.d.) called for support of the Registered Nurse Safe Staffing Act that would create reliable nurse staffing levels. The ANA (n.d.) proclaimed that managing the RN-to-patient ratio improves job satisfaction and patient outcomes. Nurses' dissatisfaction with inadequate staffing is often supported by the research and is linked to less than satisfactory patient outcomes. This is only the beginning of the problem. In *Keeping Patients Safe: Transforming the Work Environment of Nurses*, the IOM (2004b) noted the following (**Exhibit 4–2**):

- **Loss of trust in hospital administration is widespread among nursing staff.** . . . This loss of trust stems in part from a perception that initiatives in patient care and nursing work redesign have emphasized efficiency over patient safety. . . . Poor communication practices have also led to mistrust.
- **Clinical nursing leadership has been reduced at multiple levels, and the voice of nurses in patient care has diminished**. Hospital reengineering initiatives often have resulted in the loss of a separate department of nursing. . . . At the same time, nursing staff have perceived a decline in chief nurse executives with power and authority equal to that of other top hospital officials, as well as [a decline] in directors of nursing who are highly visible and accessible to staff. . . . These changes— along with losses of chief nursing officers without replacement; decreases in the numbers of nurse managers; and increased responsibilities for remaining nurse managers for more than one patient care unit, as well as for supervising personnel other than nursing staff . . . —have had the cumulative effect of reducing direct management support available to patient care staff. This situation hampers nurses' ability to fix problems in their work environments that threaten patient safety. (p. 4)

Evidence has shown that understaffing, negative cultures, burdening nurse managers with more than 50 FTEs, 12-hour shifts, the lack of interdisciplinary shared governance, allowing physician or other staff disruptive or abusive behaviors, and moral distress issues are linked to poor patient outcomes; decreased patient, nurse, and physician satisfaction; higher staff turnover; and decreased reimbursement.

Exhibit 4–2   IOM Notes Negative Quality/Patient Safety Effects of Work Redesign

- Loss of trust in hospital administration
- Work redesign emphasized efficiency over patient safety
- Loss of a separate department of nursing
- Decline in nurse executives with the power and authority equal to the rest of the executive team
- Decrease in the number of nurse managers
- Remaining nurse managers have responsibility for more than one unit

Source: Data from Institute of Medicine. (2004b). *Keeping patients safe: Transforming the work environment of nurses.* Washington, DC: The National Academies Press.

Complexity Issues

All of the preceding problems are complexity issues. Everything is interconnected. With a sentinel event as an example, the event causes disorder. A root cause analysis restores order, *but hopefully with some small incremental change or changes in the way the work is done.*

Consider the following example of a sentinel event. During the time that the sentinel event occurred, staffing was inadequate, turnover was high because of a negative unit culture, and the nurse manager's leadership skills were inadequate. All these issues created complexity and contributed to the error. There was no single cause and "fixing" only one of the problems will not prevent the event from reoccurring. Such quick fixes increase complexity, which is counterproductive to PI work because more complexity creates more errors. This is the reason that all stakeholders are involved in review and resolution of sentinel events because what is needed is to determine ways to fix the causes and simplify processes. Sharing the learnings from root cause analyses with all staff demonstrates transparency. Secrets have a way of eventually becoming public knowledge.

Cultural Issues

Another factor related to what patients want and value is culture. Increasingly, the U.S. population is becoming more racially and culturally diverse. According to the 2010 U.S. census (U.S. Census Bureau, 2011):

- 72% were white (223.6 million) (This includes 16% Hispanic, [50.5 million])
- 13% were black or African American (38.9 million)
- 5% were Asian (14.7 million)
- 2.9%, were American Indian and Alaska Native (2.9 million)
- 0.2% were Native Hawaiian or other Pacific Islander (0.5 million)
- 6% were other races (19.1 million)

The U.S. Hispanic population almost doubled in the last decade (43% growth), yet the U.S. Asian population grew faster than any other major race for the same time period (U.S. Census Bureau, 2011). It is common to see Spanish television stations or to buy a product with instructions written in several languages. Obviously, the U.S. population is ethnically diverse.

This diversity constitutes a new perspective toward not only culturally diverse patients, but also toward culturally diverse staff. We are often unaware of specific cultural beliefs, values, and life ways and may, inadvertently, tread on those beliefs and practices as we deliver health care. Just as there is a need for improvement related to patient-centered care, quality, and safety, there is room for improvement related to culturally competent care.

As healthcare professionals, it is important to recognize the wonderful differences that exist between cultures and to support the cultural beliefs and norms of others. It is important to educate all staff regarding cultural differences, to value these differences, and to encourage everyone to respect and give radical loving care to each person based on that person's cultural beliefs. Alexander (2002) recommends that this "include the following core components: cultural/racial/ethnic identity, language/communication ability and style, religious beliefs and practices, illness and wellness behaviors, and healing beliefs and practices" (p. 32).

We have a lot of work to do to achieve better cultural understanding. Fortunately, good references are available. The following books describe different cultures and give a description of how nursing care needs to differ depending on a person's ethnic, cultural, or regional background:

- *Healing by Heart: Clinical and Ethical Case Stories of Hmong Families and Western Providers* by K. A. Culhane-Pera, D. E. Vawter, P. Xiong, B. Babbitt, and M. M. Solberg (2003)
- *Transcultural Nursing: Assessment and Intervention* by J. N. Giger (2012)
- *Transcultural Nursing: Concepts, Theories, Research, and Practice* by M. Leininger and M. McFarland (2002)
- *Transcultural Health Care: A Culturally Competent Approach* by L. D. Purnell (2012)
- *Caring for Women Cross-Culturally* by P. St. Hill, J. Lipson, and A. I. Meleis (2003)

These books are important for nurse leaders because much of the information is unknown to many healthcare providers.

Healthcare workers are ethnocentric in giving care to clients when they do not provide care based on what patients want and value. It is imperative that we take the time to learn about patients' cultural or ethnic differences. Care based on cultural differences affects nutrition, family functioning, lifestyle differences, spiritual or religious differences, biological variations, the way one relates to both health and disease, communication issues, differences in locus of control, differences in views about independence versus collectivism, and socioeconomic realities.

Additional cultural differences exist between physicians, nurses, and nonclinical administrators. In medical school, physicians often learn that they are autonomous and independent (although this is changing with group practices). This can lead to autocratic, domineering, and paternalistic behaviors because often teamwork and collaboration are not stressed nor valued. Also, nurses may determine that they are in a lower position in the hierarchy of importance because administrators tend to provide more support to physicians (who have the power to admit; thus, they affect revenue). These differences can be overcome. It is important that each member of the healthcare team is valued and respected and that everyone upholds the same organizational values to provide quality care for patients. When administrators do not support organizational values and give too much autonomy to physicians, disruptive physician behaviors may continue, creating a less effective or even hostile work environment. Patient care, as well as reimbursements, can be compromised when this occurs.

This section on cultural diversity could be an entire book because there are so many cultural differences in our world. It is of the utmost importance that cultural differences are recognized and respected within our healthcare system and that each person receives loving care specific to his or her expectations.

Disparities Issues

Significant healthcare access issues continue. The fifth *National Healthcare Disparities Report* (AHRQ, 2008) described disparities related to the quality of and access to health care. Although some progress has been made, the report highlights gaps that did not improve (**Exhibit 4–3**). A primary problem has been to decrease the identified gaps related to lack of insurance.

Exhibit 4–3   Disparities Among Races

- Blacks had a rate of new AIDS cases 10 times higher than whites.
- Asian adults aged 65 and over were 50% more likely than whites to lack immunization against pneumonia.
- Native Americans and Alaska Natives were twice as likely to lack prenatal care in the first trimester as whites.
- Hispanics had a rate of new AIDS cases over 3.5 times higher than that of non-Hispanic whites.
- Poor children were over 28% more likely than high-income children to experience poor communication with their health care providers.

Source: Agency for Healthcare Research and Quality. (2008). *National Healthcare Disparities Report: 2007.* AHRQ Pub. No. 08-0041. Rockville, MD: U.S. Department of Health and Human Services.

In a statistical brief for the Agency for Healthcare Research and Quality, Rhoades (2005) presented data that the percentage of uninsured persons varies throughout the year but as many as 13.6% Americans were uninsured for the entire year. According to the CDC (2013), 18.2% of the U.S. population was uninsured. Those without insurance often do not get needed medical care.

The good news is that almost "seven out of every ten Americans under age 65 years are covered by employment-based health insurance" (Committee on the Consequences of Uninsurance, 2001, p. 4). Nevertheless, unemployment abounds. Miller, Vigdor, and Manning (2004) claimed that lack of insurance creates hidden costs for society. These authors based this claim on data from the IOM report that estimated the cost in terms of foregone health, shorter lives, and demands on the healthcare infrastructure to be $65 billion to $130 billion a year. Using this hidden cost to provide insurance coverage would be more effective. (See the earlier discussion of the impact of the PPACA, 2010.)

Currently, the healthcare "safety net" provides care for the uninsured or underinsured, 44 million low-income Americans. The largest provider in this safety net is hospital emergency departments (EDs). Community clinics, public health departments, and hospital-based clinics, created to provide this care, cannot accommodate the demand. Hospital ED visits classified as nonurgent continue to increase, totaling 14% of total visits in 2005. Key reasons for this include difficulty obtaining timely appointments with a primary care provider, the lack of affordable transportation, and the lack of insurance. Much of this is not reimbursed; thus, hospitals incur more and more of the expense of providing this care. It will be interesting to see the impact of the PPACA (U.S. Government Printing Office, 2010) on these issues.

Regulatory Response: Restricting or Eliminating Reimbursement

As healthcare expenses rise, federal and state governments are faced with deficits. At the same time, there is a growing elderly group who is eligible for Medicare. The Centers for Medicare and Medicaid Services (CMS), which represents more than 50% of the health insurance in this country, responded by reimbursing for quality care and withholding reimbursement when quality issues were identified (*pay for performance or value-based purchasing*).

Hospitals

Acute care facilities must demonstrate compliance with the guidelines for care of certain conditions to receive the highest possible reimbursement. In this case, the CMS (the payer) specified certain patient care paths to obtain reimbursement. If the patient care path is not followed as specified, the healthcare organization does not receive reimbursement for the care. For example, if antibiotics are not given within 2 hours of a pneumonia diagnosis (the care path specification), the payer will not reimburse the hospital. This emphasizes the importance of clinician timeliness in treating the patient, or everyone loses, including the patient.

In 2008, additional indicators were put in place restricting or eliminating reimbursement for certain hospital-acquired conditions that were not present on admission (CMS, 2012d). These hospital-acquired conditions were expanded to 11 categories for fiscal year 2013 (CMS, 2012c). (See **Exhibit 4–4**.) These conditions have been termed *never events*.

The CMS (2013g) quality initiatives encompass the gamut of the healthcare system, from providers to hospital care, and include quality measures information that CMS recommends that consumers use when faced with healthcare decisions. The CMS quality initiatives span several years and are easily confused, and thus only an overview is provided here.

The Hospital Inpatient Quality Reporting Program was originally mandated by the Medicare Prescription Drug, Improvement, and Modernization Act (MMA) of 2003 (CMS, 2003). The MMA authorized CMS to pay hospitals a higher annual update on their payment rates based on reporting of identified quality measures. The initial MMA rate was a 0.4% reduction for hospitals that did not successfully report. In 2005, the Deficit Reduction Act increased the reduction to 2.0 percentage points (CMS, 2013b).

The Hospital Outpatient Quality Reporting Program was mandated by the Tax Relief and Health Care Act of 2006 (CMS, 2006). This program required hospitals to submit outpatient quality measures data. The data included process, structure, outcome, and efficiency measures. Outpatient care encompassed ED services, observation, outpatient surgical services, laboratory tests, and radiology (CMS, 2013a).

Exhibit 4–4   2013 CMS Hospital-Acquired Conditions

Foreign Object Retained After Surgery
Air Embolism
Blood Incompatibility
Stage III and IV Pressure Ulcers
Falls and Trauma
- Fractures
- Dislocations
- Intracranial Injuries
- Crushing Injuries
- Burn
- Other Injuries

Manifestations of Poor Glycemic Control
- Diabetic Ketoacidosis
- Nonketotic Hyperosmolar Coma
- Hypoglycemic Coma
- Secondary Diabetes with Ketoacidosis
- Secondary Diabetes with Hyperosmolarity

Catheter-Associated Urinary Tract Infection (UTI)
Vascular Catheter-Associated Infection
Surgical Site Infection, Mediastinitis, Following Coronary Artery Bypass Graft (CABG)
Surgical Site Infection Following Bariatric Surgery for Obesity
- Laparoscopic Gastric Bypass
- Gastroenterostomy
- Laparoscopic Gastric Restrictive Surgery

Surgical Site Infection Following Certain Orthopedic Procedures
- Spine
- Neck
- Shoulder
- Elbow

Surgical Site Infection Following Cardiac Implantable Electronic Device (CIED)
Deep Vein Thrombosis/Pulmonary Embolism Following Certain Orthopedic Procedures
- Total Knee Replacement
- Hip Replacement

Iatrogenic Pneumothorax with Venous Catheterization

Source: Centers for Medicare and Medicaid. (2012c). *Hospital-acquired conditions (present on admission indicator).* Retrieved from http://www.cms.gov/Medicare/Medicare-Fee-for-Service-Payment/HospitalAcqCond/Hospital-Acquired_Conditions.html

An example of a quality initiative is the Hospital Value-Based Purchasing Program (CMS, 2013c), effective fiscal year 2013, which provides value-based incentive payments based on the hospital's performance on quality measures (pay for performance) or based on the hospital's improvement on quality measures from the baseline period. *The higher the hospital's performance or improvement, the higher the value-based incentive payment.* If a hospital does not meet these guidelines, reimbursement will be decreased by a percentage for the following year. Thus, hospitals not only lose on a never event, but are penalized further for reimbursement the next year.

Home Health

There are three types of home health quality measures: (1) process, (2) outcomes, and (3) potentially avoidable events (CMS, 2012b). Details related to home health measures are extensive and can be found at www.cms.gov/Medicare/Quality-Initiatives-Patient-Assessment-Instruments/HomeHealthQualityInits/HHQIQualityMeasures.html.

Long-Term Care

The CMS nursing home measures are also extensive. There are 5 short-stay quality measures and 13 long-stay nursing home quality measures (CMS, 2013c). Beginning in 2009, nursing homes in Arizona (41), New York (79), and Wisconsin (62) took part in a 3-year demonstration project related to pay for performance for nursing homes (CMS, 2013e). The data are not yet available. Details related to nursing home quality measures are vast and can be found at www.cms.gov/Medicare/Quality-Initiatives-Patient-Assessment-Instruments/NursingHomeQualityInits/NHQIQualityMeasures.html.

Postacute Care

Finally, additional CMS quality initiatives are in place for postacute care (CMS, 2012e) and for end-stage renal disease (ESRD) (CMS, 2012a). The ESRD Quality Initiative, which became effective in 2012, was the first pay for performance (also known as value-based purchasing) quality initiative implemented as mandated by the Medicare Improvements for Patients and Providers Act (MIPPA) of 2008 (U.S. Government Printing Office, 2008). Its goal was to enhance the quality of care provided to ESRD patients as they battle this devastating disease (CMS, 2012a). Additional information regarding the CMS quality initiatives can be found at www.cms.gov/Medicare/Quality-Initiatives-Patient-Assessment-Instruments/QualityInitiativesGenInfo/index.html?redirect=/qualityinitiativesgeninfo/.

Quality Reporting System Mandate

In an effort to align payment incentives across the healthcare system, CMS (2013f) implemented payment incentives and adjustments to promote reporting of quality information by identified providers. The quality reporting system is mandated by federal legislation. Beginning in 2015, the program also applies to eligible providers who do not satisfactorily report quality measures data (CMS, 2013f). Details related to the Physician Quality Reporting System can be found at www.cms.gov/Medicare/Quality-Initiatives-Patient-Assessment-Instruments/PQRS/index.html.

Medicaid programs are funded at both state and federal levels; thus, these restrictions on reimbursement are being linked to Medicaid payments as well. Next, the American Hospital Association (AHA) developed guiding principles for nonpayment for all insurance companies for certain serious adverse events (that are preventable, may indicate a hospital system error, or where there are published guidelines for prevention of these errors if the hospital deems the event was preventable) from the National Quality Forum's list of 28 serious reportable events (Tennessee Hospitals & Health Systems, 2008) **(Exhibit 4–5)**.

Exhibit 4–5   The American Hospital Association Guidelines for Reimbursement Restriction

The American Hospital Association recommends that hospitals not seek payment from patients or their insurance companies for the following serious preventable adverse events if the hospital deems the event was preventable:

- Surgery on a wrong body part
- Surgery on the wrong patient
- Wrong surgical procedure
- Unintended retention of a foreign object
- Patient death or serious disability associated with an air embolism that occurs while being treated in a health care facility
- Patient death or serious disability associated with a medication error
- Patient death or serious disability associated with a hemolytic reaction due to administration of ABO/HLA incompatible blood or blood products
- Artificial insemination with the wrong donor sperm or wrong egg
- Infant discharged to the wrong person
- Death or serious disability (kernicterus) associated with failure to identify and treat hyperbilirubinemia in neonates
- Patient death or serious disability associated with a burn incurred from any source while being cared for in a health care facility

Source: Data from Tennessee Hospitals & Health Systems. (2008). *THA develops nonpayment policy on serious adverse events.* Nashville, TN: Tennessee Hospital Association.

Patient safety was of such concern to the public that The Joint Commission implemented National Patient Safety Goals in 2003 (The Joint Commission, 2013c). Accredited facilities must demonstrate compliance with the intent of these goals to maintain their accreditation status. Details regarding the 2013 National Patient Safety Goals (The Joint Commission, 2013d) can be found at www.jointcommission.org/standards_information/npsgs.aspx.

Our Reality Is Changing—Ready or Not!

Another challenge throughout society is the move from the Industrial Age to the Information Age. Many of us are still stuck in the Industrial Age that is replete with patriarchal systems and huge healthcare system dinosaurs, dominated by administrators heavily committed to the bottom line as first priority with little or no understanding of the care side (what patients want and value) of health care. These administrators think nothing of cutting costs by cutting nursing budgets, because nursing constitutes the largest operational budget item in most facilities, and by cutting registered nurses (RNs). These administrators do not understand what they have done. When the bottom line is the first priority, the organization will eventually fail and go out of business. This has already happened.

We have a lot of work to do! There are additional challenges in this new reality, the Information Age. In the midst of inadequate staffing, time has become more compressed, so time passes more quickly. Many nurses have noticed that they do not seem to have as much time as they did in the past. This exacerbates the staffing issues. In addition to not having enough time, suddenly there is too much information (another complexity issue) in our reality, and the way we perceive information has changed. The question is not necessarily how much information we can learn, retain, and use. Instead, it is how well we can *access* the needed information. Baby boomers often have difficulty with this reality, but more recent generations are already experiencing and embracing it.

Healthcare systems are moving to highly integrated computer systems, which are costly ventures. Medicare and Medicaid EHR Incentive Programs "provide financial incentives for the 'meaningful use' of certified CHR technology to improve patient care" (CMS, 2013d, para. 1). To receive incentive payments, providers must demonstrate that they are "meaningfully using" (CMS, 2013d, para. 1) EHRs through compliance with objectives. The EHR Incentive Programs consist of three stages with increasing requirements for participation (CMS, 2013d). Meeting meaningful use criteria equates to significant monies for eligible healthcare providers and hospitals. There is mounting concern regarding the cost of technology because healthcare costs are increasing at alarming and unsustainable rates (de Koning et al., 2006).

The Information Age has brought about more technology to purchase and to learn to use. As healthcare monies are curtailed or cut, we have computer systems that do not interface with one another because they are not integrated. Purchased information systems quickly become obsolete, and information system companies go out of business and leave healthcare workers without support. Sometimes technology that is purchased is incomplete, requiring staff to complete electronic charting along with a paper chart. There are major issues, including more errors, which are the result of inadequate planning and implementation of these systems. Staff forget to use their assessment and professional judgment skills; rather, they simply rely on technology. Sometimes staff develop workarounds when the technology creates problems. These workarounds can be positive or negative, if staff are in a hurry for a quick fix to circumvent the system. Some staff resist using technology. Informatics personnel and departments have been added, which further increases the cost of the U.S. healthcare system. There are downtime issues (when technology is not working) that staff must be prepared to manage. This is increasingly important because in the current workplace some staff nurses have never used a paper chart. Added to these issues is the government insistence that healthcare providers meet Health Insurance Portability and Accountability Act of 1996 requirements while managing healthcare costs related to the Balanced Budget Act. Nevertheless, computerized systems are needed for prompt payment for care that has been provided. Insurers do not always use the same systems as providers do.

The current trend for patient safety involves many technological purchases. The dilemma is that these technology purchases need to be made at a time when reimbursements are curtailed.

Technology has brought about positive care changes. Procedures are less invasive, and telehealth is becoming more predominant.

> The technology of the time is quickly moving the health professions into a context where the kind of therapies that will be used require less mechanical and manual intervention and a greater use of other innovative approaches. This transition makes it possible to treat illness at an earlier stage and either eliminate or alter the need for more mechanical (surgical) interventions that are more intensive and costly. It is quickly becoming a time of ending for the health care system as we know it. Furthermore, it is the end of the Newtonian, 20th century medical and nursing practice, and other health-related practices, as those disciplines have historically understood them. (Porter-O'Grady, 2003, p. 62)

All health professionals are facing the new reality. Payers have changed their focus to an ambulatory-oriented patient care delivery system that prevents hospitalization and to have more services available to keep patients in their homes. Healthcare administrators can choose whether to respond to this new reality, working to change behaviors and practices, or they can choose to continue with the same patriarchal practices of old. The former results in an enhanced, more satisfying healthcare environment for both patients and healthcare workers. The latter is outdated, and eventually the organization will dissolve.

Porter-O'Grady and Malloch (2007) state:

> What one does and what difference it makes are the key issues for all providers. If an organization provides 1,000 services and only 25 make a difference, then the other 975 services must be considered for elimination—even if the 975 services have billing codes that render them reimbursable.
>
> Provider accountability for contributions to patient care outcomes is a missing piece of health care. All professional care providers must focus their actions on achieving desired outcomes and implement only interventions that have a basis in science or a realistic chance of benefiting patients.

The measurement of health care outcomes is gradually becoming more meaningful and reflective of patient needs. Unfortunately, indicators are often looked at in an order that fails to take into account the basic goal of health care—health improvement. For example, productivity measures are typically examined prior to clinical outcomes. If productivity targets are exceeded, increases in productivity are mandated without consideration of their potential impact on care provision. (p.387)

The new Information Age requires different approaches and perspectives:

Moving into a new age does not mean leaving everything behind. It does mean thinking about what needs to be left behind and reflecting on what does go with us as we move into an age with a different set of parameters. (Porter-O'Grady & Malloch, 2011, p. 10)

Significant changes that affect the way patient care is provided, the current care delivery systems, and even the nurses' perspectives on the world in general are imminent. In the short term, it is easy to be complacent and not pay attention to the changes. However, they are all around us:

This is the beginning of the end of nursing care as we have all become accustomed to providing and using. . . . The hospital-based, sickness-oriented, late-stage model of nursing service delivery is no longer either appropriate or prevailing. Nurses now must determine what traditional practices and functions are no longer relevant or sustainable and let them go. At the same time, nurses must discern what is emerging on the practice horizon that must now become increasingly a part of nursing practice. Influences like genomics, nano-therapy, fiberoptics, pharmacotherapeutics, virtual care models, early-stage interventions, patient managed delivery, [alternative therapies], etc. are now pressing on the periphery of the profession and will dominate nursing adaptation for the next 2 decades. (Porter-O'Grady, 2003, p. 62)

The only constant in our present reality is that it will change. We are at a crossroads. We can lament what we are losing, or have lost, or we can look around us for clues as to what we might expect and begin to design where we need to go next. Because we are all in the healthcare box, some of these changes are hard to perceive because they are outside our view of reality.

In addition to the traditional nursing role changing, our administrative roles are changing. We are here to support giving patients what they want and value and those at the point to care to achieve this in the best way possible. The choice is ours—to remain stuck in our past, or to move into an exciting, more fulfilling, unknown future. We have an opportunity to create our new reality. It is up to us as we respond to each situation. This is an exciting, challenging time when we, as nurse professionals and as nurse (or healthcare) administrators, can forge new roles that better fit the new realities and encourage staff to do the same.

Last, but perhaps most important, the new reality is that collaborative relationships and teamwork are important and are based on listening to our patients and involving them in making decisions about their care. Nurses need to recognize (and mourn) the loss of the familiar environment but move on, welcoming the opportunity to take actions that will get us closer to the patient. Nurses will thrive if they are able to constantly value the people we serve *and* the people on our team.

The work of the time for the clinical leader is helping colleagues and patients end their attachment to the kind of healthcare system they have grown comfortable with. So many nurses are mourning the loss of something they think should not have passed or should be retained. Many nurses are mourning the loss of those very practices, sentiments, or roles that brought them to nursing in the first place. Some even wish those traditions would return. The truth is that most of what is being mourned should neither be retained nor protected. Neither the times nor yesterday's circumstances will return, nor should they. . . . Those ideals that brought many of us to nursing (enough time for good care, long stays, detailed care processes, residential models of care, heavy emphasis on manual procedures, compliant and passive patient roles, etc.) no longer exist. The question is not will these processes return but instead: what is nursing now becoming and how must I adapt?

A major role of the clinical leader in this day and time is engaging others around the reality of their own change. Complacency at this time of radical shifting is a strategy that guarantees failure. The leader must take whatever action is necessary to impress upon those he or she leads that this is a time of great mobility and shifting foundations. (Porter-O'Grady, 2003, p. 62)

Where Do We Start?

No problem can be solved from the same consciousness that created it. We must learn to see the world anew.

—*Albert Einstein*

Reframing Our Worldview

In the Information Age, the locus of control has shifted from the provider to the patient. Yet many providers act as if they have the locus of control. We do things to patients without consulting them. Many of us do not take the time to find out what our patients want and expect. Yet our world has changed. Porter-O'Grady and Malloch (2011) stress the importance of increasing the focus on patients:

It is no secret that the locus of control for healthcare services should be the patient, not the provider. Yet in spite of all the efforts to create patient-focused care delivery systems, few patients would agree that they are in fact the focus of services or in control of anything. In explanation, they could cite facts such as these:

- Providers continue to prescribe treatments without discussion with the patients.
- Visiting hours are still in effect.
- Appointment times for services are based on Monday through Friday schedules.
- Patient procedures and their scheduled times are determined by providers without input from patients or families. (p. 455)

As you read this chapter begin to think of the many ways that nurses can change how healthcare services are provided—ways that are much more effective and that involve the patient in care decisions. This leads us to something that we need to make the top priority as we give care: *finding out what the patient wants and values*.

There are opportunities all around us. Patients have access to more information about their care, yet they need our help in translating the meaning of various options available to them when they experience disease. At the same time, they are turning to healthier lifestyles so they can live longer, healthier lives. Nurses have an advantage in this environment because, although we learn about disease and how it is treated, we also learn about prevention and health. In healthcare organizations, nurses are with patients far more than are physicians, who quickly come by to see patients and then are gone. Patients value our interpersonal skills because we are more likely to listen and to help. Thus, for us, moving into this new age is not as difficult as it is for physicians who are mainly focused on disease and which medications to prescribe to deal with disease.

Nurses also have a lot to offer to bottom-line healthcare administrators who do not understand the care side unless they experience disease, at which point their perspective often dramatically shifts to a new appreciation of the care side and of what nurses have to offer. We can help them in this shift because we are closer to the patient and can bring that perspective to the table. The important place for survival is at the point of care. As administrators, we need to encourage and empower staff at the point of care to make 90% of the decisions about that care. Staff need to become leaders, helping the patients become leaders in their own care decisions. We administrators are here to facilitate staff being able to do this. We need to be sure that staffing is adequate, and more staff may be needed during peak times. We need to protect staff so that they can do their work. We need to support interdisciplinary shared governance at the bedside with everyone in the organization doing regular rounds.

One purpose of this book is to help nurse administrators to express what is needed using statistics so that linear administrators are more likely to listen. This helps make it possible for patients to get what they value while they are with us. Linear administrators understand, and need, numbers. If we format what we believe is needed in a way that shows numbers and dollars, our suggestions are more likely to be supported within an organization. Along with this we need to involve staff in budgets, sharing financial information. Transparency throughout the organization is the end goal.

Our First Priority: Discovering What the Patient Wants and Values

Value from the patient's perspective is the most important concern. Sometimes patients believe that the healthcare provider does not listen, does not care to listen to what the patient actually wants or needs. The old paternalistic medical model—we will just tell you what is best for you—is outdated, is resented, and no longer applies to most patients. Patients often feel depersonalized, experience long waits, and, worse yet, receive substandard care, as discussed in **Exhibit 4–3**, especially if they are in a lower socioeconomic group or if they are a racial or ethnic minority.

Porter-O'Grady and Malloch (2011) discuss the change in the patient–provider relationship:

- Patients now determine the parameters of the patient–provider relationship, setting the stage for a different kind of interaction than has historically occurred.
- Patients need to develop partnerships with providers to sort through the available choices and pick the best. They need providers to act as educators who are willing to assist them in making health care decisions.
- Patients need help from providers both in verifying the accuracy of the data they have independently garnered from a host of sources and in interpreting the data.
- Patients are interested in options, not an order to undergo a particular treatment. They want to be able to consider a range of options within the context of their own personal values and priorities and choose the one option that best fits these.
- Providers now need to be concerned with what patients know and can do with regard to controlling their own health decisions in a "user-driven" world. More of the responsibility for health care will be placed on patients and their loved ones. Providers must now transfer skills to others and surrender ownership of care to others. (p. 17)

It is important for the nurse manager to constantly think, *"What does the patient want and value?"* along with *"safety, safety, safety,"* *"quality, quality, quality,"* and *"cost-effectiveness, cost-effectiveness, cost-effectiveness."* The nurse manager can facilitate what is valuable to patients. The expectation is that staff at the point of care do the same thing. This is a change for most of us, who are accustomed to providing care with no consideration of the *patient's* perspective.

Administrators are not alone in needing to change their perspective. All staff, board members, physicians, and the executive team must change their perspectives. Everyone has to talk with each patient and listen to what he or she has to say. *The most important place is at the point of care, and administrators must support those who are at this point of care.* Paying attention to what the patient values as *first priority*, with safety and quality second, enables us to make better decisions, be more effective, and save money and risk to the patient. This perspective has a positive impact on the financial bottom line as well; thus, everyone wins!

Values depend on the circumstances and whose point of view is being considered. Patient perceptions, and what the patient wants, are more important than what we believe the patient *should* want when determining quality indicators. Once we have determined what evidence-based care might be necessary for a specific patient (after we have determined what the patient wants), there is still more to do. We need to then offer the patient choices in remedies and therapies that fall under that evidence-based care rubric, while ensuring that the patient is fully informed. Currently, healthcare team members fail in healthcare delivery because we often consider what we want instead of consulting the patient and finding out the patient's wishes.

Value has another implication. We all must understand the importance of including our **patients as leaders in the decision-making process of their care**. The patient has to be involved in deciding which services will be provided. This can be a challenge! Or, perhaps we should change the way we think about this: This is an opportunity! It is exciting to be part of quality health care, based on what the patient wants and values. This pivotal point will change health care as we know it.

The Consumer-Driven Health Care Institute (2013) promotes policy that empowers individuals to make decisions about their health care, advocating the following:

- Consumers will work with their physicians and health care providers to create a better health care outcome for themselves and their families.
- Health care usage is more cost efficient with empowered and knowledgeable consumers who use information tools.
- Price and quality transparency about health care professionals is a key method for effective consumer health care choices. (para. 2)

Transparency means that we share all pertinent information. Consider that if we did not share, the Internet nevertheless provides voluminous information, and CMS provides information to the general public, including facility quality ratings. We cannot stop the tide—information is accessible to the public. Some of the information is helpful and excellent; some is erroneous and misleading. We can assist patients to appropriately evaluate this information to make the best decisions. `

Another trap for nurses is to lament that improvements cannot be made because of inadequate resources. Active listening does require a lower nurse-to-patient ratio so that the nurse can take the time to determine what patients value and desire. In addition, traditionally there have been cyclical nursing shortages. But bemoaning shortages and financial constraints does not improve patient care. The excuse of inadequate resources needs to be discarded, and instead nurses must determine how to make a positive difference. However, that being said, it is important that administrators make sure that staffing *is* adequate for current patient needs. And all of us, including staff, need to be creative and make sure we are using the resources we have in the most advantageous way possible. This is important because, if nurses do not find a way to do things better, someone else will. Consider freestanding surgery centers, for example, where the same surgical procedures are completed at lower costs than in the hospital setting. This is partially the result of lower fixed costs. Thus, what is needed is to determine the reason that fixed costs are considerably higher in hospitals.

Nurses need to be innovative and encourage all staff and physicians to be innovative. When contemplating current practice, nurses must evaluate what needs to be changed. For example, are limited visiting hours really necessary? Why are most procedures scheduled Monday through Friday? It is interesting that consumer groups advocate *not* having procedures scheduled on Friday because staff are often limited on weekends and are thus less equipped to deal with patient complications. If a patient has an acute episode on Friday evening, why does the patient have to wait until Monday for most services? We must question everything that we do!

Not much has been discussed about quality and safety in this section because the issues that were reviewed are important if nurses are to deliver patient-centered quality services. It is important to emphasize listening to the patient, providing sufficient information for decision making, and supporting the patient in treatment decisions—all within a safe, cost-effective environment.

The Healing Relationship

The IOM (2001) advocates, "Care is based on continuous healing relationships" (p. 3). At times, in this chapter we mention "loving" care. Love is necessary for healing. By *love*, we mean a caring relationship. Jean Watson (2004) examined the relationship between caring and curing in her book *Postmodern Nursing and Beyond*. The author examines both the technical side of nursing and the holistic side, which is traditionally associated with caring. Over the years, a lot of emphasis has been put on the caring component of nursing practice.

Chapman (2004) made the connection between loving and healing and stressed the importance of listening to the patient. This means that as we listen to each patient, we read between the lines using our intuition. The physical diagnosis may not be the most important issue for the patient. Instead, nurses must determine what the patient wants and values and focus the patient's care on what is important to the patient.

Chapman (2004) emphasizes not seeing a patient as a stranger but as a brother or sister. He encourages us to see that what the patient needs goes beyond the physical needs to the emotions. Significant life changes are often thrust upon a patient. The patient may be in pain, and pain can be a lonely experience. The term "radical loving care" (Chapman, 2004) stresses the importance of making a significant connection with each patient. It is a trinity that is very beneficial to have present in a healthcare organization: the Golden Thread (the loving thread that connects us), the Sacred Encounter (each time we interact with a patient), and the Servant's Heart (we serve others). It is so important that we included *heart* in the title of this text!

> Loving care has a long and beautiful tradition in human history. In these pages the heritage of loving care is symbolized by the image of a Golden Thread, which is also a symbol of faith in God. It represents the positive tradition of healing versus the negative tradition of transaction-based behavior. (Chapman, 2004, p. 10)

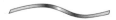

> A second symbol, a pair of intersecting circles, signifies the merging of love and need in the Sacred Encounter, which is the fundamental relationship between caregiver and patient. This symbol also signifies hope—the hope that comes into our hearts when we experience loving encounters. (Chapman, 2004, p. 10)

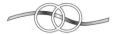

> The third symbol, a red heart, signifies the nature of the Servant's Heart. It also symbolizes love and is love's greatest expression. This expression, although it specifically references the heart, assumes the full involvement of our best thought processes. Loving care is not loving if it fails to engage the best skills and competency of caregivers. (Chapman, 2004, p. 10)

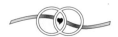

Patient and Family Advisory Councils

One way to find out what patients want and value is to conduct focus groups with patients and families. For example, Pointe and colleagues (2003) established two Patient and Family Advisory Councils, one for pediatrics and one for adults (it would be helpful to establish one for elderly adults as well):

> At Dana-Farber Cancer Institute in Boston, we have been engaged for more than 5 years in a process of rethinking and redesigning many of our most critical operations in order to integrate the voices of patients and families into virtually everything we do. Although this work is far from complete, we believe we have made significant progress in crafting a new paradigm of care: one that places the patient and family in an entirely new position within the organization's operational and care structures. . . . By working through the councils, the voices of patients and families are blended with those of clinicians, administrators, and other staff as the processes and systems of care are designed and delivered. Patients provide input on organizational policies, are placed on continuous improvement teams, and are invited to join search committees and develop educational programming for staff. Members of the councils also sit on the Joint Committee on Quality Improvement and Risk Management, a board-level committee that approves the institute's quality improvement plan, evaluates outcomes of quality improvement activities, and reviews reports regarding sentinel events.
>
> Creating this level of integration requires important preliminary work within the organization. There must be a shared understanding of the critical components of patient-centered care. There must be strong advocacy for the concept at the highest levels of the administrative leadership team. And there must be in place a strong, interdisciplinary work team, for it is premature to think about integrating patients and families into a team if the underpinnings of effective teamwork are not yet in place. (pp. 82–83)

Focus groups or patient advisory councils can be very beneficial in determining what patients and families value and want related to health care. Many organizations find that focus groups augment other forms of feedback. Consumers Advancing Patient Safety (2012) has a step-by-step guide with examples on how to partner with patient groups to enhance value and safety (Leonhardt, Bonin, & Pagel, 2007). Additional information regarding Consumers Advancing Patient Safety can be found at www.patient-safety.org.

In addition, it is important to include the patient and family in interdisciplinary rounds and shift reports *at the patient's bedside*. In some organizations, interdisciplinary rounds and shift reports are completed just outside the patient's room. This is disrespectful to the patient, who is the leader of his or her plan of care, and these conversations may also pose confidentiality issues. Often, the healthcare workers focus on their needs rather than the needs and values of the patient. Of course, the patient's acuity and state of rest may preclude report at the bedside.

Replace Patient Compliance with What the Patient Wants and Values

Recall that the patient is the leader in his or her care. Value is based on what the patient wants and needs; thus, the phrase *patient compliance* should be eliminated from our healthcare vocabulary. The term originates from the patriarchal medical system. *Patient compliance* assumes that healthcare workers know better than the patient what the patient wants and values. This term has negative connotations, and thus many healthcare workers use the term *adherence* instead of *compliance*.

The ethical principle of autonomy applies here. Special pause is needed related to this issue because the ANA *Code of Ethics with Interpretive Statements* (2001) upholds the patient's right to self-determination, or *autonomy,* specifically:

> **Patients have the moral and legal right to determine what will be done with their own person; to be given accurate, complete, and understandable information in a manner that facilitates informed judgment; to be assisted in weighing the benefits, burdens, and available options in their treatment, including the choice of no treatment; to accept, refuse, or terminate treatment without deceit, undue influence, duress, coercion, or penalty; and to be given necessary support through the treatment and decision-making process.** Such support would include the opportunity to make decisions with family and significant others and the provision of advice and support from knowledgeable nurses and other health professionals. Patients should be involved in planning their own health care to the extent they are able and choose to participate. (Provision 1.1.4)

The patient has a right to choose and what is termed "noncompliant" may be due to what the patient wants and values, or it may result from a lack of knowledge. Thus, it is the healthcare worker's responsibility to educate the patient related to current evidence-based care. Then the patient is equipped to make decisions based on what is valued and needed.

Longtin and associates (2010) found that the nurse–patient relationship was based on a "paternalistic model" (**Exhibit 4–6**) in which the patient was a "passive recipient of care" (p. 54). The authors stated that patients who participate in the decision-making process are exercising and exemplifying their right to self-determination. Consider these findings:

- Only 73% of patients filled their prescriptions within 1 week of leaving the hospital. Patients filled 82% of their heart-related prescriptions and only 35% of those not related to the heart (Jackevicius, Li, & Tu, 2008).
- Only 60% of patients discharged from the hospital filled their prescriptions within 2 days. Patients reported difficulties in understanding why they needed the medications, concerns about costs, transportation challenges, and wait times as reasons for noncompliance (Kripalani, Henderson, Jacobson, & Vaccarino, 2008).
- The Mayo Clinic published a study finding that only 86% of patients recently discharged from the hospital realized that a new medication(s) had been prescribed. Of those, only 22% could name at least one adverse effect (Maniaci, Heckman, & Dawson, 2008).

To further understand "patient noncompliance," consider the side effects that can occur with medications. When the physician or nurse practitioner prescribes a medication, for example, a steroid, and the patient decides that the harmful side effects outweigh the benefits and does not take the medication, perhaps being "noncompliant" is smart and safe.

Exhibit 4–6   Paternalist Model of a Patient–Health Care Worker Relationship

Only experts (health care workers) are qualified to diagnose and treat disease.
All decisions rely entirely on the knowledge of the health care worker.
The health care worker is the guardian of the patient's interest and must respect the principle of beneficence.
The patient is a passive recipient of care.

Source: Longtin, Y., Sax, H., Leape, L. L., Sheridan, S. E., Donaldson, L., & Pittet, D. (2010). Patient participation: Current knowledge and applicability to patient safety. *Mayo Clinic Proceedings, 85*(1), 53-62. doi: 10.4065/mcp.2009.0248

Health literacy has come to light as a problem that influences patient adherence to recommended treatment. The U.S. Department of Health and Human Services (n.d.) defined *health literacy* as the "degree to which individuals have the capacity to obtain, process, and understand basic health information and services needed to make appropriate health decisions" (para. 1). This includes the individual's basic reading levels. Poor health literacy is associated with poor health outcomes. The IOM (2004a) reported that 90 million people in the United States "have difficulty understanding and acting upon health information" (p. 1). An inability to understand medical language and printed instructions affects the individual's ability to follow recommended treatments. Clear communication in plain language is imperative. It is important to determine that the patient understands the provided education.

Another pervasive "noncompliance" issue is the cost of healthcare services. Again, using a medication example, consider a scenario in the local pharmacy. An elderly woman waits line for her prescriptions, and the pharmacist tells her that her medications total $568. She says, "I am on a fixed income. I don't have that much money." The pharmacist says, "Well, your doctor insists on not using generic medications, so there is nothing I can do to bring the cost down." They finally agree for her to pay for a week's worth of medications and to wait for her next Social Security check. If this woman uses her Social Security check to pay for medications, how will she pay for other necessities, such as rent and food? Her physician considers the generic medications less effective. However, did the physician take into account *value* as defined by the patient (what she needs)? Would it have been better for the pharmacist to call the physician to discuss the possibility of using generic drugs to save costs for the client? And even if generic drugs were used, can this woman afford to buy the medications and still have money for rent and food? Were *all* of these drugs necessary? Why do the drugs cost so much?

Larger societal issues add to the problem of patient "noncompliance." Consider the difficulties that many patients encounter in seeing their physician when they experience problems. They are charged for an office visit. If they need to be transferred to a specialist, in a health maintenance organization system they may or may not be able to get beyond the gatekeeper to obtain the care they need. The public deals with "compliance" issues by surfing the Internet and reading literature related to their health condition or illness—sometimes becoming better informed than healthcare providers—and by turning to alternative medicine. Perhaps the most important adherence issue is that nurses and other healthcare providers forget that patients have the right to make choices.

It is important to discuss treatments, including medications, with patients. Nurses need to do a better job of patient (and family) education. Healthcare workers must encourage the patient (and family) to ask questions and to understand how to best deal with health problems. Nurses need to have time to do this activity to teach patients in ways that patients understand. When the patient compliance patriarchal system is gone, it will be replaced with what the patient wants and values.

The Quality Dimension

Consider quality with the recollection that what the patient wants and values comes *first*. In addition to listening to the patient and involving the patient in decision making about treatments and care from the patient's value perspective, quality (including safety) is paramount. When nurses are effective in the quality arena, our decisions and actions provide care that is needed in the safest, most effective way. What exactly is quality?

This chapter describes a fundamentally different perspective in defining quality and what quality is really all about. Quality has many definitions. Quality can mean different things to different people. Many organizations have chosen to identify quality indicators that can be measured and compared.

The IOM (2001) calls for quality through the redesign of health care based on 10 rules. The Joint Commission (2013a) expects quality through compliance with prescribed standards. Nursing standards and scope of practice define our practice as well. The CMS (2013g) touts:

> Quality health care for people with Medicare is a high priority for the President, the Department of Health and Human Services (HHS), and the Centers for Medicare and Medicaid Services (CMS). HHS and CMS began Quality Initiatives in 2001 to assure quality health care for all Americans through accountability and public disclosure. (para. 3)

Definitions of quality have been inadequate. In fact, most definitions do not consider the patient's perspective but rather rely heavily on the perspective of the healthcare professional or that of the payer or regulator. Nurses have forgotten the most important person in the equation—our *patient,* our *client,* our *resident.* Most often healthcare professionals do not consult the patient to find out what the patient wants, needs, or values. Perhaps this is best captured in the definition of quality in the book *Through the Patients' Eyes* (Gerteis, Edgman-Levitan, Daley, & Delbanco, 1993):

> Quality . . . has two dimensions. One has to do with technical excellence: the skill and competence of professionals and the ability of diagnostic or therapeutic equipment, procedures, and systems to accomplish what they are meant to accomplish, reliably and effectively. Borrowing the language and conceptual models of industrial engineering, we speak in this sense of "quality control," "quality assurance," and "quality improvement."
>
> The other dimension is related to subjective experience—its texture and substance, its sentient quality. In this sense, we speak of the quality of a sensation or experience or the quality of human relationships. In health care, it is quality in this subjective dimension that patients experience most directly—in their perception of illness or well-being and in their encounters with health care professionals and institutions. (p. xi)

For this new century, the IOM (2001) recommends that healthcare workers commit to six aims for improvement that will change the perspective of care to one that focuses on what the patient wants and values:

> Advances must begin with all health care constituencies—health professionals, federal and state policy makers, public and private purchasers of care, regulators, organization managers and governing boards, and consumers—committing to a national statement of purpose for the health care system as a whole. In making this commitment, the parties would accept as their explicit purpose "to continually reduce the burden of illness, injury, and disability, and to improve the health and functioning of the people of the United States." The parties also would adopt a shared vision of six specific aims for improvement. These aims are built around the core need for health care to be:
>
> - *Safe*: avoiding injuries to patients from the care that is intended to help them.
> - *Effective*: providing services based on scientific knowledge to all who could benefit, and refraining from providing services to those not likely to benefit.
> - *Patient-centered*: providing care that is respectful of and responsive to individual patient preferences, needs, and values, and ensuring that patient values guide all clinical decisions.
> - *Timely*: reducing waits and sometimes harmful delays for both those who receive and those who give care.
> - *Efficient*: avoiding waste, including waste of equipment, supplies, ideas, and energy.
> - *Equitable*: providing care that does not vary in quality because of personal characteristics such as gender, ethnicity, geographic location, and socioeconomic status.

A health care system that achieves major gains in these six areas would be far better at meeting patient needs. Patients would experience care that is safer, more reliable, more responsible to their needs, more integrated, and more available, and they could count on receiving the full array of preventive, acute, and chronic services that are likely to prove beneficial. Clinicians and other health workers also would benefit through their increased satisfaction at being better able to do their jobs and thereby bring improved health, greater longevity, less pain and suffering, and increased personal productivity to those who receive their care. (pp. 2–3)

Patient-centered means listening to each patient. The patient might value something entirely different from the care that is provided. It is important to understand what the patient values. It is best to ask the patient. Often, patients value different things at different times. For example, when a patient is in critical condition, the patient may want a highly skilled, prompt, technologically advanced, yet kind caregiver, whereas a nonacute patient may prefer a rapid turnaround with a kind, personable caregiver. Nevertheless, it is more than that. The answer to the value question depends on how the patient defines quality of life.

Performance Improvement

It must be determined whether the total organization is achieving quality. Of course, all workers can improve. All organizations need PI work to examine quality and safety issues as well as to identify opportunities to improve processes and outcomes. It is a proactive process, meaning that everyone identifies problems and contributes to improvement efforts. Performance improvement has been implemented with varying success in many healthcare organizations and businesses.

Performance improvement is referenced by several terms, for example, continuous improvement, continuous quality improvement, total quality measurement, and quality management, to name a few. Several methods are used to improve performance; however, many healthcare organizations use some form of "plan, do, study, act," or PDSA, to address quality improvement. The IHI (2012a) outlined a model that includes questions the organization must answer followed by the PDSA cycle to test the change to determine whether improvement was made (**Exhibit 4–7**). This is an efficient practice model that results in increased patient satisfaction and quality.

Six Sigma (Smith, 2003) is a popular approach to performance that was previously used in businesses other than health care. Six Sigma provides a systematic approach to improve patient outcomes. The elements of Six Sigma (**Exhibit 4–8**) have been implemented in many hospitals to reduce patient safety events through reduction of process variation. This PI tool incorporates data analysis to identify and reduce variation. By reducing variability and promoting standardization, the potential for errors is greatly decreased, resulting in increased patient safety and better outcomes. Standardization is an important concept. For example, many individuals interact with patients in our healthcare service industry. The aim is for all staff to be cognizant of and use certain customer service behaviors and scripted responses. This means that customer service is standardized so that regardless of the patient contact, these customer service behaviors are present.

Although it is helpful to have standardization in processes, this approach does not take into account individual patient differences and can increase complexity. When complexity increases more errors occur. Some advocate making small incremental changes at the bedside, rather than standardization. Each patient's expectations are different because patients want and value different things. Thus, nurses need to listen to patients about what they want and value.

Scripted responses (another part of Six Sigma) can be helpful when a staff member is not sure how to respond to a patient. However, many professionals resent scripted responses, especially experienced staff who have the judgment to respond appropriately to patients.

Although *Lean* and *Six Sigma* are separate entities, there is a current effort in health care to combine these two methods into a single approach to performance quality improvement (Glasgow, Scott-Caziewell, & Kaboli, 2010). Using both approaches provides processes focused on measuring and eliminating errors

---

Exhibit 4–7 Model for Improvement

The Model for Improvement, developed by Associates in Process Improvement, includes three fundamental questions and Plan-Do-Study-Act (PDSA) cycles to conduct small-scale tests of change.
Questions to answer:
- *What are we trying to accomplish?* Set aims and time specific measurable goals.
- *How will we know that a change is an improvement?* Establish measures, compare with a baseline measure for evaluating results.
- *What changes can we make that will result in improvement?* Brainstorm ideas and test one at a time in a pilot setting. The idea is to fine-tune the process before fully implementing it across the organization. Prioritize which change should be tried first.

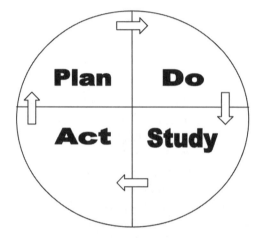

Plan the test of change. Activities, actions, task, or process step.
Do implement the change.
Study the change results. Is the result or outcome better? Was the defined goal met?
Act keep the change or go back to planning. Is fine-tuning needed or start from scratch? Revisit the fundamental questions.

Source: Adapted from the Institute for Healthcare Improvement (IHI). The Model for Improvement, as seen on IHI's website (www .IHI.org), was developed by Associates in Process Improvement [Langley, Nolan, Nolan, Norman, Provost. *The Improvement Guide.* San Francisco: Jossey-Bass Publishers; 2009].

Exhibit 4–8 Critical Elements of Six Sigma

- Genuine focus on the customer.
- Data and fact driven management: the numbers speak.
- Processes are where the action is; processes are the key vehicle to success.
- Proactive management: acting in advance of a problem rather than reacting.
- Boundaryless collaboration: break down barriers between departments, organize work teams across the organization.
- Drive for perfection but tolerate failure.

Source: Data from Smith, B. (2003). *Lean and Six Sigma—a one-two punch.* Quality Progress, 37–41.

(Six Sigma) while ensuring efficient work flow and value-added time (Lean) (Glasgow et al., 2010). Combining these two approaches also balances the regulatory need to maintain process performance (Six Sigma) while supporting rapid continuous improvement (Lean), and thus also easing the tension between the need for incremental changes and system changes.

An important part of the role of an administrator is to pay attention to, and promote, ways the healthcare team can reframe their work to better achieve each patient's goals. This is complicated because it is a new concept for many individuals in health care. In *On the Mend: Revolutionizing Healthcare to Save Lives and Transform the Industry* (Toussaint & Gerard with Adams, 2010)—a must read—the authors describe how various stakeholders (including physicians and patients/families) used the Lean approach, but determined the *value* component by going to the "gemba," or the bedside, where the value is created. They made sweeping changes in the way the continuum of care was delivered by the multidisciplinary team:

> We have learned that every medical act is a series of steps that can be examined and improved. By investigating these steps, and the path that patients take through our hospitals and clinics, we have learned to identify value from the patient's point of view and to start getting rid of the waste that clogs the system of healthcare delivery. In doing this work, we have made life better for our patients. (p. 2)

As they did this process they identified three core principles: (1) *Focus on the patient* (not the hospital or staff) and design care around them. (2) *Identify value* for the patient and get rid of everything else (waste). (3) *Minimize time* to treatment and through its course (p. 14). They designed a *collaborative care unit* where the interdisciplinary team saw the patient within 90 minutes of admission to determine a plan of care, including the anticipated discharge date. As the teams worked together, they trod on sacred cows that, if they did not have value to the patient, were called "waste." Conflicts occurred. It was a difficult process. As they planned for large changes in the way they were doing things, people began to dread the day they would start the change. Yet better care resulted.

> In 2002 for instance, mortality rate for coronary bypass surgery at ThedaCare was nearly 4%—about 12 deaths per year. After several improvement projects in cardiac surgery over seven years, in which we typically removed 40% of wasted time and effort with each pass, cardiac mortality was reduced to near zero. Also, a patient's average time spent in hospital fell from 6.3 days to 4.9 and the cost of a coronary bypass declined 22%. Teamwork like this has saved us more than $27 million and ThedaCare has passed those savings along, becoming the overall lowest-price healthcare provider in Wisconsin. (p. 3)

Paying attention to value, along with quality and safety, puts us in an interesting dilemma. Value, quality, and safety are somewhat elusive because they can never be totally achieved. Yet nurses need to constantly improve patient care processes. It is important to dedicate time and effort to striving to achieve value, quality, and safety. When nurses believe that they have done their best, they have satisfying work experiences. When excellent, safe care is delivered, and the patient values the service, everyone on the healthcare team feels good about his or her work, and, most important, the patient benefits by experiencing the best possible care.

Input and participation by staff are essential to the success of PI teams. Front-line staff are most familiar with the problems and opportunities and can be instrumental in identifying and implementing change or in orchestrating sabotage when they are not consulted. Involvement in PI programs is often mandated in annual employee evaluations and reflected in bonuses for incentive plans.

Former patients are particularly valuable members of PI teams. Improvement efforts are meant to improve patient care, and input from these stakeholders may reveal what was important to them during their encounters with the healthcare system. It is also helpful if project members include patients' family or significant others because these individuals experienced the difficulties inherent in a healthcare crisis or in encounters with the healthcare system. Input from all stakeholders related to the project is invaluable. They have the best ideas about what needs to be done, or changed, to achieve value.

Performance improvement efforts must involve all stakeholders to critically evaluate current practice, processes, potential environmental hazards, and other unsafe situations before incidents occur. Again, the goal is to be proactive rather than reactive. The PI plan should be integrated with the organization's operations and financial plan, as well as education and strategic plans to provide enhanced safety for patients.

It is imperative that administrators focus on safety when considering budget requests. Nurses need to be assertive and consistently tout the importance of these expenditures.

This means that all healthcare workers must look around with "new eyes" to see potential issues that, if recognized, could be prevented. Consider the following list:

- Drug packaging looks the same for different drugs or drug names are similar. Bar coding is critical.
- Errors involve a breakdown in communication. High-risk communications include times of transition such as shift change, patient transfer to another area, or transfer to another facility. Adopting a standard communication method is helpful. **Exhibit 4–9** provides an example of an effective communication method that resulted in 96% to 100% retention of information.
- When staffing is inadequate, more safety issues occur. It may be better to employ more staff, close beds, merge units, or use other planned strategies so that everyone knows what to do when this occurs.
- It is important for every RN routinely to make rounds and talk with the patients. These activities provide opportunities to discover what the patient wants and values.
- It is equally important for nursing assistants to make regular rounds and make sure patients are routinely turned and given important care.
- Poor teamwork and ineffective leadership bring on a multitude of safety issues.
- Sometimes an RN does not assume leadership of a team, for example, a new graduate RN. This brings to light the importance of mentors and preceptors.
- Woods and Doan-Johnson (2002) analyzed 21 disciplinary case files from nine boards of nursing to develop a taxonomy of nursing practice errors (**Exhibit 4–10**). In an effort to raise awareness, it is important to share this information with staff. These errors must be addressed through staff education and PI efforts.
- Lack of critical thinking can cause errors. Staff members need to be educated to go beyond "task orientation" to understand systems thinking before they select actions.
- Interdisciplinary miscommunication is a serious safety issue. Markey and Brown (2002) noted that a team of RNs, physical therapists, occupational therapists, patient care assistants, and physicians, when working together on teams, discovered that each discipline had a different vocabulary for the same activities:

Each department had its own activity and mobility vocabulary and because staff members' duties for mobilizing patients were not defined, creating a common language and clarifying responsibilities were essential to ensuring effective patient mobility plans. The group developed seven standard descriptions of mobility and activity levels ranging from "Total 100%/Be prepared to do everything" to "Independent/No assistance needed." With dressing, for instance, a patient who needs "total assistance" would meet the description, "Patient needs to be dressed," while a patient who needs "moderate" assistance would be noted as "Get dressing articles ready. Can put limbs in clothing but can't pull on completely." (p. 1)

Exhibit 4–9   SBAR Communication

S situation (the current issue)
B background (brief, related to the point)
A assessment (what you found/think)
R recommendation/request (what you want next)

Source: Data from Haig, K., Sutton, S., & Whittington, J. (2006). SBAR: A shared mental model for improving communication between clinicians. *Journal on Quality and Patient Safety, 32*(3), 167–175.

Exhibit 4–10   Categories of Nursing Errors

- Lack of attentiveness
  Attentiveness refers to the nurse's ability to find out and remember assessment data on each patient "paying attention to the patient's clinical condition and response to therapy, as well as potential hazards or errors in treatment" (p. 46).
- Lack of agency/fiduciary concern
  Lack of agency/fiduciary concern gets back to what the patient values. Here the nurse needs to be an advocate for the patient, by questioning physician orders, calling physicians, and paying attention to patient/family requests.
- Inappropriate judgment
  The nurse's judgment and clinical expertise is important if the nurse is to intervene on the patient's behalf.
- Medication errors
  A medication error is any preventable event that may cause or lead to inappropriate medication use or patient harm while the medication is in the control of the health care professional, patient, or consumer. Such events may be related to professional practice, health care products, procedures, and systems, including prescribing; order communication; product labeling, packaging, and nomenclature; compounding; dispensing; distribution; administration; education; monitoring; and use (p. 47). Many medication errors are never reported.
- Lack of intervention on the patient's behalf
  Often, symptoms that the nurse does not recognize or respond to in a timely manner result in a complication or death that could possibly have prevented.
- Lack of prevention
  Teach all employees to identify any potential problems and rectify them as soon as the problems are noticed. Infection control, immobility hazards, and a safe environment are areas of concern.
- Missed or mistaken physician or health care provider orders
  Use of a provider order entry and a computerized documentation system could more effectively prevent this occurrence.
- Documentation errors (p. 46)
  Additional documentation errors are problematic in two areas:

  1. *Charting procedures or medications before they were completed.* Such a documentation error can cause a patient to miss a dose of medication or a treatment and can confuse, misrepresent, or mask a patient's true condition.
  2. *Lack of charting of observations of the patient* causes serious harm when a nurse fails to chart signs of patient deterioration, pain, or agitation or particular signs of complications related to the illness or therapies (p. 48).

Source: Data from Woods, A., & Doan-Johnson, S. (2002, October). Executive summary: Toward a taxonomy of nursing practice errors. *Nursing Management,* 45–48.

These authors found that specific guidelines were most helpful in carrying out the activities specified by nurses, patient care assistants, physicians, physical therapists, or occupational therapists. These guidelines were also shared with patients and families, which accomplished better consistency when working with patients. For example, the patient care assistants understood specifically what to have the patient do as well as what the aide should do for the patient. These guidelines provided a set of scripted behaviors that achieved a more consistent approach. As previously mentioned, scripted formats are popular in healthcare settings because scripted formats provide more consistent care regardless of the provider.

Performance improvement work that resulted in healthcare improvements includes Kalisch and associates (2007), who reported interventions that resulted in lower patient fall rates, lower turnover and vacancy rates, and improved teamwork. Likewise, Hall and colleagues (2008) designed a workplace intervention that resulted in higher perceptions of participants' work and work environment. Finally, Shermont and associates (2008) suggested a 10-minute huddle in the middle of a shift to quickly update nurses on current conditions and to establish priorities regarding next steps. There is a lot of work to be done related to PI efforts. These are only examples. Interestingly, *when PI work is effective, it most often decreases expenses as well.*

Evidence-Based Practice

When contemplating quality patient care, consider whether the most appropriate, up-to-date care is provided. Research has shown that both physicians and nurses plan care and treatment based on what they learned in school, even if that was 20 years ago. In addition, the nurse may not know what is best for a certain individual with a particular need. Nurses must have access to the latest research related to the problem, and/or treatment of the problem, and must use that information and professional judgment to determine the most appropriate approach. Evidence-based practice is a synthesis of research and clinical expertise that has demonstrated to be successful related to particular conditions. This is a challenge because there is so much information available. Knowing where to find the best information, how to evaluate the information to determine what is the best or most appropriate research, and how to apply it to practice is complicated.

The Internet and technology systems are powerful resources. For example, a lot of research on patient outcomes is available. When a physician or nurse practitioner writes a medication order, he or she may not know which of several drugs might be most effective. Evidence-based decision-support systems can quickly determine the best available research for specific topics. These systems also provide evidence-based plans of care and therapy recommendations. Zynx Health (2013) is a decision-support system that provides this service as well as those databases discussed in Chapter 5.

Evidence-based practice is important, but only 15% of the nursing workforce consistently implements practice based on evidence (Shirey, 2006). One problem is that nurses and providers do not realize how easily information can be accessed or they do not take the time to look up current research results. Many lack the skills to translate research knowledge into practice. Obtaining the information is only the first step. Administrators can encourage evidence-based practice by removing barriers to access, by providing technology (such as a computer or handheld device), and by establishing the expectation that practice must be based on current evidence. Sometimes evidence is available in the EMR system. Additionally, administrators and leaders must use evidence to guide our leadership and management practices.

To help close the gap between what is known as evidence and what is practiced, a national consensus committee has convened, identifying appropriate competencies for basic, advanced, and doctoral-level nursing education. Use of competencies to evaluate and build nursing skills is essential in promoting practice based on evidence. Kathleen Stevens and her team developed the ACE Star Model of Knowledge Transformation that provides a framework for moving research study findings to bedside practice, creating a positive impact on health outcomes. The model and additional information about evidence-based competencies can be found the Academic Center for Evidence-Based Practice at the School of Nursing UT Health Sciences Center in San Antonio, Texas; the website is www.acestar.uthscsa.edu.

Clinical Pathways and Protocols

When delivering care, evidence-based practice can be achieved by using clinical pathways, order sets, or clinical protocols as long as the pathways or protocols are kept current. An effective clinical pathway is the result of interdisciplinary teamwork; the team includes the physician, nurse, social worker, dietitian, and patient and may include other members such as chaplain or nurse aide or significant family members. Approved protocols can automatically be implemented without an additional order. A caution related to clinical pathways is that all caregivers must continue to take into account patient idiosyncrasies or differences (and what the patient wants and values) that might change the pathway.

Changing Administrative Practices

Variation in the success of PI programs is often related to administrative leaders who do not support the work. Thus, problem processes proliferate that may negatively affect the success of the organization. Often, PI endeavors are not perceived as important. This text provides information regarding how to be more effective as an administrator. For example, nurses need to examine their leadership. If that is not effective, everything else is problematic as well. The IHI (2011c) offers a free tool, *Strategies for Leadership: Hospital Executives and Their Role in Patient Safety*, that can be downloaded from its website (www.ihi.org; you must register to download the guide, but it is free). The IHI (2012b) also presents eight steps for leaders to follow to achieve patient safety. These steps are presented in **Exhibit 4–11**.

Nurses need to complete an organizational assessment and learn how to identify and make systems changes effectively. Note that the most effective changes are small, incremental, and at the point of care. Little by little better quality is achieved. This is better than adding to the complexity with quick fixes, which create more issues to be dealt with later. As complexity increases, errors increase. Nurses need to know how to find information related to their administrative work to remain up-to-date in administrative practices and must encourage staff and physicians to use these resources.

As we move into the Information Age, we need to leave behind many administrative practices and pursue other practices that traditionally have not been part of our role. Porter-O'Grady and Malloch (2011) define what they see as major administrative tasks in the twenty-first century:

- Deconstructing the barriers and structures of the 20th Century,
- Alerting staff about the implications of changing what they do,
- Establishing safety around taking risks and experimenting,
- Embracing new technologies as a way of doing work,
- Reading the signposts along the road to the future,
- Translating the emerging reality into language the staff can use,
- Demonstrating personal engagement with the change effort,
- Helping others adapt to the demands of a changing health system,
- Creating a safe milieu for the struggles and pain of change,
- Enumerating small successes as a basis for supporting staff
- Celebrating the journey and all progress made. (p. 19)

Exhibit 4–11   Process for Achieving Patient Safety and High Reliability

1. Address strategic priorities, culture, and infrastructure.
2. Engage key stakeholders.
3. Communicate and build awareness.
4. Establish, oversee, and communicate system-level aims.
5. Track/measure performance over time, strengthen analysis.
6. Support staff and patient/families impacted by medical errors.
7. Align system-wide activities and incentives.
8. Redesign systems and improve reliability.

Source: Reprinted from the Institute for Healthcare Improvement. (2006). Botwinick L, Bisognano M, Haraden C. *Leadership Guide to Patient Safety.* IHI Innovation Series white paper. Retrieved from http://www.ihi.org/knowledge/Pages/IHIWhitePapers/LeadershipGuidetoPatientsSafetyWhitePaper.aspx

Add the following questions to this list:

- Is the care up-to-date?
- Do our administrative practices reflect the Information Age, or are they stuck in the Industrial Age?
- Is consistent listening to the patient a priority? Do we share information with patients and involve them in making treatment decisions?

Accomplishing the items on this list is important to work toward the goal of listening to our patients and involving them in their treatment decisions.

The IOM (2001) provides the best signpost, to date, for us to use as our ultimate goal. It advocates the redesign of our healthcare delivery systems based on 10 fundamental rules. *Redesign* has been so mismanaged in health care that the word has negative connotations. The difference here is that *redesign* as described by the IOM uses the administrative practices discussed in this text. It is *not* a bottom-line approach to downsize. The 10 rules of redesign are as follows:

1. **Care is based on continuous healing relationships**. Patients should receive care whenever they need it and in many forms, not just face-to-face visits. This implies that the healthcare system must be responsive at all times, and access to care should be provided over the Internet, by telephone, and by other means in addition to in-person visits.
2. **Care is customized according to patient needs and values**. The system should be designed to meet the most common types of needs but should have the capability to respond to individual patient choices and preferences.
3. **The patient is the source of control**. Patients should be given the necessary information and opportunity to exercise the degree of control they choose over healthcare decisions that affect them. The system should be able to accommodate differences in patient preferences and encourage shared decision making.
4. **Knowledge is shared and information flows freely**. Patients should have unfettered access to their own medical information and to clinical knowledge. Clinicians and patients should communicate effectively and share information.
5. **Decision making is evidence-based**. Patients should receive care based on the best available scientific knowledge. Care should not vary illogically from clinician to clinician or from place to place.
6. **Safety is a system property**. Patients should be safe from injury caused by the care system. Reducing risk and ensuring safety require greater attention to systems that help prevent and mitigate errors.
7. **Transparency is necessary**. The system should make available to patients and their families information that enables them to make informed decisions when selecting a health plan, hospital, or clinical practice, or when choosing among alternative treatments. This should include information describing the system's performance on safety, evidence-based practice, and patient satisfaction.
8. **Needs are anticipated**. The system should anticipate patient needs rather than simply react to events.
9. **Waste is continuously decreased**. The system should not waste resources or patient time.
10. **Cooperation among clinicians is a priority**. Clinicians and institutions should actively collaborate and communicate to ensure an appropriate exchange of information and coordination of care. (pp. 8–9)

Provider Accountability in the Cost–Quality Dilemma

The linear healthcare administrator, heavily committed to the bottom line, may question, "Where is the money coming from for all this?" Reframing is in order. Recall that nurses are now in the Information Age and the rules have changed. The bottom line-oriented administrator may not have realized this yet, so we must be patient and keep on persistently creating the new healthcare environment. Porter-O'Grady and Malloch (2011) suggest that nurses should reframe the cost–quality dilemma by asking a value question.

> It is not uncommon for leaders to be unsure of the real value of the services provided by healthcare providers in their organizations. Some providers are not sure of this themselves. Evidence must show that resources are being used efficiently to bring about clear improvements in patient conditions, increase the ability of the patients to manage their own health, and add to the patients' knowledge of their conditions and/or healthy behaviours. This is quite different from providing services as defined in a standards manual.
>
> Determining the value of healthcare services is an integral part of quantum leadership. This value, which is defined by means of an equation containing the three elements of cost, quality, and service, is never simply a matter of dollars . . . . Instead, its calculation takes into account what is actually gained and what are the real costs. The exact equation is expressed thus: healthcare value = resources (funds and labor and supplies) + quality (appropriateness of interventions) + service (satisfaction and effective relationships).
>
> Finding the value of a healthcare service requires healthcare leaders and care providers to ask the following questions:
>
> - What is the actual service provided?
> - How do organizational processes support this service?
> - What are the interactions between these processes?
> - What impact does the service have on the patients and the community?
>
> The answers to these questions guide leaders and healthcare providers toward wise choices—toward clinical decisions that are the most cost-effective and result in the highest quality care being provided at the lowest cost. The challenge for leaders is to reframe the healthcare quality issue as a value question. Again, value is defined as the result of an interactive process involving cost, quality, and service. (p. 300–301)

Striving for value will make a difference. The nurse manager is situated between senior leaders and staff and thus is in a pivotal position to influence change. The nurse manager is a teacher for staff and role model for all healthcare workers. Focusing on what the patient values and wants is a wise choice as opposed to focusing on those things that do not make a difference for patients. Often, this is a new concept for patients and families as well. A proportion of patients will not accept the new role, some because of culture, others because of health literacy, lack of knowledge, or a host of additional reasons (Longtin et al., 2010).

This brings the nurse back to the foundational document, the ANA *Code of Ethics with Interpretive Statements*, which demands that nurses provide the patient with the needed knowledge. Patients have the moral and legal right "to be given accurate, complete, and understandable information in a manner that facilitates informed judgment" (ANA, 2001). Habitually seeking what the patient wants and values is *not optional*; rather it is our mandate. The issue is a serious one.

A "bottom-line" administrator simply on the basis of salary alone may deem that RNs are more expensive to employ. To save money the administrator may demand the staffing mix be changed by decreasing the number of RNs and adding licensed practical nurses (LPNs) or nursing assistants. This demand is not supported by evidence. Melberg (1997) examined budgets and staffing at five hospitals, documenting that a hospital budget with a 96% RN staff mix is *less expensive* than another hospital budget with a 64% RN mix. In fact, the hospital with the highest costs had the *lowest* RN skill mix (64%). Melberg (1997) noted:

> A high RN mix [96%] does not correlate with higher nursing costs per patient day in acute or critical care. Diluting the RN mix does not always reduce staffing costs. Although hospital A has a 96 percent RN-skill mix, the highest in the system, total nursing salary per patient day falls exactly in the middle. The highest costs occurred at hospital C where, in fact, the 64 percent RN mix is the lowest in the system. This finding is consistent in acute care, in critical care and on the orthopedic units—specialty nursing areas found in all five hospitals and therefore used for comparison. This difference is not explained by regional variations in RN salary, since RN salary at hospital A during the period of study was higher than at any hospital in the system except hospital E. (p. 48)

Likewise, a study by Lindrooth, Bazzoli, Needleman, and Hasnain-Wynia (2006) corroborates that it is more cost-effective to provide a higher RN ratio. Thus, cost may be *higher* with a higher ratio of LPNs and nurse aides.

This is only the beginning of the cost issue because RNs save costs in other areas in addition to salaries. Consider patient outcomes and the cost of patient safety events. Recall earlier in this chapter that the IOM (2004a) documented that each patient safety event added an additional $8,750 to each hospital stay. Also recall research that notes higher RN ratios are linked to better patient outcomes. When lower RN staffing leads to death or injury, it is a *very high cost*. Thus, determining the appropriate nursing skill mix requires analysis of the care environment, population served, patient acuity, patient turnover, the type and manner in which care is delivered, culture, budget, staff competencies, and evidence-based findings. There are no easy answers. What works best in one setting (for example, in a step-down unit) may not be best in another (for example, a skilled unit). Thus, the nursing skill mix is determined by the current circumstances and changes to meet new situations as they occur.

Administrators must critically analyze issues of adequate staffing and the RN staffing mix. Research supports the fact that increased RN staffing affects patient safety. This provides the impetus for administrators to focus on RN recruitment and retention efforts. Recall from earlier in this chapter that the ANA (2013b) cited, "*each additional patient care RN employed (at 7.8 hours per patient day) will generate over $60,000 annually in reduced medical costs and improved national productivity*" (para. 5).

What Does It Mean to Be in the Information Age?

Performance improvement in the Information Age means that nurses must use technology effectively. In the past, many computer systems were not integrated. The transition to a fully integrated computerized system moves the organization to a more viable state that enables improved access and use of information. Integration allows use of clinical decision support at the point of care, which is crucial to implement evidence-based practice. This presents a major financial undertaking because computer systems are expensive. Costs extend beyond the walls of the organization, which brings about additional challenges. Physicians and other providers need to be able to access the system from multiple locations, not just when they are in the facility. For true point-of-care access, computers must be mobile or at every point of care.

Online Clinical Documentation Systems

The Leapfrog Group (2013) identified the importance of CPOE. There are entire online clinical documentation systems that are even better with physician order entry. This is especially pertinent in large healthcare systems. Online documentation provides integration of documentation from all disciplines. All disciplines chart together, and thus there is immediate access to relevant information, as well as better continuity of care. In addition, preformatted charting presents an easy, time-saving format for the clinician to follow. Patient safety is enhanced through decision support. Built-in clinical alerts identify abnormal results, allergies, stop dates on medicines, incompatible medicines, times to administer medications and provide a variety of other safeguards that promote patient safety and quality.

Online systems also provide immediate and virtual access to laboratory and radiology results in both the healthcare facility and the physician's office. In addition, physicians can interact with the CPOE system from their office location. Prescriptions and discharge instructions can be generated. From a safety standpoint, the liability related to legibility problems is decreased.

In these systems, documentation is thorough and better reflects patient status, resulting in enhanced safety and increased reimbursement as a result of accurate coding for billing. The systems can also link cost and quality data.

An alert to clinicians using computers in the patient's presence is that patients may erroneously think that providers are using the computer in a way unrelated to patient care. Thus, it is important for providers to explain computer work to clarify their actions for patients.

Bar Coding

A closed-loop system comprising a scanner to bar-code the medication, the clinician administering the medication, and the patient's armband has proven very successful in reducing medication errors related to the five rights of medication administration: right patient, right route, right dose, right time, and right medication. Medication-dispensing systems such as Pyxis and Omnicell are available in many facilities to assist with medication administration. The medicine is categorized in drawers, and the appropriate drawer opens when the patient name and medication name are entered. Some facilities have implemented robotics to assist with medication identification in the pharmacy as well as with delivery from the pharmacy. In this era of healthcare shortages at crisis proportions, robotic help is needed. These strategies also decrease the possibility of error. Although costs are significant, the savings realized from diverted errors, increased patient satisfaction, and promotion of quality more than makes up for the expense.

Portable Electronic Devices

Portable electronic devices are used to promote efficiency and decrease transcription errors. Access is available from remote locations, for example, during the admission process to retrieve demographic and insurance information. In addition, clinicians can retrieve information about medications, diagnoses, and other health data immediately as needed.

Recognition of Value and Quality

A number of programs in health care focus on value and quality. Some have gained national awareness.

The Planetree Model

The Planetree model acknowledges the importance of environment, providing a more humanistic, personalized, patient-centered experience. The delivery is holistic, encompassing mental, social, and emotional dimensions as well as physical symptoms. The goal is to maximize health care by combining medical therapy with complementary alternatives and use architectural and environmental designs in the process. Planetree embraces a novel concept in that the provision of compassionate, nurturing, personalized care is designed not only for patients and patient families, but also for staff. Thus, using the Planetree approach, the organization must embrace a culture that nurtures staff as well as patients (Planetree, n.d.).

Planetree partners with providers across the continuum. The Planetree philosophy promotes innovative, patient-centered healthcare models, which focus on healing and nurturing the body, mind, and spirit in a thoughtful environment (**Exhibit 4–12**). Planetree also provides a framework for assessment of the structure and processes needed to sustain the patient-centered culture.

Exhibit 4–12   Planetree Components

- **Humanness:** Human beings are cared for by human beings in a healing environment in which care is personalized and directed by patients, residents, and families based on their unique values and desires. The healing environment is created within a culture that also nurtures the human caregiver.
- **Family, Friend, and Social Support:** Social support is fostered throughout the continuum with involvement of family and friends when possible. Support includes visitation, the option of presence of family and friends during invasive procedures, and extends to pet therapy.
- **Education and Information:** Illness is viewed as an educational and enlightening opportunity. Patients and residents are provided access to and are encouraged to read their medical record. Educational resources are provided to patients and residents in order to foster active participation in their care and well-being. Education opportunities, for example libraries and Internet access, are extended to families and the community.
- **Design of the Healing Environment:** The physical environment is designed to foster healing and well-being. The design values humans and provides the comforts of home across the continuum of care. Examples of the healing environment include gardens, rooms for social activities, chapels, accommodations for families, and so forth.
- **Nutrition:** Nutrition is viewed as essential for health and well-being. The organization provides a role model for delicious and healthy eating. Preparing food, dining, and food choices are flexible based on the patient's preference.
- **Arts and Entertainment:** Creativity, camaraderie, and fun are nurtured through art, classes, music, movies, and so forth.
- **Spirituality and Diversity:** Patient, resident, family, and staff spirituality is supported in the healing environment through means which provide connections with their inner resources; examples include chapels, gardens, and meditation rooms.
- **Human Touch:** Touch is used to decrease anxiety, pain, and stress. Training programs are provided for families, staff, and volunteers.
- **Complementary Therapies:** Therapy choices are extended beyond traditional western care. Complementary therapies such as Reiki, guided imagery, and acupuncture are used. Additional therapies include exercise and wellness programs.
- **Healthy Communities:** The health and wellness of the larger community is redefined and includes schools, senior citizen centers, churches, and others in the community.

Source: Adapted from Planetree. (n.d.). About Planetree. Retrieved from http://www.planetree.org/ABOUT/ABOUT.html

The Eden Alternative

A philosophy similar to the Planetree model that has been instituted in long-term care is the Eden Alternative (2009), developed by Dr. William Thomas, geriatrician. This philosophy is based on the belief that the focus of long-term care should be care and not treatment. Thomas further elaborates that the major problems in nursing homes are loneliness, boredom, and helplessness; the residents are overmedicated, deprived of the enjoyment of a pleasant meal by unnecessary dietary restrictions, and subject to endless activity programs developed to meet regulatory compliance rather than provide entertainment for the residents. Thomas's solution was the creation of an environment that allowed people to flourish by inundating them with life in the form of plants, animals, and children. The Eden Alternative offers a more humanistic, home-like environment; it offers residents opportunities to maintain and control the environment and encourages interaction and compassion (Eden Alternative, 2009).

The Leapfrog Group

Organizations have implemented voluntary programs that measure and report safety data and outcomes. An example is the Leapfrog Group, which supports pay for performance. The Leapfrog Group is a

> consortium of major companies and other large private and public healthcare purchasers. . . . Members and their employees spend tens of billions of dollars on health care annually. Leapfrog members have agreed to base their purchase of health care on principles that encourage quality improvement among providers and consumer involvement. (Leapfrog Group, 2013, para. 3)

Its primary focus is to improve and implement best practices.

Magnet Recognition Program

Earning the esteemed designation of a Magnet facility has become a renowned indicator of quality. This is an expensive process in terms of both money and resources for the facility. Magnet recognition is a voluntarily process encompassing strenuous evaluation of nursing excellence and innovation in nursing practice (American Nurses Credentialing Center [ANCC], 2013). The Magnet Recognition Program has three goals:

- Promote quality in a setting that supports professional practice
- Identify excellence in the delivery of nursing services to patients/residents
- Disseminate best practice in nursing services (ANCC, 2013, para. 7)

The National Database of Nursing Quality Indicators

The NDNQI was developed by the American Nurses Association (ANA, 2013a) to collect and report nurse-sensitive outcomes data in an effort to show how nursing care promotes quality and patient safety. Participation is voluntary, and thus data may not provide an accurate picture of nursing care across the nation. Nevertheless, the NDNQI data provide nurse administrators a tool to compare outcomes, staffing, and other nurse-sensitive measures. Some of the data include incidents of hospital-acquired pressure ulcers, fall rates, and restraint use in relation to nursing hours per patient day and skill mix.

Performance Measurement

In an effort to contain costs, performance measurement became popular in the early 1990s when companies purchasing health plans needed to examine cost and quality data to determine which plan was best for the dollars spent. At first, these efforts were called report cards and only summary performance data were included. Later, report cards were used internally by healthcare organizations to improve services. (Details can be found at www.healthgrades.com/.)

The idea behind performance measurement is that patient outcomes could be used to determine the effectiveness of organizational performance. Although this measurement is an improvement on past practices, there are several problems with this measurement: (1) future performance cannot be determined from historical data; (2) no one asked the patient what the patient wanted or valued; (3) organizations are inundated with data, leaving little time to analyze or use the data effectively; and (4) sometimes the data were used punitively when outcomes were poor, which only impeded future improvements.

The following are examples of how report card data are used:

1. The ANA (2013a) used NDNQI data as a report card to compare voluntarily reported nursing-sensitive outcomes such as fall rates related to nurse staffing and other organizational characteristics.
2. Hospital Compare uses a report card format to compare outcomes for specific measures for Medicare beneficiaries (Medicare.gov, n.d.). These data are available for patients and families and can be used for selecting the facility of choice based on outcomes. (Details can be found at www .hospitalcompare.hhs.gov.)

As report card data became available, The Joint Commission (2013b) expanded performance measurement to include two sets of measures, core or standardized measures and noncore measures. In 2003, The Joint Commission joined forces with CMS to align efforts and required organizations to report on certain measures depending on the populations served (The Joint Commission, 2013b). Measures are identified for hospitals, long-term care facilities, and home care. The results are available to the public at www.qualitycheck.org (The Joint Commission, 2013e).

Sentara Healthcare established performance improvement goals and then tied them to the incentive plan (Grayson, 2002). Taking it one step further would entail a link for all staff to achievement of the established goals.

> Our chief medical officer, who has worked in four institutions, said that this is the only place he's worked where he actually gets calls from the non-medical managers asking if we are making progress in the clinical quality indicators because their compensation is tied to these improvements. So it's a system to foster innovation with built-in accountability aimed at increasing the quality of care. . . . A good example is our remotely monitored electronic ICU. Intensive care specialists monitor ICU patients 19 hours a day for timely intervention. [From 7 AM to noon, physicians make rounds in the actual units.] The physician has computer access to the patient's records, including lab or radiographic tests, and can view the patient and talk with staff via in-room, high-resolution video cameras. The system enhances traditional rounds and on-site monitoring. Patient mortality rates have dropped 25 to 35 percent and it's achieved a 155 percent payback. (Grayson, 2002, p. 36)

Benchmarking

Many healthcare organizations benchmark quality measures. Often, when benchmarking, the organization sets a goal, for example, to be in the top 25th quartile. However, benchmarking can be fraught with problems. Rudy, Lucke, Whitman, and Davidson (2001) reported the following:

> Benchmarking is a common approach to establishing quality. However, the conclusions drawn from benchmarking depend heavily on whether the benchmark is obtained from the literature, from hospital-specific sources, or from an integrated hospital system. Benchmarking using the literature may appear the simplest, but often a literature-based benchmark is not available, is not sufficiently relevant, or differs in definitions, populations, or clinical practice. . . . An important but rarely addressed issue in literature-based benchmarking is assessing uncertainty, such as the standard error, in the benchmark itself.
>
> Internal benchmarking is available to hospitals with the relevant databases and statistical expertise, but it can provide an invalid assessment of performance when compared to other institutions. . . .
>
> System benchmarking appears to avoid the pitfalls of these other two methods, but it requires coordinated database resources and sophisticated statistical analyses. System-based benchmarks without adequate adjustments for acuity put hospitals with higher acuity at a disadvantage. Hospitals with smaller censuses may have larger differences between hospital-specific and system-based estimates than do those with larger censuses. (p. 189)

There is an additional problem with benchmarking. Comparisons do not take into account what has value from the patient's perspective. For example, when benchmarking the wait time for an ED visit, a wait time of 1 hour might compare favorably with other ED wait times. Nevertheless, consider this statement from the patient's perspective: The patient does not enjoy experiencing an hour wait in the ED to be seen by the provider. From the patient value perspective, it is better to eliminate the wait time and have the patient seen by the provider immediately. Some EDs already use 30 minutes as the benchmark; even a 30-minute wait is not as valuable to the patient as no wait time. Recall, if healthcare workers do not fix it, someone else will!

Patient Satisfaction

Patient satisfaction is one early performance measure that focuses on what the patient values. Patient satisfaction instruments are a beginning measurement of value, although they take place *after* the healthcare experience. Hospitals have used patient satisfaction measurements for some time because measuring patient satisfaction has been an important core outcome measure for Joint Commission accreditation.

Examples of companies that provide patient satisfaction instruments and services to healthcare organizations include Gallup® (2013) and Press Ganey Associates® (2013). Generally, hospitals pay these companies to collect and tabulate the data. This is considered more effective because patients are more likely to be forthright with an outside vendor as opposed to those providing their care. There are other advantages to using an outside vendor: The organization's results are ranked among similar organizations, thus providing benchmarking opportunities.

To adequately assess patient satisfaction, both the patient's and the provider's expectations must be clearly identified. In the past, patients were seen as customers in need of health care; now they are viewed as informed consumers looking for quality care. Health care has become a competitive business. Many facilities are using contract agencies to market their services and measure their success, and they have implemented service excellence initiatives to improve patient satisfaction. Some even have scripted behaviors and protocols to standardize dialogue in difficult situations. This is an example of standardization previously discussed.

It is important to remember that nurses deal with people. What has value to one individual may not have value to another. For example, one individual may welcome talking about emotions with a healthcare provider, whereas another individual may find this invasive. One individual may respond to pain by being stoic, whereas another who experiences even mild pain may scream and yell.

Staff evaluations may be directly linked to satisfaction results. Results from patient satisfaction surveys can be very useful and can be used to do the following:

- Improve and measure the quality of care
- Manage complaints
- Implement strategic planning and marketing decisions
- Evaluate and/or provide bonuses to departments or individual (physician and nonphysician) staff
- Enhance public relations
- Meet accreditation standards
- Monitor for risk management
- Link survey results to clinical data
- Use survey results for contract payer negotiations
- Compare the results for benchmarking
- Link the results to financial data

Performance Measurement and Patient Value

It is questionable as to whether these measures reflect what patients want and value. The CMS Quality Initiatives (CMS, 2013g) and the Joint Commission's National Patient Safety Goals (The Joint Commission, 2013d) are patient-centered, but, again, it is uncertain whether these measure the patient's perception of value. Outside vendors measure patient satisfaction, but, again, do the operational definitions capture the patient's perception of value?

Empirical data have dominated the healthcare system. What is needed in addition to quantifiable data is capture of the complexity of healthcare work (Porter-O'Grady & Malloch, 2011). Porter-O'Grady and Malloch further note that qualitative data, for example, "patient–provider relationships, effectiveness of the procedure, patient satisfaction, and health behaviors practiced is not considered in the reimbursement categories" (p. 85). This links to the patient and family advisory focus groups discussed earlier in this chapter. The data received from these groups provide rich information for PI work.

Administrators must maintain the focus on what patients want and value. If leaders lose sight of this goal, statistics are useless. The organization may be profitable and have stellar patient outcomes, but if patients are not getting what they need, want, and value, they have a choice as to whether or not to return to the facility. As organizations collect data from focus groups, or even as they organize the groups, they must consider the data in terms of populations served because voluminous qualitative data can become overwhelming. The emphasis must move from individuals to populations. As nurses examine patient populations, their focus should move beyond identified diseases or problems. For example, parents of young children have concerns that are different from those of older adults who are experiencing chronic diseases and who are on fixed incomes. Focus group participants may need to be organized to better identify these populations.

Balanced Scorecard: Best Approach to Performance Measurement

Balanced scorecards are the best way to conduct improvement work (IHI, 2012c). Metrics captured in the organization's balanced scorecard are tied directly to the strategic plan. A primary utility of the balanced scorecard is the tie between strategic management and performance management. Measurement of key financial, quality, market, and operational indicators provides management with an understanding of performance in relation to established strategic goals and graphically displays a snapshot of the institution's overall health (Health Care Advisory Board, 1999). Plotting the data for these measures using a run chart (then a control chart when sufficient data points are collected) is a simple and effective way to determine whether changes are leading to improvement or whether the gains are sustained (IHI, 2012c). Run charts and control charts are graphs of data over time and are important tools for assessing effectiveness of change (IHI, 2011b). Benefits of run charts include the following:

- They help improvement teams formulate aims by depicting how well (or poorly) a process is performing.
- They help in determining when changes are truly improvements by displaying a pattern of data that you can observe as you make changes.
- They give direction as you work on improvement and information about the value of particular changes. (IHI, 2011b, para. 2)

It is vital that administrators and managers understand the type data collected and the correct type of chart to be used. This information is beyond the scope of this chapter.

Utilization Review

Another measurement related to the care provided is *utilization review*. The Utilization Review Accreditation Commission (URAC, 2011) reviews healthcare operations to ensure business is conducted in a manner consistent with national standards. The URAC (2013) is the leader in Health Utilization Management Accreditation (HUM). Similar to The Joint Commission, URAC evaluates organizations to determine whether they meet defined standards in one or more programs such as disease management, case management, or credentialing. The URAC's standards address the following:

- Medical necessity criteria that are evidence based and promote consumer safety;
- Specialty matched clinical peers for medical necessity review;
- Requirements for consistency in maintaining the highest confidentiality in utilization management (UM) processes as we approach a new age with electronic health records (EHR) and health information exchanges;
- The need for flexibility for stand-alone UM organization and UM functions within health benefit programs such as indemnity insurance, health maintenance organizations (HMOs), preferred provider organizations (PPOs), consumer-directed healthcare plans, and third-party administrators (PAs);
- Specialty UM organizations, such as mental health, dentistry, physical medicine rehabilitation, genetic testing, and hospitals. (URAC, 2013, para. 2)

Utilization management has a quality dimension in that the primary purpose is to ensure appropriate use of available services and resources. Many organizations integrate utilization management into the case management role, creating a more complete system of quality management. Historically, healthcare organizations established a person or department to complete utilization review through the relay of clinical information to payers so that the payers could determine whether they would pay for additional care for patients. In the managed care climate, providers cannot provide the care and then submit the bill; rather, they must get preapproval for the care. The payers determine whether the care is allowable. Once the payers determine that the care meets their criteria, the patient is certified for payment.

Employee Issues

When discussing value and quality, it is important to remember employees. When administrators value employees, employees value patients. Thus, this section describes value and quality related to employees.

OSHA Standards for Employee Safety

The first issue is employee safety. There are many possible hazards in the healthcare industry. The Occupational Safety and Health Administration (OSHA) provides nationally mandated standards for the workplace (U.S. Department of Labor, n.d.). Detailed information is available at the U.S. Department of Labor OSHA website (at www.osha.gov). Administrators and other leaders must be regularly oriented to OSHA standards. In addition, OSHA has record-keeping requirements that mandate that organizational leaders keep records updated to document compliance with OSHA standards. In larger healthcare systems, both quality and infection control personnel are often concerned with workplace compliance with OSHA standards. In smaller systems, OSHA compliance often becomes an additional responsibility of staff who already have many other roles and responsibilities. Regardless, the nurse manager must be aware of the current standards, ensure that employees are oriented to these standards, and ensure that the unit environment is in compliance with the standards.

Promoting a Healthy Workplace

Achieving a healthy workplace includes examining the environment. This can be quite complicated. For example, a sharps injury from a needle used by a patient who has AIDS or hepatitis is a major hazard.

> Of the nearly 14 injury cases per 100 long-term-care employees, a significant number are related to patient lifting or repositioning tasks. OSHA recommends "that manual lifting of residents be minimized in all cases and eliminated when feasible." . . . Possible solutions . . . include using mechanical lifts and ceiling-mounted lift systems. . . . For patients with the ability to assist, or who are able to bear weight completely, equipment such as sit-to-stand devices, ambulation-assist devices, transfer boards, and lift cushions or chairs can minimize assistance needed in transferring. [This includes height-adjustable beds with electric controls rather than cranks and showering and bathing assistive devices.] (Weber, 2008, p. 30)

The general public, patients, employees, and administrators frequent healthcare facilities. The volume of people who have access to healthcare facilities presents a number of ways that employees and others could be put at risk (infectious diseases, violence, and so forth). Administrators are responsible for maintaining a safe environment for staff as well as patients.

Disaster Planning and Preparedness

Disaster planning and preparedness has assumed new significance. With the many weather-related events, facilities must be prepared to deal with theses issues, even when the facility has been decimated. In addition, the issue of bioterrorism must be addressed for patients and employees. The intentional introduction of anthrax, smallpox, or other disease entities as a biological weapon would certainly play havoc on already short-staffed, financially burdened healthcare facilities. Procedures to address the identified emergency are dictated by the Federal Emergency Management Administration (FEMA, n.d.), but facility-related issues such as lack of available nurses and methods to contain or quarantine are facility specific and should be addressed in policy. Sadly, these issues must be considered at budget time to designate appropriate funds for protective apparel, vaccinations, preparation and training for staff, and public education.

Chaos Theory

Another scientific field of thought is chaos theory. In this theory, the world all around us seems chaotic, but when all of this seeming chaos "is plotted over millions of iterations," it creates a perfectly proportioned picture. This offers great hope for us. Even when it seems that total chaos surrounds us, we must rise above it and look down to find the order and perfection.

> Chaos is an essential constituent of all change. It works to unbundle attachment to whatever is impeding movement. Chaos challenges us to simultaneously let go and to take on. It reminds us that life is a journey of constant creation. (Porter-O'Grady & Malloch, 2011, p. 22)

Sometimes when unexpected events happen or setbacks or difficult situations occur, it is comforting to know that these experiences accomplish good things for us. Nurses can learn from such situations and become better persons. In addition, these experiences can lead to something different or new that we would probably never have tried if the difficulties had not occurred.

When considering planning for change, chaos theory tells us that we cannot possibly plan, or map out, all of the details of the change because of chaotic occurrences. As these occurrences happen, they necessitate adjustments in the plan. This is why all staff need to be involved in understanding the plan and need to be empowered to accomplish it—because the final product, or components of the final product, will ultimately be different from what was planned. Really, there is no final product. Chaos continues to change what was implemented. No one can stop change; rather, it continually moves on into uncharted territory.

Many administrative leaders do not understand the concept of constant change. Instead, they try to cling to the Industrial Age idea that everything is rational and can be planned out in minute detail. It is as if they think they can just order others to follow through on their plan, and then they become frustrated when people do not follow through. This is not the new reality. Continuing to believe this opens us up to unnecessary frustration, and employees will be frustrated as well.

Instead, all of us must be open to the reality around us, see the changes that are occurring, and help interpret the chaos for one another. Although everyone has their own views of reality, chaotic reality happens, and changes will occur and leave us behind, obsolete and unfulfilled.

Leaders now must incorporate the vagaries of complexity and chaos into the process of anticipating and planning for the future. Detailing the specifics of some future state is no longer a viable means of planning. Discernment and signpost reading are better skills to have than are those related to defining and direction setting. Leaders must realize that no real-time insight is sustainable, nor is it entirely accurate. It is simply a reflection of the particular point a person or organization is at in their continuous and relentless unfolding and becoming.

A good leader is one who can read the signposts suggesting that a change is imminent and can discern the direction of the change and the elements indicating its fabric. The good leader synthesizes rather than analyzes and views the change thematically and/or relationally, drawing out of it what kind of action or strategy should be applied—the response, that is, that best positions for the organization to thrive in the coming circumstances.

For a leader to act as a strategist today means not detailing the organization's future actions, but analyzing the relationship of the system to its external environment, determining the ability of the system to respond and adapt in a sustainable way, and translating that relationship and ability into language that has meaning for those who must do the work of the organization. Translating the signposts into understandable and inspiring language is more critical than almost any other strategic task. It is vital that a change have implications for those who are doing the work. Another way of saying this is that it must have meaning to them within the framework of their work activities so that they can commit to it, which they must do if they and the organization are to adapt to the change successfully. The leader's job is to describe the change in a way that allows the workers to understand its value and how it will affect their own efforts.

In this new era, leaders need insights about contextual themes rather than step-by-step guidance on how to implement a minutely defined vision. They must understand that their organization is on a journey and that they need to continuously peruse the landscape for guidance rather than create a list of steps through which the organization will move on its way to a preset future. Becoming aware of the themes and undercurrents and reading the contextual signposts regularly is a wiser and more effective strategy for the new age leader than laying out an itemized plan that may or may not correspond with future conditions. (Porter-O'Grady & Malloch, 2011, pp. 23–24)

See **Exhibit 4–13**.

Exhibit 4–13   Interdependence

In nature everything is interdependent. There is an ebb and flow between all the elements of life. Leaders must see their role from this perspective. Most of the work of leadership will be managing the interactions and connections between people and processes. Leaders must remain aware of these truths:

- Action in one place has an effect in other places.
- Fluctuation of mutuality means authority moves between people.
- Interacting properties in systems make outcomes mobile and fluid.
- Relationship building is the primary work of leadership.
- Trusting feeling is as important as valuing thinking.
- Acknowledging in others what is unique in their contribution is vital.
- Supporting, stretching, challenging, pushing, and helping are part of being present to the process, to the players, and to the outcome.

Source: Porter-O'Grady, T., and Malloch, K. (2003). *Quantum leadership: A textbook of new leadership.* Sudbury, MA: Jones and Bartlett, p. 22.

Discussion Questions

1. Describe strategies used by the nurse administrator that provide patients with what they want and value.
2. What administrative practices support PI efforts?
3. Provide examples of the 10 IOM (2001) rules for redesign applied to your healthcare setting.
4. State five ways that administrators promote patient safety.
5. Why is it important to provide evidence-based care? Discuss some of the challenges nurse administrators face in creating an environment in which bedside nurses use evidence-based care.
6. Discuss the use of run charts and control charts to improve quality.
7. Discuss how Lean thinking and Six Sigma can be used together to improve healthcare quality.
8. What are ways to promote employee safety?
9. Describe how complexity theory applies to your practice.
10. Explain reasons that chaos theory offers hope for the future of health care.

Glossary of Terms

Balanced Scorecard—a tool used to measure key financial, quality, market, and operational indicators which provides management with an understanding of performance in relation to established strategic goals and graphically displays a snapshot of the institution's overall health.

Benchmarking—comparison of quality measures with quality measures from a different source, for example, a similar unit or organization or from the literature.

Bioterrorism—term first used in 1991; terrorism which involves biological weapons.

Bureaucracy—organizations with specializations, adherence to rules, and a hierarchy of authority.

Chaos Theory—recognizes that human and organizational systems are self-organizing; there is constant tension between stability and chaos.

Complexity Science—scientific ideas derived from quantum physics, chaos theory, and systems theory which recognize that human and organizational systems are self-organizing; acknowledges that everything is related at some level.

Complexity Theory—recognizes that behavior is nonlinear and that order is found in seemingly random complexity.

Ethnocentric—the belief that one's own faction is superior.

Health Literacy—the ability of individuals to obtain, process, and understand health information and services in order to make appropriate health decisions.

Healthcare Disparity—health care that is markedly less in regard to access and availability of facilities or services.

Healthcare-Associated Infections—infections associated with the delivery of health care; caregiver-to-patient, environment-to-patient, or patient-to-patient.

Institute of Medicine—an independent, nonprofit, nongovernmental organization which provides advice to decision makers and the public.

Kaizen Blitz—collaborative work held over 3–5 days in which staff evaluate, develop, and redesign identified processes followed by monitoring to measure whether the gains are sustained.

Lean—uses standard solutions to common problems with a focus on the customer; processes assure efficient work flow and value-added activities; the primary analytic tool is value-stream mapping.

Malcolm Baldrige National Quality Award—the highest level of national recognition for performance excellence in the United States.

Meaningful Use—in order to receive incentive payments from CMS, providers must demonstrate that they are "meaningfully using" electronic health records (EHRs) through compliance with objectives; organizations must "meaningful use" certified computerized health record (CHR) technology to improve patient care.

Missed Care—the omission of vital care tasks such as turning, ambulating, feeding, mouth care, and toileting, which can lead to patient complications, for example, decubitus ulcers and pneumonia.

National Database of Nursing Quality Indicators (NDNQI)—consists of nurse-sensitive indicators; the only database of indicators at the nursing unit level.

National Patient Safety Goals—actions that organizations accredited by The Joint Commission are required to take in order to prevent medical errors.

National Quality Forum—a nonprofit, public service organization committed to the transformation of health care to a safe, equitable, and high value system.

Non-Value-Added Time—excessive amounts of nursing time being spent on support activities.

Outcome Measures—the effects of healthcare practices and interventions.

Patient Care Quality—the determination of what the patient wants and values; to make the patient the leader of his/her care.

Patient-Centered Care—care that is focused on the patient's experience of illness and health care and on systems needed to meet the individual patient's needs.

Patient Safety Officer—position which promotes safety through education; examines issues to determine better, safer organizational processes; discover the root cause; create system changes to prevent future incidents of the same kind; and then involvement in implementing programs designed to foster safety.

Positive Deviance—proposes that within organizations some individuals or groups have different "deviant" practices that produce better "positive" outcomes; holds that staff at the point of care are best equipped to solve the problem.

Quality—definitions have been inadequate; most importantly to determine what the patient wants and values; consists of two dimensions, technical excellence and the subjective experience measured by the patient.

Rapid Improvement Events (RIEs)—collaborative work held over 3–5 days in which staff evaluate, develop, and redesign identified processes followed by monitoring to measure whether the gains are sustained.

Risk Management—role which has historically been to identify, manage, and reduce risk in order to support the delivery of safe health care while reducing organizational legal risks.

Root Cause Analysis—a tool used to identify process variation by asking "Why?" related to each finding in order to drill down to discover why a portion of the process occurred or did not occur.

Six Sigma—a popular approach to performance improvement; focus is on measuring and eliminating errors; used to reduce patient safety events through reduction of process variation; tools incorporate data analysis to identify and reduce variation; provides a systematic approach in order to improve patient outcomes.

Sentinel Event—an unexpected occurrence including death or serious physical or psychological injury (or the risk thereof).

The Joint Commission (TJC)—an independent, not-for-profit organization that accredits more than 20,000 healthcare organizations in the United States; TJC accreditation symbolizes an organization's commitment to meeting identified performance standards.

Transparency—the availability (free flow) of information that allows informed decisions.

Value-Based Reimbursement—reimbursement based on quality rather than quantity; incentive payments based on performance measures or improvement of performance from the baseline.

Value-Stream Mapping—the primary analytical tool in *Lean* activities which can be used effectively to identify interruptions in order to make improvements in work flow; this tool is an extended process flowchart which focuses on speed, continuity of flow, and work in progress in order to identify non-value-added steps and bottlenecks.

Voice of the Customer—the process for capturing patient- and other customer-related information which are intended to be proactive and continuously innovative so that they capture customers' stated, unstated, and anticipated requirements, expectations, and desires.

Volume-Based Reimbursement—reimbursement based on quantity rather than quality.

References

Agency for Healthcare Research and Quality. (n.d.). *Patient safety and quality: Duplicate medication order errors increase after computerized provider order entry is implemented*. Retrieved from http://www.ahrq.gov/legacy/research/jan12/0112RA12.htm

Agency for Healthcare Research and Quality. (2008). *National healthcare disparities report: 2007*. AHRQ Pub. No. 08-0041. Rockville, MD: U.S. Department of Health and Human Services.

AHC Media. (2008). Change the culture, protect the patient using "positive deviance" to prevent MRSA. *Hospital Infection Control, 35*(9), 97–101.

Aiken, L., Clarke, S., Sloane, D., Sochalski, J., & Silber, J. (2002). Hospital nurse staffing and patient mortality, nurse burnout, and job dissatisfaction. *Journal of the American Medical Association, 288*(16), 1987–1993.

Alexander, R. (2002). A mind for multicultural management: Foster an environment that celebrates patient diversity. *Nursing Management, 33*(10), 30–34.

American Hospital Association 2011 Committee on Performance Improvement. (2011, September). *Hospitals and care systems of the future.* Chicago, IL: Author.

American Nurses Association. (n.d.). *Safe staffing: The Registered Nurse Safe Staffing Act.* Retrieved from http://www.nursingworld.org/SafeStaffingFactsheet.aspx

American Nurses Association. (2001). *Code of ethics for nurses with interpretive statements.* Silver Spring, MD: Author.

American Nurses Association. (2008). *Nurse staffing impacts quality of patient care.* Retrieved from http://www.nursingworld.org/FunctionalMenuCategories/MediaResources/PressReleases/2008PR/NurseStaffingImpactsQualityofPatientCare.aspx

American Nurses Association. (2013a). *NDNQI: National Database of Nursing Quality Indicators.* Retrieved from https://www.nursingquality.org/

American Nurses Association. (2013b). *Nursing staffing plans and ratios.* Retrieved from http://www.nursingworld.org/MainMenuCategories/Policy-Advocacy/State/Legislative-Agenda-Reports/State-StaffingPlansRatios

American Nurses Credentialing Center. (2013). *Program overview.* Retrieved from http://www.nursecredentialing.org/Magnet/ProgramOverview

Bargmann, J. (2002). The top hospital in America. *AARP, 77*(8), 44–53.

Biron, A., Lavoie-Tremblay, M., & Loiselle, C. (2009). Characteristics of work interruptions during medication administration. *Journal of Nursing Scholarship, 41*(4), 330–336.

Boev, C. (2012). The relationship between nurses' perception of work environment and patient satisfaction in adult critical care. *Journal of Nursing Scholarship, 44*(4), 368–375.

Brackett, T., Comer, L., & Whichello, R. (2013, March/April). Do Lean practices lead to more time at the bedside? *Journal for Healthcare Quality, 35*(2), 7–13.

Centers for Disease Control and Prevention. (2012). *Falls among older adults: An overview.* Retrieved from http://www.cdc.gov/HomeandRecreationalSafety/Falls/adultfalls.html

Centers for Disease Control and Prevention. (2013). *Fast facts: Health insurance coverage.* Retrieved from http://www.cdc.gov/nchs/fastats/hinsure.htm

Centers for Medicare and Medicaid Services. (2003). *Medicare Prescription Drug, Improvement, and Modernization Act (MMA) of 2003.* Retrieved from http://www.cms.gov/Medicare/Demonstration-Projects/DemoProjectsEvalRpts/downloads/MMA649_Legislation.pdf

Centers for Medicare and Medicaid Services. (2006). *Tax Relief and Health Care Act of 2006.* Retrieved from http://www.cms.gov/Medicare/Quality-Initiatives-Patient-Assessment-Instruments/PQRS/downloads/PQRITaxReliefHealthCareAct.pdf

Centers for Medicare and Medicaid Services. (2011, April). *Fact Sheets: Details for: CMS issues final rule for first year of hospital value-based purchasing program.* Retrieved from http://www.cms.gov/apps/media/press/factsheet.asp?Counter=3947

Centers for Medicare and Medicaid Services. (2012a). *End-stage renal disease (ESRD) quality initiative.* Retrieved from http://www.cms.gov/Medicare/End-Stage-Renal-Disease/ESRDQualityImproveInit/index.html

Centers for Medicare and Medicaid Services. (2012b). *Home health quality initiative: Quality measures.* Retrieved from http://www.cms.gov/Medicare/Quality-Initiatives-Patient-Assessment-Instruments/HomeHealthQualityInits/HHQIQualityMeasures.html

Centers for Medicare and Medicaid Services. (2012c). *Hospital-acquired conditions.* Retrieved from http://www.cms.gov/Medicare/Medicare-Fee-for-Service-Payment/HospitalAcqCond/Hospital-Acquired_Conditions.html

Centers for Medicare and Medicaid Services. (2012d). *Hospital-acquired conditions (present on admission indicator).* Retrieved from http://www.cms.hhs.gov/HospitalAcqCond/01_Overview.asp#TopOfPage

Centers for Medicare and Medicaid Services. (2012e). *Post acute care reform plan.* Retrieved from http://www.cms.gov/Medicare/Medicare-Fee-for-Service-Payment/SNFPPS/post_acute_care_reform_plan.html

Centers for Medicare and Medicaid Services. (2013a). *Hospital inpatient quality reporting program.* Retrieved from http://www.cms.gov/Medicare/Quality-Initiatives-Patient-Assessment-Instruments/HospitalQualityInits/HospitalRHQDAPU.html

Centers for Medicare and Medicaid Services. (2013b). *Hospital outpatient quality reporting program.* Retrieved from http://www.cms.gov/Medicare/Quality-Initiatives-Patient-Assessment-Instruments/HospitalQualityInits/HospitalOutpatientQualityReportingProgram.html

Centers for Medicare and Medicaid Services. (2013c). *Hospital quality initiative.* Retrieved from http://www.cms.gov/Medicare/Quality-Initiatives-Patient-Assessment-Instruments/HospitalQualityInits/index.html

Centers for Medicare and Medicaid Services. (2013d). *Meaningful use.* Retrieved from http://www.cms.gov/Regulations-and-Guidance/Legislation/EHRIncentivePrograms/Meaningful_Use.html

Centers for Medicare and Medicaid Services. (2013e). *Nursing home quality initiative: Quality measures*. Retrieved from http://www.cms.gov/Medicare/Quality-Initiatives-Patient-Assessment-Instruments/NursingHomeQualityInits/NHQIQualityMeasures.html

Centers for Medicare and Medicaid Service. (2013f). *Physician quality reporting system*. Retrieved form http://www.cms.gov/Medicare/Quality-Initiatives-Patient-Assessment-Instruments/PQRS/index.html

Centers for Medicare and Medicaid Services. (2013g). *Quality initiatives—general information*. Retrieved from http://www.cms.gov/Medicare/Quality-Initiatives-Patient-Assessment-Instruments/QualityInitiativesGenInfo/index.html?redirect=/QualityInitiativesGenInfo/

Chapman, E. (2004). *Radical loving care: Building the healing hospital in America*. Nashville, TN: Baptist Healing Hospital Trust.

Committee on the Consequences of Uninsurance. (2001). *Coverage matters: Insurance and health care. Institute of Medicine report brief*. Retrieved from http://www.iom.edu/Reports/2001/Coverage-Matters-Insurance-and-Health-Care.aspx

Commonwealth Fund. (2013). *Why not the best? Results from the National Scorecard of U.S. Health Systems Performance, 2011*. Retrieved from http://www.commonwealthfund.org/Publications/Fund-Reports/2011/Oct/Why-Not-the-Best-2011.aspx?page=all

Consumer-Driven Health Care Institute. (2013). *Our mission*. Retrieved from http://www.cdhci.org/index.php

Consumers Advancing Patient Safety. (2012). *How to develop a community-based patient advisory council*. Retrieved from http://patientsafety.org/page/109387/

Cookson, D., Read, C., Mukherjee, P., & Cooke, M. (2011). Improving the quality of emergency department care by removing waste using Lean Stream Mapping. *International Journal of Clinical Leadership, 17*, 25–30.

Crowell, D. M. (2011). *Complexity leadership: Nursing's role in health care delivery*. Philadelphia, PA: F. A. Davis.

Culhane-Pera, K., Vawter, D., Xiong, P., Babbitt, B., & Solberg, M. (2003). *Healing by heart: Clinical and ethical case stories of Hmong Families and Western providers*. Nashville, TN: Vanderbilt University Press.

de Koning, H., Verver, J. P. S., van den Heuvel, J., Bisgaard, S., & Does, R. J. M. M. (2006, March-April). Lean Six Sigma in healthcare. *Journal for Healthcare Quality, 28*(2), 4–11.

Dunton, N., Gajewski, B., Klaus, S., & Pierson, B. (2007). The relationship of nursing workforce characteristics to patient outcomes. *Online Journal of Issues in Nursing*. Retrieved from http://www.nursingworld.org/MainMenuCategories/ANAMarketplace/ANAPeriodicals/OJIN/TableofContents/Volume122007/No3Sept07/NursingWorkforceCharacteristics.aspx

Eden Alternative. (2009). *About us: The Eden Alternative*. Retrieved from http://www.edenalt.org/about/index.html

Federal Emergency Management Agency. (n.d.). *Home page*. Retrieved from http://www.fema.gov/

Gallup. (2013). *Home page*. Retrieved from http://www.gallup.com/home.aspx

Garcia, R. (2006). Five ways you can reduce inappropriate prescribing in the elderly: A systematic review. *Journal of Family Practice, 55*, 305–312.

Gerteis, M., Edgman-Levitan, S., Daley, J., & Delbanco, T. (1993). *Through the patients' eyes: Understanding and promoting patient-centered care*. San Francisco, CA: Jossey-Bass.

Giger, J. N. (2012). *Transcultural nursing: Assessment and intervention* (6th ed.). New York, NY: Mosby.

Glasgow, J. M., Scott-Caziewell, J. R., & Kaboli, P. J. (2010, December). Guiding inpatient quality improvement: A systematic review of Lean and Six Sigma. *Joint Commission Journal on Quality and Patient Safety, 36*(12), 533–540.

Gravlin, G., & Bittner, N. (2010). Nurses' and nursing assistants' reports of missed care and delegation. *Journal of Nursing Administration, 40*(7/8), 329–335.

Grayson, M. (2002, October). Forward motion. *Hospital and Health Services Networks*, 34–38.

Haig, K., Sutton, S., & Whittington, J. (2006). SBAR: A shared mental model for improving communication between clinicians. *Journal on Quality and Patient Safety, 32*(3), 167–175.

Hall, L., Doran, D., & Pink, L. (2008). Outcomes of interventions to improve hospital nursing work environments. *Journal of Nursing Administration, 38*(1), 40–46.

Hay, L. (1988). *Heal your body*. Carson, CA: Hay House.

Health Care Advisory Board. (1999). *Balanced scorecards*. Retrieved from http://www.advisory.com

Institute for Healthcare Improvement. (2011a). *Designate a patient safety officer*. Retrieved from http://www.ihi.org/knowledge/Pages/Changes/DesignateaPatientSafetyOfficer.aspx

Institute for Healthcare Improvement. (2011b). *Run chart tool*. Retrieved from http://www.ihi.org/knowledge/Pages/Tools/RunChart.aspx

Institute for Healthcare Improvement. (2011c). *Strategies for leadership: Hospital executives and their role in patient safety.* Retrieved from http://www.ihi.org/knowledge/Pages/Tools/StrategiesforLeadershipHospitalExecutivesand TheirRoleinPatientSafety.aspx

Institute for Healthcare Improvement. (2012a). *How to improve.* Retrieved from http://www.ihi.org/knowledge/Pages/ HowtoImprove/default.aspx

Institute for Healthcare Improvement. (2012b). *Leadership guide to patient safety.* Retrieved from http://www.ihi.org/ knowledge/Pages/IHIWhitePapers/LeadershipGuidetoPatientSafetyWhitePaper.aspx

Institute for Healthcare Improvement. (2012c). *Measures.* Retrieved from http://www.ihi.org/knowledge/Pages/ Measures/default.aspx

Institute for Healthcare Improvement. (2013a). *Falls prevention.* Retrieved from http://www.ihi.org/explore/falls/ Pages/default.aspx

Institute for Healthcare Improvement. (2013b). *Transforming care at the bedside.* Retrieved from http://www.ihi.org/ offerings/Initiatives/PastStrategicInitiatives/TCAB/Pages/default.aspx

Institute of Medicine. (1999). *To err is human: Building a safer health system.* Washington, DC: National Academies Press.

Institute of Medicine. (2001). *Crossing the quality chasm: A new health system for the 21st century.* Washington, DC: National Academies Press.

Institute of Medicine. (2004a). *Health literacy: A prescription to end confusion.* Washington, DC: National Academies Press.

Institute of Medicine. (2004b). *Keeping patients safe: Transforming the work environment of nurses.* Washington, DC: National Academies Press.

Institute of Medicine. (2006). *Preventing medication errors.* Washington, DC: National Academies Press.

Institute of Medicine. (2007). *Creating a business case for quality improvement research: Expert views, workshop summary.* Washington, DC: National Academies Press.

Jackevicius, C., Li, P., & Tu, J. (2008). Prevalence, predictors, and outcomes of primary nonadherence after acute myocardial infarction. *Circulation, 117,* 1028–1036.

The Joint Commission. (2013a). *About our standards.* Retrieved from http://www.jointcommission.org/standards_ information/standards.aspx

The Joint Commission. (2013b). *Core measures sets.* Retrieved from http://www.jointcommission.org/core_measure_ sets.aspx

The Joint Commission. (2013c). *National patient safety goals.* Retrieved from http://www.jointcommission.org/ standards_information/npsgs.aspx

The Joint Commission. (2013d). *2013 national patient safety goals.* Retrieved from http://www.jointcommission.org/ standards_information/npsgs.aspx

The Joint Commission. (2013e). *Quality check.* Retrieved from http://www.qualitycheck.org/consumer/search QCR.aspx

Kalisch, B., Curley, M., & Stefanov, S. (2007). An intervention to enhance nursing staff teamwork and engagement. *Journal of Nursing Administration, 37*(2), 77–84.

Kalisch, B., & Lee, K. (2012). Congruence of perceptions among nursing leaders and staff regarding missed nursing care and teamwork. *Journal of Nursing Administration, 42*(10), 473–477.

Kane, R., Shamliyan, T., Mueller, C., Duval, S., & Witt, T. (2007). *Nursing staffing and quality of patient care. Evidence Report/Technology Assessment No. 151.* AHRQ Publication No. 07–005. Rockville, MD: Agency for Healthcare Research and Quality.

Klevens, R. M., Edwards, J. R., Richards, C. L., Horan, T. C., Gaynes, R. P., Pollock, D. A., & Cardo, D. M. (2007, March-April). Estimating health care-associated infections and deaths in U.S. hospitals, 2002. *Public Health Reports, 122,* 160–166.

Kripalani, S., Henderson, L., Jacobson, T., & Vaccarino, V. (2008). Medication use among inner-city patients after hospital discharge: Patient-reported barriers and solutions. *Mayo Clinic Proceedings, 83*(5), 529–535.

Leape, L. L., & Berwick, D. M. (2005). Five years after *To Err is Human*: What have we learned? *Journal of the American Medical Association, 293*(19), 2384–2390. doi:10.1001/jama/293.19.2384

Leapfrog Group. (2013). *The Leapfrog Group fact sheet.* Retrieved from http://www.leapfroggroup.org/about_us/ leapfrog-factsheet

Leininger, M., & McFarland, M. (2002). *Transcultural nursing: Concepts, theories, research, and practice.* New York, NY: McGraw-Hill.

Leonhardt, K., Bonin, D., & Pagel, P. (2007). *How to develop a community-based patient advisory council. Aurora Health Care and CAPS Toolkit.* Retrieved from http://patientsafety.org/page/109387/;jsessionid=7vhlrvtobuim2

Lindberg, C., & Clancy, T. R. (2010). Positive Deviance: An elegant solution to a complex problem. *Journal of Nursing Administration, 40*(4), 150–153.

Lindrooth, R., Bazzoli, G., Needleman, J., & Hasnain-Wynia, R. (2006). *The effect of changes in hospital reimbursement on nurse staffing decisions at safety net and nonsafety net hospitals.* Retrieved from http://www.pubmedcentral.nih.gov/articlerender.fcgi?tool=pubmed&pubmedid=16704508

Longtin, Y., Sax, H., Leape, L.L., Sheridan, S. E., Donaldson, L., & Pittet, D. (2010). Patient participation: Current knowledge and applicability to patient safety. *Mayo Clinic Proceedings, 85*(1), 53–62. doi:10.4065/mcp.2009.0248

Maniaci, M., Heckman, M., & Dawson, N. (2008). Functional health literacy and understanding of medications at discharge. *Mayo Clinic Proceedings, 83*(5), 554–558.

Markey, D., & Brown, R. (2002). An interdisciplinary approach to addressing patient activity and mobility in medical-surgical patient. *Journal of Nursing Care Quality, 16*(4), 1–12.

Medicare.gov. (n.d.). *Hospital compare.* Retrieved from http://www.medicare.gov/hospitalcompare/?AspxAutoDetect CookieSupport=1

Melberg, S. (1997). Effects of changing skill mix. *Nursing Management, 28*(11), 47–48.

Miller, W., Vigdor, E., & Manning, G. (2004, January-June). Covering the uninsured: What is it worth? *Health Affairs,* W4157–W4167.

National Institute of Standards and Technology. (2012). *Baldrige and health care: New survey reaffirms a proven partnership for success.* Retrieved from http://www.nist.gov/baldrige/baldrige-120412.cfm

National Institute of Standards and Technology. (2013). *Healthcare criteria for performance excellence.* Gaithersburg, MD: Author.

O'Grady, E. (2009). Acknowledge the paradoxes and advance the profession. *Nursing Economic$, 27*(5), 337, 347.

Pape, T. (2008). *Checklists with medication vest or sash reduce distractions during medication administration.* Retrieved from http://www.innovations.ahrq.gov/content.aspx?id=1799

Planetree. (n. d.). *About us.* Retrieved from http://planetree.org/?page_id=510

Pointe, P., Conlin, G., Conway, J., Grant, S., Medeiros, C., Nies, J., et al. (2003). Making patient-centered care come alive: Achieving full integration of the patient's perspective. *Journal of Nursing Administration, 33*(2), 82–90.

Porter-O'Grady, T. (2003). Of hubris and hope: Transforming nursing for a new age. *Nursing Economic$, 21*(2), 59–64.

Porter-O'Grady, T., & Malloch, K. (2003). *Quantum leadership: A textbook of new leadership.* Sudbury, MA: Jones and Bartlett.

Porter-O'Grady, T., & Malloch, K. (2007). *Quantum leadership: A resource for health innovation* (2nd ed.). Sudbury, MA: Jones and Bartlett.

Porter-O'Grady, T., & Malloch, K. (2011). *Quantum leadership: Advancing innovation, transforming health care* (3rd ed.). Burlington, MA: Jones & Bartlett Learning.

Press Ganey Associates. (2013). *Home page.* Retrieved from http://www.pressganey.com/index.aspx

Purnell, L. D. (2012). *Transcultural health care: A culturally competent approach* (4th ed.). Philadelphia, PA: F. A. Davis.

Radnor, Z. J., Holweg, M., & Waring, J. (2012). Lean in healthcare: The unfilled promise? *Social Science & Medicine, 74,* 364–371.

Reed, K., & May. R. (2011). HealthGrades patient safety in American hospitals study. *HealthGrades.* Retrieved from https://www.cpmhealthgrades.com/CPM/assets/File/HealthGradesPatientSafetyInAmericanHospitalsStudy 2011.pdf

Relihan, E., O'Brien, V., O'Hara S., & Silke, B. (2010, October). The impact of a set of interventions to reduce interruptions and distractions to nurses during medication administration. *Quality & Safety in Health Care, 19*(5), 52–57.

Rhoades, J. (2005). *The uninsured in America, 1996–2004: Estimates for the U.S. civilian noninstitutionalized population under age 65. AHRQ Statistical Brief #84.* Retrieved from http://meps.ahrq.gov/mepsweb/data_files/publications/st84/stat84.pdf

Rudy, E., Lucke, J., Whitman, G., & Davidson, L. (2001). Benchmarking patient outcomes. *Journal of Nursing Scholarship, 33*(2), 185–189.

School of Nursing, UT Academic Health Science Center, San Antonio. (2012). *Academic Center of Evidence-Based Practice*. Retrieved from http://www.acestar.uthscsa.edu/

Scott, R. D. (2009). *The direct medical costs of healthcare-associated infections in U. S. hospitals and the benefits of prevention*. Retrieved from http://www.cdc.gov/HAI/pdfs/hai/Scott_CostPaper.pdf

Shermont, H., Mahoney, J., Krepcio, D., Baccari, S., Powers, D., & Yusah, A. (2008). Meeting of the minds: Ten-minute "huddles" offer nurses an opportunity to assess unit workflow and optimize patient care. *Nursing Management, 39*(8), 38–44.

Shirey, M. (2006). Evidence-based practice: Impact on nursing administration. *Nursing Administration Quarterly, 30*(3), 252–265.

Simonson, W., & Feinberg, J. (2005). Medication-related problems in the elderly: Defining the issues and identifying solutions. *Drugs and Aging, 22*(7), 559–569.

Smith, B. (2003, April). Lean and Six Sigma—a one-two punch. *Quality Progress,* 37–41.

Stevens, J., Corso, P., Finkelstein, E., & Miller, T. (2006). *The costs of fatal and non-fatal falls among older adults*. Retrieved from http://injuryprevention.bmj.com/content/12/5/290.full

St. Hill, P., Lipson, J., & Meleis, A. (2003). *Caring for women cross-culturally*. Philadelphia, PA: F. A. Davis.

Storfjell, J., Ohlson, S., Omoike, O., Fitzpatrick, T., & Wetasin, K. (2009). Non-value added time: The million dollar nursing opportunity. *Journal of Nursing Administration, 39*(1), 38–43.

Storfjell, J., Omoike, O., & Ohlson, S. (2008). The balancing act: Patient care time versus cost. *Journal of Nursing Administration, 38*(5), 244–249.

Tennessee Hospitals & Health Systems. (2008). *THA develops nonpayment policy on serious adverse events*. Nashville, TN: Tennessee Hospital Association.

Toussaint, J., & Gerard, R., with Adams, E. (2010). *On the mend: Revolutionizing healthcare to save lives and transform the industry*. Cambridge, MA: Lean Enterprise Institute.

Trbovich, P., Prakash, V., & Stewart, J. (2010). Interruptions during the delivery of high-risk medications, *Journal of Nursing Administration, 40*(5), 211–218.

URAC. (2011). *Home page*. Retrieved from https://www.urac.org/

URAC. (2013). *URAC's Health Utilization Management Accreditation*. Retrieved from https://www.urac.org/programs/prog_accred_HUM_po.aspx?navid=accreditation&pagename=prog_accred_HUM

U.S. Census Bureau. (2011). *Overview of race and Hispanic origin: 2010*. Retrieved from http://www.census.gov/prod/cen2010/briefs/c2010br-02.pdf

U.S. Department of Health and Human Services. (n.d.). *Quick guide to health literacy: Fact sheet*. Retrieved from http://www.health.gov/communication/literacy/quickguide/factsbasic.htm

U.S. Department of Labor. (n.d.). *Occupational Health and Safety Administration*. Retrieved from http://www.osha.gov/

U.S. Government Printing Office. (2008). *Medicare improvements for Patients and Providers Act of 2008*. Retrieved from http://www.gpo.gov/fdsys/pkg/PLAW-110publ275/pdf/PLAW-110publ275.pdf

U.S. Government Printing Office. (2010). *Patient Protection and Affordable Care Act of 2010*. Retrieved from http://www.gpo.gov/fdsys/pkg/PLAW-111publ148/pdf/PLAW-111publ148.pdf

Vanhey, D., Aiken, L., Sloane, D., Clarke, S., & Vargas, D. (2004). Nurse burnout and patient satisfaction. *Medical Care, 42*(2 Suppl.), II57–II66.

Watson, J. (2004). *Postmodern nursing and beyond*. New York, NY: Elsevier.

Weber, S. (2008, July). Ergonomics standards: An overview. *Nursing Management,* 28–31.

Wetterneck, T. B., Walker, J. M., Blosky, M. A., Cartmill, R. S., Hoonakker, P., Johnson, M. A., et al. (2011). Factors contributing to an increase in duplicate medication order errors after CPOE implementation. *Journal of the American Medical Informatics Association, 18,* 774–782.

Whitman, G., Kim, Y., Davidson, L., Wolf, G., & Wang, S. (2002). The impact of staffing on patient outcomes across specialty units. *Journal of Nursing Administration, 32*(12), 633–639.

Woods, A., & Doan-Johnson, S. (2002, October). Executive summary: Toward a taxonomy of nursing practice errors. *Nursing Management,* 45–48.

World Health Organization. (2013). *Health financing: Health expenditure per capita by country (latest year)*. Retrieved from http://apps.who.int/gho/data/node.main.78?lang=en

Zynx Health. (2013). *Home page*. Retrieved from http://www.zynxhealth.com/

Pinpointing Evidence-Based Information: How to Find the Needle in the Information Haystack

Rick Wallace, MA, MDiv, MAOM, MSLS, EdD, AHIP,
Nakia Joye Woodward, MSIS, AHIP, and Kelly Loyd, MSIS

OBJECTIVES

- To understand the foundations of evidence-based practice and how EBP relates to nursing practice.
- To develop an understanding of the information resources available to nurses through the Web, handheld devices, and electronic health records.
- To understand the different study designs and their relationship to the evidence pyramid.

Introduction

Practicing financial management without evidence is like doing surgery blindfolded. So, do not skip this chapter. This is an important one.

Much of health care, both in clinical practice and financial management, is practiced without evidence. John E. Wennberg (2010) in his book *Tracking Medicine* describes how clinical procedures are performed across the United States with no rhyme or reason. Wennberg found that communities with similar demographics had highly variant surgical rates. The only reason for the differences was physician preference. Wennberg developed the *Dartmouth Atlas of Health Care* (http://www.dartmouthatlas.org), which details the distribution of health services across the United States.

The PBS program entitled *The Good News in American Medicine*, produced by T. R. Reid, highlighted Wennberg's work. Reid, a journalist with the *Washington Post*, is known for another PBS program, *Sick Around the World*, which described health care in five wealthy nations around the world (France, Germany, Japan, the United Kingdom, and Canada). The program, along with Reid's bestselling book, *The Healing of America*, points out that all five of these countries provided universal health care at about *half* the cost of healthcare in the United States (Palfreman & Reid, 2008; Reid, 2010). The key to cutting costs is that they spend a small fraction of healthcare costs on financial administration compared to the United States. In Wennberg's work detailing unnecessary clinical procedures, and Reid's book describing the efficiency of healthcare practices in other wealthy countries, evidence plays a major role.

When we searched a major nursing literature database on the terms *finances* or *costs,* limited the results to the years 2010–2012, and limited the publication type to *systematic review*—a very high level of evidence (more on publication types later)—we received a return of 185 abstracts of journal articles. Titles from the search results included:

> "Quality of Life and Economic Costs Associated with Post-Thrombotic Syndrome"
> "Incident and Costs of Corticosteroids-Associated Adverse Events"
> "Midlevel Health Providers Impact on ICU Length of Stay, Patient Satisfaction, Mortality, and Resource Utilization"
> "Costs of Hospital-Acquired Infection and Transferability of the Estimates"
> "Economic Evaluation of Nurse Staffing and Nurse Substitution in Health Care"
> "Hospital Nurse Staffing Models and Patient and Staff-Related Outcomes"

In the journal article "Health Care in Crisis! Can Nurse Executives' Beliefs About and Implementation of Evidence Based Practice Be Key Solutions in Health Care Reform?" Sredl and associates (2011) revealed how evidence is used in practice by nurses:

> In the nursing milieu, rife with change, perhaps the most significant change encountered by the nursing profession in the last decade is EBP [evidence-based practice]. . . . Studies have indicated that its use improves the quality of care and patient care and lowers health care costs. . . . For the Institute of Medicine's goal that 90% of health care decisions be evidence based by 2020, health care institutions must provide their staff with appropriate resources to create a culture that creates evidence-based care.
>
> There is little published evidence that CNEs (Chief Nursing Executives) actually value and understand, much less use, EBP. When CNEs fully understand, believe in, and implement EBP, they can be in a position to mentor their staff so that they also understand, believe in, and implement EBP to improve the quality of health care and patient outcomes as well as help to lower health care costs. (pp. 73–74, 78)

What exactly is evidence-based practice? The classic definition is derived from David Sackett's 1996 definition of evidence-based medicine as "The conscientious, explicit, and judicious use of current best evidence in making decisions about the care of individual patients" (Sackett, et al., 1996, p. 72).

The problem is that much of healthcare practice is based on tradition, the local environments, clinical preferences, and factors *other than* the best scientific literature that exists for a clinical practice. Clinicians do not use the evidence for several reasons: too much evidence exists, they do not have access to new evidence, it is time-consuming, they have never been instructed to find evidence, and they are uncertain about assessing the strength and quality of one piece of evidence versus another. We hope that through this chapter, readers embark on the pathway of becoming *information masters* and overcome the aforementioned barriers of using evidence.

Some points need to be highlighted to clarify Sackett's definition. It in no way excludes the clinician's experience or the patient's preferences. As a matter of fact, evidence-based practice encourages the integration of best evidence, clinical experience, and patient preferences. The definition states the need to use the best evidence available. It does not say each decision must be supported by a meta-analysis. Often there is not a higher level of evidence for a particular problem, so clinicians have to use the highest level available based on the hierarchy of evidence, which we cover later.

It is important to note that even though evidence-based practice leads to a reduction in cost and an improvement in morbidity and mortality, nurses do not always follow best practice. This is where nurse managers can play a crucial role. Nurse managers have been found to be more confident evidence users. This confidence would be put to good use if they would serve as evidence-based practice mentors for other nurses in the organization. For evidence-based practice to succeed, nurse managers need to help provide an organizational culture that supports it (Melnyk et al., 2012).

A practical way to implement evidence-based practice is by using a framework commonly referred to as the *five A's*, which are assess, ask, acquire, appraise, and apply.

Assess

Assessment is routine in the clinic. What is the diagnosis of this patient? What therapy should the person receive? Assessment is also part of the financial management role of nurse managers. How much will this procedure cost? How can we improve clinical outcomes of patients and reduce costs or hold costs steady?

Ask

The ongoing, even unconscious, process of assessment naturally leads to asking questions. A hallmark of being a professional is to be curious. No matter how well we apply ourselves in our education, we have gaps in our knowledge. A mnemonic device was created to help people focus their clinical questions. A focused clinical question is much more answerable than an unfocused one is.

PICO represents the patient/population/problem, intervention being considered, comparative/contrasting intervention being considered, and outcomes(s) of interest. Consider the following:

(P) **Patient/population/problem:** What is the patient population of interest? *Be specific.* If it is a clinical question, the P might be elderly patients in nursing homes with urinary tract infections

(UTIs) as opposed to just UTI patients. If it is a managerial question, an example of the P is "hospital nursing staffs where staff morale is a problem."

(I) Intervention: The intervention is the primary course of action that seems plausible as a solution to the problem.

(C) Comparative intervention: The comparative intervention is an alternative solution to the problem that is causing uncertainty in the decision-making process. More than one comparative intervention may exist. Examples of intervention/comparative interventions for the morale problem are as follows:

a. Intervention—setting staff work time to 8-hour shifts.
b. Comparative intervention 1—setting staff work time to 12-hour shifts.
c. Comparative intervention 2—having options to work an 8-hour shift or a 12-hour shift.

At this point, this question could be feathered out into multiple questions. Realizing that one question might actually be several questions is an advantage of using the PICO process. For example, the I and C could be increased wages versus no increased wages, better benefits versus maintaining current benefits, or morale-building exercises versus no exercises.

(O) Outcome(s): This part is the most important component of the question-asking process. In the preceding nurse staffing example, the desired outcome is improved morale. When possible, the outcome should be *SMART*: specific, measureable, achievable, realistic, and timely. Questions should be focused on specific outcomes that can lead to improvements in clinical outcomes, costs, patient satisfaction, and employee growth.

However, the PICO process only works with *foreground questions*. Foreground questions are practice or management questions in which there is indecision between two or more options. *Background questions*, in contrast, are questions that are fact based, such as the incidence of breast cancer in women aged 20 to 30 years.

Examples of PICO:

P: In nursing home patients
I: Supervised exercise programs
C: Bed exit alarm
O: Decrease in falls

Resultant question: In nursing home patients, do supervised exercise programs versus a bed exit alarm lead to a decrease in falls?

P: In registered nurses
I: Team-building exercises
C: No team-building exercise
O: Increased job satisfaction

Resultant question: In registered nurses, do team-building exercises lead to increased job satisfaction?

Exhibit 5–1, Clinical Question Worksheet, can be helpful in deciding on a question to ask. In addition, the University of Minnesota Libraries has an excellent guide to the PICO process, "Evidence Based Practice: An Interprofessional Tutorial" (http://hsl.lib.umn.edu/learn/ebp/).

Exhibit 5–1   Clinical Question Worksheet

The Clinical Question & Information Resources
Construct your question

Patient, Population or Problem	Intervention, Prognostic Factor, Exposure	Comparison Intervention (if appropriate)	Outcome you would like to measure or achieve	Type of question you are asking	Type of study you would want to find
How would I describe a group of patients similar to mine?	Which main intervention, exposure, prognostic factor am I considering?	What is the main alternative to compare with the intervention?	What can I hope to accomplish, measure, improve, affect?	How would I categorize the question?	What would be the best study design in order to answer this question?

Source: Adapted from http://eno.duhs.duke.edu/sites/eno.duhs.duke.edu/files/public/guides/pico-worksh.pdf

Acquire

The acquisition of the appropriate evidence resources is the next step in the evidence-based practice cycle. As you are searching for evidence, it is imperative to remember that unless you are writing an exhaustive systematic review, you need to find just enough evidence to answer your question. It is very easy to get lost in the maze of resources, so we give you some tools to guide your way. Resources may be primary or secondary. *Primary resources* are original research such as individual journal articles. *Secondary literature* is multiple primary resources combined into a new unit such as a systematic review or a meta-analysis. Many secondary resources can be used on a smartphone or tablet at the point of care.

Exhibit 5–2, Evidence Ratings and Grade of Recommendations, is a useful tool for evaluating evidence. It breaks down evidence into research levels and grades recommendations based on these levels.

One important concept to consider when acquiring evidence is that all evidence is not created equal. Different study types exist that can be placed in a hierarchy according to the strength of the evidence. This hierarchy is commonly referred to as the evidence pyramid (**Exhibit 5–3**). The most common study types are systematic reviews, meta-analyses, randomized controlled trials, cohort studies, case-control studies, cross-sectional studies, case series, and case studies. You should have a basic knowledge of the types of studies, how each one is designed, when each one is appropriate, and which ones yield the strongest evidence.

> **Systematic reviews:** Systematic reviews are covered later.
>
> **Meta-analyses:** A *meta-analysis* is a mathematical process in which the statistical results of several similar studies are combined. Often, studies have small sample sizes, which reduces their power. Power is a statistical concept. A low-powered study may not have statistical significance.
>
> **Randomized controlled trials (RCTs):** A *randomized controlled trial* is a type of individual study in which the researcher carefully controls the subjects in the trial and the exposures the subjects receive. It is an experimental design and is considered high-level evidence. The higher *levels of evidence* (*LOE*) produce the more trustworthy results. Of course, at any evidence level for this to be true the study must be well designed and well executed with attention to potential bias, sample size, and other methodological issues. We cover critical appraisal later.

Exhibit 5–2 Evidence Ratings and Grade of Recommendations from the Oxford Centre for Evidence-Based Medicine

Oxford Centre for Evidence-Based Medicine—Levels of Evidence (March 2009)

What are we to do when the irresistible force of the need to offer clinical advice meets with the immovable object of flawed evidence? All we can do is our best: Give the advice, but alert the advisees to the flaws in the evidence on which it is based.

The CEBM 'Levels of Evidence' document sets out one approach to systematising this process for different question types.

Level	Therapy/ Prevention, Aetiology/ Harm	Prognosis	Diagnosis	Differential diagnosis/ symptom prevalence study	Economic and decision analyses
1a	SR (with homogeneity*) of RCTs	SR (with homogeneity*) of inception cohort studies; CDR" validated in different populations	SR (with homogeneity*) of Level 1 diagnostic studies; CDR" with 1b studies from different clinical centres	SR (with homogeneity*) of prospective cohort studies	SR (with homogeneity*) of Level 1 economic studies
1b	Individual RCT (with narrow confidence interval"¡)	Individual inception cohort study with >80% follow-up; CDR" validated in a single population	Validating** cohort study with good" " " reference standards; or CDR" tested within one clinical centre	Prospective cohort study with good follow-up****	Analysis based on clinically sensible costs or alternatives; systematic review(s) of the evidence; and including multi-way sensitivity analyses
1c	All or none§	All or none case-series	Absolute SpPins and SnNouts" "	All or none case-series	Absolute better-value or worse-value analyses " " " "
2a	SR (with homogeneity*) of cohort studies	SR (with homogeneity*) of either retrospective cohort studies or untreated control groups in RCTs	SR (with homogeneity*) of Level >2 diagnostic studies	SR (with homogeneity*) of 2b and better studies	SR (with homogeneity*) of Level >2 economic studies
2b	Individual cohort study (including low quality RCT; e.g., <80% follow-up)	Retrospective cohort study or follow-up of untreated control patients in an RCT; derivation of CDR" or validated on split-sample§§§ only	Exploratory** cohort study with good" " " reference standards; CDR" after derivation, or validated only on split-sample§§§ or databases	Retrospective cohort study, or poor follow-up	Analysis based on clinically sensible costs or alternatives; limited review(s) of the evidence, or single studies; and including multi-way sensitivity analyses

Level	Therapy/ Prevention, Aetiology/ Harm	Prognosis	Diagnosis	Differential diagnosis / symptom prevalence study	Economic and decision analyses
2c	"Outcomes" research; ecological studies	"Outcomes" research		Ecological studies	Audit or outcomes research
3a	SR (with homogeneity*) of case-control studies		SR (with homogeneity*) of 3b and better studies	SR (with homogeneity*) of 3b and better studies	SR (with homogeneity*) of 3b and better studies
3b	Individual case-control study		Non-consecutive study; or without consistently applied reference standards	Non-consecutive cohort study, or very limited population	Analysis based on limited alternatives or costs, poor quality estimates of data, but including sensitivity analyses incorporating clinically sensible variations.
4	Case-series (and poor quality cohort and case-control studies§§)	Case-series (and poor quality prognostic cohort studies***)	Case-control study, poor or non-independent reference standard	Case-series or superseded reference standards	Analysis with no sensitivity analysis
5	Expert opinion without explicit critical appraisal, or based on physiology, bench research or "first principles"	Expert opinion without explicit critical appraisal, or based on physiology, bench research or "first principles"	Expert opinion without explicit critical appraisal, or based on physiology, bench research or "first principles"	Expert opinion without explicit critical appraisal, or based on physiology, bench research or "first principles"	Expert opinion without explicit critical appraisal, or based on economic theory or "first principles"

Produced by Bob Phillips, Chris Ball, Dave Sackett, Doug Badenoch, Sharon Straus, Brian Haynes, Martin Dawes since November 1998. Updated by Jeremy Howick March 2009.

Grades of Recommendation

A	consistent level 1 studies
B	consistent level 2 or 3 studies *or* extrapolations from level 1 studies
C	level 4 studies *or* extrapolations from level 2 or 3 studies
D	level 5 evidence *or* troublingly inconsistent or inconclusive studies of any level

Source: From http://www.cebm.net/index.aspx?o=1025

Exhibit 5–3   Evidence Pyramid

Evidence-Based Practice in the Health Sciences, Information Services Department, Library of the Health Sciences-Chicago, University of Illinois at Chicago. Available online at: http://ebp.lib.uic.edu. Reprinted by permission.

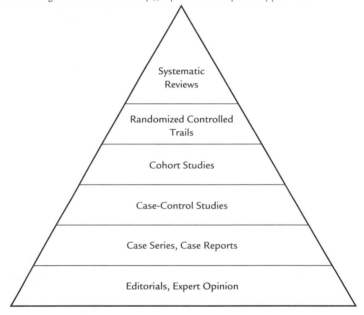

Source: Evidence-Based Practice in the Health Sciences, Information Services Department, Library of the Health Sciences-Chicago, University of Illinois at Chicago. Available online at: http://ebp.lib.uic.edu. Reprinted by permission.

An example of an RCT is to take a group of nurses and keep them on their current rotation. Take a similar group of nurses and put them on a new rotation system in which you hypothesize their morale and productivity will increase. You use a validated survey instrument to measure the results after a period of time. An example of a RCT like this is "Evaluation of an Open-Rota System in a Danish Psychiatric Hospital: A Mechanism for Improving Job Satisfaction and Work-Life Balance" (Pryce, Albertson, & Nielsen, 2006).

Cohort studies: A *cohort study*, as are all the remaining studies discussed, is an observational study. A cohort study is a prospective study that starts with two groups, one exposed to the study area of interest, and the other not. Both groups are followed over time and outcomes are recorded and compared between the two groups. The researcher does not control the exposure.

Turnover is a costly problem. A hospital could track all new RNs hired over a 5-year period. They might do a survey at the point of hiring to gain basic demographic information of interest and one at the point any of the newly hired RNs leave during the 5-year study period. The exit interview could inquire into the reasons the RN left, such as management issues, salary, family issues, hours, and problems with coworkers. The data could be analyzed to determine why RNs left. An example of a cohort study done on this topic is "Turnover of New Graduate Nurses in Their First Job Using Survival Analysis" (Cho, Lee, Mark, & Yun, 2012).

Case-control studies: A *case-control study* is a retrospective study. It looks back in time. The researchers start with people who already have the outcome of interest. They then look for exposures that led to the outcome by using medical records, surveys, phone interviews, personnel records, and so forth. The cases are matched to controls who are similar to the cases but do not have the outcome of interest.

A case-control study could be performed on a group of clinics experiencing major financial problems with "no-shows." A group of no-shows is identified from the past 2 years. These patients are interviewed to discover the reasons for missing an appointment. A similar group of patients who made their appointments is also identified. The two groups are chosen so that they are demographically similar. The control group is also interviewed. Factors examined in the structured interview include transportation, work status, and others. Both groups are then analyzed and compared to determine underlying causes of nonattendance. An example of a case-control study similar to this is "Reasons for Non-Attendance: Audit Findings from a Nurse-Led Clinic" (Wilkinson & Daly, 2012).

Cross-sectional studies: A *cross-sectional study* looks at exposures and outcomes at one point in time. It is useful for exploring research ideas, but not in determining causality. Suppose we obtained the names and addresses of all RNs in a three-county region. They are all surveyed in regard to exposures—work satisfaction, stress, coworker conflicts, pay satisfaction, and so forth—and outcomes—current work status, number of job changes in the last 5 years. The data are then analyzed for correlation among the various factors.

In the study "Hospital and Unit Characteristics Associated with Nursing Turnovers Include Skill Mix but Not Staffing Level: An Observational Cross-Sectional Study" (Staggs & Dunton, 2012), data on RN and total nursing staff turnover were analyzed with factors such as Magnet status and location to see if any correlation existed.

Case series: A *case series* uses data from several individual cases. An example is gathering information about cases in which a nurse implemented a course of action that saved money. Five such scenarios could be described in one research study.

Case studies: Although *case studies* are a popular study type, they rank on the bottom level of the evidence pyramid. However, this does not mean they are not valuable. In management, the case study is a time-honored methodology. Case studies are featured in the *Harvard Business Review* and used for examples in training. The case study "Improving Nurse Retention in a Large Tertiary Acute Care Hospital" (Hinson & Spatz, 2011) describes how "5 change consults . . . resulted in a 91% reduction in voluntary nurse turnover, yielding a savings of $655, 949" (p. 103).

All the study types described here can be searched in the large citation databases PubMed and CINAHL. PubMed (**Exhibit 5–4**) is free and is produced by the U.S. government. CINAHL is proprietary.

Haynes developed a five Ss description of evidence resources: systems, summaries, syntheses, synopses, and studies (Haynes, 2006, p. A8). The five Ss description can also be organized into a strong to weak hierarchy, like the methodology pyramid (**Exhibit 5–5**).

Systems: *Systems* are evidence resources that are incorporated into the *electronic health record* (*EHR*). They are mapped to a subject vocabulary in the EHR such as International Classification of Diseases (ICD) codes and are automatically retrieved and placed in the patient's record by the system.

Summaries: *Summaries* are reviews such as the Cochrane Database of Systematic Reviews (http://www.thecochranelibrary.com). Large numbers of studies on a topic are collected and then accepted or rejected based on predetermined inclusion/exclusion criteria. The included studies are analyzed and then synthesized into a focused answer to a clinical question. The Cochrane Database of Systematic Reviews at the Cochrane site provides just the summary, but that usually yields adequate information. The full Cochrane Database of Systematic Reviews (**Exhibit 5–6**) can be purchased through OVID, EBSCO, or John Wiley and Sons.

Exhibit 5–4   PubMed Database

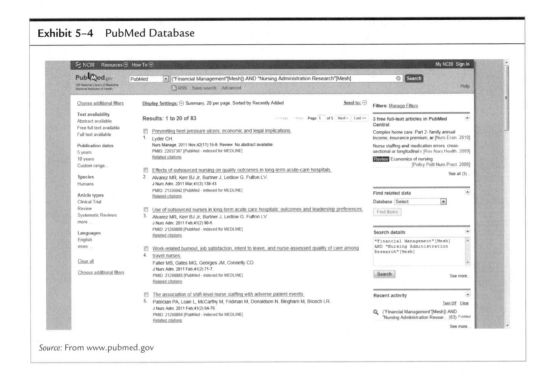

Source: From www.pubmed.gov

Exhibit 5–5   The 5S Pyramid

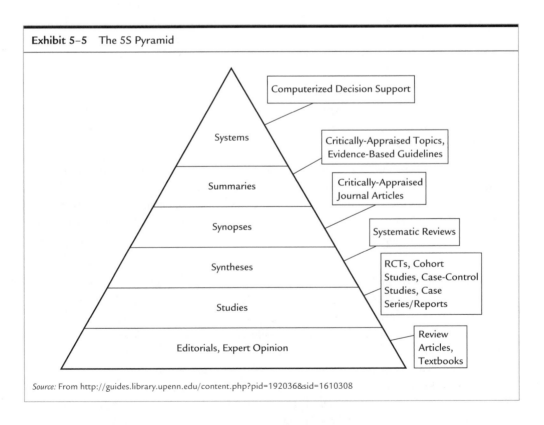

Source: From http://guides.library.upenn.edu/content.php?pid=192036&sid=1610308

Exhibit 5–6   Cochrane Summaries

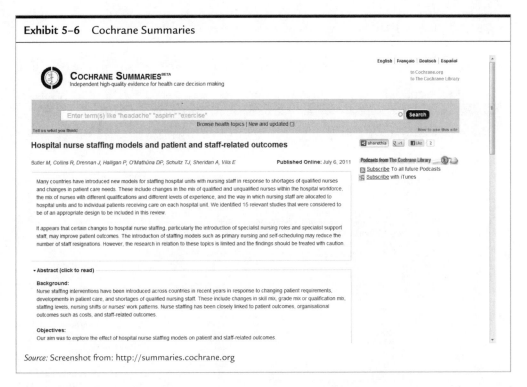

Source: Screenshot from: http://summaries.cochrane.org

Another way to search systematic reviews is through PubMed Health (www.ncbi.nlm.nih.gov/pubmed-health). PubMed Health searches 20,000 systematic reviews, including those in the Cochrane Database of Systematic Reviews and Database of Abstracts of Reviews of Effects (DARE). The large citation databases PubMed and CINAHL can be limited to systematic reviews when searched. In PubMed, users can specify the limits on the left side bar, choose *Article Type,* and then find *Systematic Reviews.* **Exhibit 5–7** shows PubMed results using the systematic review filter. In CINAHL, in the limits section, users can select *Publication Type* in the drop-down menu and choose *Systematic Reviews.*

Syntheses: *Syntheses* are referred to as *critically appraised topics (CATs).* Products that fit into this category are Dynamed (http://dynamed.ebscohost.com/), Clinical Evidence (http://clinicalevidence.bmj.com), ACP Pier (http://pier.acponline.org), and First Consult (www.firstconsult.com). These resources identify the best evidence on a disease topic from multiple sources and synthesize the evidence into one document. Usually they include an evidence ranking.

Synopses: Some of the commercial products in this category are ACP Journal Club (http://acpjc.acponline.org/), Essential Evidence Plus Daily POEM Alerts (www.essentialevidenceplus.com/product/features_dailyip.cfm), and Journal Watch (www.jwatch.org). Instead of synthesizing all of the best evidence on a disease topic, these products identify journal articles that have clinical significance and produce a critical appraisal synopsis of the individual article. It is a great way to keep up with the literature without having to read hundreds of journals.

All the product types listed so far are filtered for their methodological quality. For the following product types you need to use your own critical appraisal skills. We discuss critical appraisal later.

Studies: The next three levels of the evidence product pyramid are *randomized controlled trials, cohort studies,* and *case-control studies/case series/case reports.* All of these can be found in the large

Exhibit 5–7   PubMed Results Utilizing the Systematic Review Filter

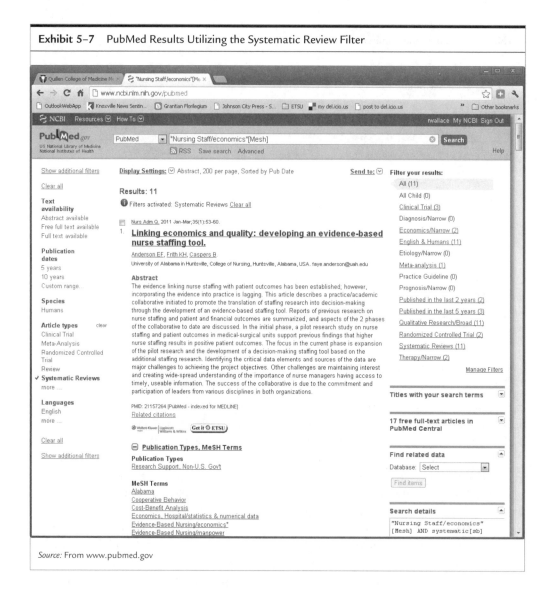

Source: From www.pubmed.gov

citation databases PubMed and CINAHL. Randomized controlled trials and case studies/reports are choices under *Article Type* in PubMed and *Publication Type* in CINAHL. *Case-control study* is a subject heading in both products. *Cohort study* is a subject heading in PubMed; CINAHL uses *prospective study* instead.

Another valuable free resource is the *National Guideline Clearinghouse* (guidelines.gov), shown in **Exhibit 5–8**. The information in this database fits into different levels of the evidence resource pyramid, depending on the quality of the guideline. Look for guidelines that have explicit evidence ratings such as the one that was used in the guideline "Prevention of Falls in the Elderly" by the Hartford Institute for Geriatric Nursing (**Exhibit 5–9**).

The bottom tier of the evidence product pyramid is *background information/expert opinion*. Products that fall into this category are textbooks and opinion journal articles.

Exhibit 5–8   Agency for Healthcare Research and Quality (AHRQ) National Guideline Clearinghouse

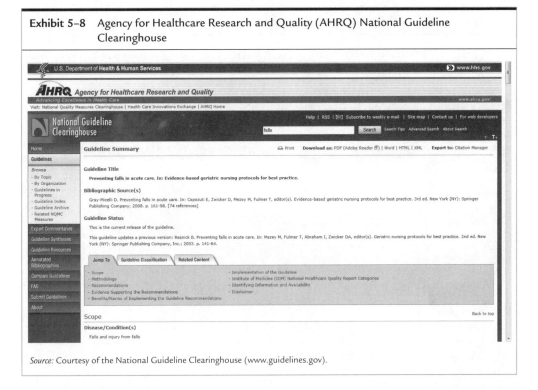

Source: Courtesy of the National Guideline Clearinghouse (www.guidelines.gov).

Exhibit 5–9   Hartford Institute for Geriatric Nursing Levels of Evidence Ratings

HIGN (2008)	**Levels of Evidence**
	Level I: Systematic reviews (integrative/meta-analyses/clinical practice guidelines based on systematic reviews)
	Level II: Single experimental study (randomized controlled trials [RCTs])
	Level III: Quasi-experimental studies
	Level IV: Non-experimental studies
	Level V: Care report/program evaluation/narrative literature reviews
	Level VI: Opinions of respected authorities/Consensus panels

Source: Reprinted by permission from Springer Publishing Company.

Complexity exists in retrieving best evidence as it does in any professional enterprise. A nurse manager definitely should acquire basic evidence-finding skills and be what David Slawson of the University of Virginia describes as an *information master* or a *YODA*, one who is "Your Own Data Analyzer" (Slawson & Shaughnessy, 2000, p. 65). The literature describes how time, access, and skill are major barriers to information retrieval. Therefore, you should develop a relationship with a professional health sciences librarian. If you are with a large healthcare system, get to know your librarian, and if you do not have one, encourage your enterprise to employ one. If you are with a smaller healthcare system, you may have an Area Health Education System (AHEC) library service that can help. AHECs are programs started with federal money that then become self-supporting or state funded or a combination of both. Their mission is to provide continuing health education, library service, and precepting opportunities for organizations that otherwise would not have access to these services. If you would like to know if there is a medical librarian in your area, contact the National Network of Libraries of Medicine (nnlm.gov) (**Exhibit 5–10**).

Exhibit 5–10   National Network of Libraries of Medicine

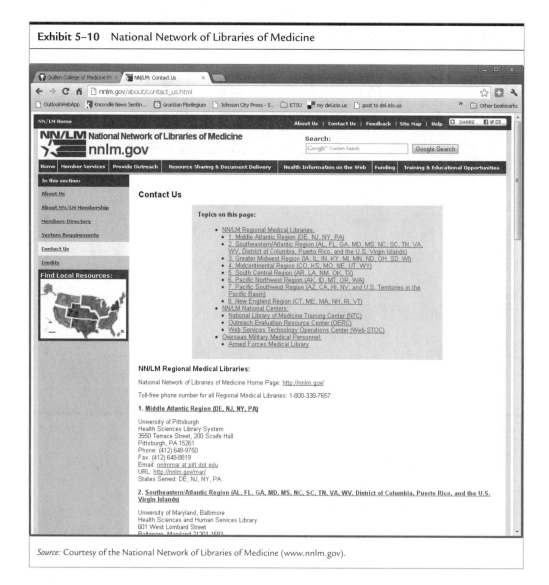

Source: Courtesy of the National Network of Libraries of Medicine (www.nnlm.gov).

A local academic health science library may also provide library services to healthcare organizations. At our organization, we provide mediated searching, delivery of journal articles and books, training, and smartphone support and obtain grants for dozens of healthcare facilities in our state.

Librarians can be helpful in selecting evidence resources for healthcare systems and for negotiating with vendors. They can efficiently do complex evidence searches for you that might take you hours to perform. Librarians have networks such as DocLine and OCLC that enable them to obtain evidence speedily from other health science libraries across the country.

ABI/INFORM is a *proprietary database* that is an excellent source for business, financial, and management information. According to the vendor website:

> Delivering over 6,800 journals, nearly 80% of which are in full-text, ABI/INFORM Complete™ is the most comprehensive business database on the market today. Offering much more than journal content, this diverse solution provides the right mix of content types to meet the needs of any business researcher. (www.proquest.com/en-US/catalogs/databases/detail/abi_inform.shtml)

The *Gale Group of databases* (infotrac.galegroup.com) is proprietary and has several business databases such as Business & Company ProFile ASAP, Business & Company Resource Center, Business & Industry, Business & Management Practices, and Business Reference Suite. Gale also has the health databases Health Reference Center Academic and Health & Wellness Resource Center.

The *Lexis/Nexis* database (www.lexisnexis.com) is another proprietary database. It is an outstanding source of legal information and news. It has information on the State Annotated Codes and is a good source for nursing board codes. *FindLaw* (www.findlaw.com) is an excellent source for finding a particular law or a case.

If you are not searching for information on a specific topic but are looking for professional reading material for nurse managers, the *Journal of Nursing Administration* (*JONA*) is an excellent publication. It is published monthly (July/August combined) by Lippincott Williams & Wilkins. Other first-rate journals include *Nursing Economic$*, *Nursing Management*, *Nursing Administration Quarterly*, *Nurse Leader*, and *Seminars for Nurse Managers*. Other appropriate nursing journals about quality, legal, education, and specific nursing clinical specialties may also be appropriate. General business journals such as the *Harvard Business Review* are also good sources, as are generic business and administration textbooks. In addition, specific professional organizations have wonderful websites, giving administrative and clinical information for their specialty.

State webpages are a superb source of statistical information. In many instances, they have the state code, health professional licensure verification, and rules and regulations from various state agencies. Another good source of statistical information is the National Center for Health Statistics, produced by the Centers for Disease Control and Prevention (cdc.gov/nchs). Also the site for phpartners.org is a quality site for health statistics (**Exhibit 5–11**).

Specific information on Medicare and Medicaid can be found at cms.hhs.gov at the Centers for Medicare and Medicaid Services. Another useful database is medicare.gov, which has a link to a site that compares nursing homes.

ERIC (eric.ed.gov) is a premier education database. According to the ERIC website:

> ERIC provides unlimited access to more than 1.4 million bibliographic records of journal articles and other education-related materials, with hundreds of new records added multiple times per week. If possible, links to full text in Adobe PDF format are included.

If you need a book, you can search for books in the subject area of your interest at Amazon.com. Copy the information and submit it to your librarian, who may be able to obtain the book on interlibrary loan. You can search the online public access catalogs of large libraries. Almost all large libraries have made their catalogs available to search freely on the Web. *LOCATORPlus*, the catalog of the U.S. National Library of Medicine, the largest medical library in the world, is available at locatorplus.gov. If you find a good title, ask your librarian to obtain it on interlibrary loan. In addition, the major publishers have very helpful websites (i.e., Jones & Bartlett Learning, jblearning.com).

Finally, you should learn to use search engines such as Google, still the search engine of choice even though other search engines do have some features not contained in Google. Take time to look around Google. The Google Images tab is a great service because it restricts your search to only images. If you wanted an image of a pressure ulcer, for example, this would be a good place to look. Google Scholar provides a way of searching scholarly material across many subject areas, from nursing to music, in many formats, such as books, papers, abstracts, and conference proceedings.

Another way to keep current and find information is through *social media*. Knowledge networks "foster social relationship or ties among people that build organizational social capital" (MacPhee, Suryaprakash, & Jackson, 2009, p. 415). Communities of practice can be formed from online collaborations that result over

Exhibit 5–11   Public Health Partners Database—Health Statistics

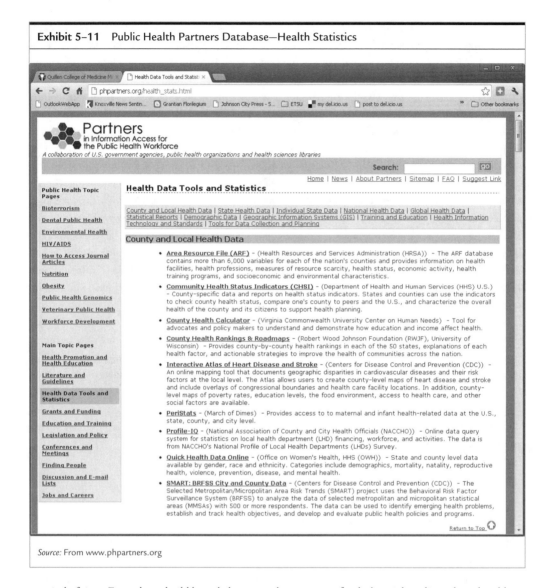

Source: From www.phpartners.org

a period of time. Examples to build knowledge networks are many of today's social media tools such as blogs, wikis, and Twitter (MacPhee et al., 2009).

The first social media tool we look at is *Twitter*. Actually, Twitter is a social networking and microblogging service that enables its users to send and read messages known as tweets. Tweets are text-based posts of up to 140 characters displayed on the author's profile page and delivered to the author's subscribers, who are known as followers. It has been used in business, churches, and schools. It can be used for research, networking, and brainstorming and to maximize classroom connections/discussions. Twitter isn't just about "I'm going to the grocery store" or "Go Giants!" Twitter is an excellent way to stay current with the latest news of your profession. By following professional organizations and leaders in your profession, you can quickly and easily keep up with the current information in your field. Examples include the following:

> http://scrubsmag.com/7-nurse-twitter-feeds-you-should-follow
> www.onlinedegreetalk.org/twitter-feeds-nursing-students
> www.lpn-to-rn.net/blog/2009/101-ways-to-use-twitter-in-your-hospital

Another social media tool of value is *blogs*. A blog is similar to an online journal. The name comes from the two words, *Web* and *log*. Blogs are written by one person, but others can comment on the blogs. There are many blogs online about and for nurses and nursing students. (As always, some will be good and some won't!)

http://blogs.nursing.jhu.edu
http://allnurses.com/nursing-news

The last social media tools we discuss are *Facebook* and *LinkedIn*. Both of these tools can be useful to professionals. Facebook focuses on building networks of friends. This aspect can be beneficial to expanding the reach of your organization or professional network. LinkedIn is a more professional website that allows the user to upload a resume, showcase skills, and build professional connections. Here are two examples:

http://megroberts.wordpress.com/2008/08/06/facebook-pages-using-them-to-benefit-your-organization
http://gigaom.com/2010/10/27/11-practical-business-uses-for-linkedin-facebook-and-twitter

One of the most important things to remember when dealing with social media is professionalism and confidentiality. The American Nurses Association's Principles for Social Networking (**Exhibit 5–12**) are included here.

The American Medical Association Council on Ethical and Judicial Affairs has published a report on professionalism in the use of social media. Some things the council feels health professionals should be aware of are the boundary that exists in the patient–health professional relationship, the perception of your professional peers of the information you post online, and the responsibility you have to report any unprofessional behavior that you see online such as violations of patient privacy. One thing you can do to protect your professional relationships is to have two separate accounts, one for personal use and one for professional use (Shore et al., 2011).

The National Council of State Boards of Nursing released a white paper in August 2011. It provides a guide including many types of scenarios to nurses who use any form of social media.

Social and electronic media possess tremendous potential for strengthening personal relationships and providing valuable information to health care consumers. [. . .] By being careful and conscientious, nurses may enjoy the personal and professional benefits of social and electronic media without violating patient privacy and confidentiality.

The Joint Commission stresses the importance of *patient education*. Where do you go for high-quality, reliable consumer health information that is not prohibitively expensive? Imagine you work for a fertility specialist. A patient's husband says to you, "My wife has been coming to this office for one year now and

---

Exhibit 5–12   American Nurses Association's *Principles for Social Networking*

1. Nurses must not transmit or place online individually identifiable patient information.
2. Nurses must observe ethically prescribed professional patient—nurse boundaries.
3. Nurses should understand that patients, colleagues, institutions, and employers may view postings.
4. Nurses should take advantage of privacy settings and seek to separate personal and professional information online.
5. Nurses should bring content that could harm a patient's privacy, rights, or welfare to the attention of appropriate authorities.
6. Nurses should participate in developing institutional policies governing online conduct.

Source: From http://www.nursingworld.org/socialnetworkingtoolkit.aspx

she is not yet pregnant. I have heard that acupuncture can help with infertility. Do you know anything about this?" What do you do?

Consumer/patient information is important, and many people are appallingly illiterate when it comes to health knowledge. "Nearly 90% of U.S. adults are less than proficient in reading, understanding and acting on medical information, according to a U.S. Dept. of Education literacy assessment of more than 19,000 Americans that was last done in 2003" (O'Reilly, 2012). Conditions such as diabetes and obesity could be greatly reduced if consumers were better educated about their health and if they would practice what they learn. We believe that this lack of availability and use of health information is a national health crisis.

Where do you begin to find unbiased, practical information? Countless consumer health information resources exist. We could give you list after list of websites, books, and organizations that provide consumer/patient health information. We have found this flood of information to be confusing to information seekers. What we prefer is to offer a limited, but manageable, number of excellent resources. By using gateways that have already been evaluated by librarians, you can save time, energy, and money.

A good starting point for finding consumer/patient information is the database *MedlinePlus* (medlineplus.gov). MedlinePlus (**Exhibit 5–13**) is maintained by the National Library of Medicine, one of the National Institutes of Health of the federal government. MedlinePlus is an aggregator of the best consumer health information on the Web. Because of its comprehensive nature, it usually makes possible "one-stop shopping" for consumer health information. When you search by topic in MedlinePlus, you retrieve a list of links from other websites that have been quality filtered. The information in MedlinePlus is grouped by topic and is easy to search. Some topics even have tutorials for those with poor reading skills as well as links to resources labeled "easy-to-read." The tutorials can be heard through computer speakers or through headphones while you watch a slideshow that explains a procedure or condition.

Exhibit 5–13 MedlinePlus Health Topics

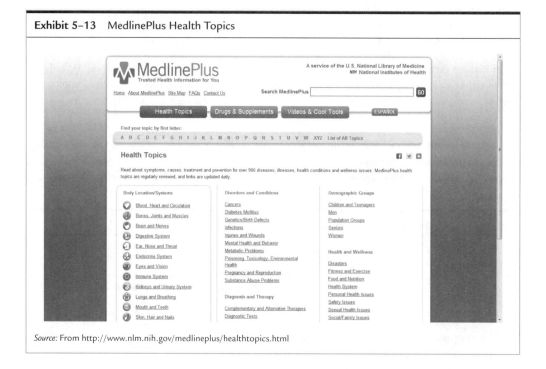

Source: From http://www.nlm.nih.gov/medlineplus/healthtopics.html

MedlinePlus is a good source of drug information and includes directories and dictionaries as well. A Spanish version of the site is also available and includes an excellent encyclopedia and Spanish-language tutorials. One of MedlinePlus's newest enhancements is the audio feature for people with low health literacy or disabilities; the website is designed to read aloud the contents of a page in either English or Spanish. MedlinePlus is now linked to consumer health information in more than 40 languages. The National Library of Medicine continually updates, expands, and improves the site.

If you cannot find an answer at MedlinePlus.gov, we recommend that you use the *Medical Library Association's Consumer and Patient Health Information Section* (*CAPHIS*) site at http://caphis.mlanet.org. The people who maintain this site are the best of the best. They are professional librarians who spend a lot of their time providing consumer/patient health information on a daily basis. The group maintains a list of the top 100 consumer/patient health information websites. According to CAPHIS:

> The purpose of the CAPHIS Top 100 List is to provide CAPHIS members and other librarians with a resource to use in their daily practice and teaching. Secondly, it is our contribution to the Medical Library Association so that the headquarters staff can refer individuals to a list of quality health web sites. Our goal is to have a limited number of resources that meet the quality criteria for currency, credibility, content, audience, etc., as described on our website.

Much fraudulent consumer/patient health information exists on the Web. A site that exposes false and misleading health information on the Web is *Quackwatch* (quackwatch.org). According to information found at the site, the mission of Quackwatch is as follows:

> Quackwatch is an international network of people who are concerned about health-related frauds, myths, fads, fallacies, and misconduct. Its primary focus is on quackery-related information that is difficult or impossible to get elsewhere. Founded by Dr. Stephen Barrett in 1969 as the Lehigh Valley Committee Against Health Fraud (Allentown, Pennsylvania), it was incorporated in 1970. In 1997, it assumed its current name and began developing a worldwide network of volunteers and expert advisors.

As a nurse manager, you should be interested in efficiency and effectiveness. *Mobile technology* (smart-phones and tablets) can assist in preventing medication errors and keep the nursing staff up-to-date in regard to clinical knowledge. Mobile devices use either the Android (Google) or Apple operating system. They can be indispensable clinical tools. The drug database *ePocrates* (epocrates.com) is a free drug reference tool. Studies have been published that demonstrate ePocrates use can reduce medication error. There are other point-of-care drug tools as well such as Lexi-Comp and Micromedex.

Point-of-care disease databases are the second main category of mobile technology resources. *Dynamed* (http://dynamed.ebscohost.com/) is a prime example of this type of resource. Dynamed has an A to Z list of diseases. Each section has a *General Information, Causes and Risk Factors, History and Physical, Diagnosis, Treatment, Prognosis,* and *Prevention* section. The information is high quality and is updated frequently. Other resources like this are Essential Evidence Plus, Clinical Evidence, Clinical Key, and UpToDate. The use of mobile technology with this type of database can overcome the attrition of knowledge clinicians experience over a lifetime.

Regular webpages are not easily viewed on smartphones. Therefore, many *smartphone webpages* are created as mobile webpages. These pages are much easier to navigate and view on a small screen. *Apps* (short for applications) are better than mobile websites. Apps are downloaded to a mobile device. Dynamed has an app. Compare the regular webpage, mobile webpage, and app for Amazon.com to see the difference between the three platforms.

Two sources for health resources on a smartphone are www.skyscape.com and www.medicalwizards .com. Just a quick perusal of Skyscape shows featured nursing texts for personal digital assistants (*PDAs*) such as RNotes (Nurse's Clinical Pocket Guide), Davis's Drug Guide for Nurses, Nursing Constellation: All-In-One Nursing Solution, and Nurse's Manual of Laboratory and Diagnostic Tests. This gives you a taste of the type of information that can be used on a smartphone or handheld device in a clinical setting.

Free downloads are available for diagnostic testing databases, screening databases, immunization databases, prognostic and therapeutic calculators, budget and scheduling information, and other useful applications. We encourage you to invest in a smartphone or tablet. They enable you to bring information with you wherever you go. They can enable you to give better care to patients. David Slawson, MD, a well-known proponent of EBP, equates a smartphone to a stethoscope as a clinical tool. In our institution, the library allows mobile technology users to drop off their device, and we load all the software for them. We install the Dynamed app and Essential Evidence Plus (essentialevidenceplus.com) mobile link. These resources are outstanding best-evidence databases. They require an annual subscription. We also install the AHRQ ePSS screening tool; Shots, which is a childhood and adult immunization schedule (immunizationed.org); Archimedes, which has more than 150 clinical calculators; and the Stat!Ref book collection (www.statref.com).

These technology tools can have a positive financial impact by reducing medication error and providing high-level evidence so that clinical practices are maintained optimally. Be an enabler by encouraging mobile technology in the clinic.

The EHR touches every aspect of health care. "The evidence suggests that the quality of nursing documentation improves after the introduction of HIT [health information technology] and that nurses spend less time on documentation than they did before HIT implementation" (Waneka & Spetz, 2010, p. 510).

Library information is no exception. For example, the consumer health database MedlinePlus can be connected to the EHR. The National Library of Medicine explains how this is done (at www.nlm.nih.gov/medlineplus/connect/overview.html): MedlinePlus Connect accepts requests for information on diagnoses (problem codes), medications, and lab tests and returns related MedlinePlus information. It is available as a web application or a web service. Upon receiving a problem code request, MedlinePlus Connect returns relevant MedlinePlus health topics and other related information. MedlinePlus has hundreds of health topic pages that bring together information from National Institutes of Health, other U.S. government agencies, and reputable health information providers. Health topic pages cover a wide range of conditions and wellness issues and include key resources to inform patients about their health: overviews, information on symptoms and treatments, recent health news, clinical trials, and much more. You can browse the list of all health topics.

For problem code requests, MedlinePlus Connect supports ICD-9-CM (International Classification of Diseases, 9th edition, Clinical Modification) and SNOMED CT (Systematized Nomenclature of Medicine, Clinical Terms). Note: MedlinePlus Connect coverage of SNOMED CT focuses on CORE Problem List Subset codes (Clinical Observations Recording and Encoding) and their descendants. MedlinePlus Connect will support ICD-10-CM when it becomes the U.S. standard. MedlinePlus Connect can also link your EHR system to drug information written especially for patients. When an EHR system sends MedlinePlus Connect a request that includes a medication code, the service returns a link or links to the most appropriate drug information. MedlinePlus drug information is the *AHFS Consumer Medication Information* and is licensed for use on MedlinePlus from the American Society of Health-System Pharmacists (ASHP, Inc.). For medication requests, MedlinePlus Connect supports RXCUI (RxNorm Concept Unique Identifier) and NDC (National Drug Code).

MedlinePlus Connect also returns information in response to laboratory test codes. This information is from the A.D.A.M. encyclopedia, which MedlinePlus licenses. For lab test requests, MedlinePlus Connect supports LOINC (Logical Observation Identifiers Names and Codes). MedlinePlus Connect supports requests for information in English or Spanish. It is intended for use within the United States healthcare system and cannot support coding systems not used in the United States.

A warning is in order: The EHR movement, along with a lot of other health information technology (HIT), is *very expensive* to install and maintain. Nurse managers are charged with being fiscally responsible. Be careful not to purchase expensive technology because a competitor purchases it. The library profession has become highly automated. As health science librarians, we try to understand the process behind any system in detail including its inputs and outputs. Then we decide whether the process would be improved by automating it, including a cost-benefit analysis. Doing the intellectual work of describing a process in detail makes shopping for automated systems much more effective. An article from the *Journal of the American Medical Informatics Association* indicated it is difficult to reach any definite conclusion as to whether the additional costs and benefits (of HIT) represent value for money (O'Reilly, Tarride, Goeree, Lokker, & McKibbon, 2012).

Nurse managers have an important role in the implementation of EHRs. An article titled "Nursing Leaders Serving as a Foundation for the Electronic Medical Record" (Edwards, 2012) from the *Journal of Nursing Trauma* stated that a nurse manager "being proactive in the reception, design, development, and implementation of an EMR plays a role in creating an organizational culture that allows for the flow of data efficiently and accurately" (p. 111). A recommended book on EHR implementation is *Connected for Health: Using Electronic Health Records to Transform Care Delivery* by L. L. Liang (2010).

The National Library of Medicine (NLM) has an excellent page of resources for *health informatics* (www.nlm.nih.gov/hsrinfo/informatics.html). Health informatics is the broader discipline that includes medical librarianship and technologies such as the electronic health record. NLM defines health informatics as "the interdisciplinary study of the design, development, adoption and application of IT-based innovations in healthcare services delivery, management and planning" (R. Procter, personal communication, August 16, 2009).

We have a great idea—use your librarian. Do not hesitate to "bother" your librarian if there is one in your facility. Librarians are one of the world's best-kept secrets. Librarians will do literature searches for you when you do not have time. They can order articles, including administrative articles, for you and your staff that the library does not have.

Some librarians are willing to come out to the clinical areas of the facility on a regular basis and interact with the staff. Librarians can find information and email it to you. One way, according to Reichel (1989), that librarians can meet the needs and obligations of the parent institution is by bibliographic instruction or teaching. Bibliographic instruction teaches library patrons how to locate and use library resources efficiently. Librarians love to teach. Schedule classes for them to work with you and/or your nursing staff. They can explain the information resources available at your facility and teach your staff how to properly use them.

You work in a rural long-term care facility. You want better information resources for your staff but cannot afford a library in the facility. What do you do? Jensen and Maddalena (1985) noted, "The results of our work show that small rural hospitals (100 beds or fewer) have extreme difficulty in maintaining adequate on-site library resources and services over a period of time" (p. 60). Thibodeau and Funk's (2009) research discovered that "about 44% of hospitals had some level of on-site library service in 1989, compared with between 33.6% and 29.1% of hospitals in 2006" (p. 274). Given the financial crunch on small hospitals, it is safe to bet that the number is much less than that now. Often, unfortunately, when a hospital makes spending cuts, the library is a victim. A solution for these hospitals may be to contract the services of an outreach librarian who would spend varying amounts of time there, depending on the size of the hospital and its information needs. The outreach librarian visits several key areas throughout the hospital including nurses' stations, the physicians' lounge, the emergency room, the pharmacy, or outlying clinics. In Gordner's (1982) experience with outreach librarianship, nurses were the largest users of the information service.

As previously noted under Acquire, there may be an AHEC program that would provide librarian services (either free for a small fee) for your geographic area. Fowkes, Campeau, and Wilson (1991) reported, "AHECs have demonstrated an ability to respond to current and emerging needs that distinguishes them from other institutions that have educational missions" (p. 219). AHECs responded better because they were more flexible than traditional academic bureaucracies and were more in touch with the communities they serve. Fowkes and colleagues continued: "Having both academic and community roots, AHECs know the needs and resources of each and how to use them in a manner that benefits both, thus strengthening and balancing the partnership between school and community" (p. 219).

The National Network of Libraries of Medicine (NN/LM) is a division of the National Library of Medicine. NN/LM has centers throughout the country. Each center has trainers who will come out to your town and teach classes on mobile technology, consumer health, public health information resources, and National Library of Medicine databases, just to name a few topics that are in their repertoire. The web address for NN/LM is nnlm.gov. To utilize the training, your organization must be an NN/LM member. Membership is free.

It is imperative that nursing leadership in rural areas provide organizational support for the enhancement of evidence-based practices. Munroe, Duffy, and Fisher (2006) reported that the overall knowledge of nurses in a rural community hospital increased significantly when evidence-based practice was promoted through personnel, education, and process interventions. An added bonus was a renewed "sense of professionalism and pride" among nursing personnel.

Florance, Giuse, and Ketchell (2002) described how Vanderbilt Medical Center librarians were trained in pharmacology, physiology, and biostatistics and actively participated in medical rounds. They not only gathered information for clinicians but also summarized it, appraised it, and offered commentary. This same practice could work with nurses. Williams and Zipperer (2003) said, "The occasional participation by the librarian in patient rounds with nurses and other clinical staff can engender trust in the relationship between the librarian and the clinical team" (p. 204). Your librarian could come on the floor once or twice every week. She could gather topics to be researched, meet new staff, update the staff about new developments in the library, and give one-on-one training. As a result, the nursing staff would save time and the librarian would become an important part of the clinical team.

We like to use the following illustration to explain why we believe librarians are an essential part of the healthcare team (Holtum, 1999):

> When health professionals request lab work, they turn to medical technologists. If an X-ray is needed, they direct the patient to a radiographic technician. The reason is simple: Even though the clinician is certainly capable of learning and performing these tasks (though at considerable time and expense), higher quality and greater cost-effectiveness are obtained by using the skills of specialists instead. Can the same not be said of the expertise and experience that librarians bring to the health care enterprise? (p. 406)?

Although you may have learned some laboratory skills in school, you still send samples to a lab for analysis. Libraries are similar. It just makes sense to give a task to those who are trained and experienced to do it. We hope you are good at finding information, but if a skilled professional is available to do it for you, you can dedicate your time to what you do best—managing the unit and working with staff who are taking care of sick people. Studies by Griffiths and King indicated that in professional organizations, having a professional librarian and library actually saved the institution money compared to what it would take for each individual to find the information they needed on their own.

Please be an advocate for libraries in your institution. Librarians need your support when budgets are cut because administrators often consider eliminating the library first as a simple cost-cutting measure. Most small hospitals and healthcare institutions do not have a library because of the expense. If this is your situation, you may want to consider contracting for the services of an outreach librarian. Of course, you can also contact a librarian by email or by telephone. Another option is to contact your local academic health sciences library for assistance.

Appraise

The next step in finding best evidence is critical appraisal. This step can be difficult, but it is doable. We should all be thankful that there are many evidence products, mentioned in an earlier section, that already preappraise the evidence for us. Critical appraisal choices depend on the type of question being asked. In healthcare, most questions are about treatment, followed by diagnosis and questions related to etiology/harm, prognosis, cost/economics, or patient education. If no summaries, syntheses, or synopses exist that answer your question, you will want to find a randomized controlled trial if you have a therapy or etiology/harm question. The best individual study type for a prognosis question is a cohort study and for a diagnosis question is a head-to-head comparison of the new diagnostic technique with the gold standard. The principle to follow is if there is not the highest evidence type available to answer your question, move down the evidence pyramid to the next level.

There are critical appraisal worksheets for different question types freely available on the Web. One list can be found at the Dartmouth Biomedical Library at www.dartmouth.edu/~library/biomed/guides/research/ebm-resources-materials.html. Another list that includes an economic analysis critical appraisal worksheet is at the Duke Medical Library at http://guides.mclibrary.duke.edu/content.php?pid=274373&sid=2262324.

A useful mnemonic device we learned from Duke to use to critically appraise therapy articles is FRISBE (follow-up, randomization, intention to treat analysis, same at baseline, blinded, equal treatment). At least 80% of those who start into a trial should be accounted for at the end (follow-up). A number less than 80% raises questions about the results. Trial enrollees should be randomly selected to be in one arm of the trial or another. The chance of ending up in one group versus another should be equal.

Intention to treat means that if a participant in one arm of the trial changes over and starts doing what is prescribed for the other arm (such as taking drug A instead of drug B), that participant should still be analyzed in the results of the group in which he or she started the trial. Both arms should have equal characteristics at the start of the trial. For example, if age and gender are important to the outcome, both groups should be similar in age and gender. You should note if the article indicated if the participants were blinded (they do not know if they are receiving exposure A or B); if the administrators were blinded, which is double blinding; and if the data analysts were blinded (triple blinding). Each arm of the trial should be treated equally. No arm should be given preferential treatment other than the exposure to which they were assigned.

Statistical measures are unavoidable in reading the research literature and give us all heartburn. You do not need to be a statistical whiz, but you should be familiar with some basic statistical procedures such as absolute risk reduction, relative risk reduction, number needed to treat, odds ratio, and correlation statistics such as Pearsons, chi-square, regression, p-values, confidence intervals, power, t-tests, and ANOVA.

Again, you do not have to be able to compute these statistics, just try to familiarize yourself with a basic definition.

Studies are critically appraised to determine their reliability (replicability in other environments) and validity (truthfulness). Various types of bias reduce the reliability and validity of evidence. Some common types of bias are selection bias, which occurs when individuals or groups are more likely to be chosen to participate in a research project than others, funding bias, which occurs when results of the study may be slanted to favor the study's financial sponsor, and publication bias, which generally applies to being inclined toward finding positive results because positive results are generally more often published in the literature.

Apply

The most important part of using evidence is applying it to a particular patient encounter or managerial problem. You must use your wisdom along with the best evidence from the research, which you now know how to find. You need to see how well the population that was studied in the research you found matches the patient or problem you are dealing with, and you must also take into consideration local norms, politics, standard practices, and so forth.

Summary

The purpose of this chapter is to teach and encourage you to practice with evidence. We have shown you some principles upon which evidence is sorted for quality, pointed you to some excellent evidence resources and some technology tools that are useful in finding evidence at the point of care, and encouraged you to use evidence professionals (librarians). Our desire is that you become lifelong evidence users and truly become information masters.

Discussion Questions

1. List five examples of practice changes based on evidence that have occurred in recent years.
2. Compare and contrast two of the nursing-specific database search sites.
3. Discuss the level of evidence scale that you would expect before changing a clinical practice at your facility.
4. What resource or resources are available to help with evaluating sites for consumer health literacy?
5. What resource or resources are available to incorporate information into the electronic health record?
6. What is the nurse manager's role in implementing evidence-based practice?
7. What are some issues that could arise from use of social media in the workplace?

Glossary of Terms

Bibliographic Database—a searchable collection of citations to publications. The publications may include books, journals, audiovisual materials, and websites. Most bibliographic databases include information about the publication, such as author, title, and copyright date. Often an abstract of the publication is included, but the full text of the article must usually be located elsewhere.

Case-Control Study—a retrospective study that collects data from charts, data sets, and patient interviews.

Case Study—a detailed analysis of a person or group from a social, psychological, or medical point of view.

Cohort Study—an observational study in which a group of people is identified in the present and followed into the future or identified from past records and followed from that time up to the present.

Electronic Health Record (EHR)—a systematic collection of health information about individual patients or populations stored in an electronic format.

Evidence-Based Information (EBI)—the melding of individual judgment and expertise with the best available external evidence to generate the kind of information that is most likely to lead to a positive outcome.

Informatics—a science that combines a domain science, computer science, information science, and cognitive science.

Levels of Evidence (LOE)—a method of ranking evidence for better decision making.

Nursing Informatics—the study of how electronic information systems are used to improve nursing systems and patient care.

PDA—personal digital assistant or handheld computer.

PICO (Population, Intervention, Comparison, Outcome)—a method of formatting a focused question resulting in a more productive search and a more relevant answer.

Proprietary Database—a privately controlled and distributed database. Access is through subscription or on a pay-per-view basis.

Randomized Controlled Trial (RCT)—a carefully designed blinded or double-blinded experiment. Randomized controlled trials are randomized in the sense that everyone who is in the population being studied has an equal chance of being chosen to be in the experimental group (arm) or control group.

Secondary Literature—articles that filter the best information from the primary literature.

Social Media—forms of electronic communication (as websites for social networking and microblogging) through which users create online communities to share information, ideas, personal messages, and other content (such as videos).

Strength of Recommendation (SOR) Ratings—guides to the trustworthiness of information.

Systematic Review—a compilation of randomized controlled trials on a single subject.

References

Cho, S. H., Lee, J. H., Mark, B. A., & Yun, S. C. (2012). Turnover of new graduate nurses in their first job using survival analysis. *Journal of Nursing Scholarship, 44*(1), 63–70. doi:10.1111/j.1547-5069.2011.01428.x

Edwards, C. (2012). Nursing leaders serving as a foundation for the electronic medical record. *Journal of Trauma Nursing, 19*(2), 111–114; quiz 115–116. doi:10.1097/JTN.0b013e31825629db

Florance, V., Giuse, N., & Ketchell, D. (2002). Information in context: Integrating information specialists into practice setting. *Journal of the Medical Library Association, 90*(1), 49–58.

Fowkes, V., Campeau, M., & Wilson, S. (1991). The evolution and impact of the national AHEC program over two decades. *Academic Medicine, 66*(4), 211–220.

Gordner, R. (1982). Riding the rural library circuit. *Medical Reference Services Quarterly, 1*(1), 59–74.

Griffiths, J-M., & King, D. W. (1991). A Manual on the Evaluation of Information Centers and Services. NATO, AGARD, New York: American Institute of Aeronautics and Astronautics. Retrieved from http://www.dtic.mil/dtic/tr/fulltext/u2/a237321.pdf

Haynes, R. B. (2006). Of studies, syntheses, synopses, summaries, and systems: The "5S" evolution of information services for evidence-based health care decisions. *ACP Journal Club, 145*(3), A8.

Hinson, T. D., & Spatz, D. L. (2011). Improving nurse retention in a large tertiary acute care hospital. *Journal of Nursing Administration, 41*(3), 103–108.

Holtum, E. (1999). Librarians, clinicians, evidence-based medicine and the division of labor. *Bulletin of the Medical Library Association, 87*(4), 404–407.

Jensen, M., & Maddalena, B. (1985). Implications of the AHEC library program evaluation: Considerations for small rural hospitals. *Bulletin of the Medical Library Association, 73*(1), 59–61.

Liang, L. L. (2010). *Connected for health: Using electronic health records to transform care delivery.* San Francisco, CA: Jossey-Bass.

MacPhee, M., Suryaprakash, N., & Jackson, C. (2009). Online knowledge networking: What leaders need to know. *Journal of Nursing Administration, 39*(10), 415–422. doi:10.1097/NNA.0b013e3181b9221f

Melnyk, B. M., Fineout-Overholt, E., Gallagher-Ford, L., & Kaplan, L. (2012). The state of evidence-based practice in US nurses: Critical implications for nurse leaders and educators. *Journal of Nursing Administration, 42*(9), 410–417. doi:10.1097/NNA.0b013e3182664e0a

Munroe, D., Duffy, P., & Fisher, C. (2006). Fostering evidence-based practice in a rural community hospital. *Journal of Nursing Administration, 36,* 510–512.

National Council of State Boards of Nursing. (2011). *White paper: A nurse's guide to the use of social media.* Chicago, IL: National Council of State Boards of Nursing. Retrieved from https://www.ncsbn.org/Social_Media.pdf

O'Reilly, D., Tarride, J. E., Goeree, R., Lokker, C., & McKibbon, K. A. (2012). The economics of health information technology in medication management: A systematic review of economic evaluations. *Journal of the American Medical Informatics Association, 19*(3), 423–438. doi:10.1136/amiajnl-2011000310; 10.1136/amiajnl-2011–000310

O'Reilly, K. B. (2012). The ABCs of health literacy. *American Medical News.* Retrieved from http://www.amednews.com/article/20120319/profession/303199949/4/

Palfreman, J., & Reid, T. R. (2008). Sick around the world (J. Palfreman, Director). In J. Palfreman (Producer), *Frontline.* Boston, MA: WGBH Educational Foundation.

Pryce, J., Albertson, K., & Nielsen, K. (2006). Evaluation of an open-rota system in a Danish psychiatric hospital: A mechanism for improving job satisfaction and work-life balance. *Journal of Nursing Management, 14*(4), 282–288.

Reichel, M. (1989). Ethics and library instruction: Is there a connection? *RQ, 28*(4), 477–480.

Reid. T. R. (2010). *The healing of America: A global quest for better, cheaper and fairer healthcare.* London, England: Penguin.

Reid, T. R. (2012). *The good news in American medicine* (L. Hartman, Producer). Arlington, VA: PBS.

Sackett, D. L., Rosenberg, W. M. C., Gray, J. A. M., Haynes, B., & Richardson, W. S. (1996). Evidence based medicine: What it is and what it isn't. *British Medical Journal, 312*(7023), 71–72.

Shore, R., Halsey, J., Shah, K., Crigger, B. J., Douglas, S. P., & AMA Council on Ethical and Judicial Affairs. (2011). Report of the AMA Council on Ethical and Judicial Affairs: Professionalism in the use of social media. *Journal of Clinical Ethics, 22*(2), 165–177.

Slawson, D., & Shaughnessy, A. F. (2000). Becoming an information master: Using POEMs to change practice with confidence. Patient Oriented Service That Matters. *Journal of Family Practice, 49*(1), 63–67.

Sredl, D., Melnyk, B. M., Hsueh, K. H., Jenkins, R., Ding, C., & Durham, J. (2011). Health care in crisis! Can nurse executives' beliefs about and implementation of evidence-based practice be key solutions in health care reform? *Teaching and Learning in Nursing, 6*(2), 73–79.

Staggs, V. S., & Dunton, N. (2012). Hospital and unit characteristics associated with nursing turnover include skill mix but not staffing level: An observational cross-sectional study. *International Journal of Nursing Studies, 49*(9), 1138–1145. doi:10.1016/j.ijnurstu.2012.03.009

Thibodeau, P. L., & Funk, C. J. (2009). Trends in hospital librarianship and hospital library services: 1989 to 2006. *Journal of the Medical Library Association, 97*(4), 273–279. doi:10.3163/1536–5050.97.4.011

Waneka, R., & Spetz, J. (2010). Hospital information technology systems' impact on nurses and nursing care. *Journal of Nursing Administration, 40*(12), 509–514. doi:10.1097/NNA.0b013e3181fc1a1c; 10.1097/NNA.0b013e3181fc1a1c

Wennberg, J. E. (2010). *Tracking medicine: A researcher's guide to understand healthcare.* New York, NY: Oxford University Press.

Wilkinson, J., & Daly, M. (2012). Reasons for non-attendance: Audit findings from a nurse-led clinic. *Journal of Primary Health Care, 4*(1), 39–44.

Williams, L., & Zipperer, L. (2003). Improving access to information: Librarians and nurses team up for patient safety. *Nursing Economic$, 21*(4), 199–201.

Workforce Management

Workload management is an integral component of hospital operations. Relying on experience, intuition, and historical usage to manage workloads is not viable in an age of plentiful information, customer expectations of value-based services, and value-based reimbursement. The focus has necessarily shifted to managing the data to guide effective decision making, specifically *evidence-based workforce management.*

Chapter 6 examines the workforce management cycle: identification of patient care needs (patient classification systems/benchmark data), core scheduling (staffing plan), daily staffing (nurse–patient assignments, skill mix, and variance management), evaluation (patient outcomes, quality), and budget management (budget and productivity monitoring) using available information systems. All this is interwoven with best evidence and technology. Nurse administrators are guided through this process and given key information on how to effectively manage our most valuable resource, the staff.

In workforce management, the nurse administrator must consider certain ethical and legal issues that guide and enhance decision making. Chapter 7 discusses organizational ethics. This chapter provides an historical perspective of ethics development in the healthcare system, presents ethical concerns of nurse administrators, and suggests insights into the development of ethical leadership.

Chapter 8 outlines some common legal issues facing nurse administrators. This chapter discusses standards of practice, nurse practice acts, laws that regulate nursing practice, how the practice standards are used as evidence in malpractice litigation, the legal significance of your nursing license, and your legal responsibility with delegation rules.

Staffing Effectiveness: Concepts, Models, and Processes

Kathy Malloch, PhD, MBA, RN, FAAN, and
Janne Dunham-Taylor, PhD, RN

OBJECTIVES

- Discover myths about staffing practices.
- Identify the components of an effective workforce management system.
- Apply a complex model for effective staffing practices.
- Describe various ways to measure patient care workload in health care and in nursing.
- Describe the staffing process.
- Explain financial implications in workforce management.
- Describe effective productivity monitoring.
- Use information technology to better manage the staffing process.

Consider this perception of staffing:

> The world of staffing is a mess. Okay, there may be exceptions, but if ever there was an area that could benefit from an overhaul, staffing is high on the list. To move staffing from its current state to one of optimal efficiency and effectiveness will not be easy. Staffing is extremely complex and the impact of our effectiveness in staffing, or lack thereof, touches almost every aspect of a care delivery system, making this a critical topic for nurse leaders. To address the challenges that staffing presents requires new levels of innovation and creativity. . . . Let's not let the barrier to uncovering the potential of excellent staffing practices be our own thinking. Approaching the topic of staffing with a sense of inquiry, letting go of mental models and constructs that are familiar and comfortable, combined with a strong understanding of the data, experience, and wisdom available to us will uncover new possibilities. (Douglas, 2009, p. 332)

Workforce Management

Effective workforce management is a key factor contributing to organizational success—better patient outcomes, better reimbursement, positive patient satisfaction scores, fewer incident reports with possible legal ramifications, greater workforce satisfaction and retention, and, of course, financial success. Thus, workforce management is an essential concept for healthcare leaders. Because nursing constitutes the majority of the workforce in healthcare facilities, nurse leaders in particular are faced with the ever-increasing demand to ensure efficient and effective service delivery, and we need to pay attention to the evidence about workforce management.

For years nurse administrators have relied on their experience, intuition, judgment, and traditions to create and justify optimal workforce management systems—systems that include an effective method to assess and predict patient care needs, a staffing plan core schedule, daily staffing processes, productivity monitoring tools, budget parameters, and quality evaluation criteria.

All this has changed; experience and traditions are not enough. This valuable knowledge must be partnered with the explosion of new evidence (**Exhibit 6–1**) and electronic clinical information system applications. Evidence-based staffing and scheduling (Hyun, Bakken, Douglas, & Stone, 2008) has become so important that *Nursing Economic$* often devotes a column to it. Clinical and financial data are now readily available in digital formats. *The emphasis is now on the integration of data from multiple sources, interpretation of the data into meaningful information, and real-time use of the information to achieve staffing effectiveness.* Necessarily, workforce management can now be *based on evidence* as well as experience and expertise.

The availability of digital data and sophisticated information processing systems is especially important in light of local, state, and regional initiatives and regulations to increase quality and decrease costs. Healthcare leaders have to be aware of healthcare reform targets, specific initiatives from the Centers for Medicare and Medicaid Services (CMS), the Agency for Healthcare Research and Quality (AHRQ), Robert Wood Johnson Foundation, the Institute of Medicine, the American Nurses Association (ANA), and staffing legislation. The second edition of *ANA Principles for Nurse Staffing* (American Nurses Association [ANA], 2012) provides policy direction for workforce management (Weston, Brewer, & Peterson, 2012).

The purposes of these initiatives are fourfold: to improve patient safety/quality of care, increase patient satisfaction, improve the health of the caregivers, and decrease costs/achieve reimbursements. These initiatives, along with ongoing research reports, drive the need for effective, evidence-based staffing systems (American Recovery and Reinvestment Act, 2009; Institute of Medicine, 2010).

Exhibit 6–1   Selected Staffing Effectiveness Research Evidence

Significant progress is being made in identifying the relationship between the role of the nurse and patient, provider, organization and cost outcomes. This exhibit lists the specific areas of impact and supporting references can be found within this chapter and in the Appendix at the end of this chapter. The increasingly broad range of evidence provides support for effective staffing plans and adjustments to daily staffing assignments including specific relationships between patient outcomes nurse characteristics and nurse schedules.

Patient outcomes
- Patient mortality/ failure to rescue: pneumonia, post-operative DVT/pulmonary embolism
- Patient-adverse outcomes: pneumonia, post-operative infections, urinary tract infections, acute myocardial infarction, congestive heart failure, patient falls, medication errors, pressure ulcers
- Smoking cessation counseling rates
- Pneumococcal vaccinations rates
- Length of stay
- Patient satisfaction
- Patient experience of care
- Patient
- Readmission
- Family complaints

Nurse characteristics
- Clinical Nurse Leader role
- Education level
- Percentage of registered nurse staffing
- Experience at the shift level
- Shift hours
- Number of days worked in a row
- Number of hours worked in a week
- Unit admission, discharge and transfer activity
- Nurse turnover
- Nurse fatigue and sleep cycles
- Nurse retention
- Nurse vacancy rate
- Reduction in agency rates
- Needlestick injuries
- Improved communication re: errors
- Nurse productivity

Environment of care
- Foundations for quality of care
- Nurse manager ability, leadership, and support
- Collegial nurse/physician relationships
- Improved operating margin
- Improved bond rating
- US News & World Report (Top 20)
- Magnet® status
- Support staff: Nursing assistants and secretaries
- Facility costs and reimbursements

Reese (2011, pp. 23–24) shares 10 evidence-based practices in workforce management:

1. Decrease the use of 12-hour shifts.
2. Investigate ways to ensure nurses leave on time at the end of a shift.
3. Decrease the use of overtime hours.
4. Spread the wealth in distributing overtime.
5. Know the staff members you're scheduling.
6. Define a skill mix for each shift and stick to it.

7. Vary the experience levels scheduled on each shift.
8. Evaluate the adequacy of rest periods between shifts when approving schedule changes.
9. Develop practice guidelines.
10. Monitor key performance indicator trends in staffing and scheduling.

Lorenz (2008) points out:

> Until there are regulations that restrict the number of hours that a nurse can work, . . .it is the ethical responsibility of organizational leaders to ensure that the risk of harm to patients by medical errors is reduced. It is incumbent upon the chief nurse executive to know and understand the data, analyze the effects of extended work hours in the organizations, and take steps that eliminate the possibility of a patient being harmed *because of staff scheduling.* (p. 301)

CMS now links reimbursement programs to patient outcomes and does not provide reimbursement for facility mistakes. The need for leaders to develop and sustain evidence-driven, valid, and reliable workforce management tools has never been greater. In addition, there is a pressing need to extend workforce management across the continuum of care to include not only inpatient care, but also outpatient care, office care, home care, and long-term care to meet the requirements of the Affordable Care Act using the Accountability Care Organization model (American Recovery and Reinvestment Act, 2009). Now that facilities are penalized by readmissions, it becomes more important to make sure the continuum of care from facility to home is effectively integrated.

Understanding the role of each of the elements in the workforce system is an important step in this process. Relying on experience, intuition, and historical usage to manage workload is not viable in an age of plentiful information and customer expectations for value-based services. Systematic, replicable systems to track and monitor caregiver skill mix, hours of care, costs, and outcomes are expectations for effective leadership. In this chapter, the essential components of an effective workforce management system (**Exhibit 6–2**) are discussed:

- Measuring patient care workload
- Creating core schedules
- Monitoring daily staffing
- Ensuring quality is achieved
- Managing variance
- Planning budgets
- Monitoring productivity
- Managing information systems (involved in every step of the workforce management cycle)

A Complex System

At one time, it was believed that a linear open systems model of inputs, throughputs, outputs, and feedback loops was adequate to frame a workforce management model. Although this linear model is helpful for an introductory assessment of staffing systems, the reality is that the complexity of healthcare staffing requires additional considerations. Complex model characteristics that reflect the interconnectedness of individuals, the uncertainty of events, and the unique self-organization of individuals within a complex system need to be used to solve problems in this twenty-first century. This results in the emergence of new subsystems, processes, and outcomes.

Exhibit 6–2   Workforce Management Cycle

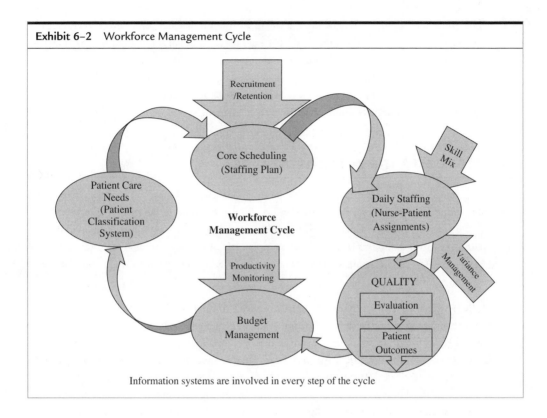

Information systems are involved in every step of the cycle

Whereas an understanding of these basic elements is essential, the dynamic interactions and ever-changing activities of the system must be considered. *Failing to consider healthcare staffing from a complex perspective and limiting the system to basic inputs, throughputs, outputs, and feedback loops render the system forever inadequate and incomplete.*

Once nurse managers understand the basic workforce management elements, they should identify and affirm assumptions specific to the dynamic interactions of the system. Examples are as follows:

- Regardless of the use of historical trend data to create schedules, *an uncertain and unknown variance from past performance is expected* (Radwin, Cabral, Chen, & Jennings, 2010) given that the future is not knowable. Thus, decisions about staffing within various scenarios, such as full census, average census, 20% below census, and seasonal changes in census, must be considered. If all staff can be involved in working out a plan for the different scenarios, when something different occurs, they can shift to the appropriate plan, making modifications as needed.
- The interconnectedness and interrelationships between and among system patients, providers, and other key stakeholders increase the numbers and types of interactions, which in turn increase or decrease the efficiency and effectiveness of the system. The more individuals are involved in a system, the greater the potential for differing interactions. Thus, as stakeholders identify events or changes, decisions need to change accordingly and must be communicated to the appropriate people. This process is most effective if all stakeholders, including staff and patients, are included in determining the next actions to be taken.

- Self-organization occurs when activities are left to themselves and new order evolves without one individual assuming leadership of the work. For example, in times of staffing challenges, numerous individuals work simultaneously without leadership direction to address the needs. In this way, even if it is the night shift or weekend, or the nurse manager is on vacation, the staffing challenges are met.
- Emergence or evolution of new ideas, processes, and structures regularly results from the interactions and interrelationships of individuals in complex systems.

Workforce Management Myths

How can we change our old perspectives and linear model about staffing? Linear thinking traps us until we realize that staffing is a complex process and that we need to pay attention to the myriad of new evidence. This chapter is crammed with evidence related to workforce management—and more is reported daily. It may help us move forward into this more effective, complex way of viewing staffing if we examine some of our old linear practices. Following are workforce management myths and evidence using a complex model to refute them (**Exhibit 6–3**).

Myth 1: We have no proof that nursing care makes a difference.
Research indicates that RN staffing has a definite and measurable impact on patient outcomes, medical errors, length of stay, nurse turnover, patient mortality, and hospital costs (Aiken, Clarke, Cheung, Sloane, & Silber, 2003; Aiken, Clarke, Sloane, Lake, & Cheney, 2008; Blegen, Goode, Spetz, Vaughn, & Park, 2011; Cho, Ketefian, Barkauska, & Smith, 2003; Frith, Anderson, Tseng, & Fong, 2012; Hickey, Gauvreau, & Connor, 2010; McCue, 2003; Needleman, Buerhaus, Mattke, Stewart, & Zelevinsky, 2002; Needleman et al., 2011; Needleman, Buerhaus, Stewart, Zelevinsky, & Mattke, 2006; Newhouse et al., 2010; Patrician et al., 2011; Reese, 2011; Rimar & Diers, 2006; Rogers, Hwany, Scott, Aiken, & Dinges, 2004; Seago et al., 2001; Sochalski, 2004; Thungiaroenkul, Cummings, & Embleton, 2007; Trinkoff et al., 2011a, 2011b; Unruh, 2003). "Research has shown that adverse events and mortality are highly dependent on nurse staffing levels and skill mix. . . . *Nursing-sensitive measures are an important component of value-based purchasing*" (Kavanagh, Cimiotti, Abusalem, & Coty, 2012, p. 385).

Myth 2: Performance doesn't change depending on whether you work 8-hour shifts or 12-hour shifts.
Research evidence shows an increase in patient care errors when nurses work 12-hour shifts compared with 8-hour shifts (Stimpfel, Lake, & Barton, 2013). In addition, needlestick injuries increase, nurses have more musculoskeletal disorders (neck, shoulders, back), more drowsy driving issues occur, and more chronic sleep deprivation problems surface—and recovery time, even after several days, does not improve these problems. When nurses worked consecutive 12-hour shifts, they got 5.5 hours sleep between shifts (Geiger-Brown & Trinkoff, 2010).

The Agency for Healthcare Research and Quality (AHRQ) has made recommendations concerning both shift duration and number of hours worked each week. Their recommendations include the following:

- Don't work more than 48 hours in a 7-day period.
- Nurse managers shouldn't schedule staff to work 12-hour shifts. (This is because they usually work beyond the end of the shift, have no breaks, and there are a high number of errors associated with 12-hour shifts.)

Exhibit 6–3 Workforce Management Myths	
If any of these myths exist in your organization, something needs to be fixed!	
Myth	**Complex System Change Needed**
Myth #1: We have no proof that nursing care makes a difference.	Research indicates that nurse staffing has a definite, measurable impact on patient outcomes, medical errors, length of stay, nurse turnover, patient mortality, and costs.
Myth #2: Performance doesn't change whether you work 8-hour shifts or 12-hour shifts.	Research shows an increase in patient care errors and nurse physical problems with 12-hour shifts.
Myth #3: All licensed nurses are equal.	Research indicates improved outcomes with the use of RNs. RNs are not the same as LPNs/LVNs.
Myth #4: RNs are more expensive than unlicensed nursing staff.	Two studies show facilities with higher RN staffing cost less.
Myth #5: Staffing is determined solely by ratios.	Ratios are incomplete as they do not consider patient differences, delegation ability, critical-thinking skills, experience, motivation, organizational skills, technical skills, or worker attitude.
Myth #6: Nurse managers should mainly work/be counted as an RN staff member.	Nurse managers should not staff the unit except in emergencies.
Myth #7: To save money nurse managers can be responsible for more than one unit.	Nurse managers are most effective when assigned 35–50 FTEs.
Myth #8: A centralized staffing model is best.	A decentralized model best suits our complex units today.
Myth #9: An open unit model is best.	A closed unit model is preferable.
Myth #10: "We have always done it this way."	There is always a better way to do/organize work.

- If nurses are scheduled to work 12-hour shifts, ensure that breaks and meals are scheduled, and that they have 10 to 12 hours off between shifts for sufficient sleep.
- If 12-hour shifts are necessary, don't schedule them consecutively so as to allow for rest between days. (Miller, 2011, p. 40)

The greatest barrier to moving away from 12-hour shifts is that many nurses like and expect this schedule because it is the norm in many institutions (Geiger-Brown & Trinkoff, 2010, p. 147). These authors suggest several strategies, including educating nurses, undergoing major organizational change, and measuring safety issues better as well as working with other facilities in the area to avoid a mass exodus.

Myth 3: All licensed nurses are equal.
This fallacy assumes the RN is the same as the LPN. This is erroneous. The literature continues to recognize improved outcomes with the use of RNs. Assuming all patients are alike and all nurses are alike is inappropriate and faulty thinking. If staffing by nurse-to-patient ratios, it is best to change it to *RN-to-patient ratios*.

Myth 4: RNs are more expensive than unlicensed nursing staff.
On the surface, we might believe RNs are more expensive because their salaries are higher than the salaries of LPNs and aides. In fact, this may not be the case (McClung, 2000). Melberg (1997) showed that a hospital budget with a 96% RN staff mix was less expensive than another hospital budget with a 64% RN mix. In fact, the hospital with the highest costs had the lowest RN skill mix (64%):

A high RN mix [96%] does not correlate with higher nursing costs per patient day in acute or critical care. Diluting the RN mix does not always reduce staffing costs. *Although hospital A has a 96 percent RN-skill mix, the highest in the system, total nursing salary per patient day falls exactly in the middle.* The highest costs occurred at hospital C where, in fact, the 64 percent RN mix is the lowest in the system. This finding is consistent in acute care, in critical care and on the orthopedic units, in specialty nursing areas found in all five hospitals and therefore used for comparison. *This difference is not explained by regional variations in RN salary, since RN salary at hospital A during the period of study was higher than at any hospital in the system except hospital E.* (p. 48)

And this does not take into account better patient outcomes that result with the use of RNs.

Myth 5: Staffing is determined solely by ratios.

In many organizations, a staffing or ratio grid is used for daily staffing. It is important to remember that staffing *solely* on ratios is incomplete. Ratios do not consider or recognize patient differences, caregiver delegation ability, critical thinking skills, experience, motivation, organizational skills, technical skills, or worker attitude. Even if the total number of care hours might be sufficient with a certain ratio, differentiation among the type of caregivers required to meet the patient needs is not identified.

Myth 6: Nurse managers should mainly work or be counted as RN staff members.

Nurse managers have many responsibilities on a unit, not only in workforce management but in making sure patient safety, quality, and budget are assured. They need to have good relationships with staff on all shifts, supporting the daily issues staff experience. They must work across interdisciplinary channels, pay attention to physician issues, do patient rounds—including talking with patients and patients' significant people, be aware of technology that benefits the unit, help staff stay updated, and more. These are important responsibilities that, if done right, take up time. Making nurse managers consistently work as an RN staff member takes away from the effectiveness of the unit. The nurse manager should be able to *occasionally* take care of patients as events occur when another hand is needed. But ***the nurse manager should not consistently be expected to be an RN staff member on the unit and should not be included in the RN staff full-time equivalents (FTEs).***

Myth 7: To save money nurse managers can be responsible for more than one unit.

This kind of thinking can be dangerous unless units are small. The industry standard has been that a nurse manager is responsible for 35 to 50 FTEs depending on unit complexity, size, patient acuity, case mix, and scope of responsibilities. One study found that the best average was 36.8 FTEs per nurse manager (Altaffer, 1998). (In business language, this is called span of control—an unfortunate term because no one controls anyone. However, the term *FTE* refers to the number of people reporting to a manager.)

In the 1990s as hospitals were facing big budget cuts, many increased the nurse manager FTEs to 150 or more. This proved to be dangerous and resulted in poorer patient outcomes, more costly legal issues, higher staff turnover, lower patient satisfaction scores, physician complaints, and so on. Nurse managers in this position were very frustrated, finding they did not have time to get to know staff, to take care of daily issues, to make sure patients were safe. Nurse manager turnover resulted with many thinking that they had been failures at their jobs.

It is even more dangerous today because CMS links reimbursement programs to patient outcomes and does not provide reimbursement for facility mistakes. Nurse managers are key to ensuring that the various CMS measures are achieved and reimbursement is not lost.

Myth 8: A centralized staffing model is best.
In fact, the opposite is true. It is always best for the people actually involved in the work to make as many decisions as possible about their work. A decentralized model is best with nurse managers and staff on a unit determining staffing. A centralized staffing meeting can be helpful at the beginning of the day to examine staffing throughout the house. In addition having a centralized float pool available can be helpful. Consider this:

> As organizations evolve they become increasingly complex over time, which means the traditional methods to measure and manage these complex systems must also evolve. By their very nature, complex systems are a dynamic network of many agents, acting in parallel, and constantly acting and reacting to what other agents are doing. The control of these *complex systems tend to be highly dispersed and decentralized*. If coherent behavior does emerge, it is typically the result of competition and cooperation among the agents themselves rather than well thought-out, planned control mechanisms. Overall, the behavior of the system is the result of a number of moment-to-moment decisions by many individuals. Not unlike living organisms, these systems strive for homeostasis and are remarkably resilient. (Clancy in Fitzpatrick & Brooks, 2010)

Myth 9: An open unit model is best.
We do not advocate *open units*, although that is the way the majority of units are organized. Here, if someone calls in sick, a nursing supervisor will have to find a replacement, either from that unit, from a staffing pool, or from another unit. The problem with open units is that they do not foster teamwork and self-responsibility. After all, someone else will worry about the staffing problem. With the open unit concept, poor leadership is rewarded—staff are found for them, while an effective nurse manager—and the staff on an effective unit—who has appropriately staffed, is penalized when staff are pulled to the unit that is not staffed appropriately. When this happens, it can eventually result in both nurse and nurse manager turnover on the effective unit because it gets so frustrating to do things right, and then always have someone pulled.

We advocate a ***closed unit model***. On a closed unit, when there is effective leadership, staff on that unit cover for each other. In this arrangement, teamwork is more likely to occur. Peer pressure—along with effective leadership—encourages staff to work together, support each other, and not call in sick unless really ill. Overtime usage decreases and staff cohesiveness increases. Patient, nurse, and physician satisfaction improves and turnover is reduced (Fertise & Baggot, 2009; Rufflin et al., 1999). Patient outcomes are positive. It's a win-win. The only problem with this arrangement is when the unit becomes drastically understaffed and occasionally needs help from outside, or when the unit census becomes very low.

In a closed unit arrangement, there is no need for a nursing supervisor. Instead, designated nurses are in charge. Staff always know who assumes the role. The nurse manager manages the unit, and when absent an assistant nurse manager, comanager, or charge nurse assumes the leadership for the shift. Staff on one shift do not leave until the next shift is appropriately staffed. The nurse manager—or another administrator—can be available by pager for emergencies. Staff figure out among themselves how to cover absences. For instance, there may be a rotation list or on-call list specifying who comes in next.

When census dips, many nurses cannot afford to take too many unpaid days off. So, in this circumstance, many closed unit staff often have an agreement with and are cross-trained for another unit(s) so that staff can be floated to that unit(s) and still get paid.

In this *decentralized model*, the unit manager has budget responsibility and the responsibility to interview and choose staff, orient staff, evaluate staff, and be there on a day-to-day basis to handle the many problems that occur.

Myth 10: "We have always done it this way."

There is always a better way to do and organize our work. As people and circumstances change, we *always* must look at practices with a fresh eye and question, "Why do we do it this way?" "Is there a better way?" Of course there is—it just has not yet occurred to us.

Rich possibilities and potential answers can be found, not only *from our own stakeholders*, but from colleagues across organizations, the *literature*, and *seminars* that discuss best practices, alternative practices, and current research in workforce management. If we all participate in dialogue about workforce management, sharing what each person has learned, thinking of different ways to organize and do the work, better practices will emerge. It is important always to question, "Is there a better way to do the work?"

Get beyond the traditional answers—question such issues as why everyone has to work every other weekend and how staff can be scheduled to accommodate their personal needs in a better way. We have an aging workforce, so consider such ideas as shorter scheduled times to cover for peak shift activities and job sharing. The sky is the limit!

Measuring Patient Care Workforce

Measuring human work is a complex process. Determining labor needs depends on a system for assessing requirements of patients and fitting these requirements to the appropriate level of staff availability and expertise. Nurse leaders are required to provide quantitative reports on workforce allocations and justify the staffing levels required. The expectation is that resources expended did indeed produce value to the patient, that there is a relationship between the nursing care provided and improvements in the patient's clinical condition. In addition, nursing workflow changes may well mean that nurses have increased work without administrators being aware this has occurred (Herdman, Burgess, Ebright, & Paulson, 2009). It is helpful if workflow can be measured.

The first step in this process is to determine patient care needs (**Exhibit 6–4**). In health care, various approaches are used to categorize patients, such as the ICD-9 (soon to be 10) or DRG systems. In nursing, methods to measure patient care needs vary between using comparative data, such as benchmarking with other units serving similar patient populations, and using patient classification system data. Using a patient classification system has become a standard management practice for healthcare leaders. A patient classification system determines patient care needs in terms of caregiver hours and skill level, providing one component of a comprehensive workforce management plan.

None of these approaches successfully captures all the nuances or degrees of care needed, nor do any totally capture the way one patient varies from another patient even when they have the same diagnosis.

However, for measuring nursing care needed, we advocate using a **valid, reliable patient classification system that is integrated with the organization's information system so that when nurses document assessments and care given, these data are automatically transferred to the patient classification system**. (Many of the current systems require more RN time to *rerecord* care data into the classification system.) Harper (2012) reports working out a way to do this for direct and indirect care given.

Exhibit 6–4   Patient Care Needs

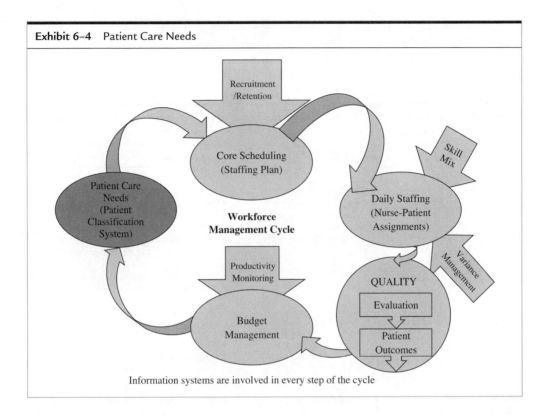

Information systems are involved in every step of the cycle

Making the Most Cost-Effective Choice

Buyers want to be assured that there is evidence and some common frame of reference for clinical decisions made throughout the health system. They want to know whether there are some normative standards of clinical practice, including price, to which all providers comply, standards that can continually be validated and replicated. Further, every provider is now under the same obligation to ensure that there is a connection between what one does and what is achieved; there is now a requirement that a clinical decision also be *the most cost-effective choice* that can be made. *It is from these mandates that the continuing need for valid and reliable patient classification systems remains relevant.*

Background on Workload Measurement Techniques

Workload measurement techniques are used to quantify the time associated with tasks performed by workers. These techniques are used to understand the nature and actual cost of work processes and to address the ongoing challenges to reduce costs, reduce effort, and improve the work environment.

The five workload measurement techniques often used in health care—motion and time study, work sampling, self-reporting, standard data setting, and expert opinion—are explained in **Exhibit 6–5**. *Motion and time study* involves continuous timed observations of a single person during a typical time period or shift of work (Burke et al., 2000).

In health care, *work sampling* forms the foundation for some computerized patient classification systems. The caregiver's work is examined for the entire shift or event of care for a selected number of times to achieve a representative range of services. Once representative data are collected, the percentage of time spent on specific activities, such as taking and recording vital signs, performing assessments, administering medications, or managing intravenous fluid therapy and discharge planning, is determined. These amounts then form the time standards for determining patient acuity on a daily basis (**Exhibit 6–6**).

Exhibit 6–5   A Comparison of the Advantages and Disadvantages of Workload Measurement Techniques

Workload Measurement	Advantages	Disadvantages
Time and Motion	• Considered the gold standard in time estimation in the industrial environment • Accuracy of time standards for selected tasks	• High cost of one-on-one observations over extended periods • Potential for observer-induced bias (changing participants' behavior when observed) • Variable task difficulty/complexity of clinical testing and procedures not considered • Multitasking events not considered • Complex interactions of physical, social, ethical, emotional, and financial dimensions of patient care not incorporated
Self-Reporting/Logging	• Simple and inexpensive • High face validity • Low cost • Minimal training required	• Inherent bias • Participants have significant burden of reporting every activity performed in a time period
Factor Evaluation/ Subjective	• High face validity and hence acceptance by operators • Most operators find it fairly easy to assign ratings	• Operators can rate changing demands of a given task but find it difficult to compare workload on qualitatively different types of tasks • No unanimous agreement on the nature of the components of workload, and hence the set of scales that should be used • Ability to capture the nursing process is questioned
Work Sampling	• Experts are hired to validate time standards making validity level high • Useful when new procedures and techniques are introduced	• Large numbers of observations are required to obtain reasonable precision in time estimates • Does not determine the duration of a work activity
Standard Data	• Quick, easy to use • Consistent and fair • Economical	• Data are unique to a specific company, and companies cannot normally use another's standard data
Expert Panel	• Easy, efficient • Can be reliable if results approximate those obtained by experts • Low cost • Considers uniqueness of situations	• Easily biased • Doesn't always reflect current conditions

Workload Measurement	Advantages	Disadvantages
Comprehensive Unit of Service	• Incorporates impact of multitasking • Relies on standardized nursing taxonomy for high validity • Includes the dynamic complexity of human phenomenon including physical, psychological, and contextual realities	• Requires use of expert or experienced nurses to develop comprehensive units of service of specific patient population • Data are unique to the setting and cannot quickly be generalized to other settings • Nurses are sometimes reluctant to give up task model for fear of not identifying work that is done

Exhibit 6–6   Example Patient Care Activity Groups: 8-Hour Shift

Activity/Time	Level 1	Level 2 Minutes/Shift	Level 3	Average Total Spent/Shift	Time (%)
Vital signs	5.0	9.5	5.0	19.5	5%
Assessments	10.0	19.0	10.0	39.0	10%
Treatments	20.0	38.0	20.0	78.0	20%
ADLs	20.0	38.0	20.0	78.0	20%
Documentation	20.0	38.0	20.0	78.0	20%
Medication administration	15.0	28.5	15.0	58.5	15%
Teaching	5.0	9.5	5.0	19.5	5%
Other	5.0	9.5	5.0	19.5	5%
Total	100	190	100	390	100%

ADLs, activities of daily living.

Self-reporting is another technique used to determine time associated with employee activities. This has high face validity (Burke et al., 2000). *Standard data setting* uses time standards developed from past experiences.

In health care, the *expert panel approach* has been used to create a comprehensive unit of service as the foundational workload unit of measure (Malloch & Conovaloff, 1999). Experienced nurses create workload standards from a comprehensive perspective of the work performed; expert nurses compile the nurse interventions, provided to a patient for an entire shift or event, and identify the time required to provide this care as a unit rather than as summation of tasks. This approach integrates the multitasking processes of nurses and avoids the risk of double counting tasks. Typically, the expert panel consists of nurses who practice in clinical, educational, research, and administrative roles such as experienced staff nurses, clinical nurse specialists, nurse managers, and associate nurse executives. The panel of nurses collaborates to estimate the amount of time and level of caregiver (*skill mix*) required to provide the total care in the comprehensive unit of service.

Healthcare Patient Classification Systems

In the healthcare industry, providers have used broader measurement approaches to classify patients. Simply stated, *classification* is the ordering of entities into groups or classes on the basis of their similarity, minimizing within-group variance and maximizing between-group variance (Gordon, 1998). *Patient classification* is a process of grouping patients into homogeneous, mutually exclusive groups to determine their dependency on caregivers or to determine patient acuity (Dunn et al., 1995; Finkler, 2001). *Acuity* is defined as the level of need or dependency of an individual patient. The process of classifying patients is an *element* of workload management (**Exhibit 6–4**), the comprehensive system that includes patient classification, scheduling, staffing, and budgeting systems.

The healthcare industry struggles to determine the best way to identify and measure effective staffing resource utilization. Healthcare costs continue to be a persistent, growing problem for both public and private healthcare funding sources. These challenges have been slowly addressed, beginning with the creation of classification systems, to better understand patient care needs in multiple settings, from inpatient hospital care to skilled nursing home care to office care. The International Classification of Diseases, Ninth Revision (ICD-9 (soon to be 10)), diagnosis-related groups (DRGs), and case mix systems are examples of classification systems, each with advantages and disadvantages. Several other classification systems, such as the Outpatient Prospective Payment System (OPPS) for ambulatory areas, *resource utilization groups (RUGs)* for long-term care, and Home HealthCare Services Payment System or *home health resource groups (HHRGs)* for home health, have emerged in recent years to address the need for classification of patient care needs (Shi & Singh, 2004).

ICD System

The *ICD system* is used to code and classify mortality data from death certificates. The International Classification of Diseases, Ninth Revision, Clinical Modification (ICD-9-CM [soon to be 10]) is used to code and classify morbidity data from the inpatient and outpatient records, physician offices, and most National Center for Health Statistics (NCHS) surveys. The NCHS serves as the World Health Organization Collaborating Center for the Family of International Classifications for North America and in this capacity is responsible for coordination of all official disease classification activities in the United States relating to the ICD and its use, interpretation, and periodic revision.

Case Mix Methods

As the industrial workload model emerged, people began to realize that there were issues with productivity measurement that involved efficiency. For example, a patient day for a normal obstetrics/gynecology unit versus a patient day for an intensive care unit requires different staffing. The same is true for home care or ambulatory visits; an initial visit usually takes longer because staff members need to get to know and assess a new patient, whereas a follow-up visit often takes less time. Somehow, this needed to be added to the productivity measurement equation.

This prompted the movement to use *case mix methods*. "Case mix is a method of clustering patients into groups that are homogeneous with respect to the use of resources. Factors used to cluster patients have included diagnosis, prognosis, resource utilization, organ system, hospital department, and patient demographic characteristics" (Sullivan & Decker, 2001, p. 120). Other clusters include clinic visits, surgical procedures, deliveries, skilled nursing facilities, home health, and other procedures.

The case mix index uses the *relative value unit* technique and refers to the overall intensity of conditions that require medical and nursing interventions. The patient's condition is assessed and an estimate of the actual amount of resources that the patient will need is determined.

Thus, Medicare began to use case mix methods, such as DRGs for hospital reimbursement, RUGs for long-term care reimbursement, OPPS for outpatient facilities, and HHRGs for home health. Each of these models attempts to identify the qualitative aspects of clinical care and translate the care into mathematical formulations.

The *DRG system* categorizes the types of patients a hospital treats based on diagnoses, procedures, age, sex, and the presence of complications or comorbidities. DRGs work by grouping the more than 10,000 ICD-9-CM codes into a more manageable number of meaningful patient categories. Patients within each category are similar clinically in terms of resource usage.

The case mix for skilled nursing facilities is driven by the *minimum data set*, which consists of a core set of screening elements used to assess the clinical, functional, and psychosocial needs of each resident. Using the data gained from the minimum data set assessment, the classification system of *RUGs* provides a per diem prospective rate based on the acuity level of residents by their use of resources. Variables include diagnosis, functional limitations, negative health conditions, skin problems, and special treatments and procedures needed. RUG-III classifies patients into 44 categories according to their healthcare needs.

OPPS uses the *ambulatory payment classification (APC)* where relative value units reflect the complexity of each procedure for the ambulatory area.

HHRGs use the Outcome and Assessment Information Set (OASIS), 80 distinct groups, to indicate the severity of the patient's condition. Reimbursement for episodes of home health services is bundled under one payment and adjusted based on the patient's HHRG.

The case mix cluster reflects patient acuity and can be integrated with budgeting information and used with staffing ratios. *The predominant problem with this is that most often the finance department does not understand the significance of the patient classification system. Patient classification systems are not traditionally covered in finance and accounting programs.*

A second issue is that *neither the ICD classification nor the case mix systems have included the fundamental work of nursing*—namely, the coordination of care, patient assessment, education, development of the plan of care, provision of a safe environment, and delegation and supervision of selected personnel.

The challenge remains to identify the real and specific work of nursing, quantify it into health care's economic equation, and create workload management systems that assure buyers they are getting value for their commitment of resources.

Patient Classification Systems in Nursing

When first introduced in the 1930s, patient classification systems were based on the industrial engineering model of nurses' time and nursing tasks. Engineers believed that patient activities could be quantified by identifying the time it took nurses to complete a task related to patient care. The identified timed tasks could then be summed to identify the number of staff needed.

Over the past 60 years, system users have identified that significant variables, ones necessary to determine accurately either the patient acuity or the staffing requirements, were omitted from these historic design structures (Van Slyck, 2000). To address these shortcomings, healthcare leaders have also integrated factor, prototype, relative value, comprehensive unit of service, and clinical pathway concepts into traditional systems to increase validity. A brief discussion of each follows.

- The *factor evaluation method* identifies selected elements of care, critical indicators, or tasks with associated times that are most likely predictors of nursing care needs. Individual patients are then assessed for the presence or absence of these critical indicators and, based on this assessment, assigned to a category. Nursing is viewed as a series of tasks performed in sequence. This method attempts to elicit a measure of overall workload. The factor evaluation system rates a number of indicators of care separately and then sums the ratings to designate the patient's acuity (Hasman, Wiersma, Halfens, & Algera, 1993). Examples of patient conditions or nursing interventions identified as critical indicators are activities of daily living, medications, monitoring, safety needs, and complex equipment. Some factor evaluation systems include as many as 400 items for the nurse to review before selecting the category that most accurately matches the patient. **Exhibit 6–7** is an example of the indicators in a patient factor classification system.

- The *prototype approach* identifies the characteristics of patients in each category. Individual patients are then assigned to the category that most closely reflects their nursing care requirements. This method generally offers profiles or descriptions of patients typical of those requiring a particular type and amount of nursing care. The system, developed by Walts and Kapadia (1996) to support their staffing algorithm, is a prototype system—it classifies patients into eight categories based on required nursing time. Examples of prototype profiles or descriptions include simple or average, above average, and high or complex patient care needs. Each profile is assigned a designated number of hours for care. Typically, no skill mix differentiation is determined in the prototype method. **Exhibit 6–8** is an example of a prototype patient classification system. Unfortunately, because patients seldom fall into all of the categories in one level, this approach does not allow for partial selection, which often leads to inconsistent and inaccurate classification of patients.

- Another concept is the *relative value unit (RVU)*. In addition to grouping patients into similar categories based on nursing care needs, a patient classification system can also quantify the workload within the categories by assigning a relative value to each category. A relative weight is assigned to each patient category; one category is assigned arbitrarily the value of 1.0 and all other categories are assigned values in relation to it. The relative value scale is then used to describe the workload for a given unit or organization.

- The *comprehensive unit of service*, developed by Malloch and Conovaloff (1999), is based on the standard data and the expert panel method. The comprehensive unit of service, an aggregate of eight categories of care, represents the total care provided by nursing during a shift or event of care and

---

Exhibit 6–7   Example of Factor Patient Classification System

Circle all that apply:

Self-care	Restraints	4–6 IV medications	Neuro check q shift
Partial care	Isolation	> 6 IV medications	Neuro check q 2 hrs
Complete bath	Wound care—simple	Telemetry monitor	Medicate for pain x3
Ambulate with assistance x2	Wound care—complex	Suction q 2 hrs	Medicate for pain > 3 times
Ambulate with two person assist x1	1 peripheral IV line	Suction > q 2 hrs	Insert foley catheter
Assistance with meals	2 peripheral IV lines	I & O q 8 hrs	Enema
Total feed	> 2 IV lines	I & O q 1 hr	Accucheck q 4 hrs
Skin care	Oral medications	Educate patient re: diabetes	Give 1 unit of blood
Heel care	1–3 IV medications	Educate patient re: surgery	Give > 1 unit of blood

integrates a multitasking factor to account for the overlap of care in identified patient situations. This model is designed to address the lack of sensitivity to the unique holistic nature of patients and fluctuations in economies of scale or the impact of nurses doing more than one task or process at a time. **Exhibit 6–9** is an example of a comprehensive unit of service. The clinical profile based on care provided to the patient determines caregiver time and skill mix required for that the patient.

- Once the standards are established using iterative summaries of expert nurse time estimations, nurses rate patients in eight categories, which represent the essence of patient care during or at the end of each shift. The hours and skill mix are generated for each patient and then summarized to identify the total unit staffing needs. Staffing hours and skill mix needed are then compared with available staff to determine adequacy of staffing or if adjustments are needed.

- Most recently, attempts have been made to quantify nurse work using the *clinical pathway*. Work efforts are identified from historical care delivery for specific diagnoses or DRGs and are used to project time and activities for the anticipated length of stay. For example, the hours and interventions required for a previous pneumonia patient become the clinical pathway for future pneumonia patients. Patient progress is tracked on the basis of patient completion of identified interventions.

Exhibit 6–8   Example of Prototype Patient Classification System: Levels 1–3

	Level 1–Average Needs	Level 2–Above Average Needs	Level 3–High Needs
ADLs	Minimal assistance	Partial bath; assistance with feeding	Total care
Medications	3–8 oral medications	9 or more oral medications 1–3 IV medications	More than 4 IV medications
Monitoring	Routine vital signs	Telemetry monitoring	Multiple monitors; telemetry, swan and/or ICP
IV Lines/Tubes	Less than 2 lines or tubes	3–6 lines and/or tubes	More than 6 lines and tubes

---

Exhibit 6–9   Comprehensive Unit of Service Example

Category	Caregiver Intervention	Rating
1. Cognitive needs	1-step commands; reorient every 2 hours	2
2. Self-care needs	Transfer with 2 staff members; 1:1 feed; complete bath	1
3. Emotional/Social/Spiritual needs	Set limits 1:1; therapeutic communication > 45 minutes; reassure every hour	2
4. Comfort/Pain management needs	Assess/Monitor q shift; medicate x1/shift	4
5. Family support needs	Update family x1/shift	5
6. Treatments	Wound care dressing change x2/shift; 8 oral medications; 2 IV medications	3
7. Interdisciplinary coordination needs	Coordinate 4 providers; delegate and supervise 2 caregivers	4
8. Transition needs time required: 3.0 hours	Assess x1/shift RN: 1.0; LPN: 1.0; NA: 1.0	5

Patient Classification System Requirements

The most effective option to measure patient care needs is to use a patient classification system. When selecting a patient classification system, the following criteria are important to consider:

- Interventions or indicator lists that provide an adequate representation of the current work of nursing
- Use of industry standardized language
- A history of validity and reliability
- Characteristics of facility geography (length of halls, available workspace, location of nurse workstations, etc.)
- Ability to determine skill mix and staff hours required for each patient
- Level of computerization and interface capability with the patient care record, patient registration systems, and scheduling systems
- Flexibility so the system can be used with all patient care delivery models
- Identification of unique patient populations of the organization
- Consistency with the organization's mission and vision

Benefits of Patient Classification Systems: Workload Measurement

Despite the challenges of creating valid and reliable patient classification systems, the benefits and rationale for valid and reliable patient classification outweigh the downsides. The reasons to implement and sustain a patient classification system include the following:

- **Understanding the relationship between patient care needs, nursing interventions, desired outcomes, and the skill level of nurses**. Determining the appropriate type and number of caregivers and support staff needed to provide safe and effective patient care is the foundation of the workforce management system (Behner, Fogg, Fournier, Frankenbach, & Robertson, 1990; Mark & Burleson, 1995).
- **Information to correlate the work of nursing and the outcomes of care**. Providing services that do not affect the outcome of patient functionality is no longer appropriate or affordable. When RN levels are low, nurses may not have time to provide essential education or prevention oversight of patients or to supervise nonlicensed staff. Further, there are documented relationships between RN staffing and levels of medication errors, patient falls, new pressure ulcers, nosocomial pneumonia, urinary tract infections, length of stay, and unplanned readmissions.
- **Determining staffing ratios**. Fixed staffing numbers (ratios) cannot be considered sufficient to manage variations in patient care and sustain quality patient care (Bolton et al., 2001). *Patient-to-nurse ratios identify the minimum staffing levels, whereas patient classification systems define the amount of staff needed for a particular situation*. Ratio-staffing levels are data derived from a valid and reliable patient classification system and from knowing the range of patient care needs. Ratio data are best used in the aggregate for budgeting and scheduling, not for day-to-day staffing. *ANA Principles for Nurse Staffing*, developed in 1998 and updated in 2008 and 2012, clearly identify and support the need for empirical data to guide decision making to identify and maintain the appropriate number and skill mix of nursing staff using valid and reliable systems. The key points in this document include the definitions, core staffing competencies, the role of the healthcare consumer, registered nurse and support staff considerations, organizational culture, practice environment, and evaluation (ANA, 2012).

- **Validation of the nursing profession**. Valid and reliable systems define and defend the work of professional nursing, increase visibility of professional nursing practice, protect patients from complications, and decrease the vulnerability of nurse staffing to budget cuts. The integration of nursing science taxonomy into practice also explicates professionalism and the ethical obligations of nursing to use resources wisely while providing skilled services.

Patient Classification System Language and Terminology

As efforts to create valid and reliable patient classification systems intensified, efforts were also made to standardize language within the systems. Discussions continue as to whether a nursing language is required or whether health system language is more appropriate because it includes all disciplines.

In 1984, the North American Nursing Diagnosis Association established the conceptual framework for a nursing diagnostic classification system. This definition and taxonomy helped to establish consistent terminology, making oral and written communication easier and more efficient. In addition, definitive nursing functions were identified and increased the nurse's accountability in assessing the patient, determining the diagnosis, and providing the treatment called for by the diagnosis.

McCloskey and Bulechek (2000) believed that the nursing process was a form of logical clinical inquiry and that the nurse made decisions about particular clinical phenomena (ANA, 1989). The nursing interventions identified and developed by the research team from the University of Iowa have become a highly regarded taxonomy for the work of nursing. *Nursing intervention classifications (NICs)* now represent an accepted and systemic approach to naming classes of nursing interventions, facilitating understanding, and communicating patient treatment plans. NIC is a comprehensive, standardized language that describes treatments that nurses perform in all settings and in all specialties. NICs include eight foundational domains: physiological (e.g., acid–base management), psychosocial (e.g., anxiety reduction), illness treatment (e.g., hyperglycemia management), illness prevention (e.g., fall prevention), health promotion (e.g., exercise promotion), interventions for individuals or for families (e.g., family integrity promotion), indirect care interventions (e.g., emergency cart checking), and interventions for communities (e.g., environmental management).

A standardized language for nursing provides the industry with tools to recognize the contributions and accomplishments of nursing. Using a standardized language is important in demonstrating contributions, influencing practice, and facilitating critical thinking. Nurses now have the necessary knowledge and instruments to clearly articulate the effects of their interventions on patient outcomes.

The increasing use of the electronic medical record has further affected the classification process. *Systematized NOmenclature of MEDicine (SNOMED)* has gained increasing support as an acceptable language that can be used by all applications. Using the standardized language provides an excellent resource for indexing, collecting, analyzing, interpreting, storing, retrieving, and aggregating clinical data.

Most recently, nurse leaders and informatics leaders created the *Technology Informatics Guiding Educational Reform (TIGER)* initiative as a mechanism to raise awareness of both the complexities and possibilities of informatics tools, principles, theories, and practices. It is believed that these efforts will support safer health care and more effective, efficient, patient-centered, timely, and equitable processes by interweaving enabling technologies transparently into nursing practice and education, making information technology the stethoscope for the twenty-first century (TIGER Initiative, n.d.). Currently, more than 500 nurses are working to bridge clinical practice quality with information technology.

Validity, Reliability, and Sensitivity of Patient Classification Systems

As previously noted, a patient classification system must be credible both to nursing staff and to those outside nursing, including executives, financial officers, and directors of healthcare plans. The validity, reliability, and sensitivity of the system must therefore be clearly established and sustained. A valid, reliable, and sensitive patient classification system that defines patient care needs is the foundation of an effective workforce management system.

Validity

A system to determine staffing needs, typically a patient classification system, is said to have a high degree of validity when it accurately represents the work of the caregivers, correctly distributes patients among distinct classes, and defines the category of caregiver required for the care (Hernandez & O'Brien, 1996a, 1996b). Nursing workload data must be accurate to make appropriate staffing and scheduling decisions and wise budget allocations. Accurate data cannot be obtained unless the patient classification system, the foundation of the workforce management system, is both valid and reliable.

Validity of the patient classification can be described as the degree to which it actually measures what it intends to measure. The patient classification system is intended to measure the work of nursing. The work of nursing includes at a minimum the general categories of physiological care, behavioral support, safety measures, family education and support, coordination of care, documentation, and community integration (McCloskey & Bulechek, 2000). Validity is a matter of degree, not an all-or-none property, and the process of validation is unending (Hernandez & O'Brien, 1996a). Validity should be monitored annually, and the method of assessing validity will vary with the type of classification system (Hernandez & O'Brien, 1996b). Several types of validity are considered in a patient classification system, including face, content, construct, internal, and external validity. Each is briefly described.

Face validity is high when nurses believe that the system accurately reflects and represents the work they do or the dependency of the patients for whom they provide care. Face validity is lost when the nurses do not fully understand the system or the assumptions that underlie it. If the nurse does not understand the philosophy of the system (i.e., task or process) and does not believe that the system captures all of the workload, face validity is lost and the instrument is no longer credible or usable.

Content validity is the extent to which the tool includes all the major elements relative to the construct being measured. The evidence is typically obtained from three sources: literature, representatives from relative populations, and content experts (Burns & Grove, 2001). Most existing tools capture the procedural work of nursing but only minimally include the coordination, monitoring, and evaluation role of the professional nurse, thus resulting in a tool with less than acceptable validity.

Construct validity is the fit between the conceptual definitions and operational definitions of variables. Conceptual definitions provide the basis for the operational definitions of variables. The measure should provide a valid inference of the construct. Does the tool measure what it claims to measure? Does the category system explain the complexity of responsibility areas and total care required (Verran, 1986)? An example is a patient assessment. The construct is the assessment and the operational definition includes those elements that comprise a nursing assessment such as body systems, psychosocial status, safety needs, family support needs, and discharge planning. Thus, the tool would necessarily include items or indicators specific to the operational definition of a nursing assessment to create construct validity.

Criterion-related validity, or predictive validity, is described as the degree to which scores on an instrument are correlated with some other characteristic. If the scoring of patient acuity is consistently associated with appropriate levels of staffing, the predictive validity would be considered high.

Internal validity, or the extent to which the measures used in the tool are a true reflection of reality (and not the result of extraneous variables), is another key characteristic of the patient classification tool. Internal validity of a patient classification system considers the credibility of the tool or system within the organization. Inclusion of scheduling and staffing requirements into a patient classification system diminishes the internal validity because the variables of staff competence levels, indirect support time, and/or regulatory requirements cloud the specific patient care requirement. Incorporating system requirements into the patient classification system decreases the internal validity.

External validity, or the extent to which the findings can be generalized beyond the sample used, is a critical issue for patient classification systems. Although the industry is desperately seeking a measurement tool that can be used in all organizations with all patient populations and with high external validity, the achievement of this goal remains a challenge. There are some commonalities in the categories of nursing care interventions from organization to organization; there can also be significant variations in the operational definitions and processes of care for the same interventions. Whereas the comparisons appear appropriate, validity is uncertain until the definitions and associated time requirements are examined. This is not to imply that some degree of external validity cannot be obtained but rather to note that when external comparisons of data from setting to setting are made, the limitations to generalizations of comparability must be noted.

Reliability

The *reliability* of the patient classification system tool addresses the consistency of rating. Different observers assessing the same patient at the same time should generate the same rating. According to Finkler (2001), prototype tools are more subjective, making this degree of reliability more difficult to achieve. Factor evaluation tools are more objective, but their reliability depends on clear definition and consistent interpretation of the critical indicators.

Ongoing measurement of reliability is necessary and generally involves two or more raters independently (*interrater reliability*) assessing a defined percentage of classified patients at a specified interval. Reliability scores of 100% (no discrepancies in ratings) are always the target. There is disagreement about the necessary frequency for interrater reliability and the number of patients to classify when doing reliability checks. Recommended frequencies span from annually to monthly. To obtain the highest degree of system reliability, annual review of 100% of system users is recommended. However, authors agree that more frequent reliability monitoring is required if a high degree of interrater reliability is not maintained (Hernandez & O'Brien, 1996a).

With prototype tools, reliability addresses only agreement of type. With the factor evaluation tools, reliability ideally is demonstrated by agreement on both patient type and individual critical indicators. Interrater reliability scores of less than 85% seriously compromise the credibility of the system.

Sensitivity

Sensitivity typically refers to physiological measures and is related to the amount of change in a parameter that can be measured precisely (Gift & Soeken, 1988). If changes are expected to be very small, the tool must be able to detect the changes. For example, infant scales that differentiate ounces are appropriate in the nursery. Truck scales that measure hundreds of pounds would not be sensitive enough for the nursery. Patient classification sensitivity is about detecting those changes that determine time and type of caregiver and is a balance between estimation of time and precise time amounts. At best, the time for patient care can be only an estimation of requirements within certain ranges because patient events are unpredictable and patient responses to care vary. Estimates within 15 minutes of actual time required for patient care are adequate for the complex phenomena of patient care.

Patient Classification Systems: Limitations and Challenges

Skepticism about patient classification systems has existed since their introduction. With the variety of patient classification systems available and the years of testing new and innovative ways of capturing time estimation, the nursing profession still struggles with the creation of credible workload management systems. To be sure, the optimal solution for measuring caregiver workload is the attachment of time and skill mix standards to clinical interventions in an electronic documentation system. With documentation driving the calculations of patient needs, the issues of reliability are decreased significantly. However, despite some advances, several sources of patient classification system mistrust still exist: low validity, misuse, failure to use the data generated, and lack of tool simplicity.

Low Validity

Task-based acuity systems do not always account for professional nursing care practices, such as patient education, interdisciplinary collaboration, family support, and delegation and supervision of other caregivers. As a result, although the system appropriately captures increasing patient severity, the assumptions used to structure staffing models are flawed (Shaha, 1995). Because much of nursing is mindwork rather than handwork, it is not surprising that the task-based methods of some systems capture only a part of nursing work. Additionally, the effects of multitasking are not captured.

At present, there is no single agreed-on patient classification system that describes the commonly accepted nursing practice components of assessment, diagnosis, intervention, and outcomes. Because there is no agreed-on system, there are few, if any, empirical data sets to describe nursing practice across clinical settings, client populations, DRGs, medical diagnoses, geographical areas, or time. The lack of standardized nursing language makes it extremely difficult to know with any degree of accuracy which type of patient classification system provides the most valid and reliable data for workforce management decisions.

Misuse of the Tool

The most common problems with classification systems relate to a phenomenon called *acuity creep*. Acuity creep occurs when the reported patient acuity increases slowly over time but the actual care does not appear to change. In other words, acuity levels creep to higher and higher levels often to justify higher resource use by managers in affected areas. Creep becomes a problem because it assumes there is an ever-increasing need for patient care resources and labor in an industry where financial resources for such care are ever decreasing (Shaha, 1995).

The use of a system with low validity makes it difficult to distinguish inappropriate acuity creep from those changes in patient care that are real. Reimbursement changes and growth in alternative areas beyond the inpatient arena have not only changed the actual acuity of inpatients but also the typical model of patient care delivery. Nurse aides, for example, were not factored into original acuity systems but provide a significant portion of care in current inpatient and outpatient settings.

The lack of trust between executives and caregivers stems in part from the belief that patient classification systems are a vehicle to decrease staffing levels. Caregivers believe that initiatives in redesigning nursing work have emphasized efficiency over patient safety. Poor communication practices between staff providing patient care and healthcare leaders have also led to mistrust. This loss of trust has serious implications for the ability of hospitals and other healthcare organizations to make the fundamental changes essential to providing safer patient care (Page, 2004).

Prospective versus Retrospective Challenges

Patient classification data are best used in planning for the next shift. Planning for the next shift requires not only information about the patient needs, but also information about the oncoming staff resources, the previous similar shift staffing (yesterday's afternoon shift to compare with the upcoming afternoon shift), facility support for housekeeping, pharmacy, transportation, teaching staff available, and anticipated admissions, discharges, and transfers.

The general consensus of nurse leaders and staff nurses is that they want a patient classification system that prospectively determines the amount of staff and skill mix that will be sufficient for meeting the patient needs on the following shift. With the advent of electronic documentation systems, the ability to both project for the next shift and document what was actually done continually increases. Specific information for prospective calculations can be extracted from several sources including orders, flow records, medication administration records, and the plan of care. Actual work performed and the associated time standards can be extracted from or mapped to orders, flow sheets, and other sources where interventions are documented.

Using electronic systems to predict and document clinical work increases the reliability and trust in the information for staffing. Although there is a core of expected care for the next shift, a minimum of 20% of the workload in most units is highly variable. New admissions, unplanned clinical condition changes, family crises, and provider rounding times make the prediction process difficult—if not impossible—without a crystal ball! And, of course, the higher the turnover of patients, the greater the variability beyond 20%. The most that a patient classification system can tell you is, on average, what the staffing should be based on history (Seago, 2002). The severity of patient illness, need for specialized equipment and technology, intensity of nursing interventions required, and the complexity of clinical nursing judgment needed to design, implement, and evaluate the patient's nursing plan are often not predictable.

Units of Measure: Total Hours and Skill Mix Required

The required skill mix for each patient is often an overlooked component of a patient classification system. An effective and useful patient classification system must identify not only the needs of the patient and the hours required for care but also the level of caregiver required to perform the work. Patient acuity or patient classification traditionally focuses on determining the time required for care; the patient acuity level is secondary information. There is indeed some correlation between acuity and amount of care required, but the correlation is not absolute. A chronic ventilator-dependent paraplegic may score high in severity of illness but not require a large number of care hours because of condition stability and established plans of care. Many systems do not differentiate between the two measurements and make the leap from quality to quantity of nursing care a significant challenge.

Failure to Use and Trust the Data Generated

The patient classification system is typically overseen by the nursing department and requires the input of staff supervisors, unit directors, and unit staff that will be affected by the data. Financial officers and leaders of other clinical services are typically not involved in the initial design and management of nursing systems. Often, the credibility of the data and the possibility of manipulating the data to the advantage of nursing are challenged, particularly if the data demonstrate increased workload and increased need for resources (Finkler, 2001). As a result, the fundamental trustworthiness of the system is questioned by non-nursing hospital leaders and the system is merely tolerated or ignored.

Lack of Tool Simplicity

To address the credibility gap, clinicians have worked to develop all-inclusive, objective lists of interventions to create a valid system. Unfortunately, these systems become lengthy and risk losing reliability very quickly. Some systems require the user to review and select from 100 or more items for each patient event, a process that seldom results in good data. Classification systems that try to list every possible intervention become overwhelming, time consuming, and not worth the effort needed to ensure accuracy. When the system is not easily integrated into the workflow, it is seen as one more thing to do and becomes a lower priority—often completed only after the shift is over. Systems that are easily misused, mismanaged, or that generate inaccurate data cannot be used by managers to defend their staffing decisions. The time it takes to complete the tool can also be a significant barrier in the collection of accurate data.

This conundrum of attempting to identify every intervention but doing so in an efficient manner sets the stage for mistrust and inaccuracy in any patient classification system. The low validity achieved when nurses attempt to identify every intervention ultimately makes the product mistrusted by nursing staff, nurse leaders, financial managers, and administration. Many of the current models of patient classification systems continue to struggle with this challenge. Resolving conflicts that arise from the use of a patient classification system for staffing have often ended up at the bargaining table and in the regulatory arena (DeGroot, 1994).

Measuring Patient Care Workload When Patient Classification Data Are Not Available

If patient classification data are not available, comparative data, such as benchmarking with other units serving a similar patient population, can be used. Benchmarking data are available from other healthcare organizations, the literature, patient classification system companies, professional organizations, or group purchasing organizations such as VHA and Premier. When benchmarking secondary data it is very important to ensure data consistency (Garry, 2000; Hall, Pink, Johnson, & Schraa, 2000). Dunham-Taylor and Pinczuk (2006) in *Health Care Financial Management for Nurse Managers: Applications in Hospitals, Long-Term Care, Home Care, and Ambulatory Care* devote a chapter to developing staffing plans for a hospital using benchmark data.

Staffing Plan Core Schedule

The second component of a workforce management system is the *staffing plan* (**Exhibit 6–10**). The staffing plan describes adherence to the ANA's *Code of Ethics*, *Social Policy Statement*, and *Standards of Practice*. The intended benefits of such a plan are: (1) improved quality of patient care; (2) positive impact on patient outcomes; (3) improved work environment; (4) increased staff satisfaction, retention, professional growth, and development; and (5) improved organizational outcomes.

Evidence supporting use of the staffing plan is abundant (**Exhibit 6–2**) and can be found throughout this chapter. *Research indicates that nurse staffing has a definite and measurable impact on patient outcomes, medical errors, length of stay, nurse turnover, patient mortality, and hospital costs* (Aiken et al., 2003; Aiken et al., 2008; Blegen et al., 2011; Cho et al., 2003; Frith et al., 2012; Hickey et al., 2010; McCue, 2003; Needleman et al., 2002; Needleman et al., 2011; Newhouse et al., 2010; Patrician et al., 2011; Reese, 2011; Rimar & Diers, 2006; Rogers et al., 2004; Seago, 2001; Sochalski, 2004; Thungiaroenkul et al., 2007; Trinkoff et al., 2011a, 2011b; Unruh, 2003). "Research has shown that adverse events and mortality are highly dependent on nurse staffing levels and skill mix. . . . *Nursing-sensitive measures are an important component of value-based purchasing*" (Kavanagh et al., 2012, p. 385).

Evidence about the *specific numerical ratio needed varies widely*. However, modification of the ratios is needed based on patient needs, nurses' level of experience, organizational characteristics, leadership issues,

Exhibit 6–10   Core Scheduling

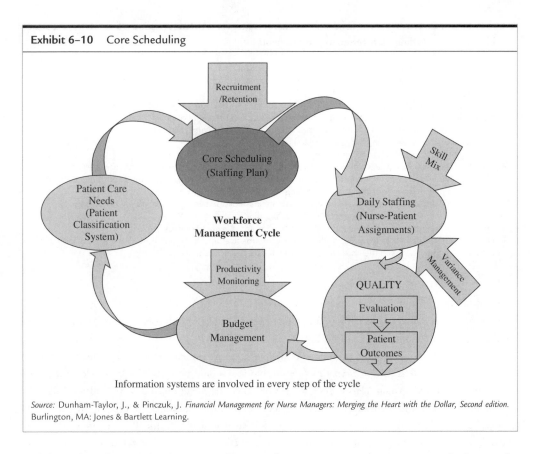

Information systems are involved in every step of the cycle

Source: Dunham-Taylor, J., & Pinczuk, J. *Financial Management for Nurse Managers: Merging the Heart with the Dollar, Second edition.* Burlington, MA: Jones & Bartlett Learning.

and the quality of interactions between and among physicians, nurses, administrators, and others on the healthcare team (Curtin, 2003).

Evidence *links health information technology (HIT) with better patient outcomes* (Waneka & Spetz, 2010). HIT improves documentation, and nurses like HIT advances.

Research is needed to identify costs of nurse-sensitive patient outcomes and adverse events *post discharge*. However, nurse staffing affects the *costs* of patient outcomes, including adverse events during a hospital stay as well as *reimbursement* (Mumolie, Lichtig, & Knauf, 2007; Pappas, 2008; Shamliyan, Kane, Mueller, Duval, & Wilt, 2009). Now that reimbursements will depend on timely nursing/medical interventions, this cost will probably rise.

The *staffing plan* (**Exhibit 6–11**) describes the structure and process by which responsibilities for patient care are assigned and how the work is coordinated among caregivers. In addition, it describes the mechanism for documenting and reporting staffing concerns. This integrated set of processes, or the *patient care delivery model*, integrates data from a valid and reliable patient classification system or, if not available, from benchmark data. For example, the patient classification system or benchmark data identify the required skill mix necessary to best manage the typical patients on any given unit. Trended data may identify a need for a change in the skill mix and staffing plan that incorporates the use of greater numbers of RNs or greater numbers of licensed practical/vocational nurses (LPNs/LVNs) and nursing assistants providing adjunctive care.

Core schedules represent an aggregated average number and skill mix required for patient care and focus on having sufficient staff to care for the population served. Components include direct, indirect, and activity time. The core scheduling is the long-range plan that becomes the organization's template for the

---

Exhibit 6–11   Staffing Plan Template Components

- Provides core schedules with aggregated average number and skill mix required
- Includes direct (including at the bedside or in the conference room), indirect (such as unit secretary), and activity times
- Incorporates the organization's goals; available staff; state and national legislation; scope of practice defined by licensure, regulations, and accreditation requirements; and planned patient demand
- Includes support hours (such as shift report, and counting supplies and medications)
- Includes the person who is in charge during a shift
- May need to temporarily change when new employees are hired
- Has several scenarios that determine when the staffing would change as patient volume increases or decreases
- Specifies that when the patient volume goes below the minimum staffing level staffing cannot be cut further
- Gives other pertinent options (such as combining services with another cost center)
- Based on patient acuity if a reliable and valid patient classification system is available. Otherwise is based on benchmark data that provides support for the staffing plan
- Includes levels of patient care needs identified in the patient classification system
- Describes the professional practice model used in the hospital and indicates how that model supports the delivery of patient care and the environment in which care is delivered

---

required number of staff. The schedule incorporates planned patient demand; scope of practice defined by licensure, regulations, and accreditation requirements; available staff; the organization's goals; state and national legislation (Gardner & Gemme, 2003).

Whenever possible, *direct care*, or interventions specific to patient care that can be directly attributed to the patient, as well as *daily planning and documentation*, should be identified in the documentation system linked with the patient classification system or benchmark data. According to O'Brien-Pallas and colleagues (1997), healthcare leaders are challenged to examine the traditional concept of direct and indirect care and to define the main constructs that may influence nursing work. Patient care work should include work that is directly attributed to the patient, whether it is at the bedside or in the conference room supporting the planning process. *Support hours such as shift report and counting supplies and medications are typically a percentage of time and are calculated for inclusion in the core schedule*. Once patient needs are determined and validated, the department director can then determine the core staffing hours and skill levels needed to run the department efficiently and effectively.

The staffing plan includes the person who is in charge during a shift (Eggenberger, 2012). This person provides leadership, makes assignments, and deals with unusual incidents or difficult situations. This person supports the management on issues as they occur during a shift or for a specified length of time.

Staffing plans may need to *temporarily change when new employees are hired*. As the new employee is oriented or if the staff member is just out of school, this person will not be able to take care of as many patients. If a preceptor is used, the preceptor will need to work the same schedule as the new employee.

The staffing plan also considers *indirect caregiver role requirements* such as the health unit secretary. Those roles that support the operations of the unit should be categorized in the schedule portion of the workforce management plan. This time, traditionally labeled as indirect time, is defined and measured in a variety of ways in organizations. Regardless of how it is defined, indirect time must be measured consistently.

Another important consideration in addition to types of caregivers is the distribution of budgeted hours across the schedule. There is a need to pattern the required numbers of nurses based on trend data. The *flaw of averages* (**Exhibit 6–12**) illustrates this point quite well. The flaw of this averaging process for health care is that the average situation *may never occur*. According to Savage (2002), the averaging process distorts accounts, undermines forecasts, and dooms apparently well-thought-out projects to disappointing results. In healthcare staffing, average caregiver needs are often used to create monthly schedules. Although this process is efficient, it may create more challenges in the long run. Consider the situation in which the average number of staff per shift is 5 and the range for each day of the week is 3 to 7 on the basis of patient activity. No shift requires 5 staff persons, yet every day is staffed with 5 persons.

Using the specific number within the range of relevant numbers, in this case a number between 3 and 7 rather than the average of 5, for each shift *results in more accurate staffing*. The wide range of time required for similar—but different—patient situations is often significant. The time required determining specific time standards for the range of patient care profiles and combinations of needs in health care would be overwhelming and cost prohibitive using motion, time, and standard data techniques.

Once basic staffing levels are determined, the nurse manager can set up several *scenarios within the staffing plan to determine when the staffing would change as patient volume increases or decreases*. The issue is matching variable demand to variable supply. For instance, Hollabaugh and Kendrick (1998) at Good Samaritan Regional Medical Center in Arizona developed a five-level pyramid to staff for peak times (winter) as well as low census/acuity times (summer), a hiring plan for the varying census times, and a more equitable cancellation policy. This plan achieved cost savings, more continuity and job satisfaction, fewer patient and physician complaints, and established a more effective way to adequately staff despite large variations in census. The amount of patient care staff, skill mix, and necessary support staff needed to assist in providing the care is adjusted based on patient needs (the daily staffing process).

When the patient volume goes *below* the minimum staffing level, staffing cannot be cut further, and other options, such as combining services with another cost center, must be considered.

Ideally, if a reliable and valid patient classification system is available, *the staffing plan is based on patient acuity*. Otherwise, it is best to have benchmark data that provide support for the staffing plan. Typically, the nurse executive, in collaboration with key stakeholders, is responsible for establishing an overall staffing plan for the division or departments of nursing and should include levels of patient care needs identified in the patient classification system. The plan describes the professional practice model used in the hospital and indicates how that model supports the delivery of patient care and the environment in which care is delivered.

Evidence for optimal, or at least adequate, staff is emerging. Research is available to substantiate *staffing plan effectiveness*. Pinkerton and Rivers (2001) identified an extensive list of contextual factors affecting staffing effectiveness (**Exhibit 6–13**). Staffing is *not* simply providing a schedule for staff so that they know when to show up for work. Effective staffing is the result of careful consideration of multiple variables and an examination of their relationship to outcomes. *Effective staffing practices* integrate historical evidence about performance from patient, family, staff, and operational perspectives. *Efficient staffing* uses the least costly level of caregiver to achieve the desired patient outcomes.

As a nurse administrator establishes a staffing plan, it is important to have this plan reflect productive hours actually worked. It is best if the budget can reflect productive hours separately from nonproductive hours.

Exhibit 6–12   The Flaw of Averages: Daily and Weekly Caregiver Staffing Requirements

S	M	T	W	T	F	S	Weekly Average
3	6	6	7	7	4	3	5.1 Caregivers

Exhibit 6–13   Understanding Contextual Variables/Factors Impacting Staffing Needs

I. Support
   A. Interdepartmental
      1. Number of support staff from other disciplines.
      2. Adequacy of support services, for example, patient transport team, volunteers.
      3. Ineffective discharge planning.
      4. Quality and/or evidence of pre-hospital patient teaching.
      5. Presence or absence of services in the hospital that support nursing care 24 hours/day.
      6. Increased ancillary service utilization.
      7. Quality of relationship with physician.
      8. Changes in other departments impacting nursing.
      9. Effectiveness of interdisciplinary teams.
      10. Effectiveness of communications.
      11. Accuracy and thoroughness of patient education by other disciplines.

   B. Intradepartmental
      1. Number of unit-based support staff.
      2. Number of orientees scheduled (training time).
      3. Teamwork or no teamwork/unit cohesiveness.
      4. Communication from patient to nurse (Is there a person answering call light who can adequately communicate problems to nurses?)
      5. Ineffective discharge planning.
      6. Full- or part-time, shift worked.
      7. Number of tasks per staff type.
      8. Health of nurse, pregnancy, work restrictions.
      9. Skill mix.
      10. Patient care modality.
      11. Consistency of patient care assignment.
      12. Staff turnover.
      13. No working preferred shift/rotating shifts.
      14. Paperwork expectation—nursing documentation.

II. Care Environment
   1. Bed turnover (combined number of admits and discharges).
   2. Environmental layout impacting efficiency.
   3. Presence of extender system (for example, tube systems, fax machines, PCs).
   4. Availability of patient safety devices (fall prevention, restraint reductions measures), or is the nurse required to have direct sight?
   5. Shift of patients from one level of care to another.
   6. Midnight census may be an outdated way of tracking workload because so many patients have early evening discharge and midnight census does not reflect work between 7 am–7 pm when most patients come and go.
   7. Medication delivery system.
   8. Having weighted factors for outpatients housed on impatient units. Most care provided in first 6 to 10 hours. If they go home at 2300, only partial credit given for intensive care.
   9. Impact of academic presence/students.
   10. Technology development: automatic blood pressure machines at bedsides, auto charting, medication dispensing, etc.
   11. User-friendly technology.
   12. Information systems: data retrieval.
   13. Information systems: order entry.
   14. Chaos factors impacting the delivery of nursing care.

III. Professional Competency
   1. Experience level of staff, new graduates, especially with diverse patient population.
   2. Organizational skills of the nurse.
   3. Delegation skills of the nurse.
   4. Level of education (degree): continuing education certifications.
   5. Charge capable (charge nurse).
   6. Philosophy and leadership style of the nursing leadership team.

7. Participation on hospital/unit/community-related activities: gets overall richer understanding of nursing.
8. Frequency of new procedures produced (learning curve).
9. Impact of generalist vs. specialist practice.
10. Number of float/temporary staff.
11. Professional attribute/professional practice model.
12. Autonomy level of the nurse.
13. Cultural competence/diverse composition of teams (correlate with diversity of patient population).

IV. Physician Driven
1. Number of consultants on case (writing excessive orders and/or conflicting orders requiring confirmation re-work).
2. Number of different physician groups, with greater impact when patients are off service.
3. Variation in physician practice/medical staff rules and regulations.

V. External
1. Changes in nursing workforce.
2. Declining nurse productivity with an aging workforce.
3. Decreased commitment to suffering.
4. Aging workforce.
5. Generational differences.
6. Regulatory requirements.
7. Legal liability for RNs.
8. Fatigue.
9. Frequency and complexity of changes.

Source: Reprinted from *Nursing Economic$*, *2001*, Volume 19, Number 5, pp. 237. Reprinted with permission of the publisher, Jannetti Publications, Inc., East Holly Avenue/Box 56, Pitman, NJ 08071-0056; (856) 256-2300; FAX (856) 589-7463; Web site: www.nursingeconomics.net; For a sample copy of the journal, please contact the publisher.

Dunham-Taylor and Pinczuk (2006) provide samples of staffing plans. Other staffing plans are available also (Douglas & Mayewski, 1996; Fralic, 2000; Schmidt, 1999; Strickland & Neely, 1995).

Last, Douglas (2010) questions how well we understand the people side of staffing:

> With staffing holding such as essential role in the success of health care delivery it makes sense that staffing be deeply understood in all its dimensions. And yet, while much attention is given to structures, processes, operations, and technology, we may be overlooking that which is perhaps, above all these things, the key to the outcomes we strive to achieve. When it comes right down to it, no matter how modern, sophisticated, or efficient staffing programs are, if the individuals who are executing the care are not qualified, engaged, and able to offer the caring necessary for healing, the whole system can unravel quickly. At its very essence staffing works because of the people who are staffed [and the administrative leadership]. (p. 415)

Considerations in Creating the Core Schedule

The following situations require adjustments in core schedules:

- Rural hospital staffing always has a greater number of RNs because patient needs vary widely.
- Patient acuity continues to increase, whereas length of stay decreases.
- The turnover of patients on one shift has increased dramatically.
- As a rule of thumb, areas where there are a lot of admissions, discharges, and transfers generally need a higher RN ratio to do the necessary assessment.

Admission, Discharge, and Transfer Patient Activity

"Norrish found that nurses reported patient turnover rates of 40 percent to 50 percent in a single shift. Lawrenz found similar unpredictability with the number of admissions, discharges, and transfers averaging from 25 percent to 70 percent of midnight census" (Mark, 2002, p. 240). Thus, staffing might be adequate at the beginning of the shift but insufficient later in the workday, causing poorer, more expensive patient outcomes, patient safety issues, and less reimbursement.

"Time constraints require nurses to share essential information quickly but nurses self-report that the information they provide and receive when a patient is transferred is highly variable from nurse to nurse" (Shendell-Falik, Feinson, & Mohr, 2007, pp. 95–104). These authors advocate using appreciative inquiry techniques to achieve better information transfer.

Although the transfer factor is generated from patient activity, these data are a component of the scheduling plan. Failure to understand and manage unit activity or unit turbulence results in chaos and frustration of even the most organized and experienced nursing staff. Specific trend data include the results of historical data from admission, discharge, and transfer activity by day of the week and time of the day. A factor for each admission is incorporated into the core schedule to minimize unit chaos and to adequately provide needed patient care services. Then, during a shift, as changes in patient volume and intensity change, huddles, additional temporary help, or other strategies may help present staff safely get through intense times.

It is interesting to note that some healthcare leaders still believe that the transfer activity is a nonissue. They believe that because staffing has been allocated for the patient being discharged, time for the admitted patient is available from the unused time of the discharged patient, that it is essentially a wash as admissions replace discharged patients. *The reality is that the admission process is significantly more intense than the discharge process and requires an additional 45 minutes of RN time and 15 minutes of unlicensed time* (Cavouras & McKinley, 1998).

As the environment becomes less stable with frequent admissions and discharges, the patient classification system becomes less accurate at predicting workload. The notion of taking data from a population (annual data) and applying it to a single point in time (shift) means that you will be correct (or nearly so) on average (Seago & Ash, 2002). Given the current healthcare turnaround time and inpatient length of stay at 3.5 to 4.0 days, the need to trend and integrate these data into the core schedule is essential (Duffield, Diers, Aisbett, & Roche, 2009).

Nursing Staff Skill Mix

An important factor in determining appropriate staffing is the *nursing staff skill mix*, the various types of nursing staff by job classification necessary to care for the patient population. To determine the skill mix the nurse manager should ask several questions: What interventions are needed by patients, and which skill level has the licensure, authorization, and ability to provide the care? How do we deliver the care? Who is best to deliver the care? How is the care divided among the various caregivers? What skill mix provides the safest care? Which is cost effective? Unfortunately, there are no ideal answers. What works best in one setting (for example, in an intermediate care unit) may not be best in another (such as a skilled unit). And, the answer to any one of these questions may depend on current circumstances such as patient acuity, turnover of patients, discharges pushed to Fridays, admissions arriving on the evening shift, staff competencies or availability, or budget deficits. Both this and the next section present further information to answer these skill mix questions. Yang and associates (2012) discuss the impact of different nursing skill mix models on patient outcomes in a respiratory care center.

Caregiver Roles: Advanced Practice Nurses

The advanced practice nurse role applies to many different kinds of nurses with advanced degrees (most often master's degrees). Acute nurse practitioners, clinical specialists, and clinical leaders can plan, educate, coordinate, and provide care for the more complicated hospitalized patients, whereas primary care nurse practitioners (NPs) and clinical specialists can see patients in various settings, prevent healthcare complications, teach patients, and encourage prevention of disease. NPs can also do admitting histories and physicals. Nurse anesthetists provide anesthesia under the guidance of an anesthesiologist. In some states, nurse midwives can actually deliver babies; in other states they function more like a clinical specialist.

Caregiver Roles: RNs

"The role of the Professional Nurse is to establish a therapeutic relationship with the patient that includes responsibility for managing the patients' care over an episode of care" (Manthey, 2001). RNs possess an extensive knowledge base and assessment capability that places them in a position of significance to the patient.

Dykes and associates (2010) found that "during 1 year, 345 CCRNs [critical care registered nurses] reported that they recovered 18,578 medical errors, of which they rated 4,183 as potentially lethal" (p. 241). As previously noted, research documents significant relationships between nurse staffing and better patient outcomes and better reimbursement.

One advantage noted with a high RN mix is that less RN time is needed to communicate with less skilled workers.

RNs presently represent four generations, creating *intergenerational* issues. *Traditional* nurses, born in 1945 or before, have a traditional work ethic, are loyal to organizations, value working well with others, are technically competent, believe in a strong chain of command, and want to win. This generation, if still working, is motivated by abbreviated work weeks and alternative work schedules.

Baby boomer RNs (born between 1946 and 1963) comprise the largest number in the present workforce, although as they retire it is estimated this will no longer be the case by 2015. Baby boomers put work first, are driven by competition and material rewards, and are always willing to "go the extra mile" and work overtime. They are hard workers, are service oriented, and seek to please. They may also be sensitive to feedback and judgmental of those who see things differently (Lavoie-Tremblay et al., 2010, p. 415). They possess expert knowledge, enjoy group process, and are staying in the workforce longer because of longer life expectancy, better health, and the poor economy. It is important to think of strategies to best utilize these nurses and deal with the eventual loss of this generation (Bleich, Cleary, & Davis, 2009; Outten, 2012), such as working fewer hours (Hill, 2010) and phased retirements. Baby boomer RNs are also motivated by financial rewards and job recognition.

Generation X RNs (born between 1964 and 1980) put their lifestyle first, see jobs as temporary, and are less loyal and more skeptical. They saw parents lose jobs as a result of downsizing. They might pick a lower-paying job if it offers less stringent work hours and allows for better work–life balance. They are motivated by meeting their own goals. Self-improvement is important to them. They don't care what others think and have a bottom-line approach, getting bored at meetings. "They value opportunities for learning. . . . Motivators [are] recognition and praise, opportunities to learn new things, individual time with manager, and high stimulation" (Lavoie-Tremblay et al., 2010, p. 415). They value rewards that give them freedom such as flexible leave policies.

Generation Y RNs (born between 1981 and 2000) are high-maintenance, highly productive people who desire jobs with flexibility, see work as only one facet of their lives, love technology, want to be able to telecommute, work part-time, and leave the workforce temporarily to have children. They also grew up with downsizing, so are more into developing their own skills. They enjoy group process. "However, they will fully engage in their work if they believe in the outcome of their work and the organizational values, . . . seek frequent feedback, and [need] leaders who are nurturing and supportive" (Lavoie-Tremblay et al., 2008, p. 290). They like jobs that have fast-track leadership programs that reward workers and will leave if this is not available. As they join the nursing workforce, they are "more likely to perceive an imbalance between effort expended on the job and rewards received, low decisional latitude, high psychological demands, high job strain, and low social support from colleagues and supervisors" (Lavoie-Tremblay et al., 2008, p. 290). They are motivated by tangible and intangible rewards that represent immediate satisfaction.

All of the generations are motivated by recognition—that pat on the back. It is important for nurse managers to meet with each employee to find out what the employee values, what his or her gifts are, and what the employee needs on the job, and then to match and provide as much of this as is possible within the workplace.

Caregiver Roles: LPNs/LVNs

The LPN/LVN provides an intermediate level of care as delegated by the RN and in accordance with state nurse practice acts. The role of the LPN is most appropriate in highly functioning teams, skilled nursing facilities, and office settings.

Caregiver Roles: Unlicensed Assistive Personnel

Unlicensed assistive personnel (UAP) assist the RN to carry out professional activities. Healthcare organizations use these workers in a variety of roles, some that are more focused on supporting the patient care environment rather than the patients themselves. The use of lower cost workers in delivering nursing care is a concept that has taken on greater significance to hospitals and other healthcare institutions grappling with real and threatened declines in reimbursement coupled with an aging nursing force. UAP have been used in a variety of roles, in addition to the traditional primary support functions at the bedside; some perform simple housekeeping or secretarial tasks, and others perform higher level clinical or technical tasks such as electrocardiograms and phlebotomy. Because there is no one accrediting body common to all types of UAP and because state laws vary regarding UAP use, hospitals have been relatively free to experiment with different care models under the guidance of their internal nursing leadership (McClung, 2000, p. 531).

The Omnibus Budget Reconciliation Act of 1987 (OBRA 87) required states to certify nursing assistants only in long-term care facilities and to define the knowledge base and competencies required for nurse assistant certification. State requirements vary.

Caregiver Roles: Volunteers

Another important role to support safe and effective staffing is the volunteer. Volunteers are used most often by hospitals but can be used in any setting or by individual units. This is a fairly untapped resource. Specific guidelines need to be developed as to their qualifications, training, and specific services they would provide.

Competency

Nurses and healthcare leaders are challenged to ensure individual nurse competency and to develop systems to address the reality of variability in caregivers and patients. Caregivers encompass a wide range of levels and achievements of skill acquisition. Incorporating the evolutionary roles of novice, advanced beginner, competent practitioner, proficient practitioner, and expert practitioner is essential to further increase the effectiveness of a workforce management system. Examples of caregiver competency indicators are listed in **Exhibit 6–14**.

Exhibit 6–14   Caregiver Competency Indicators

1. **Years of experience**
   a. In the organization
   b. In the profession
   c. In the specialty
   d. In related disciplines (LPN/VN, certified nurse assistant)
2. **Certifications**
   a. ACLS/BLS/PALS
   b. Specialty—Critical Care (CCRN), Rehabilitation (CRRN), Monitor Tech, Wound/Ostomy (Wound, Ostomy, and Continence Nursing [WOCN] and Enterostomal Therapy [ET] Nurse)
3. **Continuing education**
   a. Skills lab
   b. Course work (dialysis, chemotherapy)
   c. Inservices (internal)
   d. Workshops (external)
4. **Other**
   a. Critical thinking skills
   b. Ability to delegate effectively
   c. Manual dexterity
   d. Attitude
   e. Relationship-building skills
   f. Organizational skills

To determine how to define competency within an organization, the ANA (2003) suggests the following:

> The specific needs of various patient populations should determine the appropriate clinical competencies required of the nurse practicing in that area. . . . All institutions should have documented competencies for nursing staff, including agency or supplemental and traveling RNs, for those activities that they have been authorized to perform. (p. 5)

Other sources for establishing clinical competency are the nurses who have a great deal of experience caring for a patient population, professional nursing organizations, the literature (Kuthy, Ostmann, Gonzalez, & Biddle, 2013; LaDuke, 2000; McConnell, 2001; Taylor, 2000), benchmarking, and regulatory agencies.

Meretoja and Leino-Kilpi (2001) reviewed the available competency instruments and found that most measured "nurses' self-perception of competence. . . . It is important to have more comparative studies of nurse competence from managerial, patients', and other health e-team members' points of view" (p. 351). Within each organization, nurse administrators need to determine how to measure staff competency, document that this competency has been met, and make appropriate educational opportunities available for staff.

Specialty nurse certification (Coleman, Lockhart, Montgomery, & McNatt, 2010; Kendall-Gallagher & Blegen, 2010; Wade, 2009) is an important credential for competency and has been positively linked with patient safety.

Competency can also be linked with *career ladders* (Riley & Rolband, 2009) that provide additional opportunities and recognition for staff. Shermont and colleagues (2009) suggest *career mapping*; this not only reinvigorates careers but develops nurse leaders.

New Nurse Orientation

Orientation programs for new nurses, especially new graduates, are vital (Halfer, 2007). There are many options to achieve competency for new nurses, including internship and residency programs (Beauregard, Davis, & Kutash, 2007; Fink & Krugman, 2008; Halfer, Graf, & Sulliivan, 2008; Keller, Meekins, &

Summers, 2006; Kramer & Halfer, 2012; Mills & Mullins, 2008; Salt, Commings, & Profetto-McGrath, 2008) and having mentors work with, and supervise, staff competency (Halfer et al., 2008; Mills & Mullins, 2008). This is especially successful when mentors are selected and trained and are committed to working with new staff. These programs ease the transition for the new nurse. Attrition rates are better when such programs are in place, and patient safety outcomes are better.

The orientation process for newly licensed RNs is costly—estimated to be from $39,000 to $60,000. It takes time to orient new staff and takes time from existing staff who mentor or precept new graduates. Turnover rates of new graduates are still high (Brakovich & Bonham, 2012). (This is discussed more in the section titled "Turnover" later in this chapter.) Trepanier and associates (2012), in a cost-benefit analysis of a nurse residency program, significantly decreased turnover, reduced contract labor costs, and found a net savings between $10 and $51 per patient day. Return on investment of residency programs is excellent (Pine & Tart, 2007).

Shift Determination

There is a lot of evidence about shifts. "In a random sample of registered nurses who worked varied schedules in different environments, over half reported that their dissatisfaction with nursing was related to unreasonable employer expectations and inflexible scheduling of work hours, shifts, weekends off, and vacations" (Ruggiero & Pezzino, 2006, p. 450). *The 12-hour shift issue in Myth 7 clearly shows that, although some nurses may not want to change this practice, it is critical to do something about it if the organization is truly concerned about patient safety, nurses' health, and reimbursement. This could easily result in legal issues involving either patient or nurse injuries.*

Evidence also shows that "regardless of shift, most [nurses] expressed their dissatisfaction with working weekends and holidays, mandated overtime, irregular shift schedules, and rotating shifts. Participants like having control over their schedules, particularly . . . to meet their families' needs" (Admi, Tzischinsky, Epstein, Herber, & Lavie, 2008; Ruggiero & Pezzino, 2006, p. 451).

Schedules on some units "evolved" to use a mixture of 4-, 6-, 8-, and 12-hour shifts (Kalisch, Begeny, & Anderson, 2008). However, this can become chaotic on certain units and Kalisch and associates advocate using one shift length. Having an extra nurse for peak times makes sense and, with our aging workforce, might provide a wonderful opportunity for an older expert nurse who can no longer work 10- or 12-hour shifts.

As we discuss complexity and the need for change, several issues arise. We advocate self-scheduling within set guidelines provided by the nurse manager. This gives nurses the autonomy to determine their schedules and helps the nurse manager because staff negotiate among themselves how to cover needed shifts. Self-scheduling contributes to higher productivity and job satisfaction (Russell, Hawkins, & Arnold, 2012; Ruggiero & Pezzino, 2006). Hausfeld and colleagues (1994) reported that self-scheduling worked on a unit with a widely fluctuating census. Overtime and sick calls decreased and there was much less floating into or out of the unit. Staff autonomy and satisfaction were higher. And, staff felt that the patient care improved. A win-win situation. (The only time this fails is when there is a dysfunctional nurse manager/staff group or when parameters are not specified.)

Another option currently used is *open-shift management* where nurses can view which shifts are open and choose which ones they will work (Valentine & Nash, 2008). This occurs within systems or even can exist across a region or small state.

We need to ask: How can we do staffing more efficiently? Although we may need to provide actual shift times for a skeletal staff, why not have most nurses determine their work schedule around assigned patient needs? Let's move into the twenty-first century!

Full-Time and Part-Time Staff

To schedule most effectively, it is generally best to have both full-time and part-time staff. With too many full-time staff, not enough staff are available to cover weekends, vacations, and sick time. With too many part-time staff, continuity of care suffers. For an inpatient unit, it is preferable to have approximately 60% to 70% full-time and 30% to 40% part-time staff. This offers flexibility and still has continuity.

Part-time staff can be helpful and, in addition to working a regular schedule, may be willing to work extra shifts as long as it fits with their other life circumstances. Third seasoners (those older than 55 years) are a good source of part-time workers. Another strategy is to use job sharing between two RNs to fill a full-time position.

On-call time is another arrangement that offers more flexibility in staffing. This involves paying staff who work a regular schedule to be on call, meaning they are available to come in when needed.

Overtime

Overtime is used when understaffing occurs. Overtime is effective for occasional use and is less expensive than other options such as hiring an additional person for peak times or paying for agency staff. However, overtime can be overused and really burns out staff. If nurses have already worked a 12-hour shift, they should *not* work overtime because adverse nurse and patient outcomes occur (Bae, 2012). Too much use of overtime can also result in staff turnover. *Evidence indicates two issues: (1) it is better to fix the understaffing issues than to use overtime, and (2) "Nurses may work overtime, despite being fatigued, because they do not want to let down the people they work with"* (Bae, 2012, p. 70).

Mandatory overtime is a dangerous practice—it is a quick fix that will backfire because patient safety and staff burnout can occur. ANA, along with some states, advocates restrictions on mandatory overtime, further specifying that

> no staff member in a health care organization should be required or forced to accept work in excess of a predetermined schedule. Any employer who violates the provisions would be subject to sanctions. Nurses do not want to be forced to work overtime when they are tired or when they have other commitments. (ANA, 2001, p. 2)

Fatigue Countermeasures

Fatigue is a complicated, systems issue.

> Work-related fatigue is a major risk factor for shift-work employees and a major concern for employers. Fatigue impairment contributes to 70% of industrial accidents and injuries, as well as higher rates of divorce, domestic abuse, and chemical impairment among overworked individuals. Work-related fatigue is common among occupations that have prolonged work hours, rotating shifts, night-time work hours, excessive workload, inadequate time for rest during work, and insufficient time for recovery between shifts, all of which are characteristic of the nursing profession, particularly in acute care hospitals. (Scott, Hofmeister, Rogness, & Rogers, 2010, p. 233)

Upenieks and associates (2008) found an increase in nurse vitality—as well as an increase in satisfaction and collaboration—when staff were directly involved in planning, testing, and implementing quality/caring changes. In this study, nurses were involved in patient-centeredness activities ("whiteboards, educational materials, peace and quiet time, and change of shift introductions"); value/lean issues ("relocating supplies and medication to accessible areas including patient rooms, using computerized bedside documentation and portable phones, streamlining admission and discharge procedures, and adding a resource nurse"); and team communication activities ("enhancing team communications and transition through shift-to-shift team rounding, interdisciplinary patient rounding, and rounding with physicians") (p. 393).

Scott and colleagues (2010) found that, first, nurses may need education about "proper sleep hygiene, increased restfulness and decreased fatigue, and [having] greater confidence in their ability to control their own lifestyle issues" (p. 235). Second, nurse managers/administrators using poor staffing and scheduling methods or poor leadership practices—especially with work culture issues—can cause turmoil and staff fatigue. They need to become aware of what causes fatigue as well as what they can do to deal more effectively with this issue. Third, organizationally there are many issues to consider: education programs, changes in workplace design and technology, policies about (and compliance with) hours of service regulations, and other work-setting fatigue countermeasures such as providing policies about a designated place for staff to rest when they work too many hours.

Unhealthy Work Environments

Moral distress is "the painful psychological disequilibrium that results from recognizing the ethically appropriate action, yet not taking it, because of such obstacles as lack of time, supervisory reluctance, an inhibiting medical power structure, institution policy, or legal considerations" (Pendry, 2007, p. 217). Sometimes just the pressure of increased job demands results in higher psychological distress. Pendry cites one study where 15% of nurses who resigned did so because of moral distress. The American Association of Critical-Care Nurses (AACN) has a published a Call to Action defining organizational measures to counteract moral distress (Pendry, 2007). AACN has a free handbook on moral distress as well as a tool kit to use to deal with this issue.

Another issue that occurs in unhealthy work environments is *workplace aggression*. Nurses are at high risk for workplace aggression (Autrey, Howard, & Wech, 2013; Demir & Rodwell, 2012; Hardin, 2012; Longo & Sherman, 2007; Walrafen, Brewer, & Mulvenon, 2012; Wilson & Diedrich, 2011). This includes workplace bullying, emotional abuse, threat of or actual assault, and sexual harassment. Johnson and Rea (2009) found that 27% of nurses had experienced workplace bullying in the last 6 months and mostly by managers/directors or charge nurses. Sellers and Millenbach (2012) found that workplace aggression occurred less frequently in Magnet environments and more frequently in union environments. Workplace aggression occurs when there is low supervisory and coworker support and can occur when negative physician behavior goes unchecked (Crawford, Omery, & Seago, 2012).

Incivility issues, such as rudeness, can be a precursor to workplace aggression when they are not corrected. Stressed workers have more health problems, leave their jobs, and can make more mistakes. Increasing awareness, including both supervisor and coworker support, in the work environment and education about cognitive behavioral techniques and preventive organizational policies can help eradicate this behavior. Increasing worker resilience can lessen susceptibility to adversity in the workplace.

Turnover

Aiken and associates (2002) found that *high patient-to-nurse ratios are associated with nurse-reported job dissatisfaction and burnout*, and that if nothing is done about the resultant turnover, it becomes cyclical. This becomes very dangerous to the bottom line because with the new CMS changes, hospitals with high turnover will start to lose reimbursements. "Dissatisfaction with management, scheduling difficulties, and departmental relationships are all contributors to turnover. But an even more subtle influence is the tone of any workplace, often referred to as work environment" (Christmas, 2008, p. 5). For instance, Fraser (2010) associated issues of dissatisfaction with lack of communication, resources, and recognition.

Uncertainty and perceived lack of job security also can contribute to dissatisfaction. Applebaum and colleagues (2010) found that perceived stress is related to turnover.

New graduates are particularly vulnerable (Pendry, 2007; Spetz, Chapman, Rickles, & Ong, 2008). Pendry (2007) cites a study where one-third of new nurses left their position in the first year, and 57% left within 2 years. Their reasons fell into four areas:

> (a) patient care (acuity of patients, nurse-to-patient ratios, ability to provide safe care), (b) work environment (management issues, lack of support and guidance, too much responsibility), (c) location or nursing area move (moving to another area of nursing or physical relocation which included travel nurse positions), and (d) employment factors (salary schedule, benefits). (p. 219)

Many left nursing entirely.

Many studies have found that Generation Y new nurses have been

> expected to become competent in their area quickly and carry a large workload. . . . It is not surprising that new nurses are constantly being confronted with situations for which they feel unprepared, leading to higher work-related stress, higher job dissatisfaction, and higher intention to quit. (Lavoie-Tremblay et al., 2010, p. 419)

In fact, "the proportion of Generation Y nurses who intend to quit is almost three times higher than that of other hospital workers from Generation Y" (p. 414).

To more effectively deal with turnover, Jones (2008) suggests examining human resource management data within the organization by asking the following questions:

Turnover Information

- Who is leaving?
- When did they leave?
- Are the nurses who are leaving employees we want to keep?
- How long has each nurse worked here?
- How long has each worked in nursing (i.e., how much nursing experience does each have)?
- Why are they leaving?
- What knowledge—general nursing knowledge and organization-specific knowledge—does each nurse who leaves take with him or her?

Retention Information

- Who is staying?
- Are these the individual nurses we want and need to keep?
- Why do they stay?

Human Resource Management Practices

- Are we hiring the right people (i.e., is there a good fit between the nurse's and the organization's values and beliefs)?
- Do our orientation, training, and mentoring programs encourage new hires to stay?
- Do we offer opportunities to encourage nurses to learn and grow?
- Do we offer opportunities for nurses to assume greater responsibility and accountability?
- Are our salaries and benefits competitive in our market area?
- Do we treat our employees equitably?
- Are we a place where other nurses want to be employed? (p. 16)

Retention

Retention starts at the top. Retention of competent, effective administrators—from the CEO through the nurse managers—is as important as retention of nurses. Employees are more likely to stay and feel valued in well-run organizations (Allen, Fiorini, & Dickey, 2010; Friese & Himes-Ferris, 2013; Hirschkorn, West, & Hill, 2010) and less likely to be satisfied when in union situations (Seago, et al., 2011). Retention is important whether or not there is a staff shortage. And, it is a win-win situation because as nurse satisfaction increases, patient satisfaction increases, and the bottom line increases. Senior management and facility board members need to understand this. Likewise, patient satisfaction decreases when the nursing hours per patient decreases.

Effective administrators develop *an environment that stresses retention* (Buffington, Zwink, & Fink, 2012). Vestal (2012) and Wonder (2012) emphasized that in the present environment an additional ingredient, *engagement*, is needed. The goal is workers who "understand and are committed to the goals of top performance for the unit and the organization" (p. 10). Rivera and associates (2011) found that the nurse manager is critical in promoting employee engagement; nurses' passion for nursing was also associated with engagement. Shared governance (advocated in Magnet guidelines) enhances nurse involvement in changes that directly affect the work.

Employee retention is influenced by work environment, job security, rewards/recognition including advancement programs, mentorship, scheduling, management, pay/benefits, and fulfillment (Allen et al., 2010; Coshow, Davis, & Wolosin, 2009). Schaar and colleagues (2012) even present a cost-benefit analysis for *nurse sabbaticals*. Hill (2011) found that good relationships with peers and supervisors linked with caring behaviors were associated with job satisfaction (Amendolair, 2012) and intent to stay in the profession. Yarbrough and colleagues (2008), in a sample of 2,000 nurses, found nurses gave the highest priority to maintaining competency, accepting responsibility and accountability for practice, providing high-quality care in accordance with standards, acting as a patient advocate, and providing care without prejudice to clients of varying lifestyles.

One important factor is *resilience*. Shirey (2012) cites studies that indicate "individuals with resilience possess protective factors that assist them to recover from and thrive despite adversity" (p. 552). Resilience develops "the longer an individual stays in a challenging work environment" (p. 552). This is enhanced by support from colleagues, including the supervisor, and by individual emotional toughening. Research indicates that resilient leaders tend to cultivate resilient employees. Resilience is like leadership, it can be learned and enhanced.

Satisfied nurses report the following: collaborative interdisciplinary teamwork that includes physicians, patient progress, varied work, autonomy (Kramer, Maguire, & Schmalenberg, 2006), praise/appreciation, clinically competent coworkers, supportive nurse managers/managerial fairness, personal control of nursing practice, support for education, a perception of adequate staffing, a culture where concern for patients comes first, and experience/certification (Fraser, 2010). Satisfaction is also related to the nurse manager's leadership and, when leadership is positive, results in higher patient satisfaction (Boev, 2012).

Key retention strategies for midcareer nurses include recognition (Bryant-Hampton & Walton, 2010) as well as salary, benefits, positive working relationships, flexible scheduling, and opportunities for continued education (Hall, Peterson, Lalonde, Cripps, & Dales, 2011). In addition, boomerang recruitment can bring back nurses who have left the profession to raise families (Hart, 2009). Also, as nurses get older, enabling them to change to doing work that is less physically demanding can enhance retention.

Wieck, Dols, and Northam (2009) ranked incentives of 1,581 nurses who were Boomers, Generation Xers, and Millennials (Generation Y nurses). Older, more experienced female nurses were more likely to stay (Spetz et al., 2008; Wagner, 2009). Wagner suggests that a nonlinear model is needed to predict nurse turnover, taking into account the different needs of younger and older nurses.

Does being in a Magnet organization make a difference with retention and job satisfaction? Studies generally show that these organizations exemplify better work environments, higher nurse satisfaction, and better nurse and patient outcomes.

Kovner and associates (2009) examined intent to stay by looking at discrete variables related to 1,933 new nurses and found "perception of job opportunity is really what impacts intent to leave" (p. 89). They found that supervisory support, fewer organizational constraints (having adequate equipment/supplies), good RN–physician relationships, procedural justice, promotional opportunities, and autonomy were all factors that were associated with satisfaction.

Haeberle and Christmas (2006) found that national benchmarks on recruitment and retention are needed and suggested metrics to be measured. Gess and associates (2008) suggest an evidence-based protocol for nurse retention. Lacey and colleagues (2008) suggest using targeted interventions that enhance the work environment.

Taskforces designed to enhance the work environment are beneficial not only for nurse retention but for patient safety, patient outcomes, and achieving what patients value. *The more staff are involved with the decision making at their level—from scheduling to patient care—the more likely they will be satisfied and stay.* Everyone is a contributing, valued member. No one is more important than another. All have wonderful contributions to make. Every person has special gifts—gifts that no one else has. The manager's job is to recognize those gifts and to match an employee's gifts with the parts of the job he or she will do best.

There are many ways to improve retention. For instance, one hospital saved $65,949 by reducing voluntary turnover by 91% by implementing five changes: on-boarding strategies, rounding by team leaders and administrators, social networking by a teambuilding committee of staff, increased employee recognition efforts, and developmental "stretch" assignments (Hinson & Spatz, 2011).

Meaningful recognition that publicly honors extraordinary contributions (Lefton, 2012) strengthens the workplace.

Retention of unlicensed assistive personnel can be an enormous problem. For instance, turnover can reach 80% and up to 400% in long-term care. Kupperschmidt (2002) advocates having job reviews so that job expectations are more realistic and improve retention. Lerner and Resnick (2011) found that increased years of experience, self-esteem, and performance of exemplary nursing care were associated with job satisfaction in nursing assistants. Orr (2010) found that "the most productive collaborative working relationships appear to be focused on client needs, allow for discussion, include specifics around needs, and are full of active listening. These factors appear to help connections between support service workers and professional staff who lead" (p. 134).

Position Control

Organizationally, *position control* is the process used by human resources, computerized or on paper, that specifies actual full-time equivalents (FTEs) assigned to a unit and tracks every person in the organization. **Exhibit 6–15** shows a typical position control document that specifies the total number of FTEs and lists all staff members, their positions, and their correct FTE designation. The authors recommend that the nurse manager be sure that records are updated, noting such items as leaves of absence, vacancies, new employees, changes in FTE designations for positions, and any other issues that would affect the FTEs. If a question arises regarding actual number of FTEs, the nurse manager has the documentation to show the accurate count. Usually, a nurse manager can decide to split the FTEs differently, but the main issue is that the total number of FTEs remains the same.

Exhibit 6–15	Position Control			
Position Title	**FTE**	**Hours/Year**	**Hours/Week**	**Name**
Nurse Manager	1.0	2,080	40	S. Rutherford (8/19/82)
RN	1.0	2,080	40	J. Smith (2/14/95)
RN	0.6	1,248	24	C. Jones (0.3) (4/25/01), K. Wilson (0.3) (10/7/01)
LPN	1.0	2,080	40	T. Blair (11/17/98)
Nurse Aide	1.0	2,080	40	D. Dixon (6/3/04)
Nurse Aide	0.8	1,664	32	R. Thomas (6/18/97)
Unit Secretary	1.0	2,080	40	E. Simmons (7/15/03)

Daily Staffing Guidelines

Daily staffing (**Exhibit 6–16**) is the real-time adjustment of the schedule based on current census, acuity, and the mix of available resources (Gardner & Gemme, 2003). The increasing availability of computerized applications for data collection and analysis greatly assists nurse leaders and managers in evaluating staffing adequacy. Data from multiple sources can be quickly integrated and analyzed to optimize decision making (Hyun et al., 2008).

It is important to maintain records showing that nursing staff are working within the scope of practice determined by the state licensing board, meet current health requirements such as appropriate immunizations, and are safe, competent practitioners. The state licensing board sets minimum standards for nurse competency.

Staffing Office Center

Most often the coordination and documentation of scheduling and staffing often occur in a central location. Functions of this office vary. In a centralized model, staffing supervisors make sure that staffing is appropriate in each area. In a decentralized arrangement, each nurse manager deals with staffing for that unit, and for evening/night shifts there may be evening and/or night supervisors helping with staffing and general problems throughout the hospital.

When there is inadequate staffing on one unit, a common practice is to "float" staff from another unit. Unless part of a regular float pool, nurses hate being floated and find it to be very stressful. Good and Bishop (2011) describe having a policy where nurses are not expected to float unless they agree to it. Those who agree to float can specify the unit(s) where they will go. This, along with a staffing pool, is used for staffing.

Staffing pools may be unit specific, for the entire organization, or for several organizations in a region or state. They offer more flexibility in work schedules, and some nurses enjoy the challenge and change of working on different units with different kinds of patients. This is less costly than using agency nurses and supplies nurses who are already oriented and aware of facility policies.

Another variation on the staffing pool is having available nurses who provide extra help for a few hours when units experience heavier staffing needs.

Agency staffing can be used when all else fails—especially in larger urban areas. These nurses are more expensive (the organization must pay the agency plus the nurse) and must still meet accreditation requirements.

To accomplish daily staffing, the staffing office center may have daily staffing meetings attended by the chief nursing officer, directors of nurses, nurse managers, the shift supervisors, and other administrative

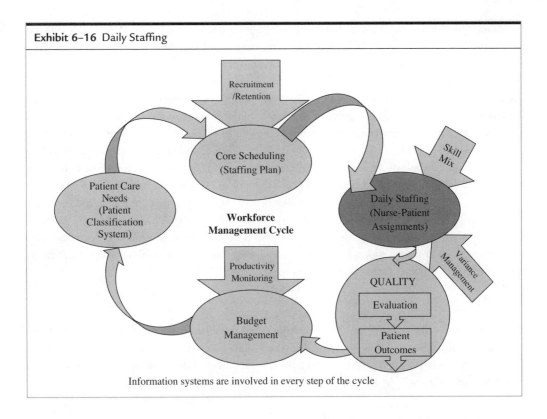

Exhibit 6–16 Daily Staffing

Recruitment /Retention

Core Scheduling (Staffing Plan)

Skill Mix

Patient Care Needs (Patient Classification System)

Workforce Management Cycle

Daily Staffing (Nurse-Patient Assignments)

Productivity Monitoring

QUALITY

Variance Management

Budget Management

Evaluation

Patient Outcomes

Information systems are involved in every step of the cycle

personnel such as the nursing office staffing person and the chief executive, operating, and financial officers. These meetings are used to identify unusual situations, to work out solutions, to find out bed availability, to share staffing concerns, and to share which positions are open or filled, along with other administrative issues.

Staffing and Scheduling Policies

As a nurse manager decides which staffing and scheduling options to use, it is helpful to have in place organizational policies such as for use of vacation time, how many staff can be on vacation at one time, how to make requests for time off, when and how to use overtime, self-scheduling guidelines, and antifatigue measures. It is important that policies enhance staffing and scheduling. However, too many policies can impede creativity and discourage someone from working. Instead, if staff are given more freedom to determine work time (this includes shift times) and time off, staff are more satisfied, retention greatly improves, and turnover decreases.

Nurse-to-Patient Assignments

The assignment of patients to specific caregivers is currently the responsibility of the nurse manager or charge nurse because multiple variables must be considered. The patient assignment process includes considering (1) the competency of caregivers; (2) yesterday's assignment (continuity of care); (3) preference of the caregiver; (4) previous shift staffing; (5) pending admissions, discharges, and transfers; and (6) geography of the unit, or proximity of patients to the central station (versus having all the resources needed at the bedside). The ultimate goal is to match patients with nurses who have the experience, qualifications, competencies, and interest required to provide the needed care and support the best possible outcomes (Cathro, 2013).

Assignment planning should also include time allotment for those indirect and administrative unit activities that support the operations of the unit, such as shift report, narcotic counts, and crash cart checks. Time devoted to the routine tasks needed to keep the department operating can be as much as 30% of the human resource time, whether there is related patient volume or not (Brady, 2001). In the NIC taxonomy, indirect care interventions are described as treatments that direct care providers perform away from the patient but on behalf of a patient or group of patients. In addition, administrative interventions are actions performed by a nurse administrator, nurse manager, or middle manager to enhance the performance of staff members to promote better patient outcomes (McCloskey & Bulechek, 2000). Failure to include time in the core schedule of the workforce management system for indirect and administrative interventions can result in feelings of inadequate staffing as a result of an undocumented but very real variance.

Nurse retention is positively affected when staff believe their assignments are doable and equitable. Experiencing a sense of accomplishment at the end of a shift and believing that appropriate care was given enhance staff satisfaction and, ultimately, retention. Recruitment becomes the result of satisfied employees who share these perceptions with other potential employees. The environment is noted for its sensitivity to quality patient care and safe staffing.

Shift Report

It is always best for staff going off duty to communicate directly with assigned staff for the next shift. Many advocate doing bedside reporting so that patients and significant others can also be involved (Cairns, Hoffmann, Dudjak, & Lorenz, 2013; Carlson, 2013; Rush, 2012). Nelson and Massey (2010) evaluated methods used and found that having a standardized, electronic report sheet facilitated report.

Variance Management

Variance data for each day should be examined to determine significance and appropriate interventions. Typically, *a variance is significant when the difference between required staff and available staff is greater than one-half of the length of a shift: 4 hours for an 8-hour shift and 6 hours for a 12-hour shift.* A variance is also significant if the classified hours and available staff are adequate but the skill mix available is not consistent with the classified skill mix. Existing staff can usually manage variances below one-half of a shift. When the variance exceeds one-half of a shift, the team should identify actions to manage the variance, and then document and address them. Examples of variance actions include postponing or rerouting admissions, calling in additional staff, floating existing staff, reevaluating the patient acuity ratings, postponing nonemergent care, and working overtime. **Exhibit 6–17** is an example of a variance management form.

This essential step is often overlooked or minimized in importance. When variance analysis is not done, the entire work of patient classification is, in fact, negated or at best ignored. The reality of the routine mismatch between patient care needs and available staff is an issue for the organization as a collective rather than the individual caregiver. Expecting caregivers to do their best in an impossible situation continues to fuel the flames of caregiver dissatisfaction, and the caregivers will ultimately exit the workforce.

Trend data for variances identify patterns and frequency of occurrences for each patient care area and define acceptable levels of variance from suggested staffing. These data are important in knowing where and when staffing problems occur and thus enabling managers to focus on fixing only problem areas rather than developing whole system changes. Analysis of aggregate variance data should be done at least quarterly and more often if significant variances occur. Variances specific to day of the week (e.g., Mondays and Fridays may require additional labor hours because of increased admissions, discharges, and transfers, or Tuesdays and Thursdays may be higher procedure days), season (e.g., winter vs. summer),

Exhibit 6–17 Calculating the Variance: Comparison of Patient Classification and Actual Staff Hours

	Patient Classification Hours	Actual Staffing Hours	Variance
RN Hours	28.0	36.0	+18.0
LPN/VN Hours	30.0	24.0	–26.0
NA Hours	35.0	24.0	–211.0
Total	93.0	84.0	–29.0

Variance Management Actions:

_____ Control of work flow by re-routing admissions

_____ Call in additional help

_____ Staff overtime

_____ Utilize Resource Nurse

_____ Reassess patient classifications for possible overestimation of staff needs

_____ Re-define the workload and eliminate or postpone nonessential tasks

_____ Other

skill mix (e.g., additional unlicensed hours needed rather than licensed hours), and shift (e.g., additional nurse aides needed on day shift vs. night shift) become readily apparent in this analysis.

Managing the daily variances between patient care needs and available staff is but one strategy and will not rectify all staffing challenges. Indeed, other essential long-term strategies are needed, including building better communication systems between leaders and staff; implementing patient classification systems, new staffing patterns, flexible scheduling, flexible benefits, technology, and new partnerships with nursing schools; and involving stakeholders in policy issues that affect patient safety and nurse staffing. These strategies are essential to address this long-standing challenge.

In **Exhibit 6–18**, seven steps are presented to describe both the flow of data and the analysis of data as patient care needs change:

> *Step 1* provides summative data from a valid and reliable patient classification system and shows the associated labor costs for direct care for RNs, LPNs, and nursing assistants. Indirect costs are factored in when direct care needs have been determined. The range of patient care needs is noteworthy because these ranges serve to guide the core scheduling process for allocation of resources on a daily basis.
>
> *Step 2* displays data using the projected volume and associated patient care need categories. Total salary dollars, average cost of care per patient day, total projected hours, total projected FTEs, and the average HPPD are identified in this step.
>
> *Step 3* identifies changing patient care needs and modifies the budget to reflect the changes.
>
> *Step 4* includes recalculated salary dollars, average cost of care per patient day, total projected hours, total projected FTEs, and the average HPPD.
>
> *Steps 5 to 7* present analyses of the changes in costs of care, FTEs, skill mix, and average HPPD.

Before finalizing changes based on these data, the impact on patient care outcomes must be examined to ensure optimal patient safety and desired clinical outcomes.

Evaluating the Core Schedule Staffing Plan

Staffing plans need to be evaluated at least annually or when significant patient or staffing issues occur (**Exhibit 6–19**). The evaluation includes examination of the numbers of staff and outcomes achieved.

Exhibit 6-18 Putting It All Together: Translating Patient Classification System Data to the Annual Budget

Step 1. Patient Classification System Summary Data: Unit A 2003

	Hours				Cost | Job Role				Notes
	RN	LPN	NA	Total Hours	RN ($25.00/hr)	LPN ($15.00)	NA ($8.00)	Total Cost	
Patient Type A	1.00	0.50	1.00	2.50	$25.00	$7.50	$8.00	$40.50	Individual patient care staffing needs form the foundation for the unit budget. The patient types A–E are used to reflect common patient care needs for calculation purposes only and do not reflect the myriad patient care needs profiles that exist on patient care units. Knowing the skill mix for each patient, the range of needs as defined by hours and skill mix are essential elements for a realistic budget. In this example, hours of care range from 2.5 to 11.0 hours per patient. The average cost per patient ranges from $40.50 to $211.00 per patient.
Patient Type B	1.50	1.00	1.50	4.00	$37.50	$15.00	$12.00	$64.50	
Patient Type C	2.00	2.00	1.50	5.50	$50.00	$30.00	$12.00	$92.00	
Patient Type D	4.00	2.50	1.50	8.00	$100.00	$37.50	$12.00	$149.50	
Patient Type E	6.00	3.00	2.00	11.00	$150.00	$45.00	$16.00	$211.00	
Range of Hours/Job Role	1.0 – 6.0	0.5 – 3.0	1.0 – 2.0	2.5 – 11.0					

Step 2. Calculating the 2004 Budget: Unit A: Dollars and FTEs

	Unit Volume	Cost/ Patient	Total Cost/ Patient Type	Hours	Total Hours	FTE's	Notes
Patient Type A	3,300	40.50	$133,650.00	2.50	8,250	3.97	The budget for 2004 is created based on actual patient care needs and skill mix experienced in the prior year. Calculations for total hours and dollars estimates for the 2004 budget year are based on the estimated volume of patient days (10,000) and percentages of patient care types expected by categories A through E.
Patient Type B	3,500	64.50	$225,750.00	4.00	14,000	6.73	The range of hours (2.5 to 11.0 hours) used by skill category provides information from which to create the daily staffing plan.
Patient Type C	1,500	92.00	$138,000.00	5.50	8,250	3.97	The total budget for RN/LPN/NA salaries for direct patient care for this unit is $782,300.
Patient Type D	1,200	149.50	$179,400.00	8.00	9,600	4.62	The average cost of care for each patient day is $78.23.
Patient Type E	500	211.00	$105,500.00	11.00	5,500	2.64	Total annual hours of care are 45,600 hours.
Projected Patient Days	10,000						Total FTE's are 21.92.
Total Projected Labor Cost			$782,300.00				Average HPPD are 4.56 hours.
Average Cost/Patient Day		$78.23					Indirect hours (e.g., unit support, employee education) are added to the core patient care needs labor budget. Typically, indirect hours range from 8–15% of the total dollars budgeted.
Total Projected Hours					45,600		
Total Projected FTEs						21.92	
Average HPPD						4.56	

Step 3. Patient Classification System Summary Data (Actual): Unit A 2004

	Hours				Cost/Job Role				Notes
	RN	LPN	NA	Total Hours	RN ($25.00/hr)	LPN ($15.00)	NA ($8.00)	Total Cost	The actual hours and skill mix used during the current year 2004 are then compared to the budgeted hours and skill mix.
Patient Type A	1.50	0.50	1.00	3.00	$37.50	$7.50	$8.00	$53.00	From 2003 to 2004 the range of hours of care increased from 2.50 to 11.0 to a range of 3.0 to 13.00.
Patient Type B	2.00	1.00	2.00	5.00	$50.00	$15.00	$16.00	$81.00	
Patient Type C	2.50	1.00	1.50	5.00	$62.50	$15.00	$12.00	$89.50	The range of direct salary cost per patient day increased from $40.50–$211.00 (as shown in Step 1) to $53.00–$247.50.
Patient Type D	4.50	2.00	2.00	8.50	$112.50	$30.00	$16.00	$158.50	
Patient Type E	7.00	3.50	2.50	13.00	$175.00	$52.50	$20.00	$247.50	
Range of Hours/Job Role	1.5 – 7.0	0.5 – 3.5	1.0 – 2.5	3.0 – 13.0					
Range of Cost/Job Role					$37.50 – $175.00	$7.50 – $52.50	$8.00 – $20.00		

Step 4. Revising the Budget for 2005: Unit A: Dollars and FTEs

	Unit Volume	Cost/Patient	Total Cost/Patient Type	Hours	Total Hours	FTE's	Notes
							The 2005 hours, skill mix, and dollars budget is revised to reflect the increase in patient care needs and skill mix changes.
Patient Type A	3,300	37.50	$123,750.00	3.00	9,900	4.76	The number of patient days remains the same at 10,000.
Patient Type B	3,500	81.00	$283,500.00	5.00	17,500	8.41	The budget increased 17% from $768,300.00 to $895,950.00.
Patient Type C	1,500	104.50	$156,750.00	5.00	7,500	3.61	The average cost per patient day increased 17% from $76.
Patient Type D	1,200	173.50	$208,200.00	8.50	10,200	4.90	The projected hours increased 26% from 45,600 to 51,600.
Patient Type E	500	247.50	$123,750.00	13.00	6,500	3.13	The total FTEs increased 24% from 21.92 to 24.81.
Projected Patient Days	10,000						The average HPPD increased 13% from 4.56 to 5.16.
Total Projected Labor Cost			$895,950.00				
Average Cost/Patient Day		$89.60					
Total Projected Hours					51,600		
Total Projected FTEs						24.81	
Average HPPD						5.16	

(continues)

Exhibit 6–19 Putting It All Together: Translating Patient Classification System Data to the Annual Budget (*continued*)

Step 5. Analysis of Annual Hours, Dollars, and Skill Mix Changes

	2003	2004	Percentage Change	Notes
Labor Cost	$768,300	$895,950	17%	From this analysis, it is concluded that both the cost and hours increased during 2004 but at differing rates. Labor cost increased 17%, while total hours increased 13%. The RN % increased 27%, the LPN % decreased 15%, and the NA % increased 19%.
Average Cost/Patient Day	$76.83	$89.60	17%	
Total Projected Hours	45,600	51,600	13%	
Total Projected FTEs	21.92	24.81	13%	
Average HPPD	4.56	5.16	13%	
RN hours	19,350	24,600	27%	
LPN hours	12,650	10,800	-15%	
NA hours	13,600	16,200	19%	

Step 6. Skill Mix Analysis 2003

	Hours					Total Hours/Skill Mix				Notes
	RN	LPN	NA			RN	LPN	NA		
3,300	1.00	0.50	1.00	2.50		3,300	1,650	3,300	8,250	The skill mix is 42.4% registered nurse, 27.7% licensed practical nurse, and 29.8% nursing assistant.
3,500	1.50	1.00	1.50	4.00		5,250	3,500	5,250	14,000	
1,500	2.00	2.00	1.50	5.50		3,000	3,000	2,250	8,250	
1,200	4.00	2.50	1.50	8.00		4,800	3,000	1,800	9,600	
500	6.00	3.00	2.00	11.00		3,000	1,500	1,000	5,500	
10,000						19,350	12,650	13,600	45,600	
						42.4%	27.7%	29.8%	100.0%	

Step 7. Skill Mix: Unit 2004

	Hours				Total Hours/Skill Mix				Notes
	RN	LPN	NA		RN	LPN	NA		The skill mix for 2004 is 47.7% registered nurse, increased from 42.4%; 20.9% licensed practical nurse, decreased from 27.7% and 31.4% nursing assistant, increased from 29.8%.
3,300	1.50	0.50	1.00	3.00	4,950	1,650	3,300	9,900	
3,500	2.00	1.00	2.00	5.00	7,000	3,500	7,000	17,500	
1,500	2.50	1.00	1.50	5.00	3,750	1,500	2,250	7,500	
1,200	4.50	2.00	2.00	8.50	5,400	2,400	2,400	10,200	
500	7.00	3.50	2.50	13.00	3,500	1,750	1,250	6,500	
10,000					24,600	10,800	16,200	51,600	
					47.7%	20.9%	31.4%	100.0%	

Exhibit 6–19 Evaluating the Core Schedule Staffing Plan

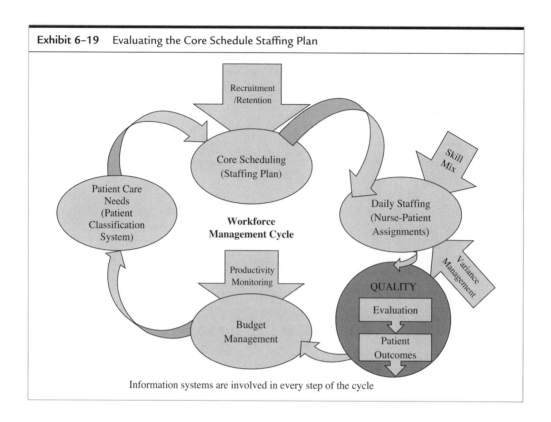

Information systems are involved in every step of the cycle

It also includes examining availability of support staff as well as the effectiveness of adjustments to changes in patient census or needs to more accurately schedule staff when needed.

Professional organizations provide further guidelines for evaluation. The American Organization of Nurse Executives *Perspectives on the Nursing Shortage* (AONE, 2000) recommends that regular evaluation reflects the value of nursing services. "Patients, providers, payers and policymakers will demand to know that changes in health care delivery in response to the diminishing size of the nursing workforce have not adversely affected patient care" (p. 15). The report stresses the importance of actual quantitative data and evidence-based policies that can be used to demonstrate the quality of the care given to patients.

The ANA, in *Principles for Nurse Staffing* (2012), drawn up by an expert panel of nurses, provides more specifics about evaluation data to be collected:

Changes in staffing levels, including changes in the overall number and/or mix of nursing staff, should be based on analysis of standardized, nursing-sensitive indicators. The effect of these changes should be evaluated using the same criteria. Caution must be exercised in the interpretation of data related to staffing levels and patterns and patient outcomes in the absence of consistent and meaningful definitions of the variables for which data are being gathered. [Thus the following data should be used to determine staffing levels.]

- Number of patients,
- Level of intensity of the patients for whom care is being provided,

- Contextual issues including architecture and geography of the environment and available technology, and
- Level of preparation and experience of those providing care (2008, pp. 5–6)

Measuring staff satisfaction provides additional data about existing issues that need to be addressed that can affect the core schedule. If staff satisfaction ratings are low, further discussion is needed with the staff group to both identify problems and potential solutions. Sometimes, the actual staffing numbers may not be the issue (for example, staff do not help each other). Or, the problem may be at a higher level where there is ineffective leadership or where there are organizational process issues that need to be resolved.

After evaluating and determining the solution(s), it might be necessary to develop a new budget, different staffing requirements, different staff mix, or better use of staff resources.

Staffing Legislation and Regulations

The Joint Commission provides standards to ensure that staffing effectiveness is achieved using an *evidence-based approach* and reinforces the need to enhance current practices. The Joint Commission standards *require organizations to assess the number, competency, and skill mix of their staff by linking staffing effectiveness to clinical outcomes*. This approach relies on the use of multiple clinical and human resource indicators rather than a single data element. Organizations collect and analyze data on multiple screening indicators, such as overtime, vacancy rates, and adverse drug events, which are believed to be sensitive to staffing effectiveness. The Joint Commission standards do not rely on arbitrary ratios but rather emphasize the need for an ongoing informed review of staffing based on credible screening indicators (The Joint Commission, 2002).

There has been increasing reliance on *legislation* to ensure adequate staffing. Regulatory issues related to national accreditation and licensure emphasize the importance of (1) adequate staff credentialing to do the assigned work, (2) policies and procedures describing how nursing assignments are completed on a shift-by-shift basis, and (3) adequacy of nurse staffing. As a required part of the regulatory process, the nurse administrator needs to demonstrate each of the preceding factors with a comprehensive workforce management system that includes accurate records of actual staffing.

The Patient Safety Act of 1999 (H.R. 1288/S. 966) requires Medicare providers (healthcare organizations) to make information on the following public:

- Number of RNs providing direct care
- Numbers of UAP
- Average number of patients per RN
- Patient mortality
- Incidence of adverse patient care incidents
- Methods used for determining staffing levels and patient care needs (AONE, 2000)

Several states have mandated all or parts of this act to be required for all healthcare organizations, even if they are not certified for Medicare. At the state level, some states have legislated staffing numbers and policies. California has implemented minimum nurse-to-patient ratios for each unit of every hospital. The impact of this legislation is emerging (Buerhaus, 2010; Tellez & Seago, 2013; Upeniks, Akhavan, Kotlerman, Esser, & Ngo, 2007).

There is a growing trend toward legislating nurse staffing to address patient safety issues. The California Assembly Bill 394 (1999) requires specific standards for UAP, patient classification systems, and minimum nurse staffing ratios. UAP cannot be assigned to perform nursing functions in lieu of RNs in acute care facilities (see www.applications.dhs.ca.gov/regulations).

According to Curtin (2003), there is some *merit* to legislatively mandated nurse-to-patient staffing ratios. Leaders of the ANA have noted that if hospitals could be trusted to staff properly, they would have done so. Mason (2003) does not believe that minimum legislated ratios will become the maximum but rather that the best hospitals will exceed those standards and the worst will be forced to stop assigning eight or more patients to the medical-surgical nurse.

Opponents to staffing ratios have been equally strident about the ineffectiveness of this approach (Buerhaus, 2010; Douglas, 2010a). Their belief is that nurse-to-patient ratios are counterproductive to evidence-based decision making and inappropriate as a staffing methodology for the complex phenomenon of patient care. Ratios assume that care is constant within each level of care, regardless of length of stay, skill mix, care delivery model, cost, competence, and unit geography. Further, some leaders may actually lower current effective RN staffing to the required minimum. Using the legislated minimum ratios is particularly ineffective in rural settings and trauma settings with wide ranges of patient care needs. The potential for failure to rescue patients in possible danger increases dramatically in these situations and can result in unplanned negative patient consequences.

Even the proponents of staffing ratio mandates recognize that *ratios do not resolve all the issues; hence, the requirement to institute a patient classification system along with the minimum ratios.* If hospitals had ensured that valid and reliable patient classification systems were used and relied on those systems as tools for determining nursing workload management, the lack of trust that historically has maligned the staff, managers, and administration would not exist. Staffing would thus be based on patient needs rather than the need to comply with mandated ratios that are arbitrary and without empirical support. Despite the best of intentions in which legislated nurse-to-patient ratios were created, the complexity of staffing is yet to be addressed adequately. Competence, experience, and education all affect productivity and patient outcomes. These variables have not been addressed in legislated staffing ratios. The debate continues regarding the staffing ratio laws enacted.

Consideration: Collective Bargaining Units

Another strategy to address safe staffing has been the use of collective bargaining (http://muse.jhu.edu/journals/lab/summary/v031/31.1clark.html). Ongoing changes in health care have subjected nurses to the effects of cost cutting, shuffled duties, and reorganization. This has prompted nurses to turn to the collective bargaining process to ensure safe staffing conditions for nurses, to correct inconsistent staffing, and to protect the patients under their care.

As long as nurses continue to feel disenfranchised, unprotected, and under siege by doctors and health-care administrators, interest in unions will grow stronger. The protection of collective bargaining and the belief that greater benefits are extracted with an intermediary provide powerful forces for healthcare workers. Increasing numbers of nurses believe that their voice in decision making is best heard through a legally binding contract between the employer and a bargaining unit. The contract prevents arbitrary decisions by the employer and enforces the right to participate in determining wages, hours of work, standards of practice, pension and benefits, and all other terms of employment.

Given the complex nature of healthcare staffing and the strident nature of collective bargaining units, new and visionary partnerships between healthcare organizations and collective bargaining units are desperately needed. Porter and colleagues (2010) suggest one method that they used in a 1,000-bed facility. The mutuality of goals for safe staffing positions incite both groups to rise to the challenge to address this pressing need and make recommendations to modify the healthcare system processes and beliefs to achieve the desired goal in a way that is beneficial to both nurses and patients.

Financial Planning

Once the patient needs and staffing plan are created, the budget (**Exhibit 6–20**) can be developed. The data collected from the workload management system provide the baseline for preparing the labor component of the nursing budget. The primary responsibility for this process belongs to the nurse executive, but nursing supervisors and unit managers are accountable for direct and worked productive hours. Resource allocation decisions begin with the assumption that the budget will be met and not exceeded. *Note Myth # 6 at the beginning of this chapter that demonstrates that using a combination of RNs, LPNs, and nurse aides are more expensive than RNs.*

Budgeting for staffing needs requires historical patient classification (or benchmarked) trend data, core scheduling staffing plans, and information from staffing variance analysis specific to the following:

- Census for each unit including averages and ranges for each shift
- Admissions, discharges, and transfer activity for each shift
- Actual direct hours and indirect hours per patient day
- RN hours as a percentage of the total hours worked

Exhibit 6–20   Budget Management

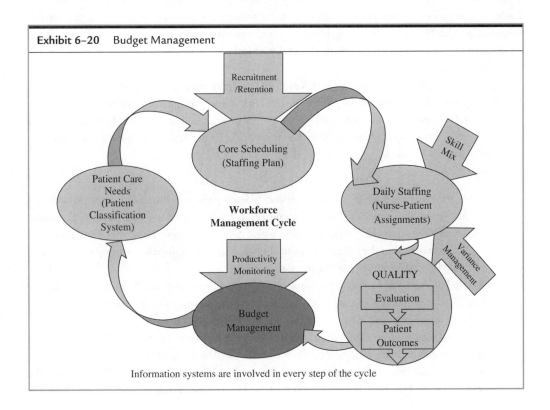

Information systems are involved in every step of the cycle

- Education hours, orientation, and training hours by unit
- Overtime hours both scheduled and incidental
- Anticipated sick time
- New staff orientation hours

The initial patient care hours estimate is adjusted for any changes in assumptions for the upcoming budget year, such as increases in expected patient volumes, new or changed patient care programs or physician coverage, or equipment purchases that would affect staffing requirements, as well as decisions made based on the previous analysis. It is also important to have *different budgets for different scenarios* such as census or seasonal changes, needs for different staffing or staff mix on certain days, or whatever has changed. It is evident that this phase cannot be achieved as planned without success at the previous levels. *Failure to respect the order of the process often results in inaccurate forecasting and financial overruns.*

Even with all that is positive in place, chaos happens. Suddenly, the census dips unexpectedly, or there is a staff shortage, or a new documentation system is implemented—all necessitating changes in the workload management plan. If scenarios have been developed beforehand, much of this can be changed quickly.

> The real issue is how administrators can balance cost, quality, satisfaction, and staffing at a time when the recession endangers their margins. . . . The intelligent use of advanced health information technology can help hospitals better match staffing to patient demand as it varied from day to day and hour to hour. (Barton, 2011, p. 37)

Effective staffing is linked to *good patient outcomes*—a critical factor in organizational financial success. We do not have good costing models to determine how much nursing time/resources or money was expended per patient for nursing care because we do not have a way to link the nurse(s) taking care of each patient. This cost, if we could measure it, could then be compared with actual reimbursement received for each patient. Hopefully, as technology improves, all this information will be captured.

It is important for the CNO to work with the CFO to figure out better costing and billing models for nursing care—linking the nurse–patient assignment, along with patient outcomes, to electronic operational databases. Then we could measure how nursing resources were expended by patient and case mix. This would also achieve another healthcare goal presented by the American Hospital Association: to have *greater billing transparency*.

Welton (2010) suggests:

- Define and price the nursing "product" separately from room and board and develop alternative accounting and billing models that allocate nursing as a variable cost and intensity to each patient, each day of stay for inpatient settings, or comparable metrics to identify nurses' contribution to care in other settings within the billing and payment system. [Welton discusses existing revenue codes that could be used for billing nursing intensity per day.]
- Directly link nurses to patients within operational and clinical databases. Then, use those data to identify the optimum mix of skill, experience, and academic preparation of nurses that provides the best value of nursing care.
- Educate nursing students, staff nurses, nurse managers, and executives on basic business and economic concepts and integrate these concepts throughout all nursing school curriculum.
- Work within the research parameters of the Patient Protection and Affordable Care Act and the Health Care and Education Reconciliation Act (P.L. 111-148) to include nursing costs and intensity

within innovative payment and delivery models that will be funded by the Centers for Medicare and Medicaid Services (CMS) Innovation. . . .

- Integrate nurses into the new accountable care organization (ACO) payment structure and explicate the nursing roles, resources, and best practices within the ACOs that achieve best outcomes of nursing care.
- Provide greater financial autonomy for nurses, such as developing separate nursing revenue centers within organizations, align nurse costing and billing practices with payment mechanisms, and allow nurses greater control over nursing revenue to achieve the best value of care. (pp. 399–400)

Meanwhile, some other important financial issues must be considered and dealt with more effectively. Within the workforce management arena, *evidence shows that turnover is very expensive for staff, patients, and hospitals and that better patient outcomes result when retention has been achieved.*

Turnover is expensive. The replacement cost of one RN is between $92,000 and $145,000 (Fraser, 2010). Jones (2008) cites a report that "estimates that organizations spend $300,000 annually in nurse turnover costs for every 1% increase in turnover" (p. 11), and that actual turnover costs are about 1.3 times a nurse's salary (p. 12). Empty positions create other costs such as overtime, temporary staff, closed beds, and patient deferrals. Other potential costs include "lapses in continuity of care, increasing patient length of stay, inefficient discharge planning, inconsistent use of policies and procedures, and communication problems" (p. 15). The cost of nurse manager turnover is even more significant.

Consider the following from the organizational finance point of view:

> Nurse turnover is bad—bad for hospitals, for patients, and for hospital employees. *Hospitals with higher turnover rates incur a higher average cost per discharge, a lower return on assets, a decreased cash flow margin* [and inadequate resource use.] . . . . High vacancy rates and continuous turnover of staff are stressing the financial and cultural fabric of health care providers.
>
> Nurse vacancy and turnover negatively affect a hospital's bottom line through (a) replacement costs that accrue from many sources, including human resource expenses on advertising and interviewing; (b) increased use of part-time employees; (c) overtime; (d) lost productivity; and (e) payouts to employees leaving the organization.
>
> *Facilities with the lowest rates of nurse turnover have the lowest rates of risk-adjusted length of stay.* (from Voluntary Hospital Association, as quoted in Coshow et al., 2009, p. 15)

The preceding fails to include the cost of lost patient reimbursement resulting from poor patient outcomes, legal costs, and resultant lower bottom lines.

Most important, consider the costs to patients when their lives or their well-being is at stake. In addition, major medical events can bankrupt patients.

Another financial issue is to achieve *value-based care*. What achieves best value to the patient? What does the patient really want? Anything else that we do creates more expense and is completed even though the patient does not want it. Many nurses do not realize this, nor do they understand how important it is to achieve only what the patient values. Educate nurses about this issue. "Optimum nursing care [providing only what the patient values] represents a balance between the intensity and quality of the delivered nursing care, including its costs, the safety, and outcomes of that care" (Welton, 2010, p. 399).

Another related financial issue for nursing staff is *non-value-added time*—or time consumed by rework and delays that could be avoided if systems and processes functioned ideally. This is time consumed with such activities as handing off, searching for supplies or equipment, fixing things, waiting, and rework often related to patient admission, transfer, and discharge; shift report; access to equipment and supplies;

access to appropriate and timely medications—especially during night shifts; scheduling—waiting for and/or transporting to diagnostic procedures; clinical record management—duplicate documentation requirements, lack of timely access to terminals, hunting for reports; interdisciplinary communication—especially with MDs; and nurse assignments and staffing (Storfjell, Ohlson, Omoike, Fitzpatrick, & Wetasin, 2009). Result: *An average of $1 million in wages is "wasted" annually on each nursing unit.*

Dealing effectively with this issue is important, not only for the patient and the bottom line, but for nurse satisfaction and retention. Many of these require the involvement of various stakeholders in the organization because organizational processes need to be improved or eliminated. AHRQ reported that "increased nursing resources in hospitals are associated with decreased patient mortality, shorter length of stays, and lower risk of adverse events" (Lacey et al., 2008)—not to mention achieving better reimbursements from CMS and other insurances. Everyone wins.

Another financial issue could be looming. *The retirement of baby boomer RNs—the largest generational workforce*—including nurse administrators, is expected to result in a nursing shortage by 2020 (Palumbo, McIntosh, Rambur, & Naud, 2009). This will constitute a significant staffing and knowledge loss for nursing. Bleich and colleagues (2009) suggest proactive strategies for knowledge transfer. Also, the recession has brought about some trends that affect the nursing workforce: Staff vacancies have plummeted; nurses are working more hours and more jobs; hospitals have experienced lower demand for new nurse graduates; and mature nurses are delaying retirement (Lawrence & Sherrod, 2010). Additionally, many nurses have not thought about their own personal retirement finances.

Last, an important financial element that cannot be ignored is to *share financial information with staff*—costs of supplies and equipment, costs when quality/safety issues are not realized, and reimbursement information about amounts actually received for care. Sharing this information is critical with the Affordable Care Act of 2010 so that staff realize how their actions directly affect the bottom line. In addition, staff can think of ways to save money and achieve better reimbursements.

Productivity Monitoring

Productivity is an important component of the workforce management system. The American Productivity and Quality Center defines *productivity* as "a process of getting more out of what you put in. It's doing better with what you have" (Health Care Education Associates, 1987). From the health care perspective, we want to achieve positive health outcomes/what the patient values at the lowest possible cost. Using these definitions is helpful in examining both the quality and quantity of the outcome, as well as the resources and processes necessary to achieve that outcome.

Enhancing productivity involves achieving more *efficiencies*—time or resources saved to deliver a service—and must be linked with *effectiveness*—the degree to which the final result achieves the desired outcome. Productivity is one of those elusive characteristics that is hard to measure and where, no matter how well it is accomplished, there is still room for improvement.

For effective organizational productivity we have to get out of our silos. Productivity is *interdisciplinary*. (This includes the finance department getting out of their silo.) All are interconnected and intersecting with each other.

> Nursing productivity must be evaluated in terms of value-added care, a vision that goes beyond direct care activities and includes team collaboration, physician rounding, increased RN-to-aide communication, and patient centeredness; all of which are crucial to the nurse's role and the patient's well being. (Upenieks, Akhavan, & Kotlerman, 2008, p. 294)

A wonderful example of breaking down silos is presented in Toussaint and Gerard's *On the Mend: Revolutionizing Healthcare to Save Lives and Transform the Industry* (2010). This is a must read!

Productivity Misconceptions

Some misconceptions about productivity can lead to viability issues if they get too far out of hand. As with all concepts, at times, *even though we all use the same words, we are actually operating under different definitions.* These differences should be identified and clarified. When allowed to continue over years, the effects of the misconceptions can be considerable. Misconceptions abound. Some common misconceptions about productivity are shown in **Exhibit 6–21**.

> Health professionals in this country are working more hours than ever before and getting less done. In fact, Americans have the dubious distinction of being first in the number of hours worked each year. The U.S. Department of Labor, Bureau of Labor Statistics, noted only a slight increase in productivity from 1960 to 1990, and the productivity increase in the last 10 years is attributed to technological advances, particularly the development of the Internet.
>
> Health care employees are burning out faster than the replacements are coming in, yet they are still being pushed to become more productive. They are working 12-hour days, are commuting up to 2 hours a day, and are held by an electronic leash to the office. Their opportunity to relax is almost nonexistent.
>
> Contrary to popular beliefs, we need to learn how to slow down our thinking at times, not speed up. Time for reflection and contemplation of ideas and issues is sorely missing in health care. The never-ending checklist is always present and demanding attention. Further, experts report that pay is not the chief motivator for productivity. In general, employees desire to do meaningful work most of all, next they desire opportunities for collaboration through group decision making, and then they want equitable pay. (Porter-O'Grady & Malloch, 2011, pp. 450–451)

To enhance productivity ask, and work on, the following questions:

- Is our work meaningful?
- Do staff have opportunities for caring activities?
- Do staff experience interdisciplinary collaboration and teamwork?
- Are the pay/benefits equitable?

Exhibit 6–21   Myths and Truths About Employee Productivity

Accepted Notions
- If employees work more hours, they will be more productive.
- If employees work faster, they will be more productive.
- If employees are paid more, they will be motivated to work harder and produce more.

The Reality
- Employees perform optimally for six to seven hours and may be able to work longer in a burst of energy or inspiration, but then they must rest.
- Employees need balance; they need a life outside of work.
- Slower, intuitive thinking is often more effective in solving problems than mental agility.
- Studies show that, in Germany, where individual performance is not rewarded with pay increases, productivity is often higher than in the United States.
- Employees are most productive when their employers pay them equitably and then do everything possible to help the employees put money out of their minds.

Source: Johnson, C. B. (2000). When working harder is not smarter. *Inner Edge, 3*(2), 18–21.

Another misconception about productivity is that *quantitative measurements are all that is needed.* Instead, these measurements need to be accompanied by *qualitative* data.

In some cases, *productivity has gotten a bad reputation with nursing staff.* This is because the word *productivity* (and now the current buzzword is *lean*) has been used synonymously with budget cuts and unrealistic layoffs.

> Slash-and-burn cost cutting brings only a series of onetime efficiencies. In the end, there's only one encore—another round of cost cutting. And that's the catch. This approach leads to increasingly hollow companies that ultimately are unable to maintain market share in an ever-expanding global economy. (Roach, 1998, p. 154)

These tactics devalue staff. If budget cuts are needed, *all stakeholders need to be involved in identifying where the cuts will occur.*

Some think that *as productivity increases, quality suffers.* This is not the case. For example, if at 7 A.M. there are too many staff but by 10 A.M. there are not enough staff, productivity could be improved by having fewer staff there at 7 with another person coming in at 10 to be there during peak load times. Here care might actually improve and staff would be less frustrated.

It is easy to think that *when a department experiences productivity problems, the department head should be directed to fix the problem.* This is silo mentality. *Although the department needs to improve, there are usually other organizational systems problems and other stakeholders who also need to work on rectifying the problem.*

The thought that *productivity improvement is the only way of improving income generation in the organization* is not accurate. *New services and changes that improve the way we deliver care are always needed.*

Sometimes we *just pay attention to internal issues.* This is another misconception. For instance, it is possible that the supply chain has malfunctioned and the organization cannot get needed supplies and equipment in a timely way, thus causing serious productivity problems. Here the problem probably lies with the supplier, and yet, chances are, staff in the organization are helping to cause the problem as well. Perhaps someone did not promptly order the needed supplies, or, as a supply becomes scarce, staff squirrel away the item—which actually worsens the shortage. Maybe the paperwork is so ponderous that it is impossible to get needed supplies quickly. To truly get to the bottom of this process issue, all stakeholders, including the suppliers, must get together to work out this problem.

We are interconnected. We are all in this together! Health care is a dynamic, complex process. Each of our actions affects the outcome.

Productivity Measurement

Productivity measurement examines such factors as staff/RN HPPD, per test, per visit, per treatment, or per procedure; FTE-to-bed ratios (sometimes written as FTE per adjusted occupied bed); and cost per unit of service (i.e., the cost per home visit, the cost per DRG, or the number of patients per overall facility budget amount), within a specific time period. When measured at regular intervals over time, these data can provide an idea of whether the productivity level has improved.

If productivity has improved, more outputs (patient days, visits, etc.) were produced, but we must also consider which resources (inputs—staff hours or FTEs) were used. If it took more FTEs to produce the patient days, productivity may not have improved. If productivity worsened, more resources were used without significantly increasing the outputs.

Measuring and managing productivity in health care presents considerable challenges. First, *our service product is not well defined.* We often don't provide cures but instead treat disease, and, as we do this, our client often experiences more discomfort. Our client may achieve better health as a final outcome, but it is possible the best outcome is to lessen pain or to achieve a peaceful death.

Second, *it is a challenge to quantify our service output.* We can measure patient days or visits, or we can say that we treated *x* number of people with pneumonia or *x* number of clients with heart disease. If there is a cure, chances are it happens after the patient no longer needs our services. However, *we often do not have enough research to know whether present practices actually affect the client outcome.* For example, which specific actions enhance or detract from healing? Why do some patients respond positively to treatment whereas others do not? How can we anticipate whether a particular patient will experience medication side effects, whereas another patient will not? Why do some patients who believe they will die actually do, whereas other patients who are expected to die live? The significant question, "Were desired patient outcome(s) achieved?" is difficult to answer at best.

Third, *did the patient get what s/he valued?* Or was something else provided and measured that the patient did not even want? Patient satisfaction is one component of what is valued. It implies client expectancy. But what the client actually valued is unknown.

A fourth issue with productivity measurement is that the measurements use *historical data,* so it is difficult to rectify problems as they occur. Also, patients may be afraid to give negative information for fear that this will adversely affect their care. Ideally, more direct feedback is needed during the actual patient experience. This is why we advocate doing regular interdisciplinary rounds.

Although not ideal, today the most effective productivity evaluation measurements combine financial, organizational, and patient outcome data and are called *performance evaluation* measured by scorecards. In performance evaluation, the outcome data (effectiveness) are compared with the processes influencing those outcomes (efficiencies). Process data measuring efficiency can include numbers and skill mix of staff; staff turnover; cost of the staffing; overhead costs; quality/safety measures implemented, including adding technology; and/or equipment and supplies consumed. Unfortunately, performance data do not yet measure whether the patient received anything of value.

As more performance data have become available on a national level through the CMS, these published summaries of various performance measures have provided performance data to regulators, payers, and consumers via the Internet. These data have prompted the changes in payment structures. Payers use these data in two ways: (1) to compare providers, choosing to have contracts only with providers who have the best performance data, and (2) to pay only for positive performance, not for problems that healthcare facilities caused for patients (pay for performance). This is called *performance-based reimbursement evaluation.*

Obtaining performance data is just the first step and, aside from the value question, brings up more questions: *Do the processes currently used and measured have an actual effect on the outcome?* For instance, does patient preoperative teaching actually result in fewer complications, quicker recovery, and higher patient satisfaction following surgery? Are there fewer medication errors when patients give themselves their own medications when possible?

There are *thousands* of these questions that we need to ask. Everyone needs to be involved in identifying questions! We may believe intuitively that we know the answers, but we must constantly be up-to-date on current evidence—and *make changes based on this information.*

Productivity Issues

Many workforce management issues affect productivity. First, productivity is affected by *staff performance factors* such as level of experience, ability or willingness to do the work, proper orientation, proper teaching of techniques, and proper information about the tasks they are expected to do. Tardiness and absenteeism, sick and vacation time, conference time, overtime, and use of agency staff can all affect productivity.

Second, the way we staff can affect productivity. Consider the following issues. When units are *under-staffed*, or nurses are working *adverse work schedules*, it creates all kinds of problems—more adverse events (Han & Trinkoff, 2011; Patrician et al., 2011), poorer patient outcomes, and nurse job stress and dissatisfaction. Stress and burnout can result in absenteeism, illness, and turnover (Tucker, Weymiller, & Cutshall, 2012). All these issues are interrelated.

Third, when *nonproductive time* (such as annual leave or administrative unit activities that support the operations of the unit) *is not included in the budget and when nonproductive time is figured into the productivity number* any time someone uses sick or vacation time, the productivity level drops. The result is enormous organizational problems—understaffing, poor patient outcomes, more legal issues, turnover, less reimbursement. It is best to have *two separate staff budgets*, one reflecting worked time and the other reflecting nonproductive time.

Fourth, Letvak and Buck (2008) identified how the *chemistry or adequacy of relationships between coworkers affects quality*. Administratively, this becomes very complicated because staff, administrators, and physicians differ in the way they respond to situations, to each other, and to patients and their families. In fact, the same person can respond differently to different patients, when part of a different work group, or when the person has a different boss.

Fifth, Kalisch (2009) found that *dysfunctional nursing teamwork* (between nurses and aides) affects missed nursing care—ambulation, turning, feeding, patient teaching, discharge planning, emotional support, hygiene, intake and output, and surveillance. Here there is a lack of essential elements of teamwork (i.e., closed-looped communication, leadership, team orientation, trust, and shared mental models). She advocates including aides in planning at the beginning of the shift (that aides also attend report) and providing debriefings during the shift so that nurses and aides can discuss the status of their work and revise the plan of care for the rest of the shift.

Teamwork also includes *working effectively with physicians and other disciplines*.

> *Improving only one component of an agency will not affect overall productivity.* Productivity improvement involves a systematic assessment of the entire organization rather than just a staffing review. For example, a physical therapist's job tasks may be tied to secretaries who answer the phones and screen calls, to data processing (records may not be transcribed and given back to the therapist for use during the scheduled visit), and to other disciplines. The therapist may have to wait for the home health aide to arrive to supervise the visit or to meet with an RN regarding the client. One provider group cannot improve or change productivity unless other components of the system are evaluated. Therefore, do not expect the RN staff to increase productivity unless productivity improvements occur in other components of the system in which RNs work. (Harris, 1997, p. 471)

Sixth, *missed care* issues plague nurses (and nurse aides) as they realize they are missing some of the work that needs to be done but just do not have time to complete it properly. Missed work often includes turning, ambulating, feeding, mouthcare, and toileting. Reasons for missed work include

> unexpected increase in volume or acuity, heavy admission or discharge activity, and inadequate support staff. . . . Disturbing findings not previously noted in the literature were that 88% of the nurse managers stated that omissions had been reported to them, with 67% reporting that these omissions occurred frequently. (Gravlin, & Bittner, 2010)

Kalisch and Williams (2009) developed a quantitative tool to measure missed care, and Kalisch and Lee (2012) reported a lack of congruence among nursing leaders and staff: "staff reported less missed care and lower teamwork than do leaders, and staff list more problems with having adequate material and labor resources than do leaders" (p. 473).

Seventh, many *workflow issues and interruptions* occur. Cornell and colleagues (2010, 2011) discuss the chaotic pace when switching activities or locations occurs. The most frequent activities nurses perform are assessment, charting, and communication. Many *interruptions* occur that detract from critical thinking (Hall, Pedersen, & Fairly, 2010). Nurses averaged more than 15 minutes on each medication pass and were at risk of an interruption or distraction with *every* medication pass (Elganzouri, Standish, & Androwich, 2009, p. 204). Cornell and associates (2010) call this *abrupt switching*—when patients or others need them or when waiting for something, they switch to something else because of a heavy workload. "The nonrepetitive flow and high amount of switching indicate nurses experience a heavy cognitive load with little uninterrupted time" (Cornell & Riordan, 2011, p. 407). This can create errors and decrease task efficiency (Biron, Lavoie-Tremblay, & Loiselle, 2009; Trbovich, Prakash, & Stewart, 2010). Thus, in many facilities the nurse giving medications is identifiable in some way (she or he wears a vest) and others know not to interrupt this person while the vest is on.

Eighth, *non-value-added time* (when staff are doing nonreal work), already discussed earlier, also decreases productivity.

Ninth, sometimes lower productivity has *environmental causes*, such as not having enough supplies, equipment, or technology to properly do the work; problems with the physical layout; or long distances for staff to travel to provide home care. Manojlovich (2010) found that "nurses may practice more professionally when the environment provides opportunities and power through resources, support, and information."

In fact, this text not only has financial implications but productivity effects. Poor leadership, poor management, unnecessary or ineffective organizational processes, and poor performance all result in productivity ineffectiveness.

At times, low productivity may be apparent overall, even when productivity seems high. For example, if not enough staff are available to work, staff may be doing as much as possible for patients yet know that more needs to be done. As staff frustration mounts, it is easy for them to start missing important things that should happen (the missed care issue). In this case, efficiency looks wonderful but effectiveness suffers. When all productivity measurements are combined, the result is actually low productivity.

Productivity Improvement

Productivity measurement in health care cannot stand alone. Productivity improvement is everyone's—all staff at all levels—responsibility. *Productivity is linked with organizational viability.* This text is designed to improve productivity.

Course Correction

Asking the questions is not enough. We need to experiment with and implement solutions. Many will fail, but some will improve how we serve our patients. Implementation is the key. And each of us can share what works with each other.

As previously mentioned, one of the best examples of productivity improvement is the interdisciplinary process used by ThedaCare in Wisconsin, which has dramatically improved patient outcomes and examined changes based on what patients value. This is described in the book *On the Mend: Revolutionizing Healthcare to Save Lives and Transform the Industry* (Toussaint & Gerard, with Adams, 2010). The authors used a process-improvement approach to create "messes" by examining the interdisciplinary steps involved in treating patients and determining whether patients even valued what they did. All this resulted in better efficiencies, better patient outcomes, and better service providing what the patient valued. The information in the book is eye-opening; it describes a much better way to achieve change. Understand that this method is fraught with difficulties because it is going to step on some interdisciplinary sacred cows! It can result in some real disagreements! Yet the outcomes (in quality, efficiencies, satisfaction) are *so* much better for both the patients and the interdisciplinary staff involved in achieving financial viability.

Information Systems

Information systems play a central role in providing efficient and effective clinical services. Information technology positively affects quality of care and nurses' daily work (DesRoches, Miralles, & Buerhaus, 2011; Waneka & Spetz, 2010). Cornell and colleagues (2010) found that computer usage has increased, but "time with patients and verbal communication remained unchanged as nurses seem to incorporate the new requirements into their normal routine" (p. 432).

We are experiencing an information and technology explosion! Douglas (2011) advocates that the nurse executive is the key to achieving the maximum benefits from staffing and scheduling technologies. Having project leaders and staff involved in choosing technologies is important, but the nurse executive, who has an overall perspective of facility staffing/scheduling issues and the strategic plan, must make sure that the workforce is headed in the best direction to achieve the best results.

Four informatics processes can support nurse staffing decisions (Hyun et al., 2008):

1. **Data acquisition from multiple data sources**. Information systems track the flow of patients, locate staff, use bar coding for patients and supplies, track call systems, process medication administration, monitor quality and safety indicators, provide documentation systems, and keep track of qualifications and competencies of staff. All this can capture nurse workload, although presently the proprietary nature of many of these systems and the lack of data integration among systems diminish effectiveness.
2. **Representation of data so that they can be reused for multiple purposes**. Scheduling, staffing, budgeting, payroll, finance, workload measurement, charging for supplies/services, and human resource management are many of the systems that, with better integration, can use the same patient information/diagnoses/care and administrative data for several purposes.
3. **Sophisticated data processing and mining**. This is being examined to determine better ways to use the information.
4. **Presentation of data in standardized and user-configurable ways**. Increasingly, decision support systems are used for evidence-based management decisions in health care. Providing automated processes that use operational report data for creating dashboards can combine indicators of clinical outcomes and resource utilization. Web-based dashboards for benchmarking, staffing and scheduling, and providing education are being developed. (pp. 154–157)

Bedside computers and clinical information systems have revolutionized hospital nursing (Shi & Singh, 2004). Software packages are available for staffing, scheduling, and budgeting actual use of staff. Integrating these systems with financial/accounting and human resource systems is still a work in progress. The use of bar coding for supply charging and medication dispensing/administration, instant test result retrieval and analysis via computer systems, hand-held charting devices, transcription options, and telemedicine technology have all affected care outcomes and the structure and processes of healthcare delivery. Technology for real-time matching of patient care needs with caregiver skill profiles from staffing and scheduling systems has emerged as an essential tool in achieving staffing excellence.

Computerized systems record the actual times of all direct and indirect nursing care activities. Currently, efforts are under way to interface documented caregiver interventions with their associated time standards and scheduling systems. Time computations and acuity ratings will be automatically calculated and updated in real time. Once all activities of caregivers can be labeled and documented, all documented activity performed for the patient can be identified. Staffing needs can then be calculated while avoiding subjectivity and information delay. With these advances, the calculation of staff hours and skill mix from documentation eliminates the need for caregivers to rate, score, or select interventions in a separate process.

Summary

Patient care leaders and managers need reliable measurement tools to determine safe and effective nurse staffing. Tools such as patient classification systems were initially developed decades ago, and much work is still needed to make these tools useful and trusted. The updates to current tools reflect some of the changes in technology, care delivery, and patient populations served and unfortunately still result in varying degrees of success.

With the development of new approaches to patient care, new parameters with corresponding methodology to measure the resources required for that care are essential to progress in the technological age. The measurement of patient care services has moved away from the specific cost accounting approaches popular 10 years ago to the analysis of data from relational databases. Collaboration with management engineers and financial experts is necessary to advance current systems.

At the patient care and caregiver level, variance from predicted, expected, or best practices provides data needed by nurse executives and financial officers, managed care plan administrators, and state and federal governments that administer health benefits. At the service and system level, data that provide insight into cause, effect, and system interactions are more useful for improving care. At the organized delivery system level, data specific to the extent to which processes and management methods influence the quality of practice can provide new insights into resource utilization, prioritization of services, and patient safety.

Discussion Questions

1. Evaluate a staffing plan for a unit.
2. If you had to choose a patient classification system for a nursing unit, which type would you choose? Give your rationale.
3. Explain how you would establish validity and reliability of a patient classification system.
4. How would you determine the skill mix for an inpatient unit? Give your rationale.
5. Do you believe there should be state legislation concerning RN staffing ratios? If so, describe what it should contain. Give a rationale for this answer.
6. How does pay for performance affect staffing?
7. How can you determine whether there is staffing adequacy?
8. Describe the components to establish competency for a staff nurse in your work area.
9. Describe staffing variances that occur. How would you deal with them effectively?

10. Give an example of productivity measurement in your facility? Evaluate it.
11. How could you improve productivity in your work unit?
12. Are any of the productivity misconceptions occurring in your workplace? If so, what are they and how could a nurse administrator more effectively influence productivity measurement in that setting?
13. Make a list of the components of a workforce management system that are based on evidence.
14. Give five examples where evidence has changed how we accomplish workforce management.
15. Why is a complexity model better than a systems model for workforce management?
16. How might generational differences affect staffing?
17. Explain why some administrators cling to the myths. How could this be changed?
18. Design a dashboard of metrics including qualitative and quantitative measures for a patient care unit.

Glossary of Terms

Acuity—the level of need or dependency of an individual patient.

Ambulatory Payment Classification (APC)—relative value units that reflect the complexity of each procedure.

Case Mix Method—a method of clustering patients into groups that are homogeneous with respect to the use of resources. Includes diagnosis-related groups (DRGs) for hospitals; resource utilization groups (RUGs) for long-term care; ambulatory payment classification (APCs) for ambulatory settings; and Outcome and Assessment Information Set (OASIS) and home health resource groups (HHRGs) for home care.

Classification—the ordering of entities into groups or classes on the basis of their similarity, minimizing within-group variance and maximizing between-group variance.

Comprehensive Unit of Service—an aggregate of eight categories of care, representing the total care provided by nursing during a shift or event of care and integrating a multitasking factor to account for the overlap of care in identified patient situations.

Construct Validity—the fit between the conceptual definitions and operational definitions of the variables.

Content Validity—the extent to which the patient classification tool includes all of the major elements relative to the construct being measured.

Core Schedules—an aggregated average number and skill mix required for patient care focusing on having sufficient staff to care for the population served; the long-range plan that becomes the template for the required number of staff.

DRG System—diagnosis-related group system; a system that categorized the types of patients a hospital treats based on diagnoses, procedures, age, sex, and the presence of complications or comorbidities. DRGs work by taking more than 10,000 ICD-9-CM (soon to be 10) codes and grouping them into a more manageable number of meaningful patient categories. Patients within each category are similar clinically in terms of resource usage.

Expert Opinion or Expert Panel—a panel of experts; individuals with a great deal of experience and ability to estimate time in their area of expertise who identify the time requirements for certain work.

External Validity—the extent to which the findings can be generalized beyond the sample used.

Face Validity—a type of validity that is high when nurses believe that the system accurately reflects and represents the work that they do or the dependency of the patients for whom they provide care.

Factor Evaluation Method—a method of identifying selected elements of care, critical indicators, or tasks with associated times that are most likely predictors of nursing care needs.

Home Health Resource Groups (HHRGs)—OASIS (Outcome and Assessment Information Set) used in home care.

ICD System—a system used to code official disease classification activities in the United States and to code and classify mortality data from death certificates.

Internal Validity—the extent to which the measures used in the patient classification tool are a true reflection of reality.

Motion and Time Studies—studies involving continuous timed observations of a single person during a typical time period or shift of work.

Nursing Intervention Classifications (NICs)—a comprehensive, standardized language that describes treatments that nurses perform in all settings and in all specialties. NICs include eight foundational domains: physiological (e.g., acid–base management), psychosocial (e.g., anxiety reduction), illness treatment (e.g., hyperglycemia management), illness prevention (e.g., fall prevention), health promotion (e.g., exercise promotion), interventions for individuals or for families (e.g., family integrity promotion), indirect care interventions (e.g., emergency cart checking), and interventions for communities (e.g., environmental management).

Patient Classification—a process of grouping patients into homogeneous, mutually exclusive groups to determine their dependency on caregivers or to determine patient acuity.

Position Control—the process used by human resources to specify actual full-time equivalents (FTEs) assigned to a unit or department.

Productivity—a process of getting more out of what you put in, doing better with what you have, and achieving more efficiencies linked with effectiveness.

Prototype Approach—identifying the characteristics of patients into categories. Individual patients are then assigned to the category that most closely reflects their nursing care requirements.

Relative Value Unit (RVU)—in addition to grouping patients into similar categories based on nursing care needs, a patient classification system can also quantify the workforce within the categories by assigning a relative value to each category.

Reliability—the consistency of rating in a patient classification system.

Resource Utilization Groups (RUGs)—used in long-term care; use the minimum data set, which consists of a core set of screening elements to assess the clinical, functional, and psychosocial needs of each resident. Using the data gained from the minimum data set assessment, RUGs differentiate residents by their use of resources.

Self-Reporting—a technique used to determine time associated with employee activities.

Sensitivity—refers to physiological measures and is related to the amount of change of a parameter that can be measured precisely.

Skill Mix—the various types of nursing staff by job classification necessary to care for the patient population.

Staffing Plan—the structure and process by which responsibilities for patient care are assigned and how the work is coordinated among caregivers.

Standard Data Setting—use of time standards developed from past experiences.

Validity—the degree to which a patient classification system actually measures what it intends to measure.

Work Sampling—a time study technique that samples work activities at systematic or random intervals.

References

Admi, H., Tzischinsky, O., Epstein, R., Herber, P., & Lavie, P. (2008). Shift work in nursing: Is it really a risk factor for nurses' health and patients' safety? *Nursing Economic$, 26*(4), 250–257.

Aiken, L., Clarke, S., Cheung, R., Sloane, D., & Silber, J. (2003). Educational levels of hospital nurses and surgical patient mortality. *Journal of the American Medical Association, 290,* 1617–1623.

Aiken, L., Clarke, S., Sloane, D., Lake, E., & Cheney, T. (2008). Effects of hospital care environment on patient mortality and nurse outcomes. *Journal of Nursing Administration, 38*(5), 223–229.

Aiken, L., Clarke, S., Sloane, D., Sochalski, J., & Silber, J. (2002). Hospital nurse staffing and patient mortality, nurse burnout, and job dissatisfaction. *Journal of the American Medical Association, 288*(16), 1987–1993.

Aiken, L., & Patrician, P. (2000). Measuring organizational traits of hospitals: The revised nursing work index. *Nursing Research, 49*(3), 146–153.

Allen, S., Fiorini, P., & Dickey, M. (2010). A streamlined clinical advancement program improves RN participation and retention. *Journal of Nursing Administration, 40*(7/8), 316–322.

Altaffer, A. (1998). First-line managers: Measuring their span of control. *Nursing Management, 29*(7), 36–39.

Amendolair, D. (2012). Caring behaviors and job satisfaction. *Journal of Nursing Administration, 42*(1), 34–39.

American Nurses Association. (1989). *Classification systems for describing nursing practice.* Kansas City, MO: Author.

American Nurses Association. (2001). *2001 ANA staffing survey.* Washington, DC: American Nurses Publishing.

American Nurses Association. (2003). *Nurse staffing plans and ratios.* Kansas City, MO: Author.

American Nurses Association. (2012). *ANA principles for nurse staffing.* Silver Spring, MD: Author.

American Organization of Nurse Executives. (2000). *Perspectives on the nursing shortage: A blueprint for action.* Monograph Series. Chicago, IL: Author.

American Recovery and Reinvestment Act of 2009, 111th U.S.H.R. § 13001–13424, 3000–3018. (2009). Retrieved from http://frwebgate.access.gpo.gov/cgi-bin/getdoc.cgi?dbname=111_cong_bills&docid=f:h1enr.pdf

Applebaum, D., Osinubi, O., Fowler, S., Robson, M., & Fiedler, N. (2010). The impact of environmental factors on nursing stress, job satisfaction, and turnover intention. *Journal of Nursing Administration, 40*(7/8), 323–328.

Autrey, P., Howard, J., & Wech, B. (2013). Sources, reactions, and tactics used by RNs to address aggression in an acute care hospital: A qualitative analysis. *Journal of Nursing Administration, 43*(3), 155–159.

Bae, S. (2012). Nursing overtime: Why, how much, and under what working conditions? *Nursing Economic$, 30*(2), 60–71.

Barton, N. (2011). Matching nurse staffing to demand. *Nursing Management, 42*(2), 36–39.

Beauregard, M., Davis, J., & Kutash, M. (2007). The graduate nurse rotational internship: A successful recruitment and retention strategy in medical-surgical services. *Journal of Nursing Administration, 37*(3), 115–118.

Behner, K., Fogg, L., Fournier, L., Frankenbach, J., & Robertson, S. (1990). Nursing resource management: Analyzing the relationship between costs and quality in staffing decisions. *Health Care Management Review, 15*(4), 63–71.

Berkow, S., Jaggi, T., & Fogelson, R. (2007). Fourteen unit attributes to guide staffing. *Journal of Nursing Administration, 37*(3), 150–155.

Biron, A., Lavoie-Tremblay, M., & Loiselle, C. (2020). Characteristics of work interruptions during medication administration. *Journal of Nursing Scholarship, 41*(4), 330–336.

Blegen, M., Goode, C., Spetz, J., Vaughn, T., & Park, S. (2011). Nurse staffing effects on patient outcomes: Safety-net and non-safety-net hospitals. *Medical Care, 49*(4), 406–414.

Bleich, M., Cleary, B., & Davis, K. (2009). Mitigating knowledge loss: A strategic imperative for nurse leaders. *Journal of Nursing Administration, 39*(4), 160–164.

Boev, C. (2012). The relationship between nurses' perception of work environment and patient satisfaction in adult critical care. *Journal of Nursing Scholarship, 44*(4), 368–375.

Bolton, L., Jones, D., Aydin, C., Donaldson, N., Brown, D., Lowe, M., et al. (2001). A response to California's mandated nursing ratios. *Journal of Nursing Scholarship, 33*(2), 179–184.

Brady. (2001). Sitting in the dark. *Organizational Effectiveness, 1*(7), 1–3.

Brakovich, B., & Bonham, E. (2012). Solving the retention puzzle: Let's begin with nursing orientation. *Nurse Leader, 10*(5), 50–53.

Brewer, C., & Frazier, P. (1998). The influence of structure, staff type, and managed-care indicators on registered nurse staffing. *Journal of Nursing Administration, 28*(9), 28–36.

Bryant-Hampton, L., & Walton, A. (2010). Recognition: A key retention strategy for the mature nurse. *Journal of Nursing Administration, 40*(3), 121–123.

Buerhaus, P. (2010). What is the harm in imposing mandatory hospital nurse staffing regulations? *and* It's time to stop the regulation of hospital nurse staffing dead in its tracks. *Nursing Economic$, 28*(2), 87–93, 110–113.

Buffington, A., Zwink, J., & Fink, R. (2012). Factors affecting nurse retention at an academic Magnet hospital. *Journal of Nursing Administration, 42*(5), 273–281.

Burke, T., McKee, J., Wilson, H., Donahue, R. M., Batenhorst, A., & Pathak, D. (2000). A comparison of time-and-motion and self reporting methods of work measurement. *Journal of Nursing Administration, 30*(3), 118–125.

Burns, N., & Grove, S. (2001). *The practice of nursing research: Conduct, critique and utilization* (4th ed.). Philadelphia, PA: Saunders.

Cairns, L., Hoffmann, R., Dudjak, L., & Lorenz, H. (2013). Utilizing bedside shift report to improve the effectiveness of shift handoff. *Journal of Nursing Administration, 43*(4), 160–165.

Carlson, S. (2013). Make it a habit: 2 weeks to bedside report. *Nursing Management, 44*(3), 554.

Cathro, H. (2013). A practical guide to making patient assignments in acute care. *Journal of Nursing Administration, 43*(1), 6–9.

Cavouras, C., & McKinley, J. (1998). Annual survey of hours. *Perspectives on Staffing and Scheduling, 17*(3), 3.

Chang, C., Price, S., & Pfoutz, S. (2001). *Economics and nursing: Critical professional issues.* Philadelphia, PA: F. A. Davis.

Cho, S., Ketefian, S., Barkauska, V., & Smith, D. (2003). The effects of nurse staffing on adverse events, morbidity, mortality and medical costs. *Nursing Research, 52*(2), 71–79.

Christmas, K. (2008). How work environment impacts retention. *Nursing Economic$, 26*(5), 316–318.

Clancy, T., in Fitzpatrick, T., & Brooks, B. (2010). The nurse leader as logistician: Optimizing human capital. *Journal of Nursing Administration, 40*(2), 69–74.

Coleman, E., Lockhart, K., Montgomery, R., & McNatt, P. (2010). Effect of certification in oncology nursing on nursing-sensitive outcomes. *Journal of Nursing Administration, 40*(Suppl. 10), S35–S42.

Cornell, P., & Riordan, M. (2011). Barriers to critical thinking: Workflow interruptions and task switching among nurses. *Journal of Nursing Administration, 41*(10), 407–414.

Cornell, P., Riordan, M., & Herrin Griffith, D. (2010). Transforming nursing workflow, Parts 1 and 2: The chaotic nature of nurse activities & The impact of technology on nurse activities. *Journal of Nursing Administration, 40*(9,10), 366–373, 432–439.

Coshow, S., Davis, P., & Wolosin, R. (2009). The "big dip": Decrements in RN satisfaction at mid-career. *Nursing Economic$*, *27*(1), 15–18.

Crawford, C., Omery, A., & Seago, J. (2012). The challenges of nurse–physician communication: A review of the evidence. *Journal of Nursing Administration*, *42*(12), 548–550.

Curtin, L. (2003). An integrated analysis of nurse staffing and related variables: Effects on patient outcomes. *Online Journal of Issues in Nursing*, *8*(3), 5.

DeGroot, H. (1994). Patient classification systems and staffing: Part 1. Problems and promise. *Journal of Nursing Administration*, *24*(9), 43–51.

Demir, D., & Rodwell, J. (2012). Psychosocial antecedents and consequences of workplace aggression for hospital nurses. *Journal of Nursing Scholarship*, *44*(4), 376–384.

DesRoches, C., Miralles, P., & Buerhaus, P. (2011). *Journal of Nursing Administration*, *41*(9), 357–364.

Douglas, D., & Mayewski, J. (1996). Census variation staffing. *Nursing Management*, *27*(2), 32–36.

Douglas, K. (2009). The naked truth: Staffing in health care needs an overhaul. *Nursing Economic$*, *27*(5), 332–334.

Douglas, K. (2010a). Ratios—If it were only that easy. *Nursing Economic$*, *28*(2), 119–125.

Douglas, K. (2010b). When caring stops, staffing doesn't really matter. *Nursing Economic$*, *28*(6), 415–419.

Douglas, K. (2011). What every nurse executive should know about staffing and scheduling technology initiatives. *Nursing Economic$*, *29*(5), 273–275.

Duffield, C., Diers, D., Aisbett, C., & Roche, M. (2009). Churn: Patient turnover and case mix. *Nursing Economic$*, *27*(3), 185–191.

Dunham-Taylor, J., & Pinczuk, J. (2006). *Health care financial management for nurse managers: Applications from hospitals, long-term care, home care, and ambulatory care*. Sudbury, MA: Jones and Bartlett.

Dunn, M., Norby, R., Cournoyer, P., Hudec, S., O'Donnell, J., & Snider, M. (1995). Expert panel method for nurse staffing and resource management. *Journal of Nursing Administration*, *25*(10), 61–67.

Dykes, P., Rothschild, J., & Hurley, A. (2010). Medical errors recovered by critical care nurses. *Journal of Nursing Administration*, *40*(5), 241–246.

Eggenberger, T. (2012). Exploring the charge nurse role: Holding the frontline. *Journal of Nursing Administration*, *42*(11), 502–506.

Elganzouri, E., Standish, C., & Androwich, I. (2009). Medication administration time study (MATS): Nursing staff performance of medication administration. *Journal of Nursing Administration*, *39*(5), 204–210.

Fertise, P., & Baggot, D. (2009). Improving staff nurse satisfaction and nurse turnover: Use of a closed-unit staffing model. *Journal of Nursing Administration*, *19*(7/8), 318–320.

Fink, R., & Krugman, M. (2008). The graduate nurse experience: Qualitative residency program outcomes. *Journal of Nursing Administration*, *38*(7/8), 341–348.

Finkler, S. (2001). *Budgeting concepts for nurse managers* (3rd ed.). Philadelphia, PA: Saunders.

Fralic, M. (Ed.). (2000). *Staffing management and methods: Tools and techniques for nursing leaders*. Chicago, IL: AHA Press.

Fraser, S. (2010). Influencing outlook: The importance of nursing staff satisfaction. *Nursing Management*, *31*(9), 12–16.

Friese, C., & Himes-Ferris, L. (2013). Nursing practice environments and job outcomes in ambulatory oncology settings. *Journal of Nursing Administration*, *43*(3), 149–154.

Frith, K., Anderson, E., Tseng, F., & Fong, E. (2012). Nurse staffing is an important strategy to prevent medication errors in community hospitals. *Nursing Economic$*, *30*(5), 288–294.

Gardner, A., & Gemme, E. (2003). Virtual scheduling: A 21st century approach to staffing. *Nursing Administration Quarterly*, *27*(1), 77–82.

Garry, R. (2000). Benchmarking: A prescription for healthcare. *Journal of Nursing Administration*, *30*(9), 397–398.

Geiger-Brown, J., & Trinkoff, A. (2010). Is it time to pull the plug on 12-hour shifts? Part 1. The evidence. Part 3. Harm reduction strategies if keeping 12-hour shifts. *Journal of Nursing Administration*, *40* (3,4,9), 100–102, 357–359.

Gess, E., Manojlovich, M., & Warner, S. (2008). An evidence-based protocol for nurse retention. *Journal of Nursing Administration*, *38*(10), 441–447.

Gift, A., & Soeken, K. (1988). Assessment of physiologic instruments. *Heart and Lung*, *17*(2), 128–133.

Good, E., & Bishop, P. (2011). Willing to walk: A creative strategy to minimize stress related to floating. *Journal of Nursing Administration*, *41*(5), 231–234.

Gordon, M. (1998). Nursing nomenclature and classification system development. *Online Journal of Issues in Nursing, 3*(2). Retrieved from http://www.nursingworld.org/MainMenuCategories/ANAMarketplace/ANAPeriodicals/OJIN/TableofContents/Vol31998/No2Sept1998/NomenclatureandClassification.html

Gravlin, G., & Bittner, N. (2010). Nurses' and nursing assistants' reports of missed care and delegation. *Journal of Nursing Administration, 40*(7/8), 329–335.

Haeberle, S., & Christmas, K. (2006, November–December). Recruitment and retention metrics: Implications for leadership. *Nursing Economic$, 24*(6), 328–330.

Halfer, D. (2007). A magnetic strategy for new graduate nurses. *Nursing Economic$, 25*(1), 6–12.

Halfer, D., Graf, E., & Sullivan, C. (2008). The organizational impact of a new graduate pediatric nurse mentoring program. *Nursing Economic$, 26*(4), 243–249.

Hall, L. M., Pedersen, C., & Fairley, L. (2010). Losing the moment: understanding interruptions to nurses' work. *Journal of Nursing Administration, 40*(4), 169–176.

Hall, L., Peterson, J., Lalonde, M., Cripps, L., & Dales, L. (2011). Strategies for retaining midcareer nurses. *Journal of Nursing Administration, 41*(12), 531–537.

Hall, L., Pink, G., Johnson, L., & Schraa, E. (2000). Development of a nursing management practice atlas: Part 2, variation in use of nursing and financial resources. *Journal of Nursing Administration, 30*(9), 440–448.

Han, K., & Trinkoff, A. (2011). Job stress and work schedules in relation to nurse obesity. *Journal of Nursing Administration, 41*(11), 488–495.

Hardin, D. (2012). Strategies for nurse leaders to address aggressive and violent events. *Journal of Nursing Administration, 42*(1), 5–8.

Harper, E. (2012). Staffing based on evidence: Can health information technology make it possible? *Nursing Economic$, 30*(5), 262–267.

Harris, M. (1997). *Handbook of home health care administration* (2nd ed.). Gaithersburg, MD: Aspen.

Hart, K. (2009). Boomerang recruitment: Bridging the gap. *Nursing Economic$, 27*(1), 56–57.

Hasman, A., Wiersma, D., Halfens, R., & Algera, J. (1993). Evaluation of a patient classification system for community health care. *International Journal of Bio-Medical Computing, 33*, 109–118.

Hausfield, J., Gibbons, K., Holmeier, A., Knight, C., Stadmiller, T., & Yeary, K. (1994). Self-staffing: Improving care and staff satisfaction. *Nursing Management, 25*(1), 74–80.

Hernandez, C., & O'Brien, P. (1996a). Validity and reliability of nursing workload measurement systems: Review of validity and reliability theory. Part 1. *Canadian Journal of Nursing Administration, 9*(3), 16–25.

Hernandez, C., & O'Brien, P. (1996b). Validity and reliability of nursing workload measurement systems: Review of validity and reliability theory. Part 2. *Canadian Journal of Nursing Administration, 10*(3), 16–23.

Herdman, T., Burgess, L., Ebright, P., & Paulson, S. (2009). Impact of continuous vigilance monitoring on nursing workflow. *Journal of Nursing Administration, 39*(3), 123–129.

Hickey, P., Gauvreau, K., & Connor, J. (2010). The relationship of nurse staffing, skill mix, and Magnet recognition to institutional volume and mortality for congenital heart surgery. *Journal of Nursing Administration, 40*(5), 226–232.

Hill, K. (2010). A business case for phased retirement: Will it work for nursing? *Journal of Nursing Administration, 40*(7/8), 302–308.

Hill, K. (2011). Work satisfaction, intent to stay, desires of nurses, and financial knowledge among bedside and advanced practice nurses. *Journal of Nursing Administration, 41*(5), 211–217.

Hill, K., Cleary, B., & Hewlett, P. (2010). Commentary: Experienced RN retention strategies: What can be learned from top-performing organizations. *Journal of Nursing Administration, 40*(11), 468–470.

Hinson, T., & Spatz, D. (2011). Improving nurse retention in a large tertiary acute-care hospital. *Journal of Nursing Administration, 41*(3), 103–108.

Hirschkorn, C., West, T., & Hill, K. (2010). Experienced nurse retention strategies: What can be learned from top-performing organizations. *Journal of Nursing Administration, 40*(11), 463–467.

Hollabaugh, S., & Kendrick, S. (1998). Staffing: The five-level pyramid. *Nursing Management, 29*(2), 34–36.

Hyun, S., Bakken, S., Douglas, K., & Stone, P. (2008). Evidence-based staffing: Potential roles for informatics. *Nursing Economic$, 26*(3), 151–173.

Institute of Medicine. (2010). *The future of nursing: Leading change, advancing health*. Washington, DC: National Academies Press.

Johnson, S., & Rea, R. (2009). Workplace bullying: Concerns for nurse leaders. *Journal of Nursing Administration, 39*(2), 84–90.

The Joint Commission. (2002). *Health care at the crossroads: Strategies for addressing the evolving nursing crisis*. Retrieved from http://www.jointcommission.org/assets/1/18/health_care_at_the_crossroads.pdf

Jones, C. (2008). Revisiting nurse turnover costs: Adjusting for inflation. *Journal of Nursing Administration, 38*(1), 16.

Kalisch, B. (2009). Nursing and nurse assistant perceptions of missed nursing care: What does it tell us about teamwork? *Journal of Nursing Administration, 39*(11), 485–493.

Kalisch, B., Begeny, S., & Anderson, C. (2008). The effect of consistent nursing shifts on teamwork and continuity of care. *Journal of Nursing Administration, 38*(3), 132–137.

Kalisch, B., & Lee, K. (2012). Congruence of perceptions among nursing leaders and staff regarding missed nursing care and teamwork. *Journal of Nursing Administration, 42*(10), 473–477.

Kalisch, B., & Williams, R. (2009). Development and psychometric testing of a tool to measure missed nursing care. *Journal of Nursing Administration, 39*(5), 211–219.

Kane, R., Shamliyan, T., Mueller, C., Duval, S., & Wilt, T. (2007). The association of registered nurse staffing levels and patients outcomes: Systematic review and meta-analysis. *Medical Care, 45*(12), 1195–1204.

Kavanagh, K., Cimiotti, J., Abusalem, S., & Coty, M. (2012). Moving healthcare quality forward with nursing-sensitive value-based purchasing. *Journal of Nursing Scholarship, 44*(4), 385–395.

Keller, J., Meekins, I., & Summers, B. (2006). Pearls and pitfalls of a new graduate academic residency program. *Journal of Nursing Administration, 36*(12), 589–598.

Kendall-Gallagher, D., & Blegen, M. (2010). Competence and certification of registered nurses and safety of patients in intensive care units. *Journal of Nursing Administration, 40*(10 Suppl.), S68–S77.

Kovner, C., Greene, W., Brewer, C., & Fairchild, S. (2009). Understanding new registered nurses' intent to stay at their jobs. *Nursing Economic$, 27*(2), 81–98.

Kramer, M., & Halfer, D. (2012). Impact of healthy work environments and multistage nurse residency programs on retention of newly licensed RNs. *Journal of Nursing Administration, 42*(3), 148–159.

Kramer, M., Maguire, P., & Schmalenberg, C. (2006). Excellence through evidence: The what, when, and where of clinical autonomy. *Journal of Nursing Administration, 36*(10), 479–491.

Kupperschmidt, B. (2002). Unlicensed assistive personnel retention and realistic job previews. *Nursing Economic$, 20*(6), 279–283.

Kuthy, J., Ostmann, J., Gonzalez, R., & Biddle, D. (2013). Predicting successful nursing performance. *Nursing Management, 44*(1), 43–52.

Lacey, S., Cox, K., Teasley, S., Bonura, A., Henion, J., & Brown, J. (2008). Enhancing the work environment of staff nurses using targeted interventions of support. *Journal of Nursing Administration, 38*(7/8), 336–340.

LaDuke, S. (2000). Nurses' perceptions: Is your nurse uncomfortable or incompetent? *Journal of Nursing Administration, 30*(4), 163–165.

Lavoie-Tremblay, M., Paquet, M., Duchesne, M., Santo, A., Gavrancic, A., Courcy, F., et al. (2010). Retaining nurses and other hospital workers: An intergenerational perspective of the work climate. *Journal of Nursing Scholarship, 42*(4), 414–422.

Lavoie-Tremblay, M., Wright, D., Desforges, N., Gelinas, C., Marchionni, C., & Drevniok, U. (2008). Creating a healthy workplace for new-generation nurses. *Journal of Nursing Scholarship, 40*(3), 290–297.

Lawrence, W., & Sherrod, D. (2010). From Wall Street to Main Street. . . to your hospital. *Nursing Management, 41*(1), 31–34.

Lefton, C. (2012). Strengthening the workforce through meaningful recognition. *Nursing Economic$, 30*(6), 331–338.

Lerner, N., & Resnick, B. (2011). Job satisfaction of nursing assistants. *Journal of Nursing Administration, 41*(11), 473–478.

Letvak, S., & Buck, R. (2008). Factors influencing work productivity and intent to stay in nursing. *Nursing Economic$, 26*(3), 159–165.

Longo, J., & Sherman, R. (2007). Leveling horizontal violence. *Nursing Management, 38*(3), 34–37, 50.

Lorenz, S. (2008). 12-hour shifts: An ethical dilemma for the nurse executive. *Journal of Nursing Administration, 38*(6), 297–301.

Malloch, K., & Conovaloff, A. (1999). Patient classification systems, Part 1: The third generation. *Journal of Nursing Administration, 29*(7), 49–56.

Manojlovich, M. (2010). Predictors of professional nursing practice behaviors in hospital settings. *Journal of Nursing Administration, 40*(10 Suppl.), S45–S51.

Manojlovich, M., & Antonakos, C. (2008). Satisfaction of intensive care unit nurses with nurse–physician communication. *Journal of Nursing Administration, 38*(5), 237–243.

Manthey, M. (2001). A core incremental staffing plan. *Journal of Nursing Administration, 31*(9), 424–425.

Mark, B. (2002). What explains nurses' perceptions of staffing adequacy? *Journal of Nursing Administration, 32*(5), 234–242.

Mark, B., & Burleson, D. (1995). Measurement of patient outcomes: Data availability and consistency across hospitals. *Journal of Nursing Administration, 25*(4), 52–59.

Mason, D. (2003). How many patients are too many? Legislating staffing ratios is good for nursing. *American Journal of Nursing, 103*(11), 7.

McCloskey, J., & Bulechek, G. (Eds.). (2000). *Nursing interventions classification (NIC)* (3rd ed.). St. Louis, MO: Mosby.

McClung, T. (2000). Assessing the reported financial benefits of unlicensed assistive personnel in nursing. *Journal of Nursing Administration, 30*(11), 530–534.

McConnell, E. (2001). Competence vs. competency. *Nursing Management, 32*(5), 14.

McCue, M. (2003). Nurse staffing, quality and financial performance. *Journal of Health Care Finance, 29*(4), 54–76.

Melberg, S. (1997). Effects of changing skill mix. *Nursing Management, 28*(110), 47–48.

Meretoja, R., & Leino-Kilpi, H. (2001). Instruments for evaluating nurse competence. *Journal of Nursing Administration, 31*(7/8), 346–352.

Miller, J. (2011). When time isn't on your side: 12-hour shifts. *Nursing Management, 42*(6), 39–43.

Mills, J., & Mullins, A. (2008). The California nurse mentor project: Every nurse deserves a mentor. *Nursing Economic$, 26*(5), 310–315.

Mumolie, G., Lichtig, L., & Knauf, R. (2007). The implications of nurse staffing information: The real value of reporting nursing data. *Nursing Economic$, 25*(4), 212–227.

Needleman, J., Buerhaus, P., Mattke, S., Stewart, M., & Zelevinsky, K. (2002). Nurse staffing levels and the quality of care in hospitals. *New England Journal of Medicine, 346*(22), 1715–1722.

Needleman, J., Buerhaus, P., Pankratz, V., Leibson, C., Stevens, S., & Harris, M. (2011). Nurse staffing and inpatient hospital mortality. *New England Journal of Medicine, 364*(11), 1037–1045.

Needleman, J., Buerhaus, P. I., Stewart, M., Zelevinsky, K., & Mattke, S. (2006). Nurse staffing in hospitals: Is there a business case for quality. *Health Affairs, 25*(1), 204–211.

Nelson, B., & Massey, R. (2010). Implementing an electronic change-of-shift report using transforming care at the bedside processes and methods. *Journal of Nursing Administration, 40*(4), 162–168.

Newhouse, R., Johantgen, M., Pronovost, P., & Johnson, E. (2010). Perioperative nurses and patient outcomes— mortality, complications, and length of stay. *Journal of Nursing Administration, 40*(10 Suppl.), S54–S66.

O'Brien-Pallas, L., Irvine, D., Peereboom, E., & Murray, M. (1997). Measuring nursing workload: Understanding the variability. *Nursing Economic$, 15*(4), 171–182.

Orr, D. (2010). Characteristics of positive working relationships between nursing and support service employees. *Journal of Nursing Administration, 40*(3), 129–134.

Outten, M. (2012). Managing a multigenerational nursing workforce. *Nursing Management, 43*(4), 43–47.

Page, A. (2004). *Keeping patients safe: Transforming the work environment of nurses: Quality Chasm series.* Institute of Medicine, National Academy of Sciences. Washington, DC: National Academy Press.

Palumbo, M., McIntosh, B., Rambur, B., & Naud, S. (2009). Retaining an aging nurse workforce: Perceptions of human resource practices. *Nursing Economic$, 27*(4), 221–227.

Pappas, S. (2008). The cost of nurse-sensitive adverse events. *Journal of Nursing Administration, 38*(5), 230–229.

Patrician, P., Loan, L., McCarthy, M., Fridman, M., Donaldson, N., Bingham, M., et al. (2011). The association of shift-level nurse staffing with adverse patient events. *Journal of Nursing Administration, 41*(2), 64–70.

Pendry, P. (2007). Moral distress: Recognizing it to retain nurses. *Nursing Economic$, 25*(4), 217–221.

Pine, R., & Tart, K. (2007). Return on investment: Benefits and challenges of a baccalaureate nurse residency program. *Nursing Economic$, 25*(1), 13–19, 39.

Pinkerton, S., & Rivers, R. (2001). Factors influencing staffing needs. *Nursing Economic$, 19*(5), 236–237.

Porter, C., Kolcaba, K., McNulty, R., & Fitzpatrick, J. (2010). The effect of a nursing labor management partnership on nurse turnover and satisfaction. *Journal of Nursing Administration, 40*(5), 205–210.

Porter-O'Grady, T., & Malloch, K. (2011). *Quantum leadership: Advancing innovation, transforming health care* (3rd ed.). Burlington, MA: Jones & Bartlett Learning.

Prestia, A., & Dyess, S. (2012). Maximizing caring relationships between nursing assistants and patients: Care partners. *Journal of Nursing Administration, 42*(30), 144–147.

Radwin, L., Cabral, H., Chen, L., & Jennings, B. (2010). A protocol for capturing daily variability in nursing care. *Nursing Economic$, 28*(2), 95–105.

Reese, S. (2011). 10 ways to practice evidence-based staffing and scheduling. *Nursing Management, 42*(10), 20–24.

Riley, J., & Rolband, D. (2009). Clinical ladder: nurses' perceptions and satisfiers. *Journal of Nursing Administration, 39*(4), 182–188.

Rimar, J., & Diers, D. (2006). Inpatient nursing unit volume, length of stay cost, and mortality. *Nursing Economic$, 24*(6), 298–307.

Rivera, R., Fitzpatrick, J., & Boyle, S. (2011). Closing the RN engagement gap: Which drivers of engagement matter? *Journal of Nursing Administration, 41*(6), 265–272.

Roach, S. (1998). In search of productivity. *Harvard Business Review*, 153–160.

Rogers, A., Hwany, W., Scott, L., Aiken, L., & Dinges, D. (2004). The working hours of hospital staff nurses and patient safety. *Health Affairs, 23*(4), 202–212.

Ruflin, P., Matlack, R., Holy, C., Sorbello, S., Nadzan, L., & Selden, T. (1999). Closed-unit staffing speaks volumes. *Nursing Management, 30*(6), 37–39.

Ruggiero, J., & Pezzino, J. (2006). Nurses' perceptions of the advantages and disadvantages of their shift and work schedules. *Journal of Nursing Administration, 36*(10), 450–453.

Rush, S. (2012). Bedside reporting: Dynamic dialogue. *Nursing Management, 43*(1), 41–44.

Russell, E., Hawkins, J., & Arnold, K. (2012). Guidelines for successful self-scheduling on nursing units. *Journal of Nursing Administration, 42*(9), 408–409.

Savage, S. (2002). The flaw of averages. Harvard Business Review, 79(11), 20–21.

Salin, S., Kaunonen, M., & Aalto, P. (2012). Explaining patient satisfaction with outpatient care using data-based nurse staffing indicators. *Journal of Nursing Administration, 42*(12), 592–597.

Salt, J., Commings, G., & Profetto-McGrath, J. (2008). Increasing retention of new graduate nurses: A systematic review of interventions by healthcare organizations. *Journal of Nursing Administration, 38*(6), 287–296.

Schaar, G., Swenty, C., & Phillips, L. (2012). Nursing sabbatical in the acute care hospital setting: A cost-benefit analysis. *Journal of Nursing Administration, 42*(6), 340–344.

Schmidt, D. (1999). Financial and operational skills for nurse managers. *Nursing Administration Quarterly, 23*(4), 16.

Scott, L., Hofmeister, N., Rogness, N., & Rogers, A. (2010). Implementing a fatigue countermeasures program for nurses: A focus group analysis. *Journal of Nursing Administration, 40*(5), 233–240.

Seago, J. (2001). Nurse staffing, models of care delivery, and interventions. In K. Shojania, B. Duncan, K. McDonald, & R. Wachter (Eds.), *Making health care safer: A critical analysis of patient safety practices, evidence report.* Technology assessment No. 43. Rockville, MD: AHRQ.

Seago, J. (2002). The California experiment: Alternatives for minimum nurse-to-patient ratios. *Journal of Nursing Administration, 32*(1), 48–58.

Seago, J., & Ash, M. (2002). Registered nurse unions and patient outcomes. *Journal of Nursing Administration, 32*(3), 143–151.

Seago, J., Herrera, C., Spetz, J., Keane, D., & Ash, M. (2011). Hospital RN job satisfaction and nurse unions. *Journal of Nursing Administration, 41*(3), 109–114.

Sellers, K., & Millenbach, L. (2012). The degree of horizontal violence in RNs practicing in new your state. *Journal of Nursing Administration, 42*(10), 483–487.

Shaha, S. (1995). Acuity systems and control charting. *Quality Management in Health Care, 3*(3), 22–30.

Shamliyan, T., Kane, R., Mueller, C., Duval, S., & Wilt, T. (2009). Cost savings associated with increased RN staffing in acute care hospitals: Simulation exercise. *Nursing Economic$, 27*(5), 302–314.

Shendell-Falik, N., Feinson, M., & Mohr, B. (2007). Enhancing patient safety: Improving the patient handoff process through appreciative inquiry. *Journal of Nursing Administration, 17*(2), 98–104.

Shermont, H., Krepcio, D., & Murphy, J. (2009). Career mapping: Developing nurse leaders, reinvigorating careers. *Journal of Nursing Administration, 39*(10), 432–437.

Shi, L., & Singh, D. (2004). *Delivering health care in America: A systems approach* (3rd ed.). Sudbury, MA: Jones and Bartlett.

Shirey, M. (2012). How resilient are your team members? *Journal of Nursing Administration, 42*(12), 551–553.

Sochalski, J. (2004). Is more better? The relationship between hospital staffing and the quality of nursing care in hospitals. *Medical Care, 42*(2 Suppl.), 1167–1173.

Spetz, J., Chapman, S., Rickles, J., & Ong, P. (2008). Job and industry turnover for registered and licensed vocational nurses. *Journal of Nursing Administration, 38*(9), 372–378.

Stimpfel, A., Lake, E., & Barton, S. (2013). How differing shift lengths relate to quality outcomes in pediatrics. *Journal of Nursing Administration, 43*(2), 95–100.

Storfjell, J., Ohlson, S., Omoike, O., Fitzpatrick, T., & Wetasin, K. (2009). Non-value added time: The million dollar nursing opportunity. *Journal of Nursing Administration, 39*(1), 38–43.

Strickland, B., & Neely, S. (1995). Using a standard staffing index to allocate nursing staff. *Journal of Nursing Administration, 25*(3), 13–21.

Sullivan, E., & Decker, L. (2001). The effect of LPN reductions on RN patient load. *Journal of Nursing Administration, 33*(4), 120.

Taylor, K. (2000). Tackling the issue of nurse competency. *Nursing Management,* 35–37.

Tellez, M., & Seago, J. (2013). California nurse staffing law and RN workforce changes. *Nursing Economic$, 31*(1), 18–26.

Thungiaroenkul, P., Cummings, G., & Embleton, A. (2007). The impact of nurse staffing on hospital costs and patient length of stay systematic review: A systematic review. *Nursing Economic$, 25*(5), 255–266.

TIGER Initiative. (n.d.). *About TIGER.* Retrieved from http://www.tigersummit.com/About_Us.html

Toussaint, J., & Gerard, R., with Adams, E. (2010). *On the mend: Revolutionizing healthcare to save lives and transform the industry.* Cambridge, MA: Lean Enterprise Institute.

Trbovich, P., Prakash, V., & Stewart, J. (2010). Interruptions during the delivery of high-risk medications. *Journal of Nursing Administration, 40*(5), 211–218.

Trepanier, S., Early, S., Ulrich, B., & Cherry, B. (2012). New graduate nurse residency program: A cost-benefit analysis based on turnover the contract labor usage. *Nursing Economic$, 30*(4), 207–214.

Trinkoff, A., Johantgen, M., Storr, C., Han, K., Liang, Y., Gurses, A., & Hopkinson, S. (2010). A comparison of working conditions among nurses in Magnet and non-Magnet hospitals. *Journal of Nursing Administration, 40*(7/8), 309–315.

Trinkoff, A., Johantgen, M., Storr, C., Gurses, A., Liang, Y., & Han, K. (2011a). Linking nursing work environment and patient outcomes. *Journal of Nursing Regulation, 2*(1), 10–16.

Trinkoff, A., Johantgen, M., Storr, C., Gurses, A., Liang, Y., & Han, K. (2011b). Nurses work schedule characteristics, nurse staffing and patient mortality. *Nursing Research, 60*(1), 1–8.

Tucker, S., Weymiller, A., & Cutshall, S. (2012). Stress ratings and health promotion practices among RNs: A case for action. *Journal of Nursing Administration, 42*(5), 282–292.

Unruh, L. (2003). Licensed nurse staffing and adverse events in hospitals. *Medical Care, 41*(1), 142–152.

Upenieks, V., Akhavan, J., & Kotlerman, J. (2008). Value-added care: A paradigm shift in patient care delivery. *Nursing Economic$, 26*(5), 294–301.

Upenieks, V., Akhavan, J., Kotlerman, J., Esser, J., & Ngo, J. (2007). Value-added care: A new way of assessing nursing staffing ratios and workload variability. *Journal of Nursing Administration, 37*(5), 243–252.

Upenieks, V., Pearson, M., Needleman, J., Parkerton, P., Soban, L., & Yee, T. (2008). The relationship between the volume and type of transforming care at the bedside innovations and changes in nurse vitality. *Journal of Nursing Administration, 38*(9), 386–394.

Valentine, N., & Nash, J. (2008). Achieving effective staffing through a shared decision-making approach to open-shift management. *Journal of Nursing Administration, 38*(7/8), 331–335.

Van Slyck, A. (2000). Patient classification systems: Not a proxy for nurse "busyness." *Nursing Administration Quarterly, 24*(4), 51–59.

Verran, J. (1986). Testing a classification instrument for the ambulatory care setting. *Research in Nursing and Health, 9,* 279–287.

Vestal, K. (2012). Which matters: Employee satisfaction or employee engagement? *Nurse Leader, 10*(6) 10–11.

Wade, C. (2009). Perceived effects of specialty nurse certification: A review of the literature. *AORN, 89*(1), S5–S13.

Wagner, C. (2009). The value of a nonlinear model in predicting nursing turnover. *Journal of Nursing Administration, 39*(5), 200–203.

Walrafen, N., Brewer, M., & Mulvenon, C. (2012). Sadly caught up in the moment: An exploration of horizontal violence. *Nursing Economic$, 30*(1), 6–13.

Walts, L., & Kapadia, A. (1996). Patient classification system: An optimization approach. *Health Care Manager Review, 21*, 75–82.

Waneka, R., & Spetz, J. (2010). Hospital information technology systems' impact on nurses and nursing care. *Journal of Nursing Administration, 40*(12), 509–514.

Welton, J. (2010). Value-based nursing care. *Journal of Nursing Administration, 40*(10), 399–401.

Welton, J., Zone-Smith, L., & Bandyopadhyay, D. (2009). Estimating nursing intensity and direct cost using the nurse-patient assignment. *Journal of Nursing Administration, 39*(6), 276–284.

Weston, M., Brewer, K., & Peterson, C. (2012). ANA principles: The framework for nurse staffing to positively impact outcomes. *Nursing Economic$, 30*(5), 247–252.

Wieck, K., Dols, J., & Northam, S. (2009). What nurses want: The nurse incentives project. *Nursing Economic$, 27*(3), 169–177.

Wilson, B., & Diedrich, A. (2011). Bullies at work: The impact of horizontal hostility in the hospital setting and intent to leave. *Journal of Nursing Administration, 41*(11), 453–458.

Wonder, A. (2012). Engagement in RNs working in Magnet-designated hospitals: Exploring the significance of work experience. *Journal of Nursing Administration, 42*(12), 575–579.

Yang, P., Hung, C., Chen, Y., Hu, C., & Shieh, S. (2012). The impact of different nursing skill mix models on patient outcomes in a respiratory care center. *Worldviews of Evidence-Based Nursing, 9*(4), 227–233.

Yarbrough, S., Alfred, D., & Martin, P. (2008). Research study: Professional values and retention. *Nursing Management, 39*(4), 10–18.

Appendix

Author(s)	Publication date	Patient mortality, failure to rescue, pneumonia, post-op DVT, pulmonary embolism	Patient adverse outcomes: pneumonia, post-op infections, UTI, AMI, CHF, falls, medication errors, pressure ulcers	Smoking cessation	Pneumoccal vaccination rates	Length of stay	Patient satisfaction	Patient experience of care	Physician satisfaction	Readmission	Family complaints	Clinical Nurse Leader role	Education level	% of RNs	Shift level experience	Shift hours
		Patient Outcomes														
Aiken & Patrician	2000	x														
Aiken et al.	2002	x												x		
Aiken et al.	2003	x	x										x			
Aiken et al.	2008	x											x	x		x
Alvarez et al.	2011		x				x									
Blegen & Goode	1997		x													
Blegen & Vaughn	1998		x								x					
Blegen et al.	2011	x	x											x		
Brewer & Frazier	1998															
Djukic et al.	2011															
Gabuat et al.	2008															
Hickey et al.	2011	x	x											x		
IOM	2004															
Kane et al.	2007	x				x								x		
Kohlbrenner et al.	2011	x						x	x							x
Kutney-Lee et al.	2009						x									
Letvak et al.	2011															
Needleman et al.	2001		x													
Needleman et al.	2006		x													
Needleman et al.	2011	x														x
Neff et al.	2011															
Patrician et al.	2011		x											x	x	x
Rogers et al.	2004															x
Salin et al.	2012						x									
Shaha	2010			x	x											
Sochalski et al.	1997															
Sochalski	2004	x	x											x		
Stanley et al.	2008		x				x	x				x				
Trinkoff et al.	2011a	x	x													
Trinkoff et al.	2011b	x	x													
Unruh	2003					x				x						
Yang	2012		x													

# of days worked in a row	# of hours worked in a week	Unit admission, discharge, transfer activity	RN satisfaction	Nurse turnover	Nurse fatigue and sleep cycles	Nurse retention	Nurse vacancy rate	Reduction in agency rates	Needlestick injuries	Improved communication re: errors	Nurse productivity	Foundation for quality of care, teamwork	Nurse manager ability, leadership, and support	Collegial nurse–physician relationships	Improved operating margin	Improved bond rating	US News & World Report (Top 20)	Magnet status	Support staff: Nursing assistants/secretaries
												Nurse Outcomes				**Organizational Outcomes**			
												x	x	x					
												x							
												x							x
												x		x				x	
												x	x	x					
											x								
		x																	
					x														
x	x																		
				x															
x	x																		

Ethics in Nursing Administration

*Lois W. Lowry, DNSc, RN, ANEF, and
Jo-Ann Summitt Marrs, EdD, RN*

OBJECTIVES

- Contrast and compare the ethical theories of deontology and utilitarianism.
- Predict how the professional codes of ethics guide the administrator's practice.
- Describe the attributes of the four ethical principles.
- Describe the delicate balance between the need to be fiscally sound and to maintain an ethical culture in healthcare organizations.
- Apply the guidelines for ethical decision making to administrative decisions.
- Explain how the Magnet hospital program supports ethical practice of the chief nursing officers.
- Interpret the six steps of ethical leadership.
- Explain how traditional professional ethics must be rethought as part of interprofessional collaboration.
- Explain how information technology has affected ethical decision making of administrators.

Introduction

Nurse executives today find themselves in rapidly changing and challenging healthcare systems where personal ethics and organizational ethics often are in juxtaposition. Whatever happened to the healthcare culture of our youth when the institutions were primarily nonprofit and the medical profession comprised the governing body? In those *good old days*, professionals employed in organizations followed codes of ethics endorsed by their respective professions to guide their behavior. Individual ethics were framed by these codes—taught in the professional schools—and governed practice. These codes, then and now, affirm the professional ideals of conduct and commit members to honor them. They have two primary functions: first, to provide an enforceable standard of minimally decent care, and second, to maintain professionals' competence to safeguard patients from incompetent or unethical practice.

If these codes were sufficient to frame the care we gave in the past, why are they seemingly inadequate in the healthcare organizations of today? This chapter provides an historical perspective of ethics development in the healthcare system, presents ethical concerns of nurse administrators, and suggests insights into the development of ethical leadership.

Setting the Stage: An Historical Overview

> We may not know what our destiny will be, but one thing we do know: the only ones among us who will be really happy are those who've sought and found how to serve.
>
> —*Albert Schweitzer*

Were there ever good old days? Probably not, except in our reverie; the days were just different and perhaps simpler than today. Nightingale exhorted her nurses to "be sober and honest … devoted … to have a respect for her own calling, because God's precious gift of life is placed in her hands" (Nightingale, 1859, p. 71). These wise words were based on the need for personal *morality* so that a high quality of life could be maintained for oneself, society, and the individuals for whom one was caring.

Concern with moral values and expectations led to the development of the discipline of *ethics*, whose focus is the systematic study of and reflection on morality. All health professions, by virtue of their fiduciary relationships with patients, have developed codes of ethics to set forth moral principles as standards for behavior.

Ethical codes have been present in societies since ancient times, originating from religious principles such as service to others without exploitation. The Hippocratic Oath is one of the earliest codes (4 BC) accepted as a covenant between physicians and patients in the ancient world. This code became the dominant ethical document for all professional medicine in the Western world and is still acknowledged by medical students.

The first code of medical ethics was drafted by the American Medical Association (AMA) in 1847 and for the next 150 years committed the AMA physician to "render service to humanity" within a paternalistic framework. The patients' rights movement in the 1960s influenced the AMA to update its *code of ethics* from a *paternalistic* to a *patient-centered focus* (Veatch, 2002). The most recent AMA code of ethics, written in 2001, addresses responsibilities to patients in six of the nine principles and responsibility to community and public health in two and professionalism in the final one (AMA, 2011–2012).

Nursing, on the other hand, established *dignity and respect for persons* as the most fundamental principle in its original code written in 1976, with *self-determination* as the second most important principle.

The American Nurses Association House of Delegates revised the *Code of Ethics for Nurses with Interpretive Statements* in 2001, setting forth the profession's values and standards of conduct for nursing practice (**Exhibit 7–1**). When nurses become administrators, they must follow the American College of Healthcare Executives (ACHE) code of ethics as a broader code for their responsibilities; primarily, serving those who seek health care, oversight of the nursing staff, and interprofessional relationships (ACHE, 2003).

Exhibit 7–1   Code of Ethics for Nurses

American Nurses Association Code of Ethics for Nurses

1. The nurse, in all professional relationships, practices with compassion and respect for the inherent dignity, worth, and uniqueness of every individual, unrestricted by considerations of social or economic status, personal attributes, or the nature of health problems.
2. The nurse's primary commitment is to the patient, whether an individual, family, group or community.
3. The nurse promotes, advocates for, and strives to protect the health, safety, and rights of the patient.
4. The nurse is responsible and accountable for individual nursing practice and determines the appropriate delegation of tasks consistent with the nurse's obligation to provide optimum patient care.
5. The nurse owes the same duties to self as to others, including the responsibility to preserve integrity and safety, to maintain competence, and to continue personal and professional growth.
6. The nurse participates in establishing, maintaining, and improving health care environments and conditions of employment conducive to the provision of quality health care and consistent with the values of the profession through individual and collective action.
7. The nurse participates in the advancement of the profession through contributions to practice, education, administration, and knowledge development.
8. The nurse collaborates with the other health professionals and the public in promoting community, national, and international efforts to meet health needs.
9. The profession of nursing, as represented by associations and their members, is responsible for articulating nursing values, for maintaining the integrity of the profession and its practice, and for shaping social policy.

Source: American Nurses Association. (2001). *Code of Ethics for Nurses with Interpretive Statements.* Washington, DC: American Nurses Foundation/American Nurses Association.

Codes of ethics imply moral duties and rights and help to define one's boundaries when acting in the professional role. All codes stem from the ethical theories of deontology.

Deontology implies that one is acting correctly when guided by rules and duties that come from universal moral principles that undergird religions, such as the Ten Commandments and the Golden Rule. The German philosopher Immanuel Kant (1724–1804) introduced the concept of "categorical imperative," implying that there is a right and wrong. Persons have an obligation to act morally based on laws (e.g., do right for right's sake). *Obeying the rules is more important than the consequences of the act.* Every individual has inherent dignity and deserves respect; thus, professionals have a duty to treat their patients as ends in themselves and never as a means to an end.

Thus, it is clear how professional codes of ethics were influenced by this theoretical perspective. The strengths of deontological thinking are that the rules are clearly stated and thus enforceable by law. Living by rules and codes of behavior maintains a high moral quality of life within communities because all humans are treated with respect and dignity. There are weaknesses within deontological thinking, however. Deontology is based on the assumption that we live in a homogeneous community and not only know what the rules and duties are but are rational and autonomous beings who can understand the rationale for them. Because there are no exceptions to the rules or any guiding principles that give instruction on what to do, we are faced with ethical dilemmas when there is a conflict between two principles (Aiken, 2004). For example, if one cannot tell a lie, should we tell the patient that he or she is getting a placebo?

Ethical problem solving at this individual level is relatively simple but does illustrate the conflicting principles of truth telling and patient autonomy. How does the deontological approach, however, enable professionals to act morally and ethically when serving in more complex systems, such as a hospital that employs many levels of workers and professionals, provides services to many types and cultures of patients, and must demonstrate fiscal responsibility in the delivery of services?

The hospital systems in the early twentieth century were managed by physicians and staffed primarily by nurses, both professions being guided by their respective codes of ethics. These codes guided physician and nurse behaviors and moral duties to the patients so that competent care could be delivered. Further, most of the hospitals of the day were operated as nonprofit entities, and many were supported financially by religious systems; thus, the professionals in charge of patient care did not have the burden of balancing the budget. Further, the age of technology had not dawned, so patient care was primarily comfort care.

Society accepted that there was a natural life span: a time to be born and a time to die. There were few dilemmas surrounding prolongation of life at either end of the age spectrum. Not only were decisions about life and death simpler but less costly. Conflicts were few between the principle of *justice* (being fair to all in the delivery of treatments) and *autonomy* (the individual's right to freely choose what he or she wants). Thus, the deontological approach was generally sufficient for guiding ethical behaviors of the healthcare professionals.

As hospitals grew into more complex systems, however, management shifted from physician models to business models. The business model gave rise to *business ethics*, that is, the application of general ethical rules to business behavior such as the *Ethical Policy Statement* issued by the American College of Healthcare Executives. If society's ethical rules say that dishonesty is unethical and immoral, then anyone in the business who is dishonest with employees or customers is acting unethically. On the other hand, recalling a defective product to avoid public harm is an example of an ethical business behavior.

As the management of hospitals shifted from physicians to business administrators, the key to ethical decision making in the hospital system rested with the business administrator. These individuals had the opportunity to set the ethical tone for the organization, depending on their personal values and ethical standards, rather than from a code of ethics (Frederick, Davis, & Post, 1988).

As hospital systems became more complex, *teleological* theories were considered more appropriate to guide ethical decision making within hospitals. These frameworks *focus on the ends or goals, and on the consequences of actions rather than the means to an end.*

The most important teleological theory for healthcare ethics is *utilitarianism*. Its premise considers that *an act or behavior is right if it promotes the best consequences overall.* Ethical decisions are based on the principle of providing the greatest good for the greatest number. Actions are right to the degree that they promote overall happiness for the majority. No act is intrinsically good or evil; only the *consequences* of the act are considered (e.g., which consequence brings the most happiness to the greatest number of people). Individual good is considered less important than aggregate.

The theory was developed by two philosophers, Jeremy Bentham (1748–1832) and John Stuart Mill (1806–1873), who were contemporaries of Kant but did not agree with his premises. The strengths of utilitarianism for hospital managers are that ethical decisions are not based on the evaluation of right and wrong behaviors but on policies that promote the general welfare (Purtilo, 2005). For example, when budgeting for scarce resources, it is more likely that purchases of equipment that will serve the most persons will be selected over that which is used by a few (e.g., a computed tomography scanner over six neonatal intensive care unit beds). It is obvious that conflicts are inevitable for healthcare professionals who are functioning by their codes of ethics based on treating all patients as equals (*deontology*) and are employed within systems that are governed by utilitarianism (*teleology*).

Organizational Ethics

The patient ideally has a right to a relationship that assures that he/she will be treated with respect and the medical knowledge will be used to further his/her own plans and values.

—Brody, *The Healer's Power*

Complexity of the organization can lead to the lure of profit over service and a temptation of reimbursement coding for the dollar and using a more expensive diagnosis. Community standards also influence appropriate ethical behavior within the hospital. For example, an administrator in a large city hospital may go to a bar after work for a drink whereas this behavior in a small community hospital may be considered unethical (Morrison, 2006).

Healthcare organizations have a dual purpose: the delivery of competent, safe care to all patients by committed professionals and faithfulness to the mission of the organization. Thus, the philosophy of *organizational ethics* in health care that has emerged since the 1990s has become the best guiding framework for healthcare institutions with its unique focus on both moral analysis of the individuals in the organization and on the moral life of the institution. For example:

All employees and staff are expected to comply with the organization's Code of Ethics that includes a mission, vision, and values statement. Administrators must adhere to their own professional code of ethics and that of the organization to maintain an environment that fosters the highest ethical and legal standards (Pozgar, 2005, p. 196).

A helpful analogy for thinking about organizational ethics is *ecology*, which considers interactions among cells, organisms, and ecosystems. Similarly, organizational ethics takes into account individuals, teams of healthcare workers, institutions, integrated delivery systems, and the entire healthcare environment. Healthcare organizations possess a distinctive organizational ecology characterized by "their mission of service to alleviate pain and restore patient health, a highly complex regulated environment, many professional cultures, and a rapidly changing healthcare market" (Boyle, DuBose, Ellingson, Guinn, & McCurdy, 2001, p. 10).

Thus, the scope and character of *organizational ethics* include consideration of the interactions between ethical theories: utilitarianism and deontology; usefulness of the principles of beneficence, nonmaleficence, justice, and autonomy in resolving ethical dilemmas; personal virtues; and formal structures to resolve ethical dilemmas. Administrative leaders must provide training for the staff regarding the organization's ethics and assist in resolving ethical issues in the workplace (Boyle et al., 2001; Pozgar, 2005).

Ethical Principles

A theory must be tempered with reality.

—*Jawaharlal Nehru*

Ethical principles, like ethical theories, represent moral considerations of healthcare professionals to respect the wishes of competent patients. Some of these, such as veracity, fidelity, dignity, and respect, listed in the professional codes of ethics, refer to attributes of the professional nurse. The four major principles that focus on the patient and family—beneficence, nonmaleficence, autonomy, and justice—are accepted by all healthcare organizations as basic guides to creating the ethical caliber of the practice environment.

Two ethical principles that undergird prevention or curing of disease and assist patients to maintain their functional abilities are *beneficence* and *nonmaleficence*. Both of these have their origin in the

Hippocratic Oath and are foundational to the duties of healthcare professionals to help persons in need and to refrain from causing harm. Beneficence occurs when the nurse administrator tries to determine what good care is. Generally, good care includes making allowances for the patient's beliefs, feelings, and wishes, as well as those of the family and significant others, and balancing benefits of a health-care decision against its harms. Nonmaleficence means that healthcare providers do no harm to their patients. In real practice, this principle is violated because the patient often suffers short-term pain for long-term treatment. This principle also extends to the healthcare provider protecting those who are vulnerable such as children, those who are mentally incompetent, unconscious persons, and elderly adults (Aiken, 2004; Morrison, 2006).

In Western culture, the principle of *autonomy* is highly valued. We believe that persons are the best decision makers in matters that affect their life and health. Even advocates of evidence-based medicine conclude that the patient can assess benefits and risks of treatment more adequately than physicians can. Under certain circumstances, the right to autonomy may be taken away, especially if there is potential harm for someone else's health, well-being, or rights (Aiken, 2004). Examples of autonomy include informed consent and proof of consent and confidentiality through Health Insurance Portability and Accountability Act (HIPAA) laws. Administrators must know their level of responsibility regarding these issues (Morrison, 2006; http://www.hrsa.gov/website.htm).

The fourth principle, *justice*, refers to a social contract among persons in society as described by John Rawls. This principle supports the obligation to treat one another fairly and to expect to be treated equally regardless of sex, race, marital status, medical diagnosis, social standing, economic level, or religious belief. This principle brings into focus the arguments for a right to health care, a subject too large for the scope of this chapter. A just administrator creates a just work environment in which there is a climate of trust between staff and administration that fosters positive decision making (Morrison, 2006).

All these principles are important to nurse administrators from the perspective of their relationship to nursing staff rather than to patients. Nurse administrators must do good for the personnel under their jurisdiction and do no harm. All nursing staff have the right to be autonomous in their decision making in matters that concern them.

The most important principle for administrators, however, is justice because they must make decisions about the delivery of services to collective groups of patients. Thus, understanding the principle of *distributive justice* is essential for nurses in management. For example, staff nurses are primarily concerned about staffing on their unit, but the administrator must consider the needs of all units and allocate staff accordingly, recognizing that there are greater and lesser needs within the institution. Perhaps some beds must be closed when there is not sufficient staff. Further, safety and quality of care for patients are the ultimate concerns of nurse administrators.

It is helpful for administrators to be familiar with the six parameters of distributive justice. Each approach embodies different values and is used in different situations that lead to different actions as described:

1. **Justice renders to each the same thing**. All persons must be treated the same way, irrespective of age, sex, race, or religion. However, all services are not unlimited, so how does one differentiate need?
2. **Justice renders to each according to his or her work**. This implies that one must discern the best approach for proportional treatment, not equal treatment.
3. **Justice renders to each according to his or her merits**. This principle bases decisions on assessments of personal excellence, such as merit raises or career ladder advancement. It is less applicable in instances of distribution of institutional resources.

4. **Justice renders to each according to rank**. This statement presupposes that "rank has its privileges" and could be applied to salary ranges based on educational preparation and experience.

5. **Justice renders to each according to his or her legal entitlement**. Although this approach requires that all persons be accorded their rights under the law and under legally binding contracts, many conflicts of legal rights are difficult to solve.

6. **Justice renders to each according to his or her need**. Considering this principle, it is fair to allocate institutional resources based on patient need, but more questionable to allocate educational resources to promote a person based on personal need only (Curtin & Arnold, 2005).

Another example that illustrates how the parameters of distributive justice can be considered involves a current issue before the American Organization of Nurse Executives. Members of AONE are recommending that hospitals unbundle inpatient nursing care from daily room and board charges, as has been suggested by the Centers for Medicare and Medicaid Services, to hospital inpatient prospective payment systems (Kerry Weems, Acting Administrator, Centers for Medicare and Medicaid Services, personal communication, June 3, 2008). By following AONE's recommendation, actual nursing care hours and estimated costs for individual patients will be assigned; thus, less complex cases will receive less compensation and more complex cases will receive greater compensation when factoring in the diagnosis-related group relative weights (Dalton, 2007).

If this proposed action is taken, there will be less tendency for hospitals to overvalue services for less complex cases, which can create unwanted incentives for hospitals to specialize in more profitable cases and eliminate admission of more complex cases. This is an obvious ethical dilemma, according to parameter 2, *Justice according to work*, and parameter 6, *Justice according to need*. First, it is ethical to give more compensation to a nurse who spends 8 intensive hours caring for a patient than to a nurse who may spend 2 hours caring for a less complex patient. Both nurses should not receive the same compensation. Further, the patient with more complex needs requires more intensive nursing care to promote healing, which may result in a shorter length of stay. This results in cost savings for the hospital in an ethical way.

When nurse administrators consider the six parameters of distributive justice, they will base their ultimate decision on meeting the greatest need for the greatest number.

The four universal ethical principles give us direction and purpose to solve ethical dilemmas. None is absolute, but principles do help us to organize our thoughts, justify our actions, and formulate resolutions to competing claims. Sometimes there are conflicts between the principles. For example, a father feels a moral obligation to donate one of his kidneys to save the life of his daughter (*beneficence*). On the other hand, he desires the freedom to make his own decision because of the risk to his own health and survival (*autonomy*) (Veatch, 2002). When conflicts occur, it is essential to weigh risks and benefits in each situation, taking into account all parties involved and using a decision-making process accepted by the organization. There is not an *a priori* ranking of moral principles. **Each situation must be considered individually with input into the resolution by all persons involved in the decision**. The considerations are the stakeholders, who wins, who loses, costs, risks, and benefits.

The question arises, "Which principle takes precedence over other principles when weighing issues in an ethical dilemma?" Social workers find *the ethical principles hierarchy* helpful in listing all the principles that are common to patient-centered dilemmas (Dolgoff, Loewenberg, & Harrington, 2005). A multidisciplinary group of healthcare professional educators reprioritized the list in 2008 as a teaching tool for nurses, physicians, and social workers to read: "Do the most good and the least harm, Promote quality of life, Protect life, Promote justice, Consider autonomy and freedom, Be truthful and fully disclose, and Respect privacy and confidentiality" (**Exhibit 7–2**). Nurse administrators could benefit from using this hierarchy in their decision-making process.

Exhibit 7–2　Hierarchy of Ethical Principles

1. Do the most good and the least harm.
2. Promote quality of life.
3. Protect life.
4. Promote justice.
5. Consider autonomy and freedom.
6. Be truthful and fully disclose.
7. Respect privacy and confidentiality

Source: From DOLGOFF/LOEWENBERG/HARRINGTON. *Ethical Decisions for Social Work Practice, 7E.* © 2005 South-Western, a part of Cengage Learning, Inc. Reproduced by permission. www.cengage.com/permissions.

Clinical ethics committees function to assist families, patients, and physicians in identifying, analyzing, and resolving ethical dilemmas. Persons on the committees represent physicians, nurses, healthcare administrators, other professional disciplines, and community members, whose purpose is to foster awareness of clinical ethical issues and to provide insight into solving ethical dilemmas. These dilemmas usually fall into the following areas of consideration: conflicting rights, end-of-life decisions, prioritizing values, family conflicts, decisional-making capacity, and substituted judgment.

Ethics committees vary in their structure from formal entities that meet regularly, providing a forum for discussions, to informal meetings of physicians and nurses when an ethical dilemma is identified. Usually, the ethics committees have developed a process for ethics consults and use a decision-making model to assist in resolving ethical dilemmas. These committees, however, have a relatively narrow focus directed toward dilemmas associated with patient conditions and decisions.

Considering the range of issues within organizations at a macro level, such as employee issues, conflicts of interest, resource management, and external pressures, there is a need for *organizational ethics committees* to address the challenges of the organization. The American College of Healthcare Executives supports the development of mechanisms to deal with general ethical issues and decisions. As leaders in their respective organizations, the executives have a primary role in the development and operation of these ethical mechanisms (American College of Healthcare Executives, 1993, 2003).

The Joint Commission requires healthcare organizations to have a mechanism in place to address ethical issues present in healthcare settings (http://www.jcaho.org, 2004). *Administrative ethics* is distinct from *clinical ethics*, yet the two are interrelated. Nurse administrators are held to a higher responsibility than their employees are because they must have loyalty to aggregates of patients as well as to the nursing staff.

Charting the Direction

It is easy to catch the wave, but difficult to stay on top.

—Anonymous

Traditionally, chief nurse executives defined their ethical behaviors governing their practices based on universal values with a focus on the delivery of competent and effective nursing services to all patients. As hospitals become more complex, administrators must be concerned about both nursing ethics and business ethics. Management decisions are strongly influenced by economics, with social and legal ramifications. Administrators must size up the organizational culture or "personality" early in their tenure. Does the culture include an *ethical climate*, defined as a pervasive moral atmosphere of a social system (Bell, 2003)?

The ethical *climate* is characterized as shared perceptions of right and wrong and collective assumptions about how moral concerns should be addressed. Organizations with an ethical climate interact responsibly, model integrity, share organizational purpose and direction, and value stakeholder perspectives (Bell, 2003; Morrison, 2006; Shirey, 2012). Nurse administrators in the twenty-first century hold positions that demand knowledge (the know *what*) and skills (the know *how*) of navigating organizational cultures. Foundational to successful navigation is the development of ethical integrity within the nurse administrator role.

Ethical Leadership of Nursing Administrators

> Good quality is cheap: it's poor quality that is expensive.
>
> —*Joe L. Griffith*

Those who lead in health care must do so by their own example (virtue ethics) and through actions ensuring that core ethical principles—beneficence, nonmaleficence, honesty, and justice—are embedded into their daily work (Johnson, 2002; Pozgar, 2005).

Administrators are nurses first who are obligated to professional codes and outcomes and who are duty driven by the standards of the profession to act in the patient's best interest as advocate, to maintain competence, and to keep confidences. *Profession* (from the Latin, *profiteor*) literally means "public promises" and implies nurses' social contract. Impose business ethics onto the professional obligations and it is clear that there will be resulting tensions.

Business ethics are generally outcome oriented, stemming from utilitarian principles through the lens of results, aims, and purposes. Functioning within healthcare organizations, nurse administrators are obligated to act for the common good and to be accountable for the outcomes of their decisions. The dual role of professional and business manager sets up tensions and dilemmas in which both perspectives must be considered. How can administrators lead well in this environment? Six steps are suggested:

1. **Reflect**. Leaders must reflect on the internalized values of the profession and the values of the organization. "Taking time to reflect, taking time to be, allows for profound insights and for breakthrough ideas to arise from the stillness of the leader's being" (Cashman, 2000). Reflection accompanies goal setting, problem solving, and real action. After becoming clear on values and principles, the leader is more able to behave in ways that are more congruent with the principles.
2. **"Walk the talk."** The leader must be a role model for the organization in a visible way, living out the values and principles of the organization. Not walking the talk sends a negative message to employees that it is acceptable to stretch the limits of ethical behavior.
3. **Lead like Socrates**. Strong ethical leaders ask difficult questions and create forums in which the ethical dilemmas can be discussed openly. One who leads the way and promotes and participates in the dialogue sends an important message about the importance of ethics in the organization.
4. **Demonstrate courage**. Do the right thing for the right reasons. Foster integrity and fear will be driven from the organization.
5. **Create processes to ensure ethical integrity**. An example is to initiate a review of all operations from an ethical viewpoint.
6. **Search for simplicity**. Consciously move past the complexity to simpler analysis and reflection. Each decision can be broken down into parts, each of which can be analyzed. Maintain one set of values for life and work (Johnson, 2002, pp. 6–8).

Organizations with integrity have truly learned that there is no choice but to walk the talk of their values and to be accountable for them (Boyle et al., 2001; Pozgar, 2005). The leader's task is to embody the principles and then to help the organization to understand and become the standard that it has declared. If leaders do not practice what they preach, there is a breakdown of ethical integrity.

Several studies support the fact that top management establishes the ethical tone for the organization. If transgressions are ignored or rewarded in the organization, others are more likely to take advantage in the future (Kronzon, 1999; Morrison, 2006). If corporate ethics are more transparent, employees are more perceptive of situations with ethical undertones (Marta, 1999). Leaders can develop moral virtues or character by managing their own motivations and developing integrity (Torres, 2001). An ethical leader must first "know thyself."

Ethical Principles of Nurse Administrators

> Contribute to life at this time in the world. Know that you make a difference.
>
> —*Beverly Malone*

Administrators frequently must deal with their own ethical dilemmas as a result of their concomitant duty to patients and to the employing institution. When patient and corporate goals are not congruent, administrators face difficult choices (Seifert, 2002). Leah Curtin (2000) proposes 10 principles for ethical administration that can align the dual roles and duties as patient advocates and organizational managers. These principles reflect universal values and include both utilitarian and deontological points of view:

1. **Frugal and therapeutic elegance:** Promotes the right degree of economy of means with the right amount of resources necessary to ensure competent care (respect for life, wisdom, stability, and fairness)
2. **Clinical credibility through organizational competence:** Requires disciplining professional practice through the application of current practice guidelines, regular self and peer evaluations, mutual teaching and counseling, and promoting *organizational competence* through consistent policies that advance the welfare of employees and provide discriminating and flexible staffing and scheduling patterns designed to safeguard patient care (tolerance, responsibility, freedom, women's place, and equity)
3. **Presence:** Promotes mutually trusting and beneficent relations with peers, collaborating professionals, patients, families, and members of the general public through communicating decisions in person and monitoring and altering decisions as necessary (love, responsibility, and unity)
4. **Responsible representation:** Ensures that the clinical and ethical concerns of nurses are heard at the highest level of organizational decision making (courage, truthfulness, and justice)
5. **Loyal service:** Forbids exploiting the organization or the staff to advance one's own career (justice, responsibility, love, and stability)
6. **Deliberate delegation:** Demands that the delegation of tasks and duties includes enough authorization to accomplish them; requires an act of trust (fairness, unity, and courage)
7. **Responsible innovation:** Requires that organizational change be examined before it is implemented for its impact on patient care and employee morale (respect for life, love, and tolerance)
8. **Fiduciary accountability:** Provides value for the dollar in terms of the safety, quality, and relevance of services offered to the community (justice, truthfulness, freedom, responsibility, and hospitality)
9. **Self-discipline:** Ensures that decisions made and actions taken are based on careful deliberation, never made in anger or fear, and never for retribution or vengeance (love, tolerance, and responsibility)

10. **Continuous learning:** Recognizes that time and resources must be invested in self and staff to ensure continued competence of care and excellence in organizational performance (love, truthfulness, and fairness) (**Exhibit 7–3**)

Exhibit 7–3   Curtin's Ten Ethical Principles for Nurse Administrators

1. Frugal and therapeutic elegance.
2. Clinical credibility through organizational competence.
3. Presence.
4. Responsible representation.
5. Loyal service.
6. Deliberate delegation.
7. Responsible innovation.
8. Fiduciary accountability.
9. Self-discipline.
10. Conscious learning.

Source: Curtin, L. (2000). The first ten principles for the ethical administration of nursing services. *Nursing Administration Quarterly,* 25(1), 7–13. Reprinted by permission.

These principles are not commands so much as they are guides to decision making. When times are difficult, they serve as the voice of conscience within each of us.

Typical Ethical Issues of Nurse Administrators

Nurse administrators incur ethical responsibilities for their organization, patients, nursing staff, and the profession. Their obligation is to make decisions within the limited resources available; thus, closing beds may be the right thing to do when staffing level is unsafe, even though this action may adversely affect the organization's bottom line. Nurse administrators are faced with the same type of problems that other organizational executives have, namely, problems with human relations, potential injustices to minorities, resource management, conflicts between the right thing to do and organizational policy, failure to speak up when unethical practices occur, and supporting the corporate hierarchy as opposed to doing the job well (Boyle et al., 2001; Morrison, 2006).

Studies of administrator dilemmas in the decade of the 1990s focused on the use or allocation of resources and concerns about the quality of care (Borawski, 1995; Cumunas, 1994; Harrison & Roth, 1992; Sietsema & Spradley, 1987; Silva & Lewis, 1991). Demands to decrease budgets "no matter what" led to nurse-to-patient ratios that were unsafe, the use of less skilled personnel for patient care rather than registered nurses, hiring traveling nurses, inadequate salaries, greater workloads, and other economic pressures. Management decisions are strongly influenced by economic, social, and political factors. Riley (n.d.) found that *nurse administrators experienced three types of ethical conflict—professional role conflict, organizational conflict, and interpersonal conflict.*

In a study by Redman and Fry (2003), the six most frequently experienced issues by New England nurse administrators (in order of frequency) were as follows:

Protecting patient rights and human dignity (62.7 percent); respecting/not respecting informed consent to treatment (41.4 percent); use/nonuse of physical/chemical restraints (31.7 percent); providing care with possible risks to the registered nurses' health (TB, HIV, violence) (28.3 percent); following/not following advance directives (25.5 percent); and staffing patterns that limit patient access to nursing care (21.9 percent). Note that five of these are patient rights issues, and the sixth is a patient care issue, demonstrating that the influence of one's professional ethics are so imprinted that they often take precedence over organizational ethics. (p. 152)

The six least frequently encountered ethics issues reported by New England nurse administrators were the following:

Participating/not participating in euthanasia/assisted suicide; reporting unethical/illegal practices of health professionals or agencies; caring for patients/families who are uninformed or misinformed about treatment, prognosis, or medical alternatives; ignoring patient/family autonomy; discriminatory treatment of patients; and breaches of patient confidentiality or privacy. The first issue is an end-of-life issue; the remaining issues are patient care issues (Redman & Fry, 2003, p. 152).

In organizations where there are ethics committees, the patient care dilemmas are usually addressed within these structures, thus freeing administrators to focus on the broader issues that affect the organization.

A more extensive survey of 4,000 members of AONE, conducted about the same time, revealed that *quality of service* continued to be the most pressing issue. For example, more than 50% of the respondents agreed that the organization failed to provide quality service consistent with professional standards, failures were to the result of economic restraints, and failures in quality were acknowledged by the healthcare providers in the organization.

Despite its importance as a causative agent, *economic constraints were not the key cause of the widespread disappointment in quality; it was the conflict between the organizational philosophy and the professional philosophy and standards.* The lack of knowledge or skills to competently perform one's duties (reflecting resource limitations on continuing education and the hiring of less qualified nurses as a result of the nursing shortage) was ranked higher by nurse executives than by the healthcare organization. The authors of this study concluded that the quality issues were present because of the conflict between clinical and organizational ethics and the lack of ethics committees to provide input into these dilemmas (Cooper, Frank, Gouty, & Hansen, 2002). Nurse executives were cautioned, however, to manage costs effectively because if this was not done, their organizations would not be in business and there would be no worry about quality and outcomes.

A qualitative research study by Gaudine and Beaton (2002) identified four themes of ethical conflict between nurse managers and their organizations. *Voicelessness* was a major concern. Nurse managers were invited to administrative meetings yet were treated as "invisible" members of the group. Comments of the managers included the following:

- Nursing is not valued.
- Nursing is not understood.
- No effort is made to understand nursing.
- Nurse managers are hired because they are perceived to "toe the party line."
- Nurse managers are not present during decision making on issues that affect nursing.
- Nurse manager positions are radically decreased, resulting in minimal nursing input.

Fiscal allocation for resources was the second area of conflict as demonstrated by the following comments:

- Money is spent on acute care instead of long-term care.
- There is a failure to invest in staff development; the focus is on short-term issues instead of the quality of nurses' work life.

- Quality is sacrificed (e.g., substandard patient care or patient/family rights are secondary to a balanced budget).
- Crisis management occurs rather than long-term budgetary planning.

Third, *rights of individuals were less valued than operational needs*. Nurse managers must be concerned with all nursing staff, not only their workloads but personal concerns such as salary, benefits, and opportunities for career advancement. The managers interviewed in this study stated the following:

- Policies support the hospital's legal needs as opposed to patients' and nurses' needs as perceived by the nurse manager.
- The nurse manager is forced to make decisions that serve the needs of the organization but have negative implications for nurses.

The fourth theme reflected *unjust practices* on the part of senior administration and/or the organization. Interestingly, more comments were made on this issue than on the other issues:

- There are unfair policies used for the promotion and termination of nurse managers.
- Workloads for direct-care nurses and nurse managers are unfair.
- Senior administration fails to act even when aware of a problem.
- Decision making is centralized rather than decentralized.
- Non-nurses are given priority over nurses for first-line supervisory positions.
- There is a punitive absenteeism policy.
- There is a punitive medication-error policy.
- Nurse managers are underpaid.
- The hospital's stated values (e.g., integrity, consultation) are not upheld by the administration and the board.
- There seems to be a lack of interest and lack of information on the part of the board of directors. (Gaudine & Beaton, 2002, p. 22)

When nurse administrators did submit suggestions to resolve some of the preceding dilemmas, they claimed there was negative fallout with the organizational administrators. There was an inability to resolve issues surrounding poor and unsafe patient care, treatment of patients' friends and relatives, and issues of downsizing nursing management.

The nurses claimed that their inability to resolve ethical dilemmas was the result of personal factors, situational factors, and issues related to the nurse manager:

Personal Factors
- Inability to speak out or to act
- Unwillingness of staff nurses to speak out, often because of fear
- Inability to make the needs of nursing understood
- Knowing that senior management is aware of a problem but will do nothing
- Knowing that documenting required changes has been a waste of time

Situational Factors
- Fear that the situation will escalate if the nurse manager speaks out
- Poor communication with senior administration, either because of the organization's size or because the administration does not value nursing management

- Some people refusing to negotiate
- Opinions of physicians more valued than those of nurses
- Uninformed board of directors
- Salary inequities among nurse managers
- New nurses for whom nursing is just a job
- Difficulty in recruiting and retaining nurses
- Nurses complain instead of taking constructive action
- Unfair comparisons with other hospitals regarding staffing levels
- Staff aware that other hospitals have better resources or have eliminated their deficits
- Staff aware that other hospitals go beyond the contract
- Staff see money spent on physician retention
- Silence on the part of professional associations and other directors of nursing on an issue of which they are aware
- Staff aware that nurse manager's situation is not unique and that nursing in Canada is in trouble
- Smear campaign against a nurse manager

Factors Relating to the Nurse Manager
- The nurse manager is unable to identify what is right and what is wrong.
- Staff remember when nursing used to be valued.
- Staff need to have a mentor.
- Nurse managers feel trapped because of their number of years in nursing management.
- Nurse managers do not know if they are doing the right thing.
- Nurse managers feel responsibility to improve a situation.
- Nurse managers fail to inform staff nurses of one's efforts to resolve issues of concern to nurses. (Gaudine & Beaton, 2002, p. 26)

In this study, nurses provided some insight into factors that would mitigate the nurse managers' ethical conflicts with hospitals: support, problem solving, and refocusing. Actual comments included the following:

Support
- Support from other nurse managers, hospital administrators, physicians, hospital ethics committees, staff nurses, family, and public
- Internal strength gained from knowing that one is morally right
- Internal strength gained from knowing that one is following the Canadian Nurses Association's Code of Ethics

Problem Solving and Growth
- Problem solving with other nurse managers, hospital administrators, physicians, hospital ethics committee, staff nurses
- Learning to separate personal values from professional responsibilities
- Developing and presenting a proposal to senior administrators

Refocusing
- Hoping that the next generation (of better-educated nurses) will improve nursing
- Focusing on one's own goals and on what one can do
- Focusing on the high quality of care that nurses do provide
- Dwelling on the positive when senior administration begins to address a problem (Gaudine & Beaton, 2002, p. 27)

Negative feelings, such as frustration, anger, fear, resentment, stress, loneliness, demoralization, lack of fulfillment, and powerlessness, arise from being in conflict. Managers may develop a poor self-image because they are undervalued and unsupported. They are concerned about patient safety and the well-being of the staff. Many times they are torn between viewpoints of staff nurses and those of senior administration (Gaudine & Beaton, 2002). These study results are disturbing and have implications for nurse retention.

When conflict exists between managers and the organization, the initial reaction is disappointment from the *moral dilemma* (recognizing more than one right thing to do). If the conflicts are not resolved, nurses experience *moral distress* (knowing the right thing to do but being prevented from doing it). Some may choose the road of being silent, whereas others may leave the institution, contributing to nursing shortage and the lack of problem resolution. The helplessness, hopelessness, powerlessness circle continues. Some administrators are empowered to acknowledge the problems and address them through better work hours, increased salaries, implementing shared governance, and increased autonomy for their staff. Nurse administrators claim they are supported by their professional organizations and look to them for strategies for preventing or coping with ethical conflicts.

Fast forward to 2014 and a snapshot of the healthcare arena of today. What situations in health care have influenced ethical decision making of nurse administrators? In the classic publication *To Err Is Human* (Kohn & Donaldson, 1999), issues of hospital errors, unsafe practices, and risks to patients were candidly presented.

Although institutional changes such as the government requirement of hospital accreditation standards (JCAHO) (http://www.jcaho.org) and the formation of ethics committees helped to emphasize patient safety and quality care within healthcare institutions, articles addressing patient safety and quality care by nurses and nurse administrators continue to be published in nursing journals. Administrators are the final defense to ensure integration of the six competency domains, that is, patient-centered care, patient safety, evidence-based practice, quality improvement, informatics, and teamwork and collaboration within their organizations (Brody, Barnes, Ruble, & Sakowski, 2012; Debourgh, 2012; Disch, Dreher, Davidson, Sinieris, & Waino, 2011). The Magnet hospital program, originated by the American Nurses Credentialing Center (ANCC, 2003), has also contributed to the delivery of quality patient care, emphasizing transformational leadership with empowered, accountable clinician staff (Brody et al., 2012; Luzinski, 2012b). Nurse administrators are key players in establishing innovative environments within their institutions in which empowered nurses can practice autonomously, thus rendering safe and quality care (Luzinski, 2012a).

Organizational chief executive officers must demonstrate evidence that the nurse administrators serve as influential members of the organization's highest decision-making body for strategic planning and operations. In other words, chief nursing officers (CNOs) may not be voiceless. They must be part of the planning team. They must give proof of their contributions to decisions that affect staffing, fiscal, and administrative decisions. Their role is vital in decentralized, shared governance, multidisciplinary, and collegial working relationships.

Interprofessional collaborative practice is increasing each year and reflects a shared commitment among the professions to create safer, more efficient, and more effective systems of care. Interprofessional ethics is an emerging aspect of this domain in which administrators are responsible for fostering trust, communication, and team behavior among health professions (Interprofessional Education Collaborative Expert Panel, 2011).

Information technology has become an integral part of clinical practice. Evidence exists that the electronic medical record (EMR) has reduced the numbers of medical errors, lowered costs, and improved quality of care and patient safety (Kutney-Kelly, 2011). Ethically based administrators have an important role in the organization to emphasize the capabilities of EMRs with the staff and to create a seamless transition for patient care while the system is being implemented. Further, CNOs must take an active role instituting a successful orientation program for the workforce to learn these systems (Kutney-Kelly, 2011; Mustain, Lowry, & Wilhoit, 2008).

Our digital world of smart phones, palm pilots, computers at the bedside has spawned an *antiprincipalism movement*. That is, too much technological change too quickly tends to erode ethical considerations of what we ought to do when technology shows us new ways to do things (Gastmans, 2002, p. 8). The development of eHealth Code of Ethics is an attempt to provide guidelines surrounding technological communication (iHealthCoalition.org, n.d.). With the growth of information systems an ethical concern that continually presents itself to the administrator is confidentiality of information. Administrators must orient staff about the guidelines regarding the profession's expectations for professionalism, confidentiality, and privacy (American Nurses Association, 2010; Badzek et al., 2012). They must set policies governing employee use of social media in the workplace; for example, personal use of computers in the workplace, mismanagement of patient records, and breaches of patient confidentiality (National Council of State Boards of Nursing, 2011).

The only way for administrators to be prepared for the rapid change of events is to read, surf, and conference to keep knowledge at the cutting edge. Consider "what-if" situations before faced with a "must do" decision.

Outcomes, Opportunities, and Challenges

> The need is not only to call attention to the conflicts and problems facing us as a profession and confronting us personally, but also to offer a process for examining these confusing areas and a new way to view change and growth.
>
> —*Diann Ustal*

What Has Research Revealed That Can Assist the Nurse Administrator?

Cooper and colleagues (2004) found that quality of service continues to be an issue and that the perception of the concern extends beyond the nursing profession to include other providers as well. To overcome the problem in quality, nurse administrators need to examine their own personal contributions to the problem by asking the following questions:

1. Am I taking all appropriate steps necessary to help work through key ethical problems?
2. Am I seeking more information regarding problems that have been identified by staff?
3. Am I helping staff to see the need for the changes in nursing practice, and am I providing them with resources needed for the change?
4. Am I encouraging staff to take risks?
5. Am I motivating staff to focus on new opportunities created by change?
6. Am I participating in and encouraging others to participate in ethics committees?
7. Am I advocating changes to senior managers to improve productivity and job stability?
8. Am I advocating changes to senior managers that I believe are essential to provide the best quality patient care?

Shared governance can serve as a starting point to change the work environment to one that more closely resembles both organizational ethics and professional ethics. Being knowledgeable about the organizational culture and the ethics of the organization is a good place to begin. Nurses in administrative roles tended to report that *39% of the time they had experienced ethical issues*; this was more frequent than that for the staff nurses. The most distressing issue for the nurse administrators was the lack of patient access to nursing care, followed by that of prolonging the dying process with inappropriate measures.

Guidelines for Ethical Decision Making

There is little doubt that addressing ethical issues consumes a large amount of the nurse administrator's time and energy and that making these decisions is very difficult. When an ethical leader must grapple with the "rightness" of a decision, he or she must look at possible solutions from all points of view. The best leaders realize that there are few "best" decisions. There will always be those who disagree with the course of action decided upon. For a decision to be good, it must be subjected to analysis and must consider all the stakeholders.

Most ethical leaders choose their battles wisely. There may be times that accepting a less than optimal decision saves political capital and power for issues of significance. This does not mean that a leader should accept actions that are unethical; however, it does mean that ethical decisions are often in the gray area, not black and white. Competent decision-making skill is needed to differentiate between when flexibility is acceptable and when "right is right" without compromise (Sanford, 2006). Taft (2000) proposes the following guidelines for making decisions in ethical dilemmas:

- Consciously acknowledge the separate but related domains of philosophy, religion, economics, law and government regulation, culture, industry and disciplinary effects, and individual context as they contribute to ethical decision and action.
- Understand that conflicting obligations are the rule, not the exception. In any presenting situation, differentiate one's personal from societal values.
- Identify the ethical value hierarchy of authority that should prevail. Unless a compelling likelihood of immediate or future harm to others is present, the principles of law, government regulation, and explicit organizational policy should rule—in that order.
- When a compelling likelihood of harm to others does exist that is insufficiently addressed by law, regulation, or organizational policy, identify and discuss the ethical situation with trusted peers and managers. Consider both present and future scenarios, and acts both of commission and omission.
- Identify the process and people to engage in addressing the ethical challenge. Marshall peer support and initiate action.
- Understand the contingencies of the situation, including inherent risks for you, the nurse. Know what risks you can assume and what actions you personally are prepared to take as the situation moves toward a valid, or flawed, resolution. (pp. 18–19)

These guidelines can be used by the nurse administrator as personal principles to consider on the job. In addition to these considerations, Sanford (2006) suggests seven steps to ethical management decision making.

1. Identify the issue/question.
2. Identify the stakeholders who will be affected by the solution/answer.

Consider:

a. Customers/patients

b. Staff/employees

c. The organization

d. The community

e. Medical staff

f. Others

3. List possible solutions/answers.

4. Evaluate each solution from each stakeholder's viewpoint.

5. Identify the organization's decision-making rules.

a. Do the values and mission of the organization specify or imply greater weight to the good of certain stakeholders? Example: Is individual patient welfare given greater weight than individual employee welfare?

b. Which solution(s) best serve the common (rather than individual) good?

6. Make a decision.

a. Are you able to explain why you chose this solution?

b. Would you feel proud of the decision if it was reported on the front page of your local newspaper (along with your rationale)?

7. Act and reflect on the action.

a. Evaluate the results of the decision.

b. Learn from the evaluation to improve ethical decision making in the future.

Note that these steps take into account all stakeholders and the perspective of each. Choices made by the hospital have economic and social effects on the entire community. The moral imperative may not be clear in all cases. All solutions must be considered to ascertain which is most beneficial or least harmful to the organization, the community, the staff, and the individuals involved.

The best decision-making criteria for an organization are often determined before a final decision is made. The leadership teams who are serious about ethics in the management ranks thoroughly examine decisions for ethical content (Sanford, 2006). Institutions that manage themselves by the principles of organizational ethics add a "triple bottom line," in which the organization's effects on the environment and societal good are as important as finances (Boyle et al., 2001).

Conclusion

Leadership is a potent combination of strategy and character. But if you must be without one, be without the strategy.

—*Norman Schwarzkopf*

Into the twenty-first century, society has experienced accelerating change with increasing complexity. Ethics must be part of every decision. Ethics-based administrators require innovation and departure from doing things as usual. Just talking about the ethics and never acting on convictions put one at risk for *ethical hypocrisy*. Administrators need to assess the culture and then promote ethical consciousness and conduct among the staff. They must support an environment conducive to providing safe, high-quality, cost-effective health care that also encourages individual ethical development. It is important to seek support from internal and external sources so that success occurs. The administrator has an obligation to accomplish the organization's mission in a way that respects the values of individuals and maximizes their contributions. Implemented recommendations from *The Future of Nursing* report (Institute of Medicine, 2010) ensure that nurses at all levels are able to practice as full partners in the healthcare system. Administrators can meet the ethical challenges before them knowing that they are being supported nationally.

Discussion Questions

1. Nurse administrators must be attentive to personal codes of ethics and organizational ethics in the management of their job. How do the theories of deontology and utilitarianism inform ethical decision making?
2. Select two ethical conflicts identified in the qualitative study by Gaudine and Beaton. Describe the steps you would take to resolve each dilemma.
3. The CNO of a large community hospital is interested in applying for Magnet status, thinking that going through this process would raise the status of nurses in the hospital and the quality of nursing care. What strategies would the CNO use to move the organization in this direction?
4. The CNO of St. Elsewhere Hospital, located in a multiracial area, believes she could serve the community better if she took steps to be more sensitive to her constituents by providing translators for patients, putting up signs in Spanish, and hiring some bilingual staff. The chief executive officer (CEO) and advisory board of the hospital verbally agreed to the idea. Time passed and there was no evidence of any of the steps being taken. Then, one evening a Spanish-speaking man came to the emergency department with gunshot wounds, was turned away, and almost bled to death. The CNO expressed her ethical concerns about the situation and demanded to know why the recommendations for better cultural care had not been implemented. The CEO replied, "I agree with your concern, but the recommendations are too costly for this hospital."
   a. What are the ethical challenges for all the stakeholders? Who wins? Who loses?
   b. Which priorities are in conflict?
   c. How could the ethical principles hierarchy assist the administrators in resolving the dilemma?
   d. In what circumstances should costs outweigh benefits?
5. What ethical considerations would you, as CNO of a large medical center that supports clinical placement for students, wish to discuss with both faculty and students at the annual orientation?
6. How would you, as CNO, handle a situation in which a staff nurse sends an email with a photo of one of her pediatric patients to her friends? What ethical principles have been violated?

Glossary of Terms

Antiprincipalism Movement—too much technological change too quickly tends to erode ethical considerations of what we ought to do when technology shows us new ways to do things.

Autonomy—an individual's right to freely choose what she or he wants. In Western culture, the principle of autonomy is highly valued.

Beneficence—occurs when the nurse administrator tries to determine what good care is. Generally, good care includes making allowances for the patient's beliefs, feelings, and wishes, as well as those of the family and significant others.

Business Ethics—the application of general ethical rules to business behavior. Business ethics is primarily outcome oriented. One issue is that the goal of business is primarily economic rather than service-oriented.

Clinical Ethics Committees—groups that function to assist families, patients, and physicians in identifying, analyzing, and resolving ethical dilemmas. Persons on the committees represent physicians, nurses, other professional disciplines, and community members whose purpose is to foster awareness of clinical ethical issues and to provide insight into solving ethical dilemmas. Usually, the ethics committees have developed a process for ethics consults and use a decision-making model to assist in resolving ethical dilemmas. These committees, however, have a relatively narrow focus directed toward dilemmas associated with patient conditions and decisions.

Code of Ethics—moral principles as standards for behavior; implies duties and rights.

Deontology—an ethical framework that implies that one is acting correctly when guided by rules and duties that come from universal moral principles that undergird religions, such as the Ten Commandments and the Golden Rule.

Distributive Justice—an important principle for nurse administrators who must make judgments about the delivery of services to collective groups of patients. Understanding the principle of distributive justice is essential for nurses in management. For example, staff nurses are primarily concerned about staffing on their unit, but the administrator must consider the needs of all units and allocate staff accordingly, recognizing that there are greater and lesser needs within the institution.

Ethical Climate—a pervasive moral atmosphere of a social system; shared perceptions of right and wrong and collective assumptions about how moral concerns should be addressed.

Ethical Hypocrisy—talking about ethics but not acting upon the principles.

Ethical Principles—moral considerations of healthcare professionals to respect the wishes of competent patients. Some of these, such as veracity, fidelity, dignity, and respect, are listed in the professional codes of ethics. The four major principles are accepted by all healthcare organizations as basic guides to the ethical caliber of the practice environment, in which commitment to patients and families is primary.

Ethics—the systematic study of and reflection on morality.

Justice—being fair to all; a social contract among persons in society. This principle supports the obligation to treat one another fairly and to expect to be treated equally regardless of sex, race, marital status, medical diagnosis, social standing, economic level, or religious belief.

Moral Dilemma—recognition that there is more than one choice that is right (moral).

Moral Distress—recognition of the right thing to do and being prevented from doing it.

Morality—the lived experience of making choices.

Nonmaleficence—when healthcare providers do no harm to their patients. In real practice, this principle is violated because the patient often suffers short-term pain for long-term treatment. This principle also extends to the healthcare provider protecting those who are vulnerable such as children, those who are mentally incompetent, unconscious persons, and elderly adults.

Organizational Ethics—an ethical perspective that focuses on both moral analysis of the individuals within the organization and the moral life of the institution. The scope and character of organizational ethics include consideration of the interactions between the ethical theories of utilitarianism and deontology; usefulness of the principles of beneficence, nonmaleficence, justice, and autonomy; personal virtues; and formal structures to resolve ethical dilemmas.

Organizational Ethics Committees—groups that consider the range of issues within organizations at a macro level, such as employee issues, conflicts of interest, resource management, and external pressures; there is a need for organizational ethics committees to address the challenges of the organization. The American College of Healthcare Executives supports the development of mechanisms to deal with general ethical issues and decisions. As leaders in their respective organizations, the executives have a primary role in the development and operation of these ethical mechanisms.

Profession—from the Latin, *profiteer*, literally means "public promises" and implies nurses' social contract.

Teleology—an ethical framework that focuses on the ends and on the consequences of actions, rather than the means to an end.

Utilitarianism—when an act or behavior is right if it promotes the best consequences overall. Ethical decisions are based on the principle of providing the greatest good for the greatest number.

References

Aiken, T. (2004). *Legal, ethical and political issues in nursing* (2nd ed.). Philadelphia, PA: F. A. Davis.

American College of Healthcare Executives. (n.d.). *About ACHE*. Retrieved from http://www.ache.org/aboutache.cfm

American College of Healthcare Executives. (2003a). *ACHE code of ethics and support materials*. Retrieved from http://www.ache.org/aboutache.cfm

American College of Healthcare Executives. (2003b). *Code of ethics*. Chicago, IL: Author.

American College of Healthcare Executives. (2003c). *Ethical policy statement*. Chicago, IL: Author.

American Medical Association. (2011–2012). *AMA code of medical ethics*. Retrieved from http://www.ama-assn.org/ama/pub/physician-resources/medical-ethics/code-medical-ethics.page

American Nurses Association. (2001). *Code of ethics for nurses with interpretive statements*. Washington, DC: Author.

American Nurses Association. (2010). Nursing's social policy statement: The essence of the profession. Silver Spring, MD: Nursesbooks.org.

American Nurses Credentialing Center. (2003). *Magnet recognition program standards*. Washington, DC: American Nurses Association.

Badzek, L. A., Mitchell, K., Marra, S. E., & Bower, M. M. (1998). Administrative ethics and confidentiality/privacy issues. *Online Journal of Issues in Nursing, 3*(3). Retrieved from http://www.nursingworld.org/MainMenuCategories/ANAMarketplace/ANAPeriodicals/OJIN/TableofContents/Vol31998/No3Dec1998/PrivacyIssues.aspx

Bell, S. (2003). Ethical climate in managed care organizations. *Nursing Administration Quarterly, 27*(2), 133–139.

Borawski, D. (1995). Ethical dilemmas for nurse administrators. *Journal of Nursing Administration, 25*, 60–62.

Boyle, P., DuBose, E., Ellingson, S., Guinn, D., & McCurdy, D. (2001). *Organizational ethics in health care*. San Francisco, CA: Jossey-Bass.

Brody, A., Barnes, K., Ruble, C., & Sakowski, J. (2012). Evidence-based practice councils: Potential path to staff empowerment. *Journal of Nursing Administration, 42*(1), 28–30.

Cashman, K. (2000). *Leadership from the inside out*. Provo, UT: Executive Excellence Pub.

Center for the Study of Ethics in the Professions Codes of Ethics. Retrieved from http://ethics.iit.edu/codes/index.html.

Cooper, R., Frank, G., Gouty, C., & Hansen, M. (2002). Key ethical issues encountered in healthcare organizations. *Journal of Nursing Administration, 24*(6), 331–337.

Cooper, R., Frank, G., Hansen, M., & Gouty, C. (2004). Key ethical issues encountered in healthcare organizations. *Journal of Nursing Administration, 34*(3), 149–156.

Cumunas, C. (1994). Ethical dilemmas of nurse executives, part I. *Journal of Nursing Administration, 24*(7/8), 45–51.

Curtin, L. (2000). The first ten principles for the ethical administration of nursing services. *Nursing Administration Quarterly, 25*(1), 7–13.

Curtin, L., & Arnold, L. (2005). A framework for analysis, part II. *Nursing Administration Quarterly, 29*(3), 288–291.

Dalton, K. (2007). *A study of charge compression in calculating DRG relative weights*. RTI Project Number 0207964.012.008. Prepared for Centers for Medicare and Medicaid Services, Office of Research, Development, and Information. Baltimore, MD: RTI International.

Debourgh, G. A. (2012). Synergy for patient safety and quality: Academic and service partnerships to promote effective nurse education and clinical practice. *Journal of Professional Nursing, 28*(1), 48–61.

Disch, J., Dreher, M., Davidson, P., Sinieris, M., & Waino, J. A. (2011). Role of the CNO in ensuring patient safety and quality. *Journal of Nursing Administration, 41*(4), 179–185.

Dolgoff, R., Loewenberg, S., & Harrington, E. (2005). *Ethical decisions for social work practice*. Belmont, CA: Brooks Cole.

Gastmans, C. (Ed.). (2002). *Between technology and humanity: The impact of technology on health care ethics*. Belgium: Leuven University Press.

Gaudine, A. P., & Beaton, M. R. (2002). Employed to go against one's values: Nurse manager's accounts of ethical conflict with their organization. *Canadian Journal Nursing Research, 34*(2), 17–34.

iHealthCoalition.org. (n.d.). *eHealth code*. Retrieved from http://www.ihealthcoalition.org/ehealth-code

Institute of Medicine. (2010). *The future of nursing: Leading change, advancing health*. Washington, DC: National Academies Press.

Interprofessional Education Collaborative Expert Panel. (2011). *Core competencies for interprofessional collaborative practice: Report of an expert panel*. Washington, DC: Interprofessional Education Collaborative.

National Council of State Boards of Nursing. (2011). *White paper: A nurse's guide to the use of social media*. Chicago, IL: Author.

Nightingale, F. (1859). *Notes on nursing: What it is and what it is not*. Philadelphia, PA: Lippincott.

Nurse's role in ethics and human rights: Revised position statement. Center for Ethics and Human Rights Advisory Board. Chicago

Pozgar, G. D. (2005). *Legal and ethical issues for health professionals*. Sudbury, MA: Jones and Bartlett.

Purtilo, R. (2005). *Ethical dimensions in the health professions* (4th ed.). Philadelphia, PA: Elsevier.

Redman, B., & Fry, S. (2003). Ethics and human rights issues experienced by nurses in leadership roles. *Nursing Leadership Forum, 7*(4), 150–156.

Riley, J. (n.d.). Nurse executives' response to ethical conflict and choice in the workplace. *Nursing Ethics Network*. Retrieved from http://jmrileyrn.tripod.com/nen/research.html#anchor153522

Sanford, K. (2006). The ethical leader. *Nursing Administration Quarterly, 30*(1), 5–10.

Seifert, P. (2002). Ethics in perioperative practice: Duty to foster an ethical environment. *Association of Perioperative Registered Nurses, 76*(3), 490–497.

Shirey, M. K. (2012). Group think, organizational strategy, and change. *Journal of Nursing Administration, 42*(2), 67–71.

Sietsema, M., & Spradley, B. (1987). Ethics and administrative decision-making. *Journal of Nursing Administration, 17*(4), 28–32.

Silva, M., & Lewis, C. (1991). Ethics, policy, and allocation of scarce resources in nursing service administration: A pilot study. *Nursing Connections, 4*(2), 44–52.

Taft, S. H. (2000). An inclusive look at the domain of ethics and its application to administrative behavior. *Online Journal of Issues in Nursing, 6*(1). Retrieved from http://www.journaldatabase.org/articles/91294/An_Inclusive_Look_at_the_.html

Torres, M. (2001). Character and decision-making. (Doctoral dissertation, University of Illinois at Chicago, 2001). *Dissertation Abstracts International, 62*, 2485.

Veatch, R. (2002). *The basics of bioethics* (2nd ed.). Upper Saddle River, NJ: Prentice Hall.

Contemporary Legal Issues for the Nurse Administrator

Frances W. "Billie" Sills, MSN, RN, ARNP, LNC

OBJECTIVES

- Define law and explain how society influences the development of law.
- Describe how state nurse practice acts define the scope of nursing practice.
- Define the term *standards of care*.
- Explain the importance of defining the scope and purpose of documents that may be used as evidence of standards of care.
- State the common areas of nursing negligence and liability and the common deviations from the nursing standards of care.
- Describe how potential liability from the effects of short staffing can be minimized by determining the reasonableness of actions under the circumstances.

J. G. Holland wrote, "Laws are the very bulwarks of liberty; they define every man's rights, and defend the individual liberties of all men." These words certainly held true during his lifetime (1819–1881). But here we are in the twenty-first century and laws by their very nature are much more than memorizing a list of activities that are illegal. Law is, in fact, a policy discipline and a science of society. Laws are not cast in stone; they are subject to change as the intent of the law no longer serves the purpose for which it was written.

Law has been defined in many ways and the essence of most of the definitions is simple: *a system of principles and processes by which individuals who live in a society attempt to control human behavior in an effort to minimize the use of force as a means to enforce conflicting interests.* Through our laws, society defines the standards of behavior, the means to enforce the standards, and a system for resolving conflicts. In our democratic environment, we have the power to make changes in the laws that govern us. In 2013, we find ourselves facing many issues; one that is at the top of the list concerns the 2010 Affordable Care Act (ACA). On June 28, the U.S. Supreme Court upheld two important provisions of the ACA:

1. The requirement that individuals obtain health insurance or pay a "shared responsibility payment." This is frequently referred to as the "health insurance mandate."
2. The provisions barring all federal Medicaid funding for states opting not to adopt the ACA's Medicaid coverage expansion, that is, if states choose not to accept ACA, then those states will not be given extra ACA monies for the additional population to be served.

Since the Supreme Court decision, we have seen many law suits filed in the federal courts and in various states. What we do know is that the implementation of the ACA will require changes in the laws that regulate the healthcare system. The task ahead is to figure out how to use the law and our legal system to solve the particular identified problem by revising an existing law or create a new one.

How does this affect nursing? Because nursing is an integral part of the healthcare team in all settings from staff nurse to the head of nursing it is important for nurses to have fundamental knowledge of the laws that affect the practice of nursing. This chapter discusses: (1) the nurse practice act, the law that regulates nursing practice; (2) standards of nursing practice, how these standards are applied, and how they are used as evidence during malpractice litigation; and (3) the legal significance of the nursing license and the nurse's legal responsibility for delegation rules.

Knowledge regarding the law as it pertains to nursing practice is the best defense a nurse can have. The twenty-first century is proving to be a century of *change*. It seems that nurses are finding themselves in a constant state of chaos. The challenge of keeping up with the ongoing technological advances in equipment and procedures; acquiring knowledge on emerging diseases, medications, and diagnostic studies; and evidence-based practice becomes overwhelming. When you add to this the new push for cost containment that forces us to work faster and more efficiently, we often make immediate, crucial choices during high-pressure patient care situations. This gives the nurse little time to reflect on the legal and ethical consequences of her or his actions before performing them. Nurse managers not only have to know the law as it pertains to nursing practice, but they need to know the level of understanding each member of the nursing staff has of the law that governs their practice.

Becoming a registered nurse (RN) means that you have achieved a new status under the law. You now have a license to practice nursing. This license means that each nurse is responsible and held accountable for nursing practice. It is not only important but *essential* that the professional nurse know these standards and the scope of our practice. If we violate the standards and/or practice outside our scope of practice, the state has the authority to suspend or revoke our license to practice nursing.

As a professional you can also be sued for negligence and/or malpractice. When a professional's behavior is negligent and someone gets hurt as a result, *the stage is set for a lawsuit*. It is also important to understand that working as a *professional*, the expectations for your behavior are *higher* than that of being a "reasonable" person. You are expected to perform as a *reasonable nurse* (one that practices within the scope of practice and upholds the standards of nursing practice). If your actions are determined *not* to be what a right and reasonable nurse would do, and your actions cause someone to be injured in some way, you can be sued for malpractice.

There are four documents that each nurse should have and be familiar with:

1. The *nurse practice act* for the state in which she or he works
2. American Nurses Association's *Foundation of Nursing Practice that contains: a) Nursing's social policy statement: The Essence of the Profession, b) Guide to the Code of Ethics for Nurses: Interpretation and Application, and c) Nursing: Scope and Standards of Practice, 2nd ed. (2010 package, ANA).*
3. Specialty organizations' standards for the appropriate areas in which the nurse works
4. Nursing policy and procedures for the facility

Each individual nurse—including RNs, licensed practical/vocational nurses (LP/VNs), and advanced practice RNs—who holds a license to practice nursing is responsible and accountable for his or her own actions. In addition, supervisors are responsible for what they delegate to staff members, ensuring that it is within the individual's scope of practice and that the individual is competent to perform the task delegated.

Legal Aspects of Licensure

Receiving a license to practice nursing is a privilege, not a right. Graduation from an accredited educational program and passing the National Council Licensure Examination for Registered Nurses (NCLEX-RN) does not guarantee that a license will be granted. The state grants a license after the candidate has successfully met all the requirements in that particular state. The license is intended to guarantee public safety while the level of expertise necessary to pass the test is the minimum level needed to provide safe care. The state continues to monitor your practice and to investigate any complaints regarding your practice.

In most states, the nurse practice act does the following:

- Describes how to obtain licensure and enter practice in that state
- Describes how and when to renew your license
- Defines the educational requirements for entry into practice
- Provides definitions and the scope of practice for each level of nursing practice
- Describes the process by which individual members of the board of nursing are selected and the categories of membership
- Identifies situations that are grounds for discipline, or circumstances in which a nursing license can be revoked or suspended
- Identifies the process for disciplinary actions, including diversionary techniques
- Outlines the appeal steps if the nurse believes the disciplinary actions taken by the board are not fair or valid

The practice acts vary from state to state; some are very specific and detailed, and others simply grant the board of nursing authority to declare the rules and regulations (administrative law) and to establish the details. To understand the scope of practice within the state that you wish to practice in, you must obtain a copy of the state's nurse practice act that includes the law, rules, and regulations that the board or administrative agency has established in that state.

Remember, *knowledge is the best defense against any lawsuits*. Each nurse on your staff has the individual responsibility to know the parameters of practice and the rules and regulations that govern practice that will pay off in the long run.

The power of the board to discipline is power that can have an adverse effect on your ability to practice. Boards of nursing have the authority to censure, suspend, revoke, or deny licensure. *You can avoid liability by using caution and common sense and by maintaining a heightened awareness of your legal responsibilities.*

Change can be frightening, and there is a tendency to behave like an ostrich and bury one's head in the sand. Although this may seem like a good solution to some who believe "What I don't know cannot hurt me," nothing could be further from the truth. Ignorance of the law is no excuse when you find yourself in the middle of a lawsuit. A much safer approach is to learn all you can about how the law can affect your ability to practice. The law can be a very helpful tool in ensuring safe nursing practice with positive outcomes. When you know about the law you are in a better position to protect yourself should you find yourself dealing with legal issues. It is also important to remember, like everything else in health care, the law is always changing, and it takes effort and continuous vigilance to keep up. The first step is to learn what the law is, where it comes from, and the implications of each type.

Definition of the Law

The most common type of law that affects nurses is *statutory law*, or *statutes* or *laws*. These are documented rules that govern living in your state (state laws) or the United States (federal laws) that are passed by state legislatures and Congress. Statutes cover the rules for our relationships with each other and can be viewed as the ethics of our society written down. *The most important part of a statute is the section on definitions.* Here the authors of the statute explain what they mean when they use a certain word. This is very useful because we all use words differently, but in reading the law a more precise understanding is necessary. (Example: *Reasonable care* is defined as the level of care or skill that is customarily rendered by a competent health care worker of similar education and experience in providing services to an individual in the community or state in which the person is practicing.) The issue comes up frequently in lawsuits when the question is asked, "What is the difference between the RN and the LPN?" The answer lies in the nurse practice act of the state in the scope of practice definition.

The nurse practice act of each state is an example of *state statutory laws* and can be found at the state board of nursing, in the public library, or online on the state government's website. It is imperative to see how your state defines a *registered nurse*, an *advanced practice nurse*, and a *licensed practical nurse*. In the majority of cases, the definition will provide you with what the state says a nurse can or cannot do. It is important, however, to keep in mind that as a rule these laws are quite general and may or may not answer a specific question. When in doubt, the best rule of thumb is to contact the state board of nursing and get an answer to your specific question.

Constitutional law refers to the rights, privileges, and responsibilities that are stated in, or have been inferred from, the United States Constitution, including the Bill of Rights. States may not pass laws or institute rules that conflict with these constitutionally granted rights or rules because the Constitution is the highest law of our country. Examples of these rights are freedom of speech and religion. The right to privacy is a right that is inferred from the Constitution.

Administrative law is that in which the body of law is made by administrative agencies that have been granted the authority to pass rules and regulations and render opinions, which explain in more detail the state statutes on a particular subject. Rules and regulations passed by the state board of nursing to control the practice of nursing are an example of administrative law.

Common law is a type of law that includes decisions made by judges in court cases or established by rules of custom and tradition.

Case law is composed of the decisions rendered in court cases by appeals courts. When a decision is reached by an appeals court, a record of the court's opinion and reasoning is recorded. Cases that are appealed to a higher court are ones that involve an issue of statutory law. When a case is appealed and there is a recorded court opinion, the result is the legal principle of *stare decisis*. This means that if an issue has been decided, all other cases concerning the same issue should be decided the same way. This is also known as a *precedent*. Each state has its own body of case law and it differs from other states because it is based on decisions of individual judges who base their decisions on differing state statutes and may resolve issues in a different way.

Classifications of Legal Action

There are two major classifications of legal actions that can occur as a result of either deliberate or unintentional violations of legal rules or statutes. The first category is *criminal actions*. A criminal action occurs when an individual has done something that is considered harmful to society as a whole. These cases involve a trial with a *prosecuting attorney*, who represents the interests of the state or the United States (the *public*), and a *defense attorney*, who represents the interests of the individual accused of the crime (*defendant*). These actions can usually be identified by the title, which will read *State v. (name of the defendant)*. Examples of criminal action are murder, drug violations, and some violations of the nurse practice act such as misuse of narcotics, abuse, and neglect. Felonies and misdemeanors are the two types of criminal action. *Felonies* are serious crimes that result in the perpetrator's imprisonment. A *misdemeanor* is a crime that results in a fine with no jail time.

The second category of legal claims is *civil actions*. These actions concern private interests and rights between the individuals involved in the case. Civil actions are also known as *torts*. A tort is a civil wrong or injury resulting from a breach of a legal duty that exists by virtue of society's expectations regarding interpersonal conduct or by the assumption of a duty inherent in a professional relationship (as opposed to a legal duty that exists by virtue of a contractual relationship). *Malpractice* refers to a tort committed by a professional acting in a professional capacity.

The law broadly divides torts into two categories: unintentional and intentional. An *unintentional tort* is a civil wrong resulting from the defendant's negligence. An *intentional tort* is a deliberate invasion of someone's legal right. In a malpractice suit involving an intentional tort, the *plaintiff* doesn't need to prove that you owed him or her a duty. The duty at issue (for example, not to touch an individual without his or her permission) is defined by law, and you are presumed to owe him or her this duty. The plaintiff still must prove that you breached this duty and this breach caused him or her harm. **Exhibit 8–1** shows the actions that can lead to claims in the two categories of tort claims.

The most common unintentional tort action brought against nurses is a malpractice claim. The National Practitioner Data Bank 2003 report stated that 16,339 nurse and nurse-related practitioners had a report made against them between the years 1990 and 2003 (National Practitioner Data Bank, 2004). This number represents claims where payment is made on behalf of a specifically named nurse and so does not touch on the number of claims in which a specific facility or corporation was named, yet involved nursing actions. Recent reports show an increasing trend in reports against nurses. As a nurse you may worry about being sued for something when, in the eyes of the law, no malpractice has occurred. Not every poor outcome is a case of malpractice. Healthcare professionals can make an error in judgment. For this reason it is important to know the basic elements that must be proven before malpractice can occur.

Exhibit 8–1   Tort Claims and Actions That Lead to Tort Claims

Unintentional Tort
Negligence
- Leaving foreign objects inside a patient after surgery
- Failing to observe a patient as ordered by the physician
- Failing to obtain informed consent before a treatment or procedure
- Failing to report a change in a patient's vital signs or status
- Failing to report a staff member's negligence that you witnessed
- Failing to provide for a patient's safety
- Failing to provide the patient with appropriate teaching before discharge

Intentional Tort
Assault
- Threatening a patient

Battery
- Assisting in nonemergency surgery performed without the consent of the patient
- Forcing a patient to ambulate against his or her wishes
- Forcing a patient to submit to injections
- Striking a patient
- Inappropriately restraining a patient

False imprisonment
- Confining a patient to a psychiatric unit without a physician's order
- Refusing to let a patient return home

Invasion of privacy
- Releasing private information about a patient to third parties
- Allowing unauthorized person to read a patient's medical record
- Allowing unauthorized persons to observe a procedure
- Taking pictures of a patient without his or her consent

Slander
- Making false statements about a patient to a third party, which causes damage to the patient's reputation

---

Our legal system's view of malpractice evolved from the premise that each person is responsible, or liable, for the consequences of his or her actions. *Malpractice law deals with a professional's liability for negligent acts, omissions, and intentional harm.*

An unintentional tort is a civil wrong resulting from the defendant's *negligence*. If you are sued for negligence, *the plaintiff must prove four things*:

1. You owed him or her a specific duty. In nursing malpractice suits, this duty is equivalent to the standards of care.
2. You breached this duty.
3. The plaintiff was harmed (the harm can be physical, mental, emotional, or financial).
4. Your breach of duty caused harm.

Using a hypothetical case, let us look at the four elements to determine whether there is a case of malpractice.

Case Study

You are working the 3 to 11 PM shift in an acute care hospital and it is time to give one of your patient's his 8 PM hydrocortisone IM injection. You make sure that the physician's order in the medical record has not been changed, and when you remove the drug from the medication cart, you check it against the physician's order and find it to be correct. You go to the patient's room, call the patient by name, and check his hospital ID bracelet to ensure that it is the right patient. You give the injection in the patient's left upper outer quadrant of the buttocks and document this on the medication administration record in the medical chart.

The patient leaves the hospital and a year later you are notified by Risk Management that a lawsuit has been filed against the hospital. The patient is claiming that the injection you gave him has caused sciatic nerve damage and his whole leg is numb. Who may have malpractice liability in this situation and why? Is it the nurse, the physician, the hospital? What defenses may be available to you? *Remember the four basic elements that must be present in each malpractice case.* The plaintiff's attorney needs to prove to a jury that each element has occurred. Your attorney defends you by proving that *all, or even just one, element did not happen.* It is important to understand that this is not always a black-and-white process, which can often be frustrating and confusing. It is important for the nurse to be able to evaluate the events using the four elements and know how they are proven in court.

1. **Do you have a professional duty?** To make a claim of malpractice against a nurse the plaintiff must establish a nurse–patient relationship or, stated in legal terms, that you had a professional duty to the patient. A *duty* implies that you are employed by and rendered services at a healthcare facility—such as a hospital, clinic, long-term care facility, or home health company—as a school nurse, or in a physician's office. The first element has been proven. In cases where a nurse has given aid at the scene of an accident or volunteers at sports events or other activities where professional services may be needed, it is important to know what your status would be under such circumstances in your state and/or if you have immunity and/or are covered by malpractice insurance. The contents of a Good Samaritan Act in the state you are working are good information to have.

2. **What was the professional duty owed?** Once it has been established that a professional duty was owed, the question then becomes what is that duty? A nurse's duty owed is different from that of a physician or a nursing assistant. The duty of the nurse is to act as a reasonable nurse under the same or similar circumstances. How does the attorney prove that the nurse acted as a reasonable nurse? Several factors are considered when attempting to establish duty using evidence about what the standard of care for that nurse might be:

   a. **Nurse practice act:** The nurse practice act is probably the most important guideline for what nurses do. Most acts outline the activities, or scope of practice, that the nurse can legally perform within the jurisdiction. These tend to be described in fairly general terms. Behaviors and acts that are considered unprofessional conduct are generally more specific. A violation of any of these acts means that you have fallen below the standard of care set by the state for nurses. It can also mean that you risk action against your license. Not knowing the contents of the practice act of your state puts you in jeopardy. Therefore, it is in your best interest to keep up with the licensing standards of the state.

   b. **Expert witnesses:** The most common method to establish the duty owed by a nurse is by the testimony of a registered nurse, with training and background similar to yours. The expert nurse will testify regarding what a reasonable nurse in the same or similar circumstances would be expected to do and that you did not do it. Testimony by experts is an essential ingredient in malpractice cases for both the plaintiff and defendant in lawsuits involving nursing care issues.

   The court's position is that *a nurse is the most appropriate expert witness when dealing with the action or decisions made by a nurse.* Before 1980, it was common for physicians to testify about the standards for nursing care. In the case of *Young v. Board of Hospital Directors, Lee County*

(#82-429 [FL 1984] p. 212), the court concluded that physicians may not determine nursing standards of care. The physician, being unfamiliar with the daily practices of nurses, is unable to set a standard or to testify as to deviation from common nursing practice. The nurse expert witness can explain technology or nursing care in the language jurors can understand. This type of testimony is important to dispel common misconceptions and/or to explain scientific facts as they pertain to nursing care and the care at hand.

There is a type of malpractice case in which an expert is not required. This type of claim is called *res ipsa loquitur*, or *the thing speaks for itself*. This claim is very difficult to prove because the patient must have enough evidence to show that (1) the injury would not have occurred unless someone was negligent, (2) the instrumentality causing the injury was within the exclusive control of the defendant, and (3) the incident was not owing to any voluntary action on the part of the plaintiff. *If an individual can prove that all these exist, the burden then shifts to the defendant to prove that malpractice did not take place.* Cases in which a sponge or instrument was left in a patient or a wrong body part was operated on fall into this category of claims.

c. **Established policies and procedures:** Next to the nurse practice act, established policies and procedures of the institution in which you work are the most crucial pieces of evidence for establishing a *standard of care*. In the case study, the attorney would request the hospital's or facility's policies on documentation and administration of medications. If you did not follow the policy of the institution, you fell below the standard of care set by the institution. It is important that you know and read the policies of your healthcare facility or corporation. These policies are an important resource when you have questions about how to do a certain procedure or what your rights are in certain situations. *Policies* are the laws under which you work. It is important for you as a professional to participate in making or changing policies so that they accurately reflect what nurses are doing in your facility. Because the policies set standards for providing quality and consistent patient care, it follows that they can be used to proactively prove that you followed the standard of care set by your institution.

d. **Accreditation and facility licensing standards:** Most healthcare facilities and other healthcare organizations such as health maintenance organizations (HMOs) must go through a process whereby they become licensed and/or accredited. The Joint Commission and the National Committee of Quality Assurance are two such organizations that set standards for healthcare organizations. State licensing requirements such as those needed for facilities to admit and treat Medicare and Medicaid recipients also define standards of care. These standards are often used as evidence of a standard of care for nurses working in such facilities.

e. **Textbooks and journals:** If you are involved in a lawsuit, either as a defendant or deposed as a witness, you may be asked about textbooks that are used in the workplace, such as the *Physician's Desk Reference* (*PDR*). You can also be asked if you subscribe to any nursing journals. Articles or portions of such publications may be used as evidence of the standard of care for nurses to follow. The fact that a *PDR* is available to the nurses on the unit might be used to demonstrate that a source for the correct dose, side effects, and the correct administration of the medication was/is immediately available to you at your workplace.

f. **Professional organization standards:** Professional organizations, such as the American Nurses Association (ANA), and nursing specialty organizations, such as the American Association of Neuroscience Nurses, have published certain standards of care and/or practice guidelines. These may be used as evidence for what a reasonable nurse should do in certain circumstances.

In summary, plaintiff attorneys use many different types of evidence to demonstrate an expected standard of care. The individual nurse and the nurse manager need to remember that these documents can be your *friend* or your *enemy* depending on your knowledge of them and the importance they play in the determination of whether or not the standard of care was met.

Looking again at our case study, the plaintiff will have to find a nurse who can testify to the correct method of giving intramuscular injections. If you did not give the injection the correct way, the jury can then infer that you did not act reasonably. However, if the correct method is to give the injection in the upper, outer quadrant of the buttocks and you have documented that you did this, the testimony of the expert will not prove anything. Also because you can demonstrate that you followed the facility's policies in the administration of medication, there will be no proof of falling below a standard of care.

3. **Was there a breach of professional duty?** The plaintiff must prove what the standard of care is in a given situation and that the nurse did not meet the standard of care. Other legal reasons that are sometimes used are "the nurse fell below the standard of care" or "the nurse breached the duty owed the patient." This means that the plaintiff must demonstrate through the evidence listed that you did not act as a reasonable and prudent nurse under the circumstances.

4. **Did the breach of duty cause the injury?** *Causation* is the element that is often overlooked by the nurse, and yet it is the issue most often hotly argued by attorneys. Was the injury caused by the nurse improperly administering an intramuscular injection, or did the patient subsequently injure him- or herself after medical care was administered? The causation requirement must be proven by the plaintiff's attorney, and this is not always easy. Certain well-documented observations will make it *impossible* for the plaintiff's attorney to show causation.

   a. Clearly document the patient's physical and mental condition upon admission through discharge from your facility. These observations can be used to demonstrate that either the patient had the symptom when she or he came and/or did not have the symptom upon discharge.

   b. After any incident, such as a patient fall, document the patient's physical and mental condition. This demonstrates that any subsequent complaints cannot be attached or caused by the incident.

   c. Document clearly any actions of a patient that demonstrate noncompliance with medical directives. When a patient is noncompliant with the prescribed treatment, it, rather than the treatment itself, can cause therapeutic failure. A documented "no show" at an outpatient clinic can dispel later claims that the complaints were ignored and therefore caused the injury.

   d. Document clearly when a patient complains and when he or she does not. Again, in the case study, if it is documented that the patient had no complaints after the injection, was resting comfortably, and was discharged home with no complaints, it would be difficult to prove that the injection caused the problem.

   e. Use caution when documenting what a patient states as opposed to what you believe may have happened. If the patient states that an injection caused the problem, the correct documentation is "patient states 'my leg has felt numb since I received the injection'" rather than "hospital injection caused patient's leg to become numb."

   f. Document clearly the discharge instructions given to the patient and/or a member of the family and the level of understanding demonstrated by the patient and/or the member of the family.

   g. The presence of or lack of allergies is another important piece of information that must be documented. Neither the nurses nor the physicians cause an individual to have allergies. They have a duty to ask about and not give any medication that has caused an individual to experience an allergic reaction in the past. The documentation of "no known allergies" can completely eliminate a claim involving an allergic reaction.

Applying Causation to the Case Study

Let us go back to the case study. The patient will have to prove that the injection given by the nurse caused the numbness in his leg. Many factors could have caused the numbness. As the defendant in the case, you do not have to prove anything because you do not have the *burden of proof*. The plaintiff may have a difficult time, especially if there are no documented complaints by the patient at the time of the injection or shortly thereafter. In the case study, you documented clearly where you administered the intramuscular injection. Your action was supported by policy and guidelines for the proper administration of an intramuscular injection. The opinion of a nurse expert would further validate this.

It is important to remember that a patient's claim that you or another healthcare provider caused a problem or injury should not automatically be assumed to be true. Untoward events, problems, and/or injuries have many causes and many stories behind them. *There are four important things to remember regarding documentation that can protect you from litigation*:

1. Document the facts.
2. Document what you see and do.
3. Your role is to provide nursing care and not to judge
4. Leave the determination of fault to the courts.

Your actions and truthful documentation will be your best defense. In the case study, the proper documentation was the evidence needed to demonstrate that the intramuscular injection was not the cause of the numbness in the patient's leg.

Did the Patient Suffer Damages or Injury?

The fourth element of negligence that must be proven is that the actual physical loss or damage was caused by the defendant's negligent conduct. In the case study, numbness of the leg may be difficult to prove. Nerve conduction studies could demonstrate that the injection could not have caused the neurological injury. Numbness does not mean lack of function and would not usually prevent any activity of daily living. The age and status of the plaintiff would play an important role, as would your documentation of the lack of patient complaints and the daily ability to ambulate.

Who Is at Risk for Liability (Responsibility) in a Claim?

Personal Liability

Many nurses have asked the question, "Who is responsible for my actions as a nurse?" The simple answer is, "You are." However, how many times have we heard a supervisor, physician, or other healthcare provider say, "Don't worry, I'll take responsibility for this." It is essential that each individual nurse understand that in the eyes of the law, *each individual is accountable for his or her own actions*. There is no defense in the statement "She made me do it." Even if you are not named in a lawsuit, you will be questioned as to your involvement in the case and you will have to be able to defend your actions under oath. "I was just following orders" does not explain why you as a professional nurse made a medication error. As a professional, you are held to a professional standard of care to know about the medication you are administering, including the correct dose, side effects, and action of the drug. If you administer the wrong dose of the medication to a patient, you are going to be held accountable for the error and would most likely have liability.

Physician and Other Independent Practitioner Liability

In the past, the physicians were seen as the "Captain of the Ship" and thus ultimately responsible for everything that happened to the patient. This doctrine is no longer true. Each professional is responsible and accountable for his or her actions under each individual's scope of practice. Many nurses are under the misconception that if they are following the "doctor's orders" they are not accountable if an error occurs. It is true that nurses do have a duty to carry out the physician's orders under most circumstances; however, if the nurse believes or has reason to believe that the order is unsafe for the patient or not within the nurse's scope of practice, it is the nurse's responsibility *to refuse* to carry out the order. For example, if the physician gives an order for the nurse to administer intravenous conscious sedation, it does not relieve the nurse of the duty of determining whether this is in her or his scope of practice.

In a situation where the nurse is hired directly by a physician to work in an office practice, the physician, as an employer, can be held liable on a theory of *respondeat superior*, meaning that the employer is responsible for acts of the employee. The physician then would be named in the lawsuit, but the nurse is still responsible for his or her actions.

Another issue in today's healthcare arena is what the nurse should accept as delegated or ordered by other independent healthcare practitioners, such as nurse practitioners (NPs) and physician assistants (PAs). States have different rules as to who can give orders to the RN, so it is important that you know what the rule is in the state where you are working. The general rule is that the RN can accept orders from other licensed healthcare providers who are working within their scope of practice. It is important to remember that with delegated duties, you should accept only those that you are competent to carry out and that are within your scope of practice.

Supervisory Liability

The standard of care for a supervisor is to act as a reasonable supervisor under the same or similar circumstances. A supervisor is expected to ensure the following:

- The task was properly assigned to a worker competent to safely perform it.
- Adequate supervision was provided should the worker need it.
- The nurse provided appropriate follow-up and evaluation of the delegated task.

The *delegation of nursing duties* to unlicensed personnel presents supervisory nurses with some special risks. Changes in our healthcare delivery system and its financing are providing us with some unfamiliar categories of unlicensed caregivers with a variety of skills and expertise. Most boards of nursing hold the position that the individual nurse remains personally liable for any task delegated to an unlicensed worker on the theory that the delegated task is considered still to be the nurse's responsibility, rather than within the scope of practice of the unlicensed worker. Certain nursing responsibilities, such as assessment, nursing diagnosis, planning, evaluation, documentation, and teaching, should not be delegated to nonlicensed staff. It is important to contact the board of nursing in your state to better understand your responsibilities in the delegation of nursing duties (see **Exhibit 8–2**).

Institutional Liability

Healthcare facilities, such as hospitals, are usually sued under the theory of *respondeat superior* for the actions of its employees. Almost all healthcare institutions carry insurance to cover the acts and omissions of their employees because the institution cannot do any act that would cause a lawsuit except through

Exhibit 8–2   Joint Statement on Delegation

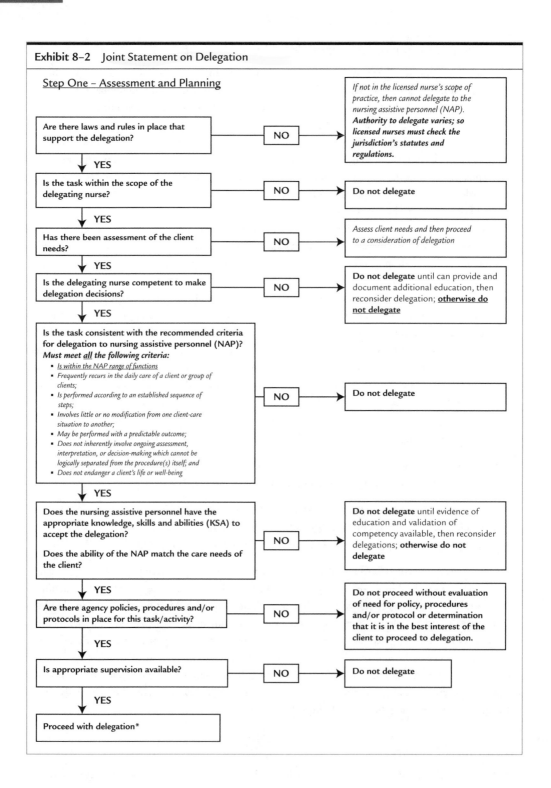

Step One – Assessment and Planning

Are there laws and rules in place that support the delegation? — **NO** → *If not in the licensed nurse's scope of practice, then cannot delegate to the nursing assistive personnel (NAP).* **Authority to delegate varies; so licensed nurses must check the jurisdiction's statutes and regulations.**

YES

Is the task within the scope of the delegating nurse? — **NO** → Do not delegate

YES

Has there been assessment of the client needs? — **NO** → *Assess client needs and then proceed to a consideration of delegation*

YES

Is the delegating nurse competent to make delegation decisions? — **NO** → **Do not delegate** until can provide and document additional education, then reconsider delegation; **otherwise do not delegate**

YES

Is the task consistent with the recommended criteria for delegation to nursing assistive personnel (NAP)? *Must meet **all** the following criteria:*
- *Is within the NAP range of functions*
- *Frequently recurs in the daily care of a client or group of clients;*
- *Is performed according to an established sequence of steps;*
- *Involves little or no modification from one client-care situation to another;*
- *May be performed with a predictable outcome;*
- *Does not inherently involve ongoing assessment, interpretation, or decision-making which cannot be logically separated from the procedure(s) itself; and*
- *Does not endanger a client's life or well-being*

— **NO** → Do not delegate

YES

Does the nursing assistive personnel have the appropriate knowledge, skills and abilities (KSA) to accept the delegation?

Does the ability of the NAP match the care needs of the client?

— **NO** → **Do not delegate** until evidence of education and validation of competency available, then reconsider delegations; **otherwise do not delegate**

YES

Are there agency policies, procedures and/or protocols in place for this task/activity? — **NO** → Do not proceed without evaluation of need for policy, procedures and/or protocol or determination that it is in the best interest of the client to proceed to delegation.

YES

Is appropriate supervision available? — **NO** → Do not delegate

YES

Proceed with delegation*

Step Two – Communication

Communication must be a two-way process

The nurse:	The nursing assistive personnel	Documentation: *Timely, complete and accurate documentation of provided care*
<ul><li>Assesses the assistant's understanding</li><ul><li>How the task is to be accomplished</li><li>When and what information is to be reported, including</li><ul><li>✓ Expected observations to report and record</li><li>✓ Specific client concerns that would require prompt reporting.</li></ul></ul><li>Individualizes for the nursing assistive personnel and client situation</li><li>Addresses any unique client requirements and characteristics, and clear expectations of:</li><li>Assesses the assistant's understanding of expectations, providing clarification if needed.</li><li>Communicates his or her willingness and availability to guide and support assistant.</li><li>Assures appropriate accountability by verifying that the receiving person accepts the delegation and accompanying responsibility</li></ul>	<ul><li>**Ask questions regarding the delegation and seek clarification of expectations if needed**</li><li>Inform the nurse if the assistant has not done a task/function/activity before, or has only done infrequently</li><li>Ask for additional training or supervision</li><li>Affirm understanding of expectations</li><li>Determine the communication method between the nurse and the assistive personnel</li><li>Determine the communication and plan of action in emergency situations.</li></ul>	<ul><li>Facilitates communication with other members of the healthcare team</li><li>Records the nursing care provided.</li></ul>

Step Three – Surveillance and Supervision

The purpose of surveillance and monitoring is related to nurse's responsibility for client care within the context of a client population. The nurse supervises the delegation by monitoring the performance of the task or function and assures compliance with standards of practice, policies and procedures. Frequency, level and nature of monitoring vary with needs of client and experience of assistant.

The nurse considers the:	The nurse determines:	The nurse is responsible for:
<ul><li>Client's health care status and stability of condition</li><li>Predictability of responses and risks</li><li>Setting where care occurs</li><li>Availability of resources and support infrastructure.</li><li><u>Complexity of the task being performed.</u></li></ul>	<ul><li>The frequency of onsite supervision and assessment based on:</li><ul><li>Needs of the client</li><li>Complexity of the delegated function/task/activity</li><li>Proximity of nurse's location</li></ul></ul>	<ul><li>Timely intervening and follow-up on problems and concerns. Examples of the need for intervening include:</li><li>Alertness to subtle signs and symptoms (which allows nurse and assistant to be proactive, before a client's condition deteriorates significantly).</li><li>Awareness of assistant's difficulties in completing delegated activities.</li><li>Providing adequate follow-up to problems and/or changing situations is a critical aspect of delegation.</li></ul>

Step Four – Evaluation and Feedback

Evaluation is often the forgotten step in delegation.

In considering the effectiveness of delegation, the nurse addresses the following questions:
- Was the delegation successful?
  - Was the task/function/activity performed correctly?
  - Was the client's desired and/or expected outcome achieved?
  - Was the outcome optimal, satisfactory or unsatisfactory?
  - Was communication timely and effective?
  - What went well; what was challenging?
  - Were there any problems or concerns; if so, how were they addressed?
- Is there a better way to meet the client need?
- Is there a need to adjust the overall plan of care, or should this approach be continued?
- Were there any "learning moments" for the assistant and/or the nurse?
- Was appropriate feedback provided to the assistant regarding the performance of the delegation?
- Was the assistant acknowledged for accomplishing the task/activity/function?

Source: Reprinted by permission from American Nurses Association.

its employees. For the most part, it is the institution, and not the individual nurse, that is named as the defendant in a lawsuit. This does not relieve the nurse from having to formally answer to the court for his or her actions or inactions. An institution's policies, or lack of them, are also common claims in a lawsuit.

Student/Instructor Liability

Nursing students have responsibility for their own actions and can be liable. The old adage that "students practice under their instructor's license" is no longer true. At the beginning of the nursing program, the student will have an instructor supervising the individual closely, but as the student progresses, the supervision lessens. Student nurses are held to the same standard of an RN for the tasks that they perform. It is important that students never accept assignments that are beyond their preparation and that they communicate frequently with their instructors for assistance and guidance. *Instructors, like supervisors, are responsible for reasonable and prudent supervision*, a standard that may be higher than that of a work supervisor because of the students' lack of experience.

Liability in Special Practice Settings

If you are a nurse manager in a specialty unit or setting, such as a critical care unit, emergency department, or labor and delivery, it is important that you know that nurses are judged by additional standards. Although errors can happen in virtually any practice setting, nurses who work in certain settings are more vulnerable to malpractice charges because the errors are more costly for the patients. The courts may also expect a higher standard of care from nurses who practice in specialty settings. The nurse manager in these settings must be familiar with the standards of practice set forth by the specialty's professional organization. It is important to remember that the newly graduated nurse has been prepared to be a generalist and not a specialist.

Critical Care Nursing

Compared with nurses who work on a general floor, nurses who work in the intensive care unit spend more time in direct care of a critical patient, whose condition can change at a moment's notice, increasing the opportunity for errors and the number of potential lawsuits. Many invasive and potentially harmful procedures are performed in this setting; critical care nurses are more vulnerable to charges of *negligence* and *battery*. If for some reason they perform duties or procedures that are outside their scope of practice, they can be accused of practicing without a license. The unilateral severance of a professional relationship with a patient without adequate notice, when the patient still needs attention, or when the nurse fails to observe the patient closely for subtle changes in condition can be charged as *abandonment*.

Two additional tort claims that can be filed against critical care nurses are the following:

- Invasion of privacy
- Failure to obtain informed consent

Emergency Department Nursing

The day-to-day practices of emergency department (ED) nurses fall into somewhat of a legal gray area because the law's definition of a true emergency is open to interpretation. For example, healthcare workers who treat a patient for what they regard as a true emergency may be liable for *battery* or *failure to obtain informed consent* if the court ultimately concludes that the situation wasn't a true emergency. One of the most common charges filed against ED nurses is *failure to assess and report a patient's condition*; however, inadequate triage may be considered *negligence*. Other tort claims that can be made against ED nurses include the following:

- Failure to instruct a patient adequately before discharge
- Discounting complaints of pain from a patient who's mentally impaired by alcohol, medication, or injury
- Failure to obtain informed consent, giving rise to claims of battery, false imprisonment, and invasion of privacy

Psychiatric Nursing

The most common tort claim against psychiatric nurses is *failure to obtain informed consent*. It is wrongly assumed that informed consent is not required, especially if the patient's condition interferes with his or her awareness or understanding of the proposed treatment or procedure. Violation of a patient's right to refuse treatment may stem from the mistaken belief that all mentally ill patients are incompetent. It is important to remember that *the right to refuse treatment is not absolute*, it can be abrogated if a drug or treatment is required to prevent serious harm to self or others. Generally, a physician, not a nurse, makes this decision, and in many cases the court makes the decision.

Malpractice claims may also stem from *failing to protect a patient from inflicting foreseeable harm to himself or herself or others*. Protecting a patient or the patient's potential victims from harm may include a duty to *warn the patient's family* that the patient is a threat to himself or herself or a duty to warn a potential victim. This duty is a standard of care in mental health practice that has been incorporated as either case law, statutory law, or both in many states. Should a nurse fail to report information given to her in confidence that could have prevented harm, she could be held liable for breaching her duty to appropriately assess the patient and for failing to comply with her duty to warn.

Obstetric Nursing

Cases that involve labor and delivery may have at least two plaintiffs: mother and child. An obstetric nurse may be held liable for the following:

- Negligence through participation in transfusion of incompatible blood, especially in relation to Rhesus factor incompatibility
- Failure to attend to or monitor the mother or the fetus during labor and delivery
- Failure to recognize labor symptoms and to provide adequate support and care
- Failure to monitor contractions and fetal heart rate, particularly in obstetric units that have internal monitoring capabilities
- Failure to recognize high-risk labor patients who demonstrate signs of preeclampsia or other labor complications

Evidence That Assists in a Lawsuit

The Medical Record

It is estimated that *one in four malpractice cases is decided on the basis of what is in the medical record* (Sullivan, 2004). You can become a nurse star or find yourself in deep trouble based on your timely and accurate documentation in the medical record. *The medical record is the first piece of evidence the plaintiff attorney asks to see.* The nurses' notes are often the first part of the medical record to be examined. The integrity, accuracy, and completeness of the medical record go a long way in making the claim defensible or indefensible.

When the nurse records the care administered, the specific time it was given, the patient's response, and the overall condition of the patient, the nurse can demonstrate that the standard of care was met. We have all heard the adage "If it is not documented, it wasn't done." In reality, simply, it is difficult to prove that it was done if there is no documentation and the plaintiff claims it was not done. The more accurate statement is "If it is documented, then it was done." Once the action has been documented at the time of the event, it is presumed that the documentation is accurate and whatever a patient says to the contrary is simply not true. This is why it is so important to document extensively, accurately, and factually in the medical record, especially when there is an adverse event.

Healthcare facilities use several documentation systems, including the following:

1. **Source oriented systems:** Documentation in this type of system stores each professional's notes in a separate system.
2. **Problem-oriented systems:** Documentation in this type of system focuses on the problems identified by all members of the treating team, and all members of the treating team document to the problem, if appropriate, on the progress notes. The notes are formulated using the acronym SOAP, which stands for subjective data, objective data, assessment, and plan.
3. **Traditional narrative formats:** In this format, the healthcare professional documents the assessment data, interventions, and patient responses in chronologic order.
4. **Focus charting:** The patient care problem(s) is the focus of concern and the documentation is specific to the focus.
5. **PIE charting:** In this system, information is grouped into three categories: problem, intervention, and evaluation.
6. **Charting by exception:** This system requires the health professional to document only abnormal or significant findings. It relies on written standards of practice that identify nurses' basic responsibilities to patients and protocols for intervention. It includes a standardized care plan based on a nursing diagnosis, in addition to several flow sheets, which enables health professionals to easily track trends.

Charting by exception (CEB) is the one system that carries with it several legal risks. Because this system relies on written standards of practice that identify the nurse's basic patient responsibilities, well-defined guidelines and standards must exist, and all staff members must clearly understand their use and use them consistently.

Lama v. Boras (1994) illustrates what can happen when nurses don't follow accepted standards of care when using CEB:

> On May 15th, 1995, R. Romero Lama had surgery for a herniated disk. Two days later, a nurse wrote in his chart that the bandage covering the surgical wound was "very bloody". An entry for the next day indicated he had pain at the incision site. On May 19th, a nurse documented the bandage was "soiled again". The next day Mr. Romero Lama began to complain of severe back discomfort; he passed the night screaming in pain. On May 21st the physician diagnosed an infection in the space between the vertebral disks, and ordered antibiotics. The patient was hospitalized for several months to treat the infection. Mr. Romero Lama sued the hospital and the physicians treating him, alleging that they failed to prepare and monitor proper medical records. The hospital did not dispute the charge that the nurses did not supply the required notes, instead they pointed out that they followed the hospital's official CEB policy.

The court ruled against the hospital on the grounds that the Puerto Rico law requires qualitative nurse's notes for each nursing skill, and the violation of this regulation caused Mr. Lama's injury. The court reasoned that a more complete picture of his evolving condition was unavailable because the hospital's CEB policy called for nurses to note qualitative observations only when needed to chronicle important clinical changes. Although objective aspects of the patient's care and condition (temperature, vital signs, and medications) were charted regularly, important details, such as the changing condition of the surgical wound and the patient's reports of increasing pain, were not. (*Lama v. Boras* [P.R. 1994], p. 75)

The medical record is presumed to be accurate if there is no evidence of fraud or tampering. Evidence of tampering can cause the record to be ruled inadmissible as evidence in court. Medical records may be corrected if the portion in error remains legible; deleting or rendering the entry illegible can impose liability. Late entries are usually acceptable if they are clearly marked "late entry" when made. Loss of the medical record raises a presumption of negligence (which can be overcome by contrary evidence). Nursing documentation must be complete, accurate, and timely to foster continuity of care. It should always include the following items:

- The initial assessment using the nursing process and applicable nursing diagnoses
- Nursing actions, particularly reports to the physician
- Ongoing assessments, including their frequency
- Variations from the assessment and plan of action
- Accountability information, including forms signed by the patient, location of patient's valuables, and patient education including patient's understanding of material taught
- Notation of care by other disciplines, including physician visits, if appropriate
- Health teaching including content and response
- Procedures and diagnostic tests
- Patient's response to therapy, particularly to nursing interventions, drugs, and diagnostic tests
- Statements made by the patient
- Patient comfort and safety measures

Many factors influence nursing documentation standards including the following:

- Federal statutes and regulations
- State regulations and statutes, including licensing statutes and nurse practice acts
- Custom
- Accrediting bodies
- Standards of practice issued by professional organizations
- Institutional policies and procedures

As a facility develops policies and procedures regarding documentation, it integrates the appropriate laws, regulations, and standards into its own policy and procedure manual. Your best assurance of following the law is to adhere to the facility's policy, which should describe who is to maintain each portion of a patient's record and by which system. A good way for the nurse manager to be aware of the quality and content of the documentation in each patient's record and the quality of the documentation done by the nursing staff is to have periodic chart audits done by the staff on randomly selected charts of the patients on the unit.

Defensive Charting: A Good Defense

All healthcare professionals should know some *simple guidelines for good defensive charting*. Defensive charting is one way to protect yourself from liability. Some tried and true guidelines include but certainly are not limited to the following:

1. All entries must be accurate and factual.
2. If a correction is needed, it should be done appropriately and according to the facility's policies.
3. Never obliterate or destroy any information that is, or has been, in the chart.
4. If you realize that you forgot to include something in your documentation, you should make a "late entry," noting the time the "late entry" charting actually occurred and the specific time the actual charting occurred. For example, (7/22/08) "2200 late entry, charting to reflect that on 7/22/08 at 1200. . . ."
4. All identified patient problems, nursing actions taken, and patient responses should be charted. A patient problem should not be documented without a nursing action and the patient response also charted
5. Document why you did not do something that you would routinely do. For example, "Pt. refused to ambulate because of . . ."
6. Be as objective as possible in your charting. Use a note that says, "Patient ambulated to the end of the hall, tolerated well, no shortness of breath noted, R-22, P rate 98, no complaints of discomfort" rather than "Patient ambulated, tolerated well."
7. In the case of a fall or some other untoward event, chart exactly what happened, what action was taken and the patient's response, the time the physician was notified, the time the physician responded, any orders given and the follow-up of those orders, and any other individuals notified, such as family members.
8. It is important that your notes are legible and clearly reflect the information you intend.
9. It is equally important to review notes from other providers because the medical record is used for communication and it should demonstrate that the team members are coordinating efforts and thought.

Situations That Put the Nurse at High Risk for a Lawsuit

Equipment Failure

In today's healthcare environment, nurses can feel that more time is spent nursing the equipment than the patient. It is true that we now practice in a very high-tech world, and with all the advances in medical technology comes more responsibility for the nurse. A certain standard of care is connected to the equipment that we use. *It must be used as directed by the manufacturer, and the nurse has a duty to know what that is and follow such directions.* There is also a duty to make sure that the equipment is free from defects.

Nurse managers are responsible for ensuring that the equipment used on their units is in correct working order and that staff understand the importance of reporting (and taking out of service, if possible) any piece of equipment that is not working properly. The hospital procedure for repairing equipment that is not working properly should be followed with the proper documentation. Nurses also need to exercise reasonable care in selecting equipment for specific procedures and patients. For example, if your patient is obese and a regular blood pressure cuff does not fit properly, you need to have available a large cuff for such patients. If a cuff does not fit properly, the reading could be inaccurate, thus placing the patient in jeopardy, which jeopardizes your practice as well because it does not meet the standard of patient care. The nurse can also be held liable for improper use of equipment that is functioning properly. This liability often occurs with equipment that cause burns.

Healthcare Facility's Responsibility for Patient Safety

Each healthcare facility shares responsibility for the patient's safety. This institutional responsibility for patient safety rests on the two most frequently used doctrines of malpractice liability.

The first doctrine, *corporate liability*, holds the healthcare facility liable for its own wrongful conduct—for breach of its duties as mandated by statutory laws, common law, and applicable rules and regulations. Over time, the courts have expanded the concept of an institution's liability for breaching its duties. In a landmark case, *Darling v. Charleston Community Hospital* (1965), the Illinois Supreme Court expanded the concept of hospital corporate liability to include the hospital's responsibility to supervise the quality of care given to its patients. In *Thompson v. The Nason Hospital* (1991), the courts went further and discussed four general areas of corporate liability:

1. A duty to use reasonable care to maintain safe facilities and equipment
2. A duty to staff the hospital with only competent physicians
3. A duty to oversee all individuals practicing medicine within the hospital
4. A duty to develop and enforce policies and procedures designed to ensure quality patient care

The second doctrine of institutional malpractice liability is *respondeat superior*. Under this doctrine the facility is liable for an employee's wrongful conduct. Basically, this means that both the employee and the facility can be found liable for a breach of duty to the patient, including the duty of ensuring the patient's safety.

Medication Errors

A study of 36 hospitals and nursing homes found that 20% of all medications administered involve some sort of mistake. All of them involved a violation of the classic five "rights" of medication administration—the failure to administer the right drug to the right patient, in the right amount, by the right route, and at the right time (Lafleur, 2004). Another study claims that 770,000 hospital patients experience an adverse drug event yearly and that almost half of these are preventable, such as those attributable to miscalculations, drug interactions, or drug allergies (Guido, 2001). The increased costs for these errors may be $2 billion for the nation as a whole (Kohn, Corrigan, & Donaldson, 2000). Claims involving medication errors are increased when the nurse fails to record the medication administration properly, fails to recognize side effects or contraindications, and/or fails to know the individual patient's allergies.

The Joint Commission's 2004 and 2005 National Safety Goals require that institutions develop bar code technology for matching patients with their medications and other treatments. Initiatives that improve patient safety also lower the chance of someone being sued. But they also set a new standard on which the standard of care may rest, and therefore they are important for every nurse to know and follow. *The nurse's ability to listen to a patient or a family member who mentions that the medication is new or to recheck when anything about the patient seems unusual may prevent a serious error.* Although many nurses believe they just don't have the time to recheck medications, making that recheck a priority will prove to be time well spent. Dealing with errors and the many consequences they can cause would take more time and can place patients and nurses in jeopardy.

Providing a Safe Environment for the Patient

Safety is being recognized more and more as a duty of healthcare institutions (The Joint Commission, 2004). The nurse manager plays multiple roles in this area. Staff must know how equipment should work and not use it if it is not functioning properly; remove obvious hazards such as chemicals, which could be mistaken for medications; and make the environment free of hazards, such as inappropriately placed furniture or equipment and spills on the floor. *An important preventive measure is knowing how to document correctly if an incident occurs* so that there can be no doubt regarding the facts of what happened and all you did to protect the patient.

Patient falls represent one of the primary risks in this category, second to medication errors, in numbers of untoward events. The following case study illustrates how inattention to the safety of your patient and the environment can not only endanger the patient but make you and the facility liable for injuries that the patient may incur:

> In *Cooper v. Rehabilitation Facility at Austin* (1998), the plaintiff, Ms. Cooper, age 71 had a history of rheumatoid arthritis but was found to be a good candidate for a knee replacement. In preparation for her upcoming surgery, she was admitted to a rehabilitation hospital to increase her mobility. While nurses attempted to transfer her from a wheelchair to a bed, she complained of pain, nausea and fainted. Eventually, she was transferred to a bed, given pain medication and O_2 by mask, while her physician was notified of the incident. Later that day, it was determined that she had a fractured right tibia and fibula. The next day, after she continued to complain of pain in her left leg, her left tibia and fibula were found to also be fractured. The patient sued the hospital, nurses, and physician. She settled her case against the physician and agreed to a non-suit regarding her claim against the nurses, but went to trial against the hospital alone on a charge of negligence. The jury found the hospital vicariously liable for the nurses' negligence in transferring her to the bed as well as for the other healthcare professionals who failed to diagnose and treat her injuries in a timely manner. They found in favor of Ms Cooper for the amount of 1,200,000 dollars. The hospital appealed but the verdict was upheld. The considerable sum of damages was based on the pain and suffering that Ms Cooper experienced as well as the change in her circumstances. Prior to the fractures, she still had the ability to perform some activities herself and hoped by having the surgery she would be able to do even more. It was obvious from the medical records that she was making progress before the fractures occurred. The court found that she entered the hospital to gain mobility and independence, not to lose it. (http://caselaw.findlaw.com/tx-court-of-appeals/123332 .html case#03-97-00057-CV)

This case is a good example of how nurses and the facility failed to protect the patient either by being involved in the patient's fall or by failing to assess a patient's risk for falling. Generally, a lawsuit is brought when the fall results in a serious injury such as a fracture and/or head injury.

Nurses are best able to defend themselves in these cases when the institution has a policy regarding the protection of patients against falls. In many facilities, it is call a "fall protocol." These policies establish levels of risk for patients, taking into account factors such as age, confusion, sedation, and/or preexisting conditions that might cause the patient to be unstable. Assessment for fall risk at the time of admission and periodically depending on the level of risk is one of the most important activities the nurse can do. The next most important thing is the documentation completed when a patient falls. The nurse's first duty when a patient falls is to the patient. This involves the following:

- Assess the patient immediately for possible injuries.
- Notify the physician about the fall and your assessment findings.
- Make sure that the patient is protected from further injury.
- Notify the family as soon as possible.

Documentation is extremely important and the following should be considered:

- Factually document how the fall was discovered, where the patient was found, and any other fact surrounding the fall.
- Document what the patient says regarding the fall.
- Document who you notified and the time.
- Document what was done for the patient, such as your assessment, the exam by a physician, any x-rays taken and the time, monitoring after the incident, and any changes in the current plan of care.

Failure to Adequately Assess, Monitor, and Obtain Assistance

There continues to be an increase in the number of cases where nursing assessment is inadequate or there is a failure to monitor and/or reuse and obtain needed medical assistance for a patient whose condition is changing or has deteriorated. Delegation of the registered nurse's responsibility of assessing and evaluating patient care is being seen more and more in the healthcare system today. If some portions of this duty are done by others (such as another RN, licensed practical nurse, or unlicensed person), the nurse primarily responsible for the care of the patient must still be aware of the findings and confirm them when they indicate a change in the patient's condition or progress.

Again, documentation of the changes and events surrounding them is critical. When it is necessary to report these changes to a physician or other healthcare professional, sometimes this involves challenging the physician or other professional staff. This can cause discomfort for you as the nurse manager or your experienced staff, not just the new graduate. The nurse must have current and accurate information. These situations require the difficult balance of assertiveness and diplomacy. These are skills that can be taught but are perfected with practice and experience.

Failure to Communicate

Communication is perhaps the most important responsibility of everyone on the healthcare team. The Joint Commission (2005) includes improved communications in its National Patient Safety Goals. The patient's total care rests on whether the communication occurs in the medical record or verbally. One of the most frequent claims against nurses in this area is the failure to communicate changes in the patient's condition to a professional with a need to know. This communication needs to be documented and should include the time, the name of the person spoken to, what was reported, and the individual's response.

Failure to Report

Several states have statutes that require healthcare professionals to report certain incidences or occurrences. If the provider fails to report as required and an individual is injured, there can be negligence per se, and no expert testimony is needed to prove the case. In addition, both institutional and professional licensure can be affected. Nurses need to be aware of the reporting statutes in the state in which they practice. In some states, it is not only a duty but the law to report certain incidents. Institutional policies and nurse practice acts on these topics are invaluable, and these guidelines make excellent topics for review at an educational meeting or seminar.

Short Staffed or Understaffing

What is adequate staffing? Unfortunately, few legal guidelines can help the nurse administrator determine the answer to this question. A few guidelines do exist; however, they vary from state to state and are limited mainly to specialty care units (such as the ICU). Even The Joint Commission offers little help. Its staffing standard sets no specific nurse–patient ratio. It just generally states, "The organization provides an adequate number of staff whose qualifications are commensurate with defined job responsibilities and applicable licensure, law, regulation, and certification."

California lawmakers took note of this and in 1999 passed a bill that required hospitals to meet minimum nurse–patient ratios in all units based on patient acuity but prohibiting nurses from being assigned to areas for which they lacked adequate orientation or clinical training. Then, in 2002 the California Department of Health Services announced nurse–patient ratios. Most other states have not followed suit. This gives the courts no reliable standard for ruling on cases of alleged understaffing. Each case has been decided on an individual basis.

There have been some important court rulings regarding understaffing. The decision in the landmark case *Darling v. Charleston Community Memorial Hospital* (1965) was based partly on the issue of understaffing. The case dealt with a young man who broke his leg playing football and was taken to Charleston's ED where the on-call physician set and casted his leg. The patient began complaining of pain almost immediately. Later, his toes became swollen and dark, then cold and insensitive, and a stench pervaded his room. Nurses checked his leg only a few times a day, and they failed to report the worsening condition. When the cast was removed 3 days later, the necrotic condition of the leg was apparent. After several surgical attempts to save the leg, it was amputated below the knee. The court found the hospital liable for failing to have enough specially trained nurses available at all times to recognize the patient's serious condition and alert the medical staff.

Since this case, several similar cases have been decided, for example, *Cline v. Lun* (1973), *Sanchez v. Bay General Hospital* (1981), and *Harrell v. Louis Smith Memorial Hospital* (1990). Almost every case involved a nurse who failed to continuously monitor the patient's condition—especially vital signs—and report changes to the attending physician. In each of these cases, the courts have emphasized the following points:

- The need for sufficient numbers of nurses to continuously monitor a patient's condition
- The need for nurses who are specially trained to recognize signs and symptoms that require a physician's immediate intervention

Hospital Liability

Courts have held hospitals primarily liable in lawsuits in which nurse understaffing is the key issue. A hospital can be found liable for patient injuries if it accepts more patients than its facilities or nursing staff can accommodate. The hospital controls the budget and, in the court's view, is the only party that can resolve the problem. That being said, many different defenses have been offered by the hospitals (for example, there were no extra nurses available or lack of funding for additional nursing staff). The courts have been hesitant to accept these defenses, particularly when the hospital has allowed the understaffing condition to exist for a long period of time.

Nurse Administrator, Nurse Manager, Charge Nurse Liability

You as the nurse administrator/nurse manager/charge nurse, for a specific amount of time, could find yourself personally liable in understaffing situations. For example:

1. You know that the unit is understaffed, but you fail to notify administration.
2. You fail to assign your staff properly and then fail to supervise their actions continuously.
3. You (or your staff) try to perform a nursing task for which you (or she or he) lack the necessary training and skills.

It is important to understand that *you are not automatically liable for mistakes made by a nurse on your staff* even though it may seem like it. Most courts won't hold the nurse administrator/nurse manager/charge nurse responsible unless that person knew or should have known that the nurse who made the mistake

1. Had previously made similar mistakes
2. Was not competent to perform the task
3. Had acted on the manager's erroneous orders

Remember, the plaintiff–patient has to prove two things: that you failed to follow customary practices, thereby contributing to the mistake, and that the mistake caused the patient's injuries.

Other staffing situations that you, as the nurse manager, can find yourself facing include the following:

1. **Sudden overload of patients:** You begin the shift and suddenly find yourself with more patients than you have staff to safely care for. What do you do?
   a. First, make every effort to protest the overload and get it reduced. Begin by asking your supervisor or director of nursing services to supply relief.
   b. If they can't or won't, your next step is to notify the hospital administration. Whether you receive help or not, it is important to write a memorandum detailing exactly what you did and the answers that you received.
   c. *Do not* walk off the job because you can be charged with *patient abandonment.* Instead, do the best you can. After the shift is over, prepare a written report of the facts and file it with the director of nursing.
2. **Floating**
   a. If a facility "floats" nurses to other units, the facility should have established policies that clearly state the competencies required of nurses asked to float to units other than where they usually work.
   b. The facility should also have a contingency plan if no such nurses are available. The policy should delineate the method of orientation for nurses who are floated to another unit.
3. **Mandatory overtime**
   a. Most nurses, and particularly nurse managers, would agree that mandatory overtime is a chronic, inappropriate response to poor staffing policies. It raises safety issues when the nurse has already worked a 12-hour shift and is too tired to continue to work safely. The practice of requiring nurses to work mandatory overtime spread throughout the country beginning in 2000 and is still continuing in some areas. In studies of mandatory overtime in other industries, the U.S. Department of Labor found that increasing scheduled work time increased time lost to absenteeism and increased injuries, and it usually required 3 hours of work to produce an additional 2 hours of productivity (Thomas, 1990).
   b. In the healthcare arena, mandatory overtime by medical residents is linked to significant numbers of patient deaths as a result of care being delivered by exhausted residents. Realistic concerns about nurses' ability to provide safe care were amplified by the release of the three Institute of Medicine (IOM) documents: *The Adequacy of Nurse Staffing in Hospitals and Nursing Homes* (Wunderlich, Sloan, & Davis, 1996), *To Err Is Human: Building a Safer Health Care System* (Kohn et al., 2000), and *Keeping Patients Safe: Transforming the Work Environment of Nurses* (Page, 2004). The number of nursing staff available to provide inpatient nursing care is linked to patient safety as shown by a substantial growing number of research studies. Recently, Aiken and associates (2002) have shown that an increased patient load is directly related to more patient

deaths, as well as higher levels of stress and burnout in nurses. These documents and additional studies provide the nurse manager with sound evidence to advocate for appropriate staffing, which improves both patient and financial outcomes.

4. **Temporary employees**
   a. The addition of agency or traveling nurses presents its own unique set of challenges for the nurse manager. Each time that you have a "temporary nurse" assigned to your unit, you must provide orientation and assess the nurse's competencies before making patient care assignments. Failure to appropriately assess the competencies of the nurse can open the door to breakdown in the standard of care, especially if the temporary nurse lacks the requisite competencies and thereby causes harm to a patient.

The mistaken belief that "a nurse is a nurse is a nurse" is constantly being disproven in this twenty-first century of high-tech patient care. The ongoing increase in potential lawsuits testifies to this. The preceding issues regarding staffing are certainly not inclusive of the multitude of problems and challenges nurse managers face on a daily basis as they and their staff struggle to provide safe, evidenced-based, high-quality clinical care to patients.

Fraud and Abuse

Unfortunately, within our current healthcare system, many examples of fraud and abuse go way beyond the nurse administrator role. Sometimes nurses do become involved, so it is important to be aware of fraud and abuse and to avoid getting involved at all costs.

The Centers for Medicare and Medicaid Services (CMS) describes fraud as "the intentional deception or misrepresentation that an individual knows to be false or does not believe to be true and makes, knowing that the deception could result in some unauthorized benefit to himself/herself or some other person" or agency (Centers for Medicare and Medicaid Services, www.medicarenhic.com/dme/dsm10.1-rev).

Fraud typically involves the following factors:

- **Overutilization:** Providing unnecessary services.
- **Upcoding:** Assigning a Current Procedure Terminology (CPT) code that reflects a higher level of service than was actually provided.
- **Billing for services not provided:** Deliberately billing for fictitious services. The issue to be resolved is whether the bill was submitted intentionally or through oversight.
- **Failing to provide necessary services:** Capitation penalizes the healthcare professional for overutilization; thus, providers may be monetarily encouraged to underserve patients.
- **Filing false cost reports:** For example, disguising an unallowable cost as an allowable cost. Typically filed by providers who are paid under Medicare Part A, including hospitals, skilled nursing facilities, and home health agencies.
- **Enrolling fictitious participants in HMOs** (Lovitky, 1997, pp. 42–44).
- **Misrepresenting the patient's diagnosis:** To justify the services or equipment furnished.
- **Unbundling or exploding:** Altering claim forms or billing for separate parts of a single procedure to obtain a higher payment or using split-billing schemes.
- **Looping:** Using insurance benefits of one member to bill for services provided for another. This is known to be more frequent when services are provided for more than one family member at the same time.

- **Double billing:** Deliberately applying for duplicate payment, that is, billing Medicare and a private insurer for the same services.
- **Phantom billing:** Billing for services rendered by an agency that is not certified as a Medicare participant through one that is certified.
- **Kickbacks:** Soliciting, offering, or receiving rebates/remunerations and bribes from other healthcare agencies or durable medical equipment companies (Tahan, 1999, p. 19).

A Medicare statute, "otherwise known as the Anti-Kickback Act" (Lovitky, 1997, p. 44) now deals with this last issue. An example of a kickback is when a physician refers a patient for laboratory tests to a lab owned by the physician or a family member.

> Several physicians have been prosecuted for accepting payment from hospitals in exchange for referring Medicare patients to those hospitals. Similar types of prosecutions have occurred with respect to illegal payments made by durable medical equipment suppliers to nursing homes and home health agencies. (Lovitky, 1997, pp. 44–45)

Furthermore:

> Distinguishing between fraud and mere negligence is imperative. Fraud generally occurs when individuals knowingly disregard the truth by submitting intentionally false claims. A mere oversight or an inadvertent error will not rise to the level of fraud; however, a pattern of oversights or errors may increase the likelihood of fraud liability. One cannot escape liability merely by intentionally not learning the truth about health claims being submitted. The government will prosecute "ostrich" behavior. Similarly, liability may not be avoided merely by outsourcing billing functions to a billing company. Typically, the government will assert its claims against both the principal and the agent in this type of circumstance. (Lovitky, 1997, pp. 42–44)

Abuse, which is not easy to prove, is billing for excessive charges, services not provided or not medically necessary, or undocumented care. CMS defines abuse as "incidents or practices . . . that are inconsistent with accepted sound medical practices, directly or indirectly resulting in unnecessary costs . . . or improper payment . . . for services that fail to meet professionally recognized standards." A familiar example is the unnecessary surgery issue with hysterectomies, tonsillectomies, caesarean sections, and coronary bypass, along with unnecessary hospitalizations, unnecessary tests, unnecessary medications, and unnecessary physician visits. Abuse can also occur when patients are denied their rights, experience verbal or physical abuse, or are restrained unnecessarily.

Estimates are that fraudulent claims probably cost billions of dollars—fraud costs both insurance companies and tax payers. Medicare fraud was found to be 14% when the federal government did the first comprehensive audit of Medicare. This finding prompted the government to start the National Health Care Anti-Fraud Association in 1985 to discover fraud and abuse and to teach about it. Several additional acts have aimed at increasing the federal government's effectiveness in this area. Meanwhile, both the Attorney General's office and the Department of Health and Human Services have begun investigating and heavily fining persons or organizations involved in fraudulent claims.

In 1998,

> as part of its Medicare fraud-busting campaign, [CMS] launched a program . . . that enlists the country's 39 million Medicare beneficiaries. As the program's 'eyes and ears in the field,' . . . seniors can report a suspected case of fraud to the agency and collect a bounty of up to $1,000. The money comes from funds recovered from providers. . . . [Seniors are doing just that, and] not all of them want money. . . . They see it as their personal responsibility. (Haugh, 1999, p. 16)

This is called the *qui tam whistleblower statute*. This law allows private individuals to sue on behalf of the U.S. government when they become aware of fraudulent activities. "The private citizen bringing the suit obtains a reward—usually 15 percent to 30 percent of any amounts collected by the government. Qui Tam suits have resulted in several large dollar awards of millions to the whistleblowers" (Lovitky, 1997, pp. 42–44).

The False Claims Act (FCA) remains the keystone of fraud and abuse prosecutions. Between the years 1987 and 2005, $15 billion was spent in FCA settlements and judgments. Health care was responsible for 33%, or $5 billion. In 2006 alone, costs were $3.17 billion, with health care in excess of $2.2 billion, or more than 70%, and we wonder why healthcare costs continue to spiral out of control.

Where does the nurse come into all this?

> The ethos of the corporation and the urgency for profit maximization place pressures on health care corporations to act in a way that may be incompatible with ethical practice. Profit-driven incentives often result in corporate deviance and criminal behavior. Nurses may be pressured to go along with schemes that may be unethical or illegal and because of shaky job markets may be unable to adhere to professional ethical guidelines. . . . Dirty hands cases are those instances in which one agent is morally forced by someone else's immorality to do what is, or otherwise would be, wrong. . . . Problems of this kind have been labeled by some as "dirty hands" situations, because the circumstances are such that the agent is left with a "moral stain" after taking an action. (Mohr & Mahon, 1996, pp. 28–29)

Conclusion

This is important background information to keep in mind when reading Chapter 7 on Ethics.

As a nurse manager in the 21st century, you are challenged to manage units that are constantly admitting and discharging higher acuity patients, to motivate and coordinate a variety of diverse health professionals and non-professionals, to embrace change that will develop work environments that are safer and more conducive to professional nursing practice, and to manage limited resources and shrinking budgets. Basic knowledge of the law as it pertains to nursing practice is another tool to add to your management skills arsenal.

Your role as a nurse manager places you in the position to effect change not only in the provision of quality patient care but in shaping a work environment that nurses want to be part of. As a role model, mentor, counselor, financial manager, and negotiator, you are one of the most important pieces of the puzzle of providing safe, quality care. Remember this:

> The law is good, if a man uses it lawfully.

> —*The First Epistle of Paul the Apostle to Timothy 1:8*

Discussion Questions

A 9-year-old boy was admitted to the emergency room with an acute asthma attack. Solu-Medrol (methylprednisolone sodium succinate), magnesium sulfate, and breathing treatments with albuterol did not open his airway so that he could breathe on his own. The boy became combative from lack of oxygen. Lidocaine and ketamine were given in preparation for a rapid-sequence intubation. Then, one of the nurses gave succinylcholine, which immediately paralyzed the respiratory muscles. It was clearly contrary to hospital policy for the nurse as opposed to the physician doing the intubation to administer succinylcholine. No one started bagging the boy for 4 minutes; then, it took almost 20 minutes longer to intubate him, during which time he went into full-blown cardiac arrest. He was successfully resuscitated but suffers from brain damage as a result of oxygen deprivation.

1. Identify what kind of constitutional law has been broken and why.
2. Using the basic elements of malpractice, discuss whether this case meets the criteria for causation.
3. In this case, who may have malpractice liability—the nurse, the physician, the hospital—and why? Discuss the defenses that may be available.
4. The medical record provides legal proof of the nature and quality of care that the patient receives. Using this case, discuss what documentation you should find in the chart regarding this incident. What finding do you believe would be key in the plaintiff's case?

Glossary of Terms

Abuse—billing for excessive charges, services not provided or not medically necessary, or undocumented care.

Administrative Law—the body of law made by administrative agencies that have been granted the authority to pass rules and regulations and render opinions that explain in more detail the state's statutes on a particular subject.

Burden of Proof—when the plaintiff has to prove that the incident occurred.

Case Law—the decisions rendered in court cases by appeals courts.

Civil Actions (Torts)—civil wrongs or injuries resulting from a breach of a legal duty that exists by virtue of society's expectations regarding interpersonal conduct or by the assumption of a duty inherent in a professional relationship (as opposed to a legal duty that exists by virtue of a contractual relationship).

Common Law—a type of law that includes decisions made by judges in court cases or rules established by custom and tradition.

Constitutional Law—the rights, privileges, and responsibilities that are stated in, or have been inferred from, the United States Constitution, including the Bill of Rights. States may not pass laws or institute rules that conflict with these constitutionally granted rights or rules because the Constitution is the highest law in our country. Examples of these rights are freedom of speech and religion. The right to privacy is a right that is inferred from the Constitution.

Criminal Actions—when an individual has done something that is considered harmful to society as a whole. These cases involve a trial with a prosecuting attorney, who represents the interests of the state or the United States (the public), and a defense attorney, who represents the interests of the individual accused of the crime (defendant). These actions can usually be identified by the title, which will read *State v. (name of the defendant)*.

Defendant—the person accused of the crime.

Expert Witness—the most common method to establish the duty owed by a nurse is the testimony of a registered nurse, with training and background similar to the nurse in question. The expert nurse testifies regarding what a reasonable nurse in the same or similar circumstances would be expected to do and whether the nurse in question did or did not do it. Testimony by experts is an essential ingredient in malpractice cases for both the plaintiff and defendant in lawsuits involving nursing care issues.

Felonies—serious crimes that result in the perpetrator being imprisoned.

Fraud—"the intentional deception or misrepresentation that an individual knows to be false or does not believe to be true and makes, knowing that the deception could result in some unauthorized benefit to himself/herself or some other person" or agency (CMS, www.medicarenhic.com/dme/dsm10.1-rev).

Intentional Tort—a deliberate invasion of someone's legal right. In a malpractice suit involving an intentional tort, the plaintiff need not prove that the defendant owed him or her a duty. The duty at issue (for example, not to touch an individual without his or her permission) is defined by law, and the defendant is presumed to owe the plaintiff this duty. The plaintiff still must prove that the defendant breached this duty and that this breach caused harm.

Malpractice—a tort committed by a professional acting in a professional capacity. Malpractice law deals with a professional's liability for negligent acts, omissions, and intentional harm.

Misdemeanor— a crime that results in a fine with no jail time.

Nurse Practice Act—probably the most important guideline for what nurses do. Most nurse practice acts outline the activities, or scope of practice, that the nurse can legally perform within the jurisdiction. These tend to be described in general terms. Behavior and actions that are considered unprofessional conduct are generally described more specifically.

A violation of any of the guidelines in a nurse practice act means that the nurse has fallen below the standard of care set by the state for nurses. It can also mean that the nurse risks action against his or her license.

Plaintiff—the injured person in a lawsuit.

Qui Tam Whistleblower Statute—a law that allows private individuals to sue on behalf of the United States government when they become aware of fraudulent activities. The private citizen bringing the suit obtains a reward—usually 15% to 30% of any amounts collected by the government. In 1998, "as part of its Medicare fraud-busting campaign, [CMS] launched a program . . . that enlists the country's 39 million Medicare beneficiaries. As the program's 'eyes and ears in the field,' . . . seniors can report a suspected case of fraud to the agency and collect a bounty of up to $1,000. The money comes from funds recovered from providers" (Haugh, 1999, p. 16).

Reasonable Nurse—a nurse who practices within the scope of practice and upholds the standards of nursing practice.

Res Ipsa Loquitur *(The Thing Speaks for Itself)*—a type of malpractice case in which an expert is not required.

Respondeat Superior—when the employer is responsible for acts of the employee.

Stare Decisis *(Precedent)*—the legal principle that requires that when an issue has been decided, all other cases concerning the same issue should be decided the same way. When a decision is reached by an appeals court, a record of the court's opinion and reasoning is recorded, and the result, also known as precedent, is the legal principle of *stare decisis*.

Statutory Law—the most common type of law that affects nurses. Statutes (laws) are documented rules that govern living in a state (state laws) or the United States (federal laws). They are passed by state legislatures and Congress. Statutes cover the rules for people's relationships with each other and can be viewed as the ethics of our society written down. The most important part of a statute is the section on definitions. Here the authors of the statute explain what they mean when they use a certain word.

Unintentional Tort—a civil wrong resulting from the defendant's negligence.

References

Aiken, L., Clarke, S., Sloane, D., Sochalski, J., & Siber, J. (2002). Hospital nurse staffing and patient mortality, nurse burnout, and job dissatisfaction. *Journal of the American Medical Association, 288*(16), 1987–1993.

American Nurses Association. (2010). Foundation of Nursing Package 2010. Silver Spring, MD: Author.

Berwick, D. (2003). Errors today and errors tomorrow. *New England Journal of Medicine, 348*(250), 2570–2572.

Brennan, J., Jr. (2007). *Update on fraud and abuse issues impacting hospitals and physicians.* Baltimore, MD: AHLA Institute on Medicare and Medicaid Payment Issues.

Cherry, B., & Jacob, S. (2005). *Contemporary nursing: Issues, trends and management* (3rd ed.). St. Louis, MO: Elsevier Mosby.

Clark A. (2003). Malpractice prevention and technology expertise. *Clinical Nurse Specialist, 17*(3), 126–127.

Guido, G. (2001). *Legal and ethical issues in nursing.* Upper Saddle River, NJ: Prentice Hall.

Harris, D. M. (2007). *Contemporary issues in healthcare law and ethics* (3rd ed.). Chicago, IL: Health Administration Press.

Haugh, R. (January 1999). *Hospitals and Health Networks,* 73:1, 1–16.

Helm, A. (2003). *Nursing malpractice: Sidestepping legal minefields.* Philadelphia, PA: Lippincott Williams and Wilkins.

Institute of Medicine. (2011). *The future of nursing: Leading change, advancing health.* Washington, DC: National Academies Press.

The Joint Commission. (2004). *Comprehensive accreditation manual for hospitals: The official handbook.* Oakbrook Terrace, IL: Author.

The Joint Commission. (2005). *National patient safety goals.* Oakbrook Terrace, IL: Author.

Kohn, L., Corrigan, J., & Donaldson, M. (2000). *To err is human: Building a safer health system.* Washington, DC: National Academy Press.

Lafleur, K. (2004). *Tackling med errors with technology. RN, 27*(5), 29–31.

Lovitky, J. A. (1997). Health care fraud: A growing problem. *Nurse Managers, 28*(11), 42–45.

Lyer, P. W. (2003). *Legal Nurse Consulting: Principles and Practice* (2nd ed.). CRC Press, Boco Raton, London, New York, Washington D.C.

McConnell, C. R. (2011). *The health care manager's legal guide.* Burlington, MA: Jones & Bartlett Learning.

Mohr, W. K., & Mahon, M. M. (1996). Dirty hands: The underside of marketplace health care. *ANS Advanced Nursing Science, 19*(1), 28–37.

National Council of State Boards of Nurses and American Nurses Association. (2006) *NSCBN and ANA issue joint statement on nursing delegation*. Retrieved from https://www.ncsbn.org/Delegation_joint_statement_NCSBN-ANA.pdf

National Practitioner Data Bank. (2004). *2004 annual report*. Washington, DC: U.S. Department of Health and Human Services.

Nurse's Legal Handbook (5th ed.). (2004). Philadelphia, PA: Lippincott Williams and Wilkins.

Page, A. (2004). *Keeping patients safe: Transforming the work environment of nurses*. Washington, DC: Institute of Medicine.

Pozgar, G. D. (2012). *Legal aspects of health care administration* (11th ed.). Burlington, MA: Jones & Bartlett Learning.

Pozgar, G. D. (2013). *Legal and ethical issues for health professionals* (3rd ed.). Burlington, MA: Jones & Bartlett Learning.

Sullivan, G. (2004). Does your charting measure up? *RN, 17*(3), 75–79.

Tahan, H. A. (1999). Home healthcare under fire: Fraud and abuse. *JONAS Healthcare Law Ethics Regulations, 1*(1), 16–24.

Thomas, H. (1990). *Effects of scheduled overtime on labor productivity: A literature review and analysis*. Document 60. Austin, TX: Construction Industry Institute.

Wunderlich, G., Sloan, F., & Davis, C. (1996). *Nursing staff in hospitals and nursing homes: Is it adequate?* Institute of Medicine Committee on the Adequacy of Nurse Staffing in Hospitals and Nursing Homes. Washington, DC: National Academy Press.

Zerwekh, J., & Claborn, J. (2006). *Nursing today: Transition and trends* (5th ed.). St. Louis, MO: Saunders Elsevier.

Health Care and the Economy

Many times, nurses do not understand how the healthcare economy affects their practice. They complain about all the administrative budget cuts or talk about the insurance companies as being the "bad guys," yet they do not realize why all this is happening to them. Thus, here in Part IV, we present a financial and economic background that helps nurses to understand how we got to our present financial situation in health care. Hopefully, using this knowledge, we can more effectively deal with our current situation.

Chapter 9 shows how we became a tertiary care, illness-based system that often does not meet the needs of our population who are lucky enough to have health insurance. Historically, when people were ill someone in the home cared for them. Amazingly, we are moving back toward that model again. Meanwhile, we can examine how insurance companies surfaced; how Social Security, Medicare, and Medicaid coverage emerged as the most prominent player in health care; how legislation like the Hill-Burton Act drove the healthcare industry to build hospitals and provided money for hospital (tertiary) care rather than for home care; and how value-based reimbursement and prospective payment have affected finances in health care. This has led to an ineffective healthcare system, which probably will not be able to pay for itself in a few years. The healthcare industry is further strained as the high cost of drugs combined with occasional healthcare personnel shortages and an aging population are having profound effects on finances. Meanwhile, state and federal governments pass legislation to achieve better quality, and insurers pay less each year for care that is given. With the present poor U.S. economy, health care is now at a crisis point.

Chapter 10 is concerned with the five stakeholders in health care: consumers, providers, payers, suppliers, and regulators. All are interrelated and complex, and this chapter gives us a better understanding of each. Our current dilemma is that we have not figured out how to achieve all three healthcare needs at once: universal coverage, quality, and cost containment.

Chapter 11 is about microeconomics. This chapter identifies four major forces that healthcare facilities face today: competition, regulation, the profit motive, and quality patient care. These key forces are examined from a microeconomic and cost accounting perspective for the nurse administrator.

How We Got to Where We Are!

*Janne Dunham-Taylor, PhD, RN, and
Joellen Edwards, PhD, RN, FAAN*

OBJECTIVES

- Understand historically how health policy has developed in this country.
- Describe how access, cost, and quality impact our healthcare payment system in this country.
- Discuss the impact of health policy on healthcare delivery systems.
- Anticipate ways in which the Affordable Care and Patient Protection Act can potentially influence health care delivery and outcomes.

How Did We Get into This Mess?

Presently, health care is a wonderful, complicated economic and quality quagmire and a lot needs fixing. The term *health care* is a misnomer; in the United States, we most frequently address "illness care." We use the term *health care* in this book but only because it is the common nomenclature for our illness system. Historically, in this country we have pursued treating illness rather than studying and implementing what brings about good health.

We know that our present piecemeal, *tertiary approach* to illness care has many serious problems. (In contrast to an emphasis on *primary care* as found in Australia, where the majority of healthcare dollars is spent on home visits and keeping individuals well.) Our dubious position as the only highly developed nation that still fails to provide basic health services to all its citizens creates unacceptable disparities in the health of our population and persistently maintains a fragmented approach to provision of health care. Research on promoting and achieving health is happening, but much larger amounts of money are spent on such pursuits as treating cancer, heart problems, and strokes—the leading causes of death—*after* they occur rather than on learning *how we can achieve health and avoid illness.*

So, how did we get into this quagmire? Examining our path can give us a better understanding of the present situation and unresolved dilemmas and offer us some idea of what may come next.

Collectively, the rules and regulations that define who gets which healthcare services, who can deliver them, and how those services are paid for are the core of the health policies that continuously affect every citizen's well-being. *Health policy* can be defined as the entire collection of authoritative decisions related to health that are made at any level of government through the public policymaking process. These decisions include those of the executive, legislative, and judicial branches of government. Over time, a number of partially successful attempts to fix the healthcare system have occurred through the development of policies at all levels of government, although they often address specific, isolated problems rather than creating a well-coordinated system that makes health care accessible and affordable to everyone.

Healthcare policies in the United States attempt to address three specific aspects related to public health concerns: (1) *access* to healthcare services, (2) *cost and cost control* of healthcare services, and (3) *quality of care* available to the population. The remainder of this chapter examines the development of healthcare policies that address these three concerns.

Foundations of Health Care: Early Days of Our Country

Early in this country's history, care was provided by women in the family who tended to health needs of relatives in the home. There was no formal education or training for these women. Instead, they relied on their personal knowledge and experience, and if they received any education or training at all, it was from other family members or neighbors who were "healers" or, if they could read, from books.

Physicians, if available, were consulted in more complicated or extreme medical situations. Formal medical education was not accessible until the 1800s. A person could become a physician by apprenticing with another practitioner, and little scientific basis for the profession existed. There was no mechanism for testing competence; anyone could hang out a shingle.

Health care was a private matter, paid for by patients or their families with cash or barter. There was no regulatory interference or supportive services from governments to protect and improve people's health. As our nation matured, governmental regulation of many aspects of health-related issues occurred.

Over time, local, state, and federal governments became more and more involved in ensuring public well-being through regulations about the direct provision of health care through agencies and hospitals, the promotion of sanitation and prevention of epidemics through formal public health departments, and health professions education and licensing, especially for physicians and nurses. Eventually, governments became involved not only in the regulation of but in actual payments for healthcare services.

The development of the public health system serves as a good example of the gradually increasing governmental regulation of health-related issues. Public health activities first began in larger cities in the early 1800s. The main focus was sanitation and prevention of epidemics of smallpox, typhoid fever, tuberculosis, and diphtheria, among other highly contagious diseases. Regulations were concerned with waste removal, swamp drainage, and street drainage. If epidemics occurred, homes or ships would be quarantined. As immunizations were developed, public health officials got involved with administering them. The first state board of health was formed in 1869 in Massachusetts. By 1900, each state had a board of health that worked on the above issues with local boards of health. Today, a myriad of public laws and regulations affects people's health, and departments of health at national, state, and local levels assess health needs, monitor compliance with health regulations, and implement programs to improve the public's health.

Policies Addressing Access to Care

Access, or the *availability of care*, is a huge issue in the U.S. healthcare system, and one that is growing rather than shrinking. *Access* can be defined as the use of personal health services in the context of all factors that impede or facilitate getting needed care (Andersen & Davidson, 2007).

Our system is unique in the developed world in that we do *not* systematically provide basic healthcare services for the entire population (*primary care*). One key factor in gaining access to services in this country is the ability to pay for them.

Medicare and Medicaid, federal and state policies that provide health programs, pay for various kinds of care for 32.2% of our citizens. The Indian Health Service offers basic health care to Native Americans living on reservations. Private insurance, most commonly obtained through employers with costs shared between employers and employees, covers 55.1% of the U.S. population, although many find themselves "underinsured" when it is time to pay the healthcare bills. Still, 15.7% of our citizens, 48.6 million individuals, have no healthcare coverage at all, leaving them to pay healthcare bills directly, in the old-fashioned way, from their own pockets or to seek care through safety net providers such as free clinics, rural health clinics, or federally qualified health centers (DeNavas-Walt, Proctor, & Smith, 2012). The number will change with the implementation of ACA. An increasing number of individuals *face bankruptcy* every year as a result of healthcare bills they cannot pay.

Access is not just about the ability to pay, however. Access also includes effective and efficient delivery of healthcare services, meaning that the services need to be culturally appropriate and geographically available, as well as delivered at a cost the user can afford.

Access to Direct Services: Hospitals and Beyond

Access to care beyond that available in the home was addressed by creating hospitals, nursing homes, and in-home care programs by trained nurses. Hospitals and nursing homes existed in the early 1800s, but in those days they existed on voluntary charitable contributions and served the indigent; were quarantine hospitals, opened and closed sporadically by public health officials to deal with epidemic diseases such as smallpox, yellow fever, or, later, tuberculosis; or were for the wealthy who could pay for the services (i.e., hiding a family member with a psychiatric illness in an insane asylum). By the mid-1800s, instruments such as the stethoscope, thermometer, sphygmomanometer, and microscope were introduced; air was viewed as a disinfectant, so good ventilation became important; antiseptic and sterile procedures were gradually introduced; better ways had been discovered to manage pain in surgery; and, later, the x-ray was invented. Hospitals, for better or worse, became accepted as tertiary treatment centers for all types of diseases.

In the early 1900s, visiting nurse agencies were started, especially in larger cities, to make health care more accessible for primarily poor residents. If able, clients paid a small fee for services provided. The visiting nurse agency board raised funds to support their work with the poor. Public health departments broadened to include maternal and child services and, in the slums of large cities, to detect tuberculosis (which had become the leading cause of death) and to control then-named venereal disease. In 1935, federal monies were made available to local and state health departments to strengthen public health departments significantly.

Social Security Act

A major societal shift occurred that dramatically affected health care in the midst of the Depression: In 1935, the Social Security Act was passed. Until this event, local and state governments and individuals and families had been responsible for services for the poor. In a landmark legislative effort, the Social Security Act shifted that responsibility to the federal government. Although not specifically intended to provide healthcare services, the Social Security Act provided funds for health-related programs for the poor in areas such as public health, maternal and child health, crippled children's programs, and benefits for elderly adults and disabled individuals.

The Social Security Act of 1935 also dramatically affected the nursing home industry. This Act specified that money be given to private nursing homes and excluded—later repealed—public institutions. Thus, for-profit and proprietary nursing homes (privately owned) proliferated to serve the welfare patient. These homes gave first priority to paying patients because the government reimbursement was substantially lower than fees for services. (Sound familiar?) A 1948 amendment made construction grants available to private and nonprofit nursing homes. Later, the proprietary homes did succeed in convincing Congress to make Federal Housing Authority (FHA) construction grants available for investor-owned facilities.

Healthcare Access Changes Post World War II

Our healthcare system as we know it today emerged after World War II. Hospitals were built as more medicines, anesthesia agents, and technologies—along with government money to build hospitals through the 1946 Hill-Burton Act—became available. National legislation emphasized *secondary/tertiary care,* highly technical hospital-based care, rather than *primary care,* defined as preventive, restorative, or medical treatment given while the patient lives at home. Hill-Burton funds focused especially on building hospitals in rural areas, creating geographical access to services that had not previously been available. Hill-Burton also required state-level planning for healthcare services.

Psychiatric treatment also changed dramatically. With the advent of psychotropic medications, more psychiatric patients could be treated in outpatient settings. In 1963, the federal government established community mental health centers for this purpose. Thus, many psychiatric patients who had been hospitalized for years were able to leave the hospitals and function in the community setting. Unfortunately, those who were more severely mentally ill suffered greatly because less money was available for their care.

Medicare and Medicaid: New Forms of Access

Until 1965, the federal government financed little in the way of direct healthcare services, concentrating only on public health issues and providing services for military personnel and Native Americans. State and local governments established and supported special facilities for mental illness, mental retardation, and communicable diseases such as tuberculosis. Less than half of elderly adults and disabled Americans had health insurance.

Then, in a wave of entitlement programming, the federal government really became enmeshed in health care by establishing Medicare and Medicaid. Naturally, this Social Security Act Amendment (Titles XVIII and XIX) benefited elderly adults and poor persons and gave them more access to health care, but providers—hospitals, other healthcare organizations, physicians, and even suppliers and the building industry—benefited as well. Medicare often became *the largest source* of revenue for healthcare providers, resulting in more hospital and long-term care building programs. As more personnel were needed for all the expansions and new building, additional federal programs were funded to supply more physicians, nurses, and allied health professionals.

Although Medicaid was (and is) particularly fraught with tension between federal regulators and states where the plan is administered, both Medicare and Medicaid opened previously unavailable access to elderly, disabled, and poor individuals. Both Medicare and Medicaid pay for hospital and long-term care, primary care, and some preventive services.

Medicare induced significant changes in long-term care. The federal government redefined who was eligible to care for Medicare patients by establishing care standards and requirements for skilled nursing facilities (SNF) and intermediate care facilities (ICF) that raised the level of care available to the public.

Medicare and Medicaid also infused the home health industry with money to expand agencies and services. Whereas there were approximately 250 home health agencies in 1960, by 1968 there were 1,328 official agencies providing home health services. Federal funding over the next 20 years gradually refocused home health on postacute services. Unfortunately, money became less available for the chronically ill client who needed longer term services. Services also changed in the home health industry as home health funding began to include rehabilitative services—physical therapy, occupational therapy, speech therapy, and social work services. This continues today.

In 1965, the Older Americans Act mandated and funded Area Agencies on Aging (AAA). These agencies fund a wide array of services for elderly adults: senior centers with nutrition and recreation programs, health promotion and screening programs, mental health evaluation and treatment, respite care, case managers to plan care for elders so that they can stay in their homes rather than be institutionalized, and services to the homebound such as meals, homemaker services, chore services, and transportation.

In 1980, the Omnibus Budget Reconciliation Act aided home care by expanding Medicare benefits to 100 visits per year, lifting a 3-day hospitalization requirement. For the first time, for-profit home care agencies could become Medicare-certified providers. In addition, advanced technology, such as ventilators, renal hemodialysis, and infusion therapy, originally found only in hospitals, all moved into the home, expanding the need for a home care nurse. This need was coupled with prospective payment for hospitals and resulted in earlier discharges and greater use of home care. The number of home care agencies increased exponentially. Battles ensued in response to the escalating cost of home care; in 1984, visits were restricted to the home bound. Later, after a 1989 court ruling (*Duggen v. Bowen*) eligibility requirements were eased once again.

Because Medicare standards required hospitals to renovate and rebuild in the 1970s, for-profit hospitals, like many other businesses, began to offer publicly traded stocks. Stockholders expected these hospitals to make a profit so stocks would increase in value and provide good dividends. In this arrangement, hospitals had to pay attention to stockholder interests. The profit-making motive applied to not-for-profit hospitals as well. They had to make profits too—using the money for pay increases, new equipment or building projects, and investments—but called it *excess of revenue over expenses* rather than profit. Investor-owned nursing homes and home care facilities also increased, creating access for those with private or public insurance.

One of the more recent changes to Medicare legislation is the Medicare Pharmacy and Modernization Act of 2003. Prior to this act, Medicare beneficiaries had no prescription drug coverage. Using elaborate eligibility and use criteria, this act provides Medicare participants with access to coverage for prescription drugs through private standalone prescription drug plans or Medicare Advantage prescription drug plans administered by approved insurance companies. Coverage actually started in 2006.

Since that time, beneficiaries have seen their premiums and copays rise and have experienced tighter utilization management. Although Medicare drug legislation has certainly provided relief for the costs of drugs, especially for lower income beneficiaries, all beneficiaries experience a gap in coverage, often called the "doughnut hole." When Medicare recipients reach a level of spending on prescriptions (adjusted yearly), coverage stops completely and resumes when the individual spends a ceiling amount (also adjusted yearly). This means that beneficiaries with limited income or no *gap insurance* may have limited access to needed drugs for a substantial portion of the year, with higher-spending (sicker) beneficiaries reaching their spending cap earlier (Stuart, Simoni-Wastila, & Chauncey, 2005).

This spending gap resulted in serious health consequences for Medicare beneficiaries and costs of more than $100 million a year in preventable hospitalizations (Morrison et al., 2012). The Affordable Care and Patient Protection Act (ACA), signed into law in March 2010, includes provisions to address the coverage gap and maintain quality outcomes for chronic illness. The U.S. Department of Health and Human Services (DHHS) reports that as of 2012, seniors had already saved more than $4 billion in prescription drug costs as a result of the coverage assistance provided by the ACA (U.S. DHHS, 2012).

Safety Net Providers

Because our system still has gaps in care, such as services for underserved and uninsured rural and inner-city populations, non-English-speaking immigrants, homeless persons, and migrant workers, modest efforts at providing what is termed *safety net* healthcare services have gradually emerged. Two examples of legislated support for the poor and uninsured can be found in the clinics and services targeted toward these populations.

The Community Health Center (CHC) Act, passed in 1965, provided funds for comprehensive health and supportive social services to be provided through clinics established to make primary care available to specific types of populations in the clinic's service area. Community health centers are funded through federal grants available through the U.S. DHHS and operate under specific rules and conditions. They are required to provide services to anyone who needs access, regardless of the person's ability to pay.

The Rural Health Clinic Act (RHC), passed in 1971, established higher rates of Medicare and Medicaid payments to rural primary care practices provided that they employ a nurse practitioner or physician assistant and meet the qualifications for federal approval as a rural health clinic. Rural health clinics can be free-standing clinics or can be associated with a rural hospital or nursing home. Although there are no specific requirements to provide care to the uninsured, most rural health clinics do strengthen the rural safety net beyond just Medicare and Medicaid patients.

As the movement toward advanced nursing practice gained momentum, schools and colleges of nursing established primary care and nursing practice centers and community health services, collectively known as *nurse-managed care*. Community nursing centers (CNCs), community nursing organizations (CNOs), and nursing health maintenance organizations (HMOs) have been sponsored by local communities, community groups, and churches and by university schools and colleges of nursing that provide the majority of these access points. Most nursing centers provide care to poor and underserved population groups (Harris, 2009). Many of these centers are also partially supported on the federal level by the Division of Nursing located within the DHHS, Health Resources and Services Administration, Bureau of Health Professions. Nursing centers are specifically targeted for funding in the ACA and should see the benefit of this funding in coming years.

Policies Addressing Cost

Cost, and controlling the cost of providing care, is one of the most perplexing issues facing the U.S. healthcare system today. The *cost* of health care can be defined as *the value of all the resources used to produce the services and expenditures* and refers to the amount spent on a particular item or service (Andersen & Davidson, 2007). Both are important concepts, but expenditures are more easily measured and tracked and thus are more commonly used to analyze financial aspects of the healthcare system.

Consumers and third-party payers have seen consistently higher rises in healthcare costs and expenditures than in other segments of the economy, with rates of increase slowing slightly for the past few years but continuing to rise (Rice & Kominski, 2007; Rice, 2007). Given that U.S. healthcare costs consume 17.9% of our *gross domestic product* (*GDP*; Martin, Lassman, Washington, & Catlin, 2012), insurance companies, employers, federal and state governments, and users of direct healthcare services are all vitally interested in payment systems and cost control.

Blue Cross/Blue Shield: Setting Trends in Paying for Care

The emergence of health insurance was a significant change in healthcare financing, moving payment for health care from personal business transactions to a third-party mediator. Initially, insurance coverage was created either to provide health care for people involved in rail or steamboat accidents or for mutual aid where small amounts of disability cash benefited members experiencing an accident or illness, including typhus, typhoid, scarlet fever, smallpox, diphtheria, and diabetes.

Then, in 1929 Justin Ford Kimball established a hospital insurance plan at Baylor University in Dallas, Texas. He had been a superintendent of schools and noticed that teachers often had unpaid bills at the hospital. By examining hospital records, he calculated that "the schoolteachers as a group 'incurred an average of 15 cents a month in hospital bills. To assure a safe margin, he established a rate of 50 cents a month.' In return, the school teachers were assured of 21 days of hospitalization in a semiprivate room" (Raffel & Raffel, 1994, p. 211). This was the beginning of the Blue Cross plans that developed across the country. Blue Cross offered *service benefits* rather than a *lump-sum payment—indemnity*—benefits that had been offered by previous insurance plans.

Following the success of Blue Cross, in 1939 the California Medical Association started the California Physicians Service to pay physician services. This became known as Blue Shield. In this plan, doctors were obligated to provide treatment at the fee established by Blue Shield, even though the doctor might charge more to patients not covered by Blue Shield. Blue Shield was in effect for people who made less than $3,000 a year. In one of many unsuccessful attempts at national healthcare reform, physicians designed and agreed to this plan to *prevent the establishment of a national health insurance plan*.

Blue Cross was quite successful. Blue Shield was not. As inflation occurred and patients made more money, the base rate was not changed, so fewer people were eligible for the Blue Shield rates. "Blue Shield made the same dollar payment for services rendered, but because the patient was above the service-benefit income level, the patient frequently had to pay an additional amount to the physician" (Raffel & Raffel, 1994, p. 213).

In many states after World War II, private insurance companies proliferated and offered health insurance policies both to individuals and to employers. Large employers were expected to offer employees healthcare benefits. Unionization played a major role. Health insurance became an *entitlement*. Soon private insurance companies (third-party payers) enrolled more than half the U.S. population. The McCarren-Ferguson Act of 1945 "gave states the exclusive right to regulate health insurance plans. . . . As a result the federal government has no agency that is solely responsible for monitoring insurance" (Finkelman, 2001, p. 188).

Federal Role in Cost Containment

To administer the complex Medicare and Medicaid programs that had been established, the federal government initiated the Health Care Financing Administration (HCFA), now the called Centers for Medicare and Medicaid Services (CMS), within the Department of Health and Human Services. Payment for Medicare and Medicaid services was based on the *retrospective* cost of the care—figured and billed to the government by healthcare organizations and by physicians seeing patients. This fee-for-service system did not limit what providers could charge for their services, and initially there was no systematic approach to fees: Providers charged what the market would bear. In the 1970s, faced with escalating healthcare expenditures, states began controlling the amount they would pay to a provider for a particular service. The rationale for setting rates that would be paid was to encourage providers to voluntarily control the costs of the care they delivered.

The federal government, along with states, was spending a tremendous amount of money on health care. In fact, the GDP for health care has grown from 6% when Medicare and Medicaid were introduced to 17.9% presently. To find money to support these programs, the government was faced with increasing taxes, shifting money from other services such as defense or education, or curbing hospital and physician costs. Curbing costs was the first choice for policymakers.

Hospital Prospective Payment: A New World for Hospitals and Providers

The next direct step by the federal government to control healthcare costs, particularly those generated in hospital settings, was the implementation of a *prospective* pricing system for Medicare patients. Before this time, hospitals and providers simply billed Medicare for their services and were paid in full. In 1983, the Health Care Financing Administration implemented a plan to pay a set price to each hospital for each diagnosis regardless of how much the facility actually spent to provide the care; this payment strategy was called *diagnosis-related groups* (*DRGs*). If hospital staff could provide care for a patient with a hip fracture, for example, at less than the DRG payment, they could keep the money and, in a sense, make a profit. If the cost of care for the patient went above the DRG payment, the hospital lost money. DRGs required hospitals to become more efficient and aware of costs. Yet, the requirements of the DRG policy induced providers to release patients from the hospital as quickly as they could and to shift costs to other third-party payers who did not engage in prospective payment, leaving doubt as to the "bottom line" in cost savings to the healthcare system overall.

Prospective payment was expanded in 1989 to include physician services outside the hospital with the introduction of the *resource-based relative value system* (*RBRVS*). This policy applied the same concept as hospital DRGs to the outpatient setting, through Medicare Part B legislation. Two goals of RBRVS were to control costs and to put more emphasis on primary care and prevention.

Health Maintenance Organizations

In another attempt to hold down healthcare costs, the Health Maintenance Organization Act of 1973 provided federal grants to develop *health maintenance organizations (HMOs)*. This act required employers with more than 25 employees to offer an HMO health insurance option to employees. HMOs had a good track record of bringing down healthcare costs because they had traditionally been serving younger, healthier populations. Thus, starting more HMOs sounded like a way to cut healthcare costs. This act provided a specific definition of what an HMO was and gave the states oversight (or licensing) responsibility.

The concept of *managed care*, as delivered by HMOs, has taken hold in the public sector as well. Both Medicare and Medicaid (in many states) have taken their own steps to promote managed care by contracting with private insurers or HMOs to take on the primary care of groups of people enrolled for healthcare coverage and to serve as gatekeepers to specialty services. These measures were intended to control healthcare costs for federal and state governments and to improve the quality of care. In actual practice, results have been mixed as the costs of health care continue to climb.

The Health Insurance Portability and Accountability Act of 1996 (HIPAA)

The *Health Insurance Portability and Accountability Act (HIPAA)* addresses several significant issues including access, quality, and cost. Major portions of HIPAA address the financing of health care. This act "establishes that insurers cannot set limits on coverage for preexisting conditions, . . . guarantees access and renewability [of health insurance], . . . [and] addresses issues of excluding small employers from insurance contracts on the basis of employee health status. In addition the law provided for greater tax deductibility of health insurance for the self-employed" (Finkelman, 2001, p. 192).

HIPAA started the *medical savings accounts,* a tax-free account provided by employers. Here the employee can annually set up an account and pay in the amount of money the employee expects to have to pay for health coverage for the year. The money paid into the account takes place before taxes are taken out by the employer. At the end of the year, if the money is not spent it goes back to the employer.

A major portion of HIPAA, and one most familiar to health professionals, mandated patient privacy procedures. This is the aspect of HIPAA that most consumers identify as well. This can vary from state to state as long as the minimum federal requirement is met (see www.hhs.gov/ocr/hipaa.). HIPAA ensures confidentiality and privacy of paper, oral (telephone inquiries and oral conversations), and electronic (computer or fax) patient health information to or from any source. Strict standards must be met.

Balanced Budget Act of 1997

The *Balanced Budget Act (BBA)* significantly lowered payments for psychiatric care, rehabilitation services, and long-term care. Because ambulatory services, SNFs, and home care services were rapidly expanding and costing more healthcare dollars, the idea was to curb spending by placing these services under prospective payment. *Prospective payment* means that the payer (led by Medicare and Medicaid) determines the cost of care before the care is given; the provider is told how much will be paid for given care. For instance, an *ambulatory payment classification system* was created, establishing a fixed dollar amount for outpatient services diagnoses; skilled nursing facilities experienced prospective payment through the *resource utilization group (RUG)* system; and home care was regulated by the *Outcome and Assessment Information Set (OASIS)* system. Even physician services changed to payments based on an RBRVS, as described previously. Hospitals, already experiencing prospective payment, had major, mandated payment reductions limiting DRG and RBRVS payment rates.

BBA reduced capital expenditures, graduate medical education, established open enrollment periods and medical savings accounts for Medicare recipients, increased benefits for children's health care, and created new penalties for fraud. BBA had a major impact on health care, causing a number of hospitals, long-term care facilities, and home care companies to fold. Profit margins were drastically reduced, and rural hospitals were disproportionately affected. This act encouraged *outsourcing*, a practice that continues today (Roberts, 2001). BBA had such profound cost-cutting effects that in December 2000, Congress passed relief legislation providing additional money for hospitals and managed care plans.

One positive aspect of BBA was the creation of the Children's Health Insurance Program, also known as CHIP, that "expands block grants to states increasing Medicaid eligibility for low-income and uninsured children, establishing a new program that subsidizes private insurance for children or combining Medicaid with the private insurance" (Finkelman, 2001, p. 398).

This act was reauthorized in 2009, after a long battle in Congress.

Another positive aspect of the BBA was a major impact on recognition of the nursing profession. Under BBA, nurse practitioners (NPs) and clinical nurse specialists (CNSs) practicing in any setting could be directly reimbursed for services provided to Medicare patients at 85% of physician fees. This occurred to both better serve populations not receiving medical care and to save costs because studies had determined that nurse practitioners could deliver as much as 80% of the medical care at less cost than primary care physicians could. This federal legislation overrode state legislation that, in some cases, required nurse practitioners to work under direct physician supervision, with reimbursement made only to physicians.

Policies Addressing *Quality*

Throughout the development of our healthcare system, the quality of care (for more detail on quality, see Chapter 4) has been assumed to be the business of individual providers, such as physicians and nurses, and specific delivery institutions, such as hospitals, long-term care facilities, and home health agencies. The blame for errors and the praise for cures were held to be between the provider or agency and patient. Outcomes of care were not collected or measured by any external, governmental organization. This is not the case today, however.

The quality care movement began in the 1980s but took a strong hold in the 1990s. In 1999, the Institute of Medicine released a shocking report, *To Err Is Human: Building a Safer Health System* (Kohn, Corrigan, & Donaldson, 2000; Richardson & Briere, 2001). This report identified multiple systematic failures in the process of delivering care. It was followed in 2001 by a second hard-hitting report, *Crossing the Quality Chasm: A New Health System for the 21st Century*, that provided specific recommendations for improvement of quality and safety. These two documents confirmed what quality experts had been saying: *Despite the enormous cost of health care in the United States, thousands of patients are injured or die as a result of errors in the course of receiving care.*

Quality in health care can be defined as "the degree to which health services for individuals and populations increase the likelihood of desired health outcomes" (Andersen, Rice, Kominski, & Afifi, 2007, p. 185). Quality of care, measured in patient or population outcomes, is now considered to be the result of the entire system of care. In many cases, aggregate results of care are public information and are readily available on the Internet (see, for instance, www.hospitalcompare.gov).

In the case of quality, a mix of public policymakers and private foundations and organizations is concerned with promoting and monitoring quality across the healthcare system. The quality movement goes much further than specific physical outcomes, such as those around outcomes of cardiac surgery, although these are critically important. Outcomes of personal, emotional, or social importance to patients are also developing, such as *patient satisfaction* or *quality of life* indices. Policy decisions at the federal level have shaped current efforts to ensure that the highest quality of care possible is provided in our healthcare system.

Governmental Agencies Concerned with Quality

The Department of Health and Human Services is the overarching federal administrative agency concerned with monitoring the quality of health care in the United States. Several components of the DHHS infrastructure assume national leadership and focus on quality issues. For instance, the Agency for Healthcare Research and Quality (AHRQ) engages in testing and reporting safety improvement strategies and makes available significant research awards to determine the best evidence for safe and effective practice guidelines. Another activity of the AHRQ is reporting disparities in health services based on race, ethnicity, and socio-economic status. AHRQ also houses the National Clearinghouse for Quality Measures, where standards and processes for measuring healthcare outcomes can be found. The AHRQ website (www.ahrq.gov/qual/measurix.htm) offers a wealth of information on measures used to assess quality in health care. AHRQ issues two reports annually to describe the quality of health care in the United States, the *National Healthcare Quality Report* and the *National Healthcare Disparities Report*, both available at the AHRQ website. AHRQ now focuses extensively on comparative effectiveness research to determine the effectiveness, benefits, and harms of different procedures, medications, and treatments in improving health outcomes. Existing and new data are examined to recommend best practices based on scientific evidence (AHRQ, 2013). Comparative effectiveness research will be increasingly important as issues of access, cost, and quality are debated.

The Centers for Disease Control and Prevention (CDC) is also concerned with safety and quality. One focus of the CDC is the promotion of health information technology systems to reduce human error. Another is the collection of disease surveillance data that track both chronic and acute infectious diseases in the private sector and in health departments. Much of the quality data is housed at the Division of Healthcare Quality Promotion, whose mission is to protect patients and healthcare personnel and to promote safety, quality, and value in the healthcare delivery system. This division has three branches that are directly linked to quality: the Epidemiology and Laboratory Branch, the Prevention and Evaluation Branch, and the Healthcare Outcomes Branch. The CDC website provides substantial information (www.cdc.gov).

The U.S. Food and Drug Administration promotes quality and safety outcomes through improving regulations for packaging and labeling of drugs and by maintaining strict reporting requirements. In addition, this administration is responsible for the regulation of biologics, cosmetics, medical devices, radiation-emitting electronic products, and veterinary products.

CMS plays a significant role in transforming healthcare delivery and financing from volume-based to value-based payments (American Hospital Association, 2011). CMS collects, monitors, and reports patient and process outcomes of the healthcare system. These performance measures are used by insurers to determine reimbursement. Hospitals technically volunteer to report critical quality outcomes. Financial incentives are offered through the Medicare program to hospitals that report their outcomes on 10 quality measures on a public website (www.cms.gov). A financial disincentive is levied against eligible hospitals that choose not to participate and contribute data. CMS publishes hospital outcomes as well as outcomes from nursing homes on its website Hospital Compare (www.hospitalcompare.hhs.gov). Other agencies and organizations publish data on health plan outcomes, medical group outcomes, and selected outcomes by individual physicians.

CMS specifies certain patient care paths for providers to obtain reimbursement. If the patient care path is not followed as specified, the healthcare organization does not receive reimbursement for the care. For example, if antibiotics are not given within 2 hours of a pneumonia diagnosis (the care path specification), the payer will not reimburse the hospital. CMS introduced what is commonly termed "pay for performance" strategies. Hospitals are now expected to prevent the development of 11 iatrogenic conditions including hospital-acquired pressure ulcers, falls with injury, catheter-associated urinary tract infections, vascular catheter infections, some surgical site infections, objects left in patients during surgery, air emboli, and blood incompatibility reactions. These conditions are commonly called "never events," meaning that they should never occur under any circumstances. Medicare no longer pays for extended hospital stays or treatment for preventable complications if they occur after admission. Four of these conditions (hospital-acquired pressure ulcers, falls with injury, catheter-associated urinary tract infections, and vascular catheter infections) are directly attributable to nursing care (Buerhaus, Donlan, DesRoches, & Hess, 2009). Therefore, nurses—especially nurse executives—are in a key position to lead improvement in this quality endeavor.

The Affordable Care and Patient Protection Act

The ACA, enacted in 2010, is the most sweeping healthcare legislation since the inception of Medicare and Medicaid in 1965. Numerous attempts literally over centuries have been made to reform U.S. healthcare but the ACA is the first to attempt to accomplish this objective. It was passed after a hard-fought battle that extended from the 2008 presidential campaign into President Barack Obama's first months in office. The ACA became a chief component of his legislative agenda, and the president used the power and influence of his office to engage support for the bill. The overall goals of the ACA are to strengthen and systematize U.S. health care and to provide near-universal coverage for American citizens and legal immigrants. The legislation is complex and multifaceted—a true attempt at system reform. Whereas this section provides a broad overview of the ACA, a useful, detailed summary of the ACA and its many components can be found at the Kaiser Family Foundation Health Reform page (http://kff.org/health-reform). The ACA seeks to strengthen patient rights and protections, make coverage more affordable and widespread, ensure access to care, and create a stronger Medicare system to care for the growing number of elderly adults in our country. Some provisions are already in force, and most of the rest will be in place in 2014 and beyond.

Specifically, to strengthen patient rights and protections, the ACA ends discrimination and denial of coverage for preexisting conditions, making it possible for individuals to transfer jobs safely and for parents of children with chronic illnesses such as asthma or diabetes to be assured they will have access to insurance coverage. The ACA ends financial limits on care for chronic, long-term conditions so that individuals who require life-long treatment can be assured they will not be denied care. Additionally, the ACA prevents insurance companies for dropping coverage when an individual uses the coverage extensively for complex conditions such as cancer care.

To make coverage more affordable, the ACA requires that 80% of insurance premiums must be used by insurance companies actually to provide care and improve quality of care rather than to pay for administrative costs. The ACA also prohibits exorbitant rate increases (those over 10%) to ensure that individuals and families can afford coverage. Small business owners are afforded tax credits for providing health insurance to their employees. The ACA requires most individuals to purchase health insurance coverage if it is not provided by their employer; but to help them manage the cost of this requirement, federal assistance is provided for individuals who earn up to 400% of the federal poverty level, and Medicaid will be extended to all individuals who earn up to 133% of the federal poverty level. States that engage with the ACA on expanding Medicaid will receive substantial federal benefits as the program is implemented. States that choose not to participate are required to present their own plan that meets federal guidelines.

To ensure better access to care, free preventive services will become available, and (already in place) parents' insurance coverage can be extended for children up to age 26 years. Insurance exchanges, publicly owned enterprises intended to offer affordable insurance coverage, are to be initiated by states; residents of states that elect not to participate in developing their own insurance exchange will have the opportunity to participate in a federal exchange. Payments for primary care services, longest the lowest paid practices, are to be enhanced, and support for federally qualified health centers increased. Fortunately for nurses and the public, the ACA includes provisions for nurse practitioner education under Title VIII and offers support for primary care through nursing centers.

A stronger Medicare system is required, including (already in process) reduction of fraud and abuse. There will be increased choices in senior health plans, and free preventive services will be made available to Medicare beneficiaries. Through a Health Care Innovations Center as part of CMS, innovations in healthcare delivery that are aimed to make a positive difference in patient outcomes will be tested and results made available as best practices. Under specific guidelines, groups of healthcare provider organizations, to be called accountable care organizations (ACOs), are in development and will incorporate and coordinate all levels of care for a population group.

The full effects of the ACA are yet unknown. The Government Accounting Office predicts significant long-term savings to the healthcare system, while other organizations predict increased cost. Political debates about implementation continue and it appears that will be a long-lasting trend. In the meantime, there is hope that more Americans can have insurance coverage and access to care will be improved.

A Look to the Future

Issues of access, cost, and quality will remain driving forces in the healthcare world for years to come, and perhaps forever. *Ever-tightening governmental funding and regulations*, such as the value-based reimbursement issues and the requirements of the ACA, force healthcare providers and institutional leaders to pay attention to patient outcomes in ways that have never before been expected.

Our *aging population* of baby boomers, now rapidly retiring, will continue to strain our healthcare system in both private and public sectors. Shortages of healthcare professionals (such as nurses and physical therapists) to care for them and those who are newly insured through the provisions of the ACA will continue as a problem to be reckoned with. Women especially feel the impact as they live longer and as they face possibly living at the poverty level in their older years. Today, women in the workforce—and 92.5% of nurses are women—continue to be paid 75 cents to every dollar a man makes. Retirement incomes will continue to reflect this societal problem.

Economic issues continue to plague federal, state, and local budgets as all face major deficits. Increasing taxes has not been popular, although as of 2013 federal taxes have increased. Increased spending cuts are also not popular. ACA creates an additional burden for federal and state budgets, with many state governors working on ways to both cut Medicaid payments and not support ACA requirements for Medicaid (a states' rights issue as yet unresolved).

The effects of the ACA, particularly the impact of ACOs and provider payments, will bear watching, especially as they are implemented in safety net and rural areas. Hospital closures in the past have disproportionately affected safety net and rural areas, and it is possible that some provisions of the ACA may have unintended consequences for citizens. As more citizens become insured and seek primary care, a dedicated effort will need to be made to ensure there are enough primary care providers to meet the anticipated needs. Federal laws to ensure full scope of practice for NPs and other advanced practice nurses may be required to adequately meet patient needs, especially as some states continue to artificially limit advanced practice.

Alternative therapies generally focus on health promotion. In the midst of all the cost-cutting in our illness care system, alternative therapies have been enjoying increased popularity with the American public even though consumers most often pay out of pocket for the services. As patients visit physicians and receive medications for diseases, they often discover that this does not cure the problem. In many cases, the medications cause other medical problems. Alternative therapies provide a way to stay healthy as well as to treat disease, and bring comfort, without producing as many side effects and as much pain. They are likely to assume even greater importance in health care in the future.

Another issue affecting our future in health care is the technology explosion. As telehealth capabilities increase, healthcare availability expands to meet the demand, opening the door for increased access to care for selected populations. *Electronic medical records* (EMRs) have great potential for increasing patient safety and the efficiency of care yet hold the ethical challenge of protecting patients' personal health information. Facilities that have accepted federal monies for EMR systems will have to meet the federal "meaningful use" requirements. This is slowly being incorporated into practice settings of all kinds and has significant implications for nurse leaders and providers (Wilson & Newhouse, 2012). In addition, the Internet has vastly improved clinician information on *evidence-based practice*. Consumers continue to access the Internet to research their specific illnesses and to determine which providers are most effective. They use this information to evaluate how effectively their provider is determining their care (Meadows, 2001) and will continue to do so with even more frequency in the future.

The science of *genomics* adds a new dimension to health care that will have an ever-increasing presence in the future. Currently, scientists have joined forces with private companies that supply enormous funds to map genes. With commercial enterprises involved, it has created great ethical implications because business leaders believe this information can produce future profits.

On one side of the U.S. healthcare landscape are people with excellent insurance, high levels of computer literacy, and life situations that allow them to seek the best care available, wherever it is available; they will be able to obtain the "personalized medicine" coming to us through genetic breakthroughs. On the other side of the landscape are the uninsured and those who are losing benefits, such as retirees, who may lack access to such sophisticated technologies. The growing numbers of uninsured and underinsured people, as well as the documented health disparities in health status of racial and ethnic minority populations and all populations living in poverty, will eventually force our legislators to address the inequalities of access and quality of care in our system. At the time of this writing, the American public finds healthcare cost and access concerns second only to their concern over the economy.

Another contributor to changes in the healthcare system in the future will be the effects of global warming, magnetic field decreases, solar flares, and the earth's poles changing directions. The impact of the extreme weather events, including ice-age conditions, heat waves, fires, volcano eruptions, earthquakes, floods, and storms, is predicted to lead to higher levels of insect- and water-borne illnesses and the reduction of food production and safe drinking water. Healthcare providers will need to address the physical and mental health needs that will arise from these conditions (Blashki, McMichael, & Karoly, 2007). Hospitals and other institutional providers will need to become even more focused on disaster preparedness and be ready to deal with an increasing number of patients requiring care for illness related to heat exposure and poor air quality (Longstreth, 1999). Drug-resistant organisms are predicted to increase, bringing new challenges in treatment of infectious diseases, such as the fungal meningitis outbreak in 2013. These developments require significant adaptation in healthcare delivery and are likely to disproportionately affect children, elderly adults, and poor people.

The problem is that healthcare costs are still high, with many individuals and employers finding health care unaffordable. Recent health policy changes hold promise to better manage healthcare resources but are fraught with political and economic unknowns. This is a time in the development of our healthcare system when nursing leadership is of paramount importance. Nurses represent the lived reality of the system; they see and hear on a daily basis patients' stories of both healing and unnecessary complications. Nursing knowledge and leadership are critical to improving our healthcare system and ensuring access, cost, and quality care for all.

That which is, already has been; that which is to be, already is.

—*Ecclesiastes* 3:15

Discussion Questions

1. How can you, as a nurse administrator or manager, work to identify and reduce disparities in health status among the patient groups you serve?
2. What implications does CMS pay for performance have for nurse administrators and managers? Why?
3. What changes might you anticipate in your employment setting as the effects of the ACA move forward? How can you, as a nurse administrator or manager, be involved in shaping the implementation of the legislation?
4. What implications do the increasing number of elderly and frail elderly adults hold for nurse administrators and managers across settings? What policy changes could be suggested to provide a better care situation for larger numbers of elderly people?
5. How has the HIPAA legislation affected your practice site? What implications do you see for nurse administrators and managers?

Glossary of Terms

Access—the availability of health care to the population; the use of personal health services in the context of all factors that impede or facilitate getting needed care. This includes effective (culturally acceptable) and efficient (geographically accessible) delivery of healthcare services.

Ambulatory Payment Classification System—prospective payment system for ambulatory settings giving a fixed dollar amount for outpatient services diagnoses.

Cost—the value of all the resources used to produce services and expenditures.

Diagnosis-Related Groups (DRGs)—prospective payment plan for hospitals where reimbursement is based on the diagnosis of the patient.

Entitlement—what a population expects from government (started in 1935 with Social Security).

Gross Domestic Product (GDP)—monetary value of all private or public sector goods and services produced in a country on an annual basis less imports.

Health Insurance Portability and Accountability Act (HIPAA)—legislation that ensures written, oral (telephone inquiries and oral conversations), and electronic (computer or fax) patient health information is kept confidential and private.

Health Maintenance Organizations (HMOs)—type of health insurance that provides a full range of integrated care but limits coverage to providers who are employees of or contract with the insurance organization.

Health Policy—the entire collection of authoritative decisions related to health that are made at any level of government through the public policymaking process.

Indemnity—lump-sum payment for healthcare services based on the retrospective cost of the care.

Managed Care—healthcare coverage where insurance companies and Medicare/Medicaid contract with private insurers or HMOs that assume the primary care of groups of people enrolled in a plan and serve as gatekeepers to specialty services. These measures were intended to control healthcare costs and to improve the quality of care.

Outcome and Assessment Information Set (OASIS)—prospective payment system for home care.

Outsourcing—where another organization that can provide services such as housekeeping, food service, and grounds keeping efficiently for a healthcare organization is hired to perform those services.

Primary Care—basic healthcare services provided as the first and continuing point of contact for prevention and health promotion, diagnosis and treatment, and referral.

Prospective Payment—where the payer determines the cost of care before the care is given; the provider is told how much will be paid to give the care.

Quality of Care—extent to which healthcare services provided achieve or improve desired health outcomes and are based on the best clinical evidence, are provided in a culturally competent manner, and involve shared decision making.

Resource-Based Relative Value System (RBRVS)—prospective payment system for physician services.

Resource Utilization Group (RUGs)—prospective payment system for skilled nursing facilities.

Secondary/Tertiary Care—highly technical hospital-based care or long-term care.

Utilization Review (UR)—where providers are required to certify the necessity of admission, continued stay, and professional services rendered to Medicare and other insurance beneficiaries.

References

American Hospital Association. (2011, September). *Hospitals and care systems of the future*. Retrieved from www.aha.org/about/org/hospitals-care-systems-future.shtml

Andersen, R., Rice, T., Kominski, G., & Afifi, A. (Eds.). (2007). *Changing the U.S. healthcare system: Key issues in health services policy and management* (3rd ed.). San Francisco, CA: Jossey-Bass.

Andersen, R. M., & Davidson, P. L. (2007). Improving access to care in America. In R. Andersen, T. Rice, G. Kominski, & A. Afifi (Eds.), *Changing the U.S. health care system: Key issues in health services policy and management* (3rd ed., pp. 3–31). San Francisco, CA: Jossey-Bass.

Blashki, G., McMichael, T., & Karoly, D. J. (2007). Climate change and primary health care. *Australian Family Physician*, *36*(12), 986.

Buerhaus, P. I., Donelan, K., DesRoches, C., & Hess, R. (2009). Registered nurses' perceptions of nurse staffing ratios and new hospital payment regulations. *Nursing Economic$*, *27*(6), 372.

DeNavas-Walt, C., Proctor, B., & Smith, J. (2012). *Income, poverty, and health insurance coverage in the United States: 2006*. Washington, DC: U.S. Government Printing Office. U.S. Census Bureau Current Population Reports, P60–233. Retrieved from http://www.census.gov/prod/2012pubs/p60-243.pdf

Finkelman, A. W. (2001). *Managed care: A nursing perspective*. Upper Saddle River, NJ: Prentice Hall.

Giordano, L., Elliott, M., Goldstein, E., Lehrman, W., & Spencer, P. (2010). Development, implementation and public reporting of the HCAHPS Survey. *Medical Care Research and Review*, *67*(1), 27–37.

Gottlieb, S. (2001, March). One doctor: One patient. *Cost & Quality*, 23–24.

Harris, M. D. (2009). *Handbook of home healthcare administration* (5th ed.). Sudbury, MA: Jones and Bartlett.

Kohn, L. T., Corrigan, J. M., & Donaldson, M. S. (Eds.). (2000). *To err is human: Building a safer health system* (Vol. 627). Washington, DC: National Academies Press.

Longstreth, J. (1999). Public health consequences of global climate change in the United States—some regions may suffer disproportionately. *Environmental Health Perspectives*, *107*(Suppl. 1), 169.

Martin, A. B., Lassman, D., Washington, B., & Catlin, A. (2012). Growth in US health spending remained slow in 2010; health share of gross domestic product was unchanged from 2009. *Health Affairs*, *31*(1), 208–219.

Meadows, G. (2001). The Internet promise: A new look at e-health opportunities. *Nursing Economic$*, *19*(6), 294–295.

Morrison, C. M., Glove, D., Gilchrist, S. M., Casey, M. O., Lane, R. I., & Patanian, J. (2012). *A program guide for public health: Partnering with pharmacists in the prevention and control of chronic diseases*. Atlanta, GA: Centers for Disease Control and Prevention. Retrieved from http://www.cdc.gov/dhdsp/programs/nhdsp_program/docs/pharmacist_guide.pdf

Raffel, M. W., & Raffel, N. (1994). *The U.S. health system: Origins and functions* (4th ed.). New York, NY: Delmar.

Rice, T., & Kominski, G. (2007). Containing healthcare costs. In R. Andersen, T. Rice, G. Kominski, & A. Afifi (Eds.), *Changing the U.S. healthcare system: Key issues in health services policy and management* (3rd ed.). San Francisco, CA: Jossey-Bass.

Rice, T. H. (2007). Measuring healthcare costs and trends. In R. Andersen, T. Rice, G. Kominski, & A. Afifi (Eds.), *Changing the U.S. healthcare system: Key issues in health services policy and management* (3rd ed.). San Francisco, CA: Jossey-Bass.

Richardson, W., & Briere, R. (Eds.). (2001). *Crossing the quality chasm: A new health system for the 21st century*. Committee on Quality Health Care in America, Institute of Medicine. Washington, DC: National Academy Press.

Roberts, V. (2001). Managing strategic outsourcing in the healthcare industry. *Journal of Healthcare Management/ American College of Healthcare Executives, 46*(4), 239.

Stuart, B., Simoni-Wastila, L., & Chauncey, D. (2005). Assessing the impact of coverage gaps in the Medicare Part D drug benefit. *Health Affairs, 24,* 167–179. Retrieved from http://www.ncbi.nlm.nih.gov/pubmed/15840626

U.S. Department of Health and Human Services. (2012). *News release: People with Medicare save more than $4.1 billion on prescription drugs.* Retrieved from http://www.hhs.gov/news/press/2012pres/08/20120820a.html

U.S. Department of Health and Human Services, Agency for Healthcare Research and Quality. (n.d.). *Measuring healthcare quality.* Retrieved from http://www.ahrq.gov/legacy/qual/measurix.htm

Wilson, M. L., & Newhouse, R. P. (2012). Meaningful use: Intersections with evidence-based practice and outcomes. *Journal of Nursing Administration, 42*(9), 395–398.

Healthcare Stakeholders: Consumers, Providers, Payers, Suppliers, and Regulators

Janne Dunham-Taylor, PhD, RN

OBJECTIVES

- Recognize the challenges that confront the healthcare industry.
- Define and identify where the healthcare costs are primarily used.
- Identify the major stakeholders within the healthcare system.
- Provide information on how the federal, state, and other regulatory agencies affect the industry.

The United States has the highest health care costs in the world, *with third world outcomes.*

> — *J. Storfjell, O. Omoike, and S. Ohlson, "The Balancing Act:*
> *Patient Care Time Versus Cost"*

Our current healthcare environment is a wonderful example of complexity—becoming more and more complex every year. Remember that complexity, if unchecked, grows exponentially and creates more problems and errors. This is evident in the healthcare environment, which is complicated by a major depression in the U.S. economy, a major federal budget deficit (with the states not far behind), and a dwindling middle class. We, as a country, could benefit from working to simplify the entire healthcare environment in small increments. However, this is not the case today. Instead, we continue to create more complexity.

Healthcare Dilemma

There are three major dilemmas in health care: universal coverage (*access*), paying for care (*cost*), and *quality*. According to economic theory, it is possible simultaneously to achieve any two of the three but not the third. For example, if you achieve universal coverage and can pay for it, costs will be very high. If you contain costs and pay for it, you will not be able to achieve coverage for everyone. As you can see from the quote at the beginning of this chapter, even though we are spending the most in the world, all we have achieved are third world outcomes.

The United States has struggled for some time to determine the best way to achieve reasonable, equitable distribution of health care without losing control of total spending. This struggle continues today. Most industrialized countries have chosen to focus on equitable distribution of health care by providing universal coverage; however, the United States continues to vacillate between equity and containing costs. The result has been limited success on both issues.

A definite result of this struggle has been the development of the medical-industrial complex. Health care has changed from a social good to a product. Healthcare delivery has become commercialized, and healthcare professionals, such as hospitals and physicians, have turned more toward using business techniques to survive. This pressure has led to economic problems, major quality and safety issues, spiraling costs, and new healthcare delivery approaches. Not all of these factors have been negative. For instance, technology has developed less invasive approaches in dealing with disease.

Healthcare expenditures are predominantly spent on illness care. One major issue in health care is that we are predominantly paying for tertiary illness care and spending little on prevention and primary care.

Five Stakeholders: Consumers, Providers, Payers, Suppliers, and Regulators

To better understand this complicated healthcare system, it is necessary to examine the five key stakeholders, or players, in the healthcare arena: consumers, providers, payers, suppliers, and regulators. Simplistically, *consumers* receive the health care, *providers* give the care, *payers* finance the care, *suppliers* provide materials and supplies to the providers, and *regulators* set laws, rules, and regulations that must be followed for giving and paying for care.

Yet, realistically, these terms are more complicated. First, these players are integrated in a healthcare system where actions taken by one stakeholder affect the other stakeholders. So, when the federal government passes a law establishing a set of regulations, consumers are affected, providers must make sure they meet the regulations, payers may be involved in meeting or policing the regulations, and suppliers may have to change supplies to meet the regulations. Second, at times stakeholders intermingle functions. For instance, (1) the consumer receives the care but is a payer when paying deductibles, (2) the federal government owns the Veterans Administration hospitals (is a provider) yet is a regulator through the Centers for Medicare and Medicaid Services (CMS), and (3) Kaiser Permanente provides insurance (is a payer) and owns healthcare organizations (is a provider).

Consumers

Consumers are patients in hospitals, residents in long-term care facilities, clients in home care, enrollees in insurance plans who receive health care, and people who pay out of pocket for health care. Consumers in health care are different from consumers in other industries because they are vulnerable. An insurance term for the consumer is *covered life*.

As the United States moves from a manufacturing-based economy to a service economy and employee work patterns continue to evolve, health insurance coverage becomes less stable. First, the service sector offers less access to health insurance than the manufacturing sector. Second, there is an increasing reliance on part-time and contract workers who have not been eligible for insurance, so fewer workers have access to employer-sponsored health insurance. The Patient Protection and Affordable Care Act (ACA) was passed to ensure that most people will have health insurance.

As the ACA evolves, all individuals will need to purchase health insurance. Subsidies are built in presently for those earning up to 400% of the federal poverty level. In addition to paying for insurance, many people need more extensive medical care. Additional money is needed (tax dollars so far) to cover this expense unless something is cut back, and cuts in federal (and state) budgets are already happening to deal with present deficits. With ACA, small business owners will be required to supply employees with health insurance and will get tax credits for this. *Will this force more small business owners to fail?* No one can be denied insurance regardless of preexisting conditions, and there will be no financial limits on care for chronic, long-term conditions. *Does this mean that our insurance premium costs will spiral upward even more?*

So, who pays for health care? Some consumers pay cash for care. Examples include wealthy persons (sometimes) and Amish. Employers offer what has become known as *consumer-directed health plans* where consumers pay up front in several ways:

- By sharing insurance premium costs. These continue to rise each year.
- By paying deductibles (the amount of money a consumer must pay before the insurance company will pay for healthcare services).
- By paying copayments (the amount of money a consumer must pay out of pocket for every healthcare service received). This amount can be fairly small, such as for a doctor's visit, but can be substantial, for example, 20% to 50%, for a procedure.
- By paying more if providers are not in the covered plan.
- By paying for any services not covered by the insurance plan such as alternative therapies or plastic surgery.
- By paying the amount above what the payer has established as a reasonable and customary charge, such as for outpatient services.[1]
- By choosing to pay cash for a healthcare service so it will not be necessary to go through the insurance company.

As the price of health care rises, consumers are paying more and employers are paying less. Examples include the following:

- Insurers are starting to expect consumers to have healthier habits and participate in wellness activities to obtain better premium rates.
- A reduction in explicit coverage has occurred, most notably for pharmaceutical benefits.
- Greater de facto limitations are placed on covered care, especially by *health maintenance organizations* (*HMOs*).
- The consumer may have to change providers based on the insurance plan his or her employer chooses.
- The cost of "Medigap" coverage is rising. This is insurance purchased by elderly adults to cover the 20% of costs that Medicare does not cover.
- Some employer-based plans now have a *maximum out-of-pocket* limit on the amount the employee has to pay annually for actual medical costs. For instance, say an employee experiences a catastrophic illness that costs $500,000 during the year. If the plan has specified a maximum out-of-pocket limit, once the employee has paid that amount (reached the limit), the employer pays 100% of the medical expenses until the maximum out-of-pocket as set by the employer. *Other plans, including Medicare, do not have this limit. Note here that Medicare only pays 80% of expenses.*

In addition, employers offer *cafeteria plans* for employees. In this arrangement, an employee chooses the amount and type of healthcare coverage (and other benefits) needed, within certain limits set by the employer.

Most often, employers charge employees a *monthly fee* for the health insurance benefit. If spouses each have an insurance plan, it is necessary to *delineate which plan* would first cover family healthcare needs, with the other spouse's plan picking up uncovered expenses only. If the employee's spouse had a good insurance plan, it is possible the employee would not require health insurance at all. This saves employers and employees money.

Then there is the problem of *uncompensated care* when uninsured or nonpaying patients do not pay for services. Even though more people will be covered with ACA, there will continue to be some people, such as migrant workers, who will not have insurance coverage and who may not be able to pay for services. Even with insurance, people must pay a portion of the payment themselves. When they do not or cannot, it becomes bad debt and providers lose money. In a climate where providers get less from insurers anyway, this becomes a burden.

Safety-net hospitals serve indigent and uninsured persons. Often, federal and state governments give these hospitals additional payments for uncompensated care. With the advent of ACA and more people at the poverty level being served, will these hospitals get even more payments? Is the government going to continue to provide additional payments?

One enormous problem in our current payment system is the costs incurred in the last year of life. End-of-life care costs amount to as much as a quarter of U.S. healthcare spending (Kovner & Lusk, 2012). *Nursing Economic$* (May/June 2012) devoted a whole issue to this topic. This is an area being examined closely by insurers to make sure unnecessary costs are avoided.

As the middle class dwindles, many cannot afford needed home health care. This problem results in more *uncompensated, untrained caregivers*—most often relatives with no nursing training—caring for consumers. These caregivers need basic care information such as turning the patient frequently to prevent bedsores, encouraging hydration, and providing better nutrition, education that a public health nurse could spearhead in the community if public health programs were more adequately funded.

Another consistent problem for consumers is *patient education and prevention* measures. Everyone seems to agree that more of this needs to be done, but in the past we have funded tertiary care with very little money going to prevention and keeping people in their homes. The question is how to achieve this change yet keep costs down. Enter ACA, which mandates more prevention. This will create additional CMS expenditures right when present costs need to be cut. One obvious answer, used by other countries, is to have the public health department provide more population-based education and prevention programs. However, public health continues to be drastically underfunded in the United States.

Providers

Providers are the individuals (nurses, physicians, dietitians, social workers, pharmacists, physical or respiratory therapists, dentists, and other healthcare personnel) and organizations (hospitals, outpatient facilities, long-term care facilities, home care agencies, or other healthcare organizations) providing the healthcare services. Some common provider organizational terms are *managed care organization (MCO)* or *health services organization (HSO)*. Healthcare organizations are groups of people working within an organizational structure to provide healthcare services to consumers. Healthcare services can be provided across the continuum of care, from how to achieve health, such as through alternative or preventive care, to treating disease, such as through acute, chronic, restorative, or palliative care.

The *executive group* in a healthcare organization includes the following members: the chief executive officer (CEO), the chief operating officer (COO), the chief financial officer (CFO), the chief nursing—or patient services—officer (CNO), general counsel, and other vice presidents from human resources, plant services, medical office, and/or information services. Membership depends on the size of the organization as well as on the CEO's and governing board's orientation.

Unless the medical staff is directly hired by the organization, the healthcare organization will have a *medical staff organization* in hospitals, sometimes called a *professional staff organization* in other settings. The medical staff organization is a separate association with its own bylaws and governing structure. It has a dotted line responsibility (meaning that the CEO does not have supervisory responsibility for it) to the CEO. Thus, the group members are not employees of the organization and are paid independently for their services. Although the medical staff group is mainly composed of physicians, it can also include other professionals such as dentists, clinical psychologists, podiatrists, nurse–midwives, nurse practitioners, and chiropractors. To receive *practice privileges* in the facility, the physician has to be recommended by the medical staff organization, which examines the physician's credentials and competency; the recommendation has to be approved by the governing board; the medical staff organization then extends the privilege of membership; and the physician accepts the bylaws of the medical staff organization. Another title for this group of physicians is *attending physicians*.

Providers generally have several payer contracts; each can pay differently and each uses different formats for electronic payment. Providers are concerned with *payer mix*. The issue is that different payers actually pay different amounts for the same services. For example, if most of the patient population served has Medicaid or Medicare as a payer, it is probable that the provider will lose money because neither pay the full amount needed to care for patients. In fact, Medicare and Medicaid pay less than 50 cents for every dollar spent. Providers prefer having a majority of private-pay patients who provide better reimbursement. Even with private-pay patients, generally discounts are given to payers. Discounts can be just a flat discount on all services rendered or calculated on a sliding scale based on volume. The provider must know whether the true reimbursement amount can still provide a profit or at least cover costs.

Pay for performance (also called *value-based purchasing*) has affected providers. Here, providers are reimbursed based on performance data (certain core measures that must be met to receive full reimbursement) that examine patient outcomes—length of stay, readmission rates, adverse reactions (many have become nonpay events), complications, infections, deaths, number of medications per patient, and consumer satisfaction and complaints. Note that since 2009, payers have refused to pay for hospital's mistakes and infections, called "never" events, and now a hospital readmission within 30 days may not be reimbursed.

Payers use the performance data to compare providers' performance and determine who gives the best care and who is less expensive. This is called *performance-based reimbursement* evaluation. Payers use this evaluation before contracting with providers for healthcare services. Better payments are given to hospitals that have good quality performance ratings, whereas hospitals that do not achieve as high a performance rating are penalized with lower payments the next year. The contract is for a specified time and for specified services.

With managed care, another provider issue emerged—*provider protection*. Physicians are expected to follow the rules of the HMO to continue working for that HMO. For example, they might agree not to order expensive or frequent diagnostic tests or authorize many patient hospitalizations. The idea behind the rules is to keep down expenses. Often, the HMO uses monetary incentives—withholds or bonuses—to ensure that costs do not skyrocket. *Withholds* are when the HMO holds part of the physician or hospital income until the end of the year and pays it back to the provider based on performance. Withholds may never be paid back to the provider and may be used instead to cover other expenses the HMO encounters. Year-end *bonuses* are another incentive method used by payers. Such practices have recently resulted in legislation aimed at either limiting the incentives or revealing the incentives to consumers. Providers need protection for due process in their relationship with payers in these matters because payers may expect that providers remain quiet about the incentives (*gag rules*).

Nurses are also providers, though at times they are not treated as such. Nurse practitioners and clinical nurse specialists can bill directly for services provided in a healthcare organization. However, with the exception of private duty nursing, nursing costs have been bundled into room charges. Only a few organizations have broken away from this model. It is such a problem in long-term care that the therapies receive higher reimbursement and a higher acuity level than nursing care receives. This is another example of what is wrong with healthcare reimbursement as it presently exists.

There have been ongoing nursing shortages, and with the advent of ACA, additional nurses will be needed. Because approximately 80% of nurses are ADNs (have an associate's degree in nursing), the Institute of Medicine advocates that nurses need more education to adequately care for more complicated patients.

Payers

Payers directly pay for healthcare services and can be individuals, employers, insurance companies, or the government. When insurers are the payers, they are not at the point of service. This is different from how payers operate in other businesses.

Employers are payers when they choose to provide healthcare benefits for employees. They can do this in one of two ways: (1) purchase (or make available) health insurance for employees, or (2) be self-insured (usually only larger employers are self-insured) and directly pay employee healthcare costs. In the latter case, the employer pays an insurance company (third party administrator) to administer the insurance plan. The employer sets up the limitations of the plan, including annual limits per employee; provides claim forms for employees; verifies employee claims; and pays providers from the employer budget. This arrangement can confuse employees who might believe they have insurance such as through Blue Cross, when in actuality their employer is self-insured and Blue Cross is only the intermediary administering the insurance plan. For self-insured employers, healthcare costs are listed as a line item on their budget.

This can create the need for huge midyear budget readjustments for unexpected large costs such as when an employee experiences a catastrophic illness that costs the employer $500,000. In this situation, the employer must find additional money to cover the healthcare line item in the budget.

Insurance companies provide individual or group insurance coverage for *covered lives*—the individuals included in the plan—for a contracted amount of time, often a year. The purchaser(s) pays a premium to the insurance company. In group plans, the premium payment is shared, or actually paid for, by employees. Generally, individuals, or even small business employers, pay more for insurance premiums than large employers. To counteract this problem, Hawaii established several HMOs for small businesses and aggregated the entire small business population together to get lower rates for small businesses.

A major change has been to have an *ambulatory-oriented patient care delivery system* that prevents hospitalization, and to have more services available to *keep patients in their homes* such as what is provided by the Centers on Aging and Health. Another goal of current legislation is to make a more seamless provider system so there is better planning and less duplication in the continuum of care (see the Case Management chapter).

A second major shift in the area of payers is the move from a *volume-based reimbursement* environment to a *value-based payment system* (American Hospital Association, 2011). Whereas payment systems of the past were concerned with the number, or volume, of patients, the new value-based environment rewards providers for positive patient outcomes (providing what patients value). In this new value-based environment, providers are not reimbursed for never events, for not following designated protocols of care within the required and specified time, or for having patients who need to be readmitted to the hospital in less than a month. *The better the hospital's performance, the higher the value-based incentive payment.*

This move to a value-based reimbursement system requires major changes in the healthcare environment. The American Hospital Association (AHA) recommends 10 must-do strategies for hospitals to be successful in the new value-based environment:

1. Aligning hospitals, physicians, and other providers across the continuum of care
2. Utilizing evidence-based practices to improve quality and patient safety
3. Improving efficiency through productivity and financial management
4. Developing integrated information systems
5. Joining and growing integrated provider networks and care systems
6. Educating and engaging employees and physicians to create leaders
7. Strengthening finances to facilitate reinvestment and innovation
8. Partnering with payers
9. Advancing an organization through scenario-based strategic, financial, and operational planning
10. Seeking population health improvement through pursuit of the "triple aim" (The triple aim is to simultaneously focus on population health, increased quality, and reduction in healthcare cost per capita, as identified by the Institute for Healthcare Improvement in 2007.)

Governments are the biggest force in the healthcare payer arena. The *federal government* is a major payer, covering more than 50% of total healthcare revenue. Federal government insurance programs include Medicare, part of Medicaid, the Federal Employees Health Benefit Program (FEHBP), Tri-Care, and the Civilian Health and Medical Program of the Uniform Services (CHAMPUS). *Thus, as the federal government implements a payment strategy, other insurers follow suit.* The state governments, often the largest employer in a state, have been responsible for health insurance for state employees in addition to sharing responsibilities for Medicaid programs with the federal government.

The term *third-party payers*, or *insurers*, refers to insurance companies, employers, or government agencies that provide healthcare insurance. The insurance company acts as an administrator of the pool of money collected from all its members, paying, or *underwriting*, the defined illness care coverage to a provider when the consumer has received healthcare services. With insurance, there is a risk to the insurance company. What if more people need coverage than anticipated? To determine the risk, the insurance company uses *actuarial data,* a statistical method that takes into account such factors as the age and sex of enrollees, past use, and cost of medical services, to determine both premium costs and definition of coverage. Obviously, it benefits the insurance company to serve a larger population, which reduces the risk and has the additional benefit of costing less to administer the plan. It is also better for the insurance company to have healthier people in the plan. This is especially an issue for the federal government, in Medicare, because it serves an older population that is more likely to need expensive illness care. The purchaser's perception of risk is also an issue. Insurance is only worth purchasing if people perceive that they may experience a risk, such as expensive surgery or other care.

Retrospective Payment

Historically, typical health insurance was *indemnity insurance*, where payment occurred after the care was given. This was called *retrospective payment*. The consumer chose the provider, the provider determined what was charged, and the insurance company paid it (*fee for service*). The insurance contract was with the individual or employer. Except for those who pay cash, true indemnity insurance is largely nonexistent today because health insurance plans use some form of managed care, or financial incentives, to be cost effective.

Prospective Payment

Like the name implies, *managed care* refers to any method of healthcare delivery that is designed to cut costs yet provide needed services (i.e., use the least expensive option for delivery of care, only pay for necessary services, control costs by contracting and telling providers what will be paid for services before the services are delivered, and involve consumers in paying for part of their care). In managed care, payers determine the amount they will reimburse for a medical service. Generally, the reimbursement strategy is *prospective payment*, where the payer determines the cost of care before the care is given. The provider is then told how much will be paid for the care. This is called the *prospective payment system* (*PPS*).

Service Benefit Plans

Service benefit plans, an example of both prospective payment and managed care, directly pay providers after negotiating and specifying the prices paid for each healthcare service. In service benefit plans, the patient pays part of the costs of care through deductibles and coinsurance. Medicare and preferred provider organizations (PPOs), such as Blue Cross, have service benefit plans. (This can be confusing because Blue Cross and Medicare also offer HMOs, a direct service delivery plan, discussed in the next section. In addition, Blue Cross and other insurance companies are the fiscal intermediaries for Medicare.) Because more than 50% of our country's population is covered by Medicare/Medicaid, this chapter provides more information on these two plans.

Medicare

Medicare, supported by payroll cash contributions placed in the Medicare Trust Fund, pays for healthcare services for Americans aged 65 years and older, for some people with disabilities who are younger than age 65, and for people with end-stage renal disease. Medicare covers approximately 80% of healthcare costs for these groups. (Note that Social Security has increased the age of full retirement for younger people.) There has been some debate as to whether there will be enough Medicare payroll cash contributions to cover healthcare once the baby boomers are all eligible.

Medicare is administered by the Centers for Medicare and Medicaid Services. Medicare usage is monitored by the Medicare Payment Advisory Commission (MedPAC) that independently advises Congress about more effective or less costly ways to manage Medicare. CMS pays an administrative fee to *fiscal intermediaries* to carry out the actual payment system for Medicare. Fiscal intermediaries are other insurance companies who already have experience with processing insurance claims—companies such as Blue Cross.

Medicare divides defined services and payments into four parts:

- Part A covers hospital inpatient services, blood transfusions in hospitals, skilled nursing up to 100 days in a benefit period, some home care and home use of medical equipment, and hospice care for those who have less than 6 months to live (see www.medicareconsumerguide.com/medicare-part-a .html). Most people receive Part A automatically on their 65th birthday. They do not have to pay a premium because they, or their spouse, paid Medicare taxes while they were working. However, there are deductibles and coinsurance costs for consumers. Under Part A, providers cannot bill consumers further for services.

- Part B covers physician and outpatient services, tests, and preventive treatments that are not covered by Part A (see www.medicareconsumerguide.com/medicare-part-b.html). If a person has paid Medicare taxes before age 65, that person is eligible to sign up for Part B; signing up for Part B is a choice that is left to the individual. If people choose to sign up, they pay a monthly fee for Part B and pay deductibles and copayments.

- Part C is like a Medicare HMO or PPO, called the Medicare Advantage (MA) Plan (see www .medicareconsumerguide.com/medicare-part-c.html). Private insurance companies that are approved by Medicare provide the coverage. Part C was supposed to combine Part A and Part B in a lower-cost alternative plan, but, in reality, it is more expensive. With ACA, there is a significant cut in this plan, bringing it in line with Parts A and B. In fact presently with ACA the Medicare Advantage Plan will be eliminated.

- Part D provides prescription drug coverage insurance through private companies approved by Medicare (www.medicareconsumerguide.com/medicare-part-d.html). Part D generally is where the individual pays a separate premium or yearly deductible, along with copays, coinsurance, or a deductible, when he or she actually buys a prescription. The person must have another plan of equal value or pay a penalty. Originally, if a person exceeded the limit, the person would have to pay 100% for prescriptions (called a donut hole) until he or she reached the catastrophic level where discounts were available. ACA attempts to fix this partially by offering gradually decreasing payments until a person reaches the limit, and then offers some drugs directly from drug companies at 50% of the cost.

Besides what the user is paying, federal tax dollars pay the rest of the costs. *Medicare only provides 80% coverage*. This means that additional insurance is needed. Consumers can purchase *Medigap* plans, sponsored by private insurance companies, in addition to paying for Medicare Parts A, B, C, and D. Medigap plans provide supplemental insurance for Medicare consumers. Plans vary. Some Medigap premiums are quite expensive, and many elderly adults cannot afford them.

Despite the prevalence of public and private supplemental coverage, Medicare beneficiaries face substantial out-of-pocket expenses. Medicare covers less than half of older adults' total health spending and is less generous than health plans that are typically offered by large employers. On average, older adults often spend at least 20% of their household income on health services and premiums.

Medicare's *service benefit plan uses prospective payment* mechanisms for care that set fixed rates for specific diagnoses. CMS sets the rates. In hospitals, these set rates are called *diagnosis-related groups (DRGs)* for medical/surgical and obstetric diagnoses (not for pediatric and psychiatric diagnoses) and are used for reimbursement but are not assigned until the patient is discharged. *Resource utilization groups (RUGs)* were adopted for long-term care reimbursement. *Ambulatory payment categories (APCs)* were started for ambulatory settings, and *the resource-based relative value scale (RBRVS)* was developed for physicians. Home care is regulated using the *Outcome and Assessment Information Set (OASIS)*.

As CMS established these prospective payment mechanisms, other insurance companies have also adopted them. Here is how they work. With DRGs, the physician is responsible for identifying the principal diagnosis upon discharge, which must be the reason for admission, using the International Classification of Diseases. Clinical Modification (ICD-9-CM 9th Revision, proposed 10th edition shortly). Up to four secondary diagnoses can be documented. If the physician does not adequately document all this, payment will not be forthcoming. When never events occur, when certain protocols are not met within the specified time, or when patients need to be readmitted within a month of discharge, this cannot be billed. The never events are labeled MS-DRGs (which stands for medical severity DRGs). Hospitals are still required to report these events. Hospitals cannot charge patients for never events, but some reimbursement is provided for physician care and other services the patient requires upon discharge that only became needed because the never event occurred.

In long-term care, Medicare reimbursement has been based on RUGs, now into RUG-III. RUGs measure resident characteristics and staff care time for various categories of patients. RUGs have seven categories of patient severity. Caregivers derive the classifications from assessments recorded in the resident *Minimum Data Set* (*MDS*) assessment instrument required for days 5, 14, 30, 60, and 90 during a Part A stay. Facilities must also complete a comprehensive assessment if a patient's condition changes significantly. So, in long-term care, reimbursement is determined by how effectively staff complete the MDS data.

APCs have been developed for the whole range of ambulatory services. APCs group thousands of procedure and diagnoses costs into several hundred categories, with separate classifications for surgical, medical, and ancillary services. Each group includes clinically similar services that require comparable levels of resources. A relative weight based on median resource use is assigned to each classification. Payment for each APC is determined by multiplying the relative weight by a conversion factor, which is the average rate for all APC services.

The resource-based relative value scale was started in an attempt to even out payments to specialty physicians (who were paid more) compared with family and general practice physicians (who received less). Presently, physicians are paid for each treatment, so there is an incentive to overuse services. ACA may affect payment if accountable care organizations are set up.

Home health care, driven by having to use OASIS, presently serves patients after acute care episodes. No money is allotted for chronic illness needs. This is a serious problem in our country because the greatest percentage of Medicare dollars is spent on acute tertiary care instead of health promotion, disease prevention, and primary care.

The problem with all these payment changes is that patients are often discharged too soon. For example, patients might still be medically unstable at the time they leave the hospital or may not be able to care for themselves and need medical care but have used up their home care allotment.

With ACA, the plan is to develop better ways to provide care to patients with long-term chronic illnesses. Overall,

> ACA initiated several delivery system reforms that are designed to promote coordinated, accountable, high-quality, and low-cost care. Mechanisms specified in the law to improve the delivery system include accountable care organizations (ACO), the patient-centered medical home, payment reforms (payment for care coordination, bundling of payment, and value-based purchasing), support for primary care, and reductions in hospital payments for preventable hospital readmissions. (Trautman, 2011, p. 29)

Where the money will come from for all this is unclear. Taxes have been raised, but with governments cutting budgets because of deficits, it remains to be seen how the goals of ACA will be realized.

Medicaid

Medicaid, a cost-sharing program involving both state and federal funds, provides services for medically indigent people, including children, and for people with severe and permanent disabilities who are younger than age 65—although elderly adults over 65 who receive welfare are also covered by Medicaid. The federal government mandates certain basic coverage: inpatient and outpatient hospital services; physician, midwife, and certified nurse practitioner services; laboratory and X-ray services; nursing facility and home health care; early and periodic screening, diagnosis, and treatment (EPSDT) for children under age 21; family planning; and rural health clinics/federally qualified health centers. States can add coverage for such things as prescription drugs, clinic services, prosthetic devices, hearing aids, dental care, and intermediate care facilities for people with mental retardation. Services and reimbursements vary widely from state to state. Each state has designed a different version of Medicaid and this is why Medicaid has different titles in different states, such as TennCare in Tennessee and MedCal in California.

Medicaid predominantly pays for custodial long-term care of more than 100 days, which represents 48% of Medicaid expenses. If people need custodial long-term care, they must be at the poverty level, as established by each state, before Medicaid will pay. If people are not at the poverty level, they can pay cash for care or let their long-term care insurance (including Medigap insurance) pay.

If a person does not have one of these options and is above the poverty level, it is possible to receive Medicaid benefits for custodial long-term care by *spending down* all assets (income, property, and other assets) until the patient is below the poverty level. Then, Medicaid benefits will begin. (In this case, the spouse is allowed a house, car, and a specified amount of money, but the rest must be "spent down.") The other option, used by a significant number of elderly adults who need custodial care, is to be cared for by a relative in the home. This avoids spending down life savings.

ACA is changing Medicaid in several significant ways: It will cover people at 133% of the poverty level, will specify essential benefits for newly eligible members, and will give increased funding to states if states choose to accept this. A number of states are resisting this by refusing to accept additional federal money for the ACA changes because then states will be mandated to add Medicaid services the way ACA outlines. Because ACA covers most of the U.S. population, this will enormously increase the money needed in federal and state budgets, right at a time when the country is experiencing a severe recession. The question is, Where will the money come from to pay for this? This question remains to be answered. So far, it seems that additional taxes will be the source for additional expenditures.

Medicaid is quickly becoming a federal-versus-state-rights issue. The federal government has mandated the states to support Medicaid, yet states struggle to continue to pay their share of Medicaid spending. This is nearing crisis proportions.

Direct Service Delivery Plans

A *direct service delivery plan* is another type of plan used by HMOs. This plan is different because it pays the provider in advance. Generally, there are five types of HMOs:

1. Staff HMOs that employ physicians individually.
2. Group model HMOs that contract with one multispecialty group of physicians. A per capita rate is paid to the physician, as specified in the contract.
3. Network model HMOs that operate just like group models, except that they contract with more than one group of physicians.

4. Individual practice association (IPA) members that include both individual and group practice physicians. The HMO contracts with the IPA for physician services. IPA physician members provide services for the HMO but also treat other patients.

5. Point-of-service HMOs. These came about more recently. Here an HMO patient can go to a physician or hospital outside the HMO but pays more out-of-pocket expense.

HMOs use *capitation* as the reimbursement mechanism. The word *capitation* comes from the per capita (per person) fee the purchaser pays. To purchase HMO services, the employer (or individual purchaser) pays a monthly (capitated) fee to the HMO. The HMO agrees to provide healthcare services specified in the contract for no additional costs to the employer or the individual. The HMO either contracts with, or hires, providers who agree to be paid in advance a monthly or yearly fee in return for providing all services enrollees will need for that period.

Under capitation, a provider could lose money if too many services are provided in the covered period, so providers want to provide only needed services. To better deal with this, consumers must first see a gatekeeper provider, such as a primary care physician or nurse practitioner. The *gatekeeper* determines whether care is necessary and, if so, makes the decision whether the patient should be referred to a specialist. The advantage to the patient is that there is no charge to see the gatekeeper and no insurance paperwork is necessary for reimbursement. In addition, there is no charge for specialty care, as long as the gatekeeper makes the specialty referral. The disadvantage to the consumer with an HMO is when the gatekeeper does not believe specialty care is needed. In this case, if the patient still wants specialty care, the patient has to pay for the specialty service or go without.

In the HMO system, gatekeepers are constantly under scrutiny for *practice patterns*. This includes collecting data on such factors as *bed days per thousand*, or the number of hospital inpatient bed days used by 1,000 health plan members in a year. Capitated payments have forced down patient length of stay.

HMOs use *disease management* to manage chronic, long-term illnesses. Disease management identifies the best practices to achieve fewer poor outcomes or at least to slow down the degenerative aspects of chronic diseases. The physician or provider is given a mandated, systematic, population-based approach that defines the patient diagnosis or problem and the specific intervention(s) to take with all patients who meet this definition. The HMO then collects data on the physician practice patterns and the patient clinical outcomes to determine how effectively the physician followed these mandates.

Who is the Bad Guy?

A common fallacy is to view third-party payers as the "bad guys"—the cause of our societal dilemmas: the inadequacy of healthcare coverage, limitations on healthcare coverage, the predominance of tertiary illness care, and the high cost of health care. However, who really is the bad guy? By reviewing the history of health care in this country, we can see a much larger societal problem. Employers spend large amounts of money on illness needs of employees, who expect the best tertiary care possible and want someone else to pay for and cure all their illnesses. Although the cost of care is shared with employees in the form of deductibles and copayments, the majority of the cost is passed on to the public through the price of whatever widget or service the employer sells. When consumers purchase the widgets or services, they complain about the high costs. Who is really to blame for these high costs? It turns out that finding the bad guy is really a hunt for a much larger societal dysfunction with many implications. We are all a part of this dilemma—the general public, consumers, employers, payers, providers, suppliers, and regulators. We all contribute to this complex problem, and we all must be involved in finding the solution.

Suppliers

Suppliers—individuals or companies—provide the supplies, equipment, and services used by healthcare providers. Nursing interacts with suppliers in a number of ways. For instance, the product evaluation committee determines the best deal on major equipment or supplies. The infection control nurse can become very involved with equipment and supplies that adversely affect either the patient or the healthcare worker.

In the late 1970s, in response to the importance of cutting costs, nationwide purchasing alliances—Premier Alliance, Voluntary Hospitals of America (VHA), and SunHealth—were formed. The idea was that materials and supplies could be purchased at less cost (many touted a 10% savings) because of the higher volume that could be purchased at once by the alliance. Presently, Premier Alliance and VHA contract volume includes approximately two-thirds of the nation's hospitals. This has caused other issues: Size brings big discounts, but not everyone wants to use the products. From a nursing perspective, it can be an issue when everyone is trained to use one supply, but the purchasing alliance gets a better deal on another similar supply that staff members have not been trained to use properly. The purchase itself may save money; however, staff education may cost the organization more on such purchases.

When healthcare organizations join a purchasing alliance, they still must rely on local companies for certain supplies and services such as waste removal, physician contractual services to staff the emergency room, and laundry facilities (if contracted outside the healthcare organization).

Warren Bennis calls the physician group "suppliers" for healthcare organizations. This seems to be the most appropriate term. However, sometimes physicians are referred to as *customers*. Many hospitals market to physicians for recruitment purposes. At times, the recruitment process also involves providing assistance for physicians, such as loans for office practices or homes, along with a certain amount of reimbursement for relocation expenses.

Regulators

Regulators are the organizations and agencies that set the rules, regulations, and/or standards that providers must meet to stay in business. This includes many groups, such as the federal, state, and local governments and judicial systems, accrediting bodies, regulators of professions such as medicine and nursing, and professional organizations. The standards used by regulators come from many sources including consumers, providers, payers, professional organizations, and even state or federal laws or executive orders.

Federal Regulation

In health care, the federal government, as a regulator, has the overall responsibility for both achieving quality and holding down costs. The Constitution specifies that the federal government has the authority to regulate interstate commerce and provide for the general welfare of its citizens. The main federal healthcare regulator is the CMS, established to administer Medicare and Medicaid and enforce national healthcare regulations. For example, federal legislation, in a 1972 cost reduction strategy, mandated *utilization review*, which is still in force today to assess medical necessity, efficiency, and/or appropriateness of services and treatment plans. Utilization review is accomplished using several mechanisms:

- *Preadmission certification:* The insurer approves care in advance. If this is required and certification is not obtained, the insurer can refuse to pay for the care.
- *Concurrent review:* Some insurers monitor patients' lengths of stay to ensure the patients are discharged quickly. If an insurer determines that the patient has received all the appropriate tests and treatments, the insurer will not authorize additional care and will refuse to pay for additional days.

- *Discharge planning:* Discharge planning has always been important and needs to begin at admission. It is important to keep lengths of stay as short as possible. However, now it is critical because if a patient is readmitted within 30 days, reimbursement will be lost for the readmission. The discharge plan may include additional care needed in the home or by transferring the patient quickly to long-term care, home care, and/or ambulatory care, which is less expensive than the hospital stay.
- *Case management:* Case care plans are developed for complicated patients to provide the needed care in the least expensive way. For example, perhaps a hospitalization can be prevented by providing home care 7 days a week.
- *Second surgical opinions:* For elective surgeries, insurers often require that the patient see a second physician to determine whether the surgery is necessary. Additionally, the insurer wants the surgery to be done in the least expensive way—outpatient is preferred, but if hospitalization is needed, it needs to be specified.

To accomplish quality monitoring, the federal government delegates specific responsibilities to each state's licensure and certification agency. For a facility to participate in Medicare and Medicaid programs, it must undergo this licensure and certification process. States vary as to actual requirements. In addition, healthcare organizations must be accredited to be eligible for Medicare reimbursement.

Other federal regulators affect health care:

- The Department of Justice and Federal Trade Commission enforce antitrust issues, which prohibit anticompetitive practices.
- The National Labor Relations Board regulates union organizing and collective bargaining.
- The Food and Drug Administration regulates drugs and medical devices and dietary regulations and inspections.
- The Securities and Exchange Commission regulates how investor-owned healthcare organizations can market, sell, and trade stock.
- The Nuclear Regulatory Commission regulates hazards arising from storage, handling, and transportation of nuclear materials.
- The Equal Employment Opportunity Commission enforces equal employment opportunities in hiring, equal pay, civil rights, and nondiscrimination regarding age.
- The judicial system has determined many healthcare regulations.

State Regulation

When the states delegated certain powers to a federal government and ratified the U.S. Constitution, they retained a wide range of authority known as the police powers, defined as the powers to protect the health, safety, public order, and welfare of the public. Consistent with the police powers, states have enacted legislation to regulate and license a wide variety of healthcare organizations that are required to obtain and retain a license and must submit to inspections and other regulation. (Longest, Rakich, & Darr, 2000, p. 69)

Health and safety issues include radiation safety, sanitation of food and water, and disposal of wastes. States may delegate some of the safety, sanitation, and waste disposal responsibilities to city and county governments. Therefore, the states regulate, inspect, and license healthcare organizations on physical plant safety issues and license and regulate various healthcare professionals and nursing education programs. In addition, each state has an insurance commission.

To be eligible for Medicare and Medicaid funding a healthcare organization must be licensed by the state annually. Certification is needed each year to receive Medicare reimbursement. After the inspection, the states make recommendations to CMS for Medicare certification.

Because about 50% of Medicaid funds are for long-term care, the federal government has mandated each state to do a more involved annual inspection of the long-term care given to each Medicaid-funded resident. As part of the inspection,

> a multidisciplinary survey team must ensure that the care reimbursed with Medicaid funds is necessary, available, adequate, appropriate—and of acceptable quality to maximize the physical and mental potential and well-being of the resident. The review also includes an assessment of [each] resident's continued placement in the home and the feasibility of meeting his needs through alternative institutional or non-institutional services. The survey team looks for evidence that the resident's discharge potential was evaluated. (Mitty, 1998, p. 248)

If the facility meets all the federal requirements, the state, representing CMS, then certifies or recertifies the long-term care facility on the day of the survey.

Another important state responsibility concerns individual licensing and certification of various health occupations. Perhaps, as nurses, we are most aware of the *board of nursing*. Each state has a nurse practice act that defines nursing practice and establishes the board of nursing. In addition, there are other professional boards, such as the board of medicine or the board licensing long-term care administrators. The professional boards define professional practice, license caregivers and set standards. To become licensed a person must show that he or she has achieved minimum competencies, and the board keeps an official roster of all who are licensed. Boards of nursing also license licensed practical nurses (LPNs) and nurse assistants for long-term care.

Generally, nurse practice acts specify that registered nurses can treat patients independently, whereas licensing for LPNs or nurse assistants specifies that licensees are dependent on the orders of a registered nurse or physician. In addition, the professional boards hold regular hearings, regulate practice, determine what is improper professional conduct, take disciplinary actions when infractions occur, introduce legislation to better define professional practice, license new nursing education programs, and oversee the quality of current nursing education programs. Most states have mandated that nursing education programs achieve an 85% student pass rate on the National Council Licensing Exam (NCLEX). Having representation on the board of nursing can be an important role in policymaking.

Although it is not a state regulatory body, it is important to note here that the purpose of the National Council of State Boards of Nursing (NCSBN) is to be a national organization where boards of nursing can "act and counsel together on matters of common interest and concern affecting the public health, safety and welfare, including the development of licensing examinations in nursing" (NCSBN, n.d.). NCSBN has been involved in several important issues. First, it has developed computerized licensure examinations, the NCLEX-RN and the NCLEX-PN, which are administered by a national test service to all individuals who want to be newly licensed as a registered nurse or licensed practical nurse. Second, NCSBN has established a multistate Nurse Licensure Compact. Presently, nurse practice acts are not uniform in all states. A state legislature can pass a law to become a part of this compact. Once passed, nurses can practice across state lines of states in the compact without getting licensed in another state, as long as they follow the practice provisions in place in the states in which they practice. The list of states that currently belong to the Nurse Licensure Compact is on the NCSBN website (www.ncsbn.org/nlc.htm).

Credentialing

Credentialing of healthcare occupations takes place in several ways: through licensure, registration, certification, and competency. With *licensure*, a person must show the state licensing board, such as the board of nursing, that he or she has achieved minimum competencies. *Registration* is the official roster kept by the board of nursing that lists all who are licensed. *Certification* is awarded to individual providers by a nongovernmental organization/registry when the individual has met certain educational requirements and passed an examination. For example, family nurse practitioners or certified nurse assistants are certified.

A number of nursing specialty organizations certify nurses (listed at http://medi-smart.com/cert.htm). In turn, these professional certifying organizations are certified by the American Board of Nursing Specialties, a certifier of certifiers (Bernreuter, 2001). Boards of nursing, as well as employers, require that people in certain health occupations are certified (i.e., nurse practitioners).

Voluntary certification for nurse administrators can be obtained from the American Nurses Credentialing Center (ANCC) and from the American Organization of Nurse Executives (AONE). Nurse executive certification can also be obtained by admission to the American College of Health Care Executives and for home/hospice care nurse executives through the National Association for Home Care's Executive Certification Program.

Certification can also be given to organizations that meet specified qualifications, such as the requirements of Medicare and Medicaid certification. A component of organizational accreditation includes the standard that employees are properly *credentialed* to do their assigned work. The evaluation process for this standard examines licenses, certification, educational background, and competency (evidence of current, safe practice or performance quality) of personnel, as well as that of the physicians.

Economic credentialing of physician patient volume and practice patterns, including patient outcomes, is now a common practice for hospitals. These factors are considered when renewing physician privileges.

Accreditation

> *Accreditation* is the process by which organizations are evaluated on their quality, based on established minimum standards. There are two major reasons for accrediting healthcare organizations. Healthcare purchasers want objective data to make informed decisions about health plans to support a good return on their investment. Data from accreditation, as well as accreditation status, can supply some of this objective data. In addition, consumers have become more interested in data about health plans as they make their own decisions about which plan to select from the choices available to them. Purchasers and consumers are interested in two critical elements: cost and quality. They want greater accountability for the quality of services. (Finkelman, 2001, pp. 230–231)

Generally, accreditation involves two steps: reviewing written materials (self-study), and an on-site visit from the accrediting body to determine whether the minimum standards have been met. Personnel in healthcare organizations must have ongoing education about current/new standards to maintain accreditation. There are many healthcare accrediting bodies (see http://gunston.gmu.edu/healthscience/547/MajorAccreditationAgencies.asp).

Professional Organizations

Professional organizations, such as ANA and AONE, continually examine professional scope of practice and professional standards. AONE, ANA, the American Association of Colleges of Nursing (AACN), and the National League for Nursing (NLN) have formed a national tri-council on nursing. Together, they represent nursing on certain national issues. In long-term care, directors of nursing can belong to the American Association of Directors of Nursing Administration in Long-Term Care or to the National

Conference of Gerontological Nurse Practitioners (NCGPN). The American Academy of Ambulatory Care Nursing (AAACN) focuses on ambulatory nursing practice. The National Association for Home Care (NAHC) represents home care professionals.

Nursing professional organizations are listed at http://www.nurse.org/orgs.shtml. The authors suggest that nurse managers belong to both clinical and administrative professional organizations that are appropriate for the area of practice in which they are working. In addition to nursing organizations, nurse administrators might want to consider other professional organizations that are pertinent to their work setting, such as the American College of Healthcare Executives (ACHE).

Note

1. As mentioned previously, this is true for coinsurance deductibles and what is above the reasonable and customary costs with regular insurance. However, with Medicare Part A and Medicaid, other than billing the deductible and coinsurance, it is illegal to bill the patient for the amount of reimbursement not paid by the government. In Medicare Part B, providers can bill up to 15% more for services than the cost covered by Medicare.

Discussion Questions

1. What would improve our healthcare system? Explain how this could happen.
2. As a nurse manager, how can you and your staff better care for the people you serve?
3. What are the characteristics of the consumers that you regularly see? How could they be better served?
4. What effect might ACA have on stakeholders?
5. What strategies could your healthcare organization adopt that would make it more effective?
6. What is measured for provider performance at your healthcare organization? Has reimbursement been lost as a result of never events or readmission within 30 days?
7. What percentages of various payers make up in your healthcare organization?
8. What information should nurse managers share with staff regarding payers?
9. What is prospective payment? How does it affect you?
10. Who are the various regulators that affect your healthcare organization?

Glossary of Terms

Bonuses—monetary incentives given to providers at the end of the year based on the providers' performance or the total plan performance.

Capitation—a reimbursement mechanism. *Capitation* comes from the per capita (per person) fee the purchaser pays. To purchase HMO services, the employer (or individual purchaser) pays a monthly capitated fee to the HMO.

Concurrent Review—a plan where health care is reviewed as it is provided. Some insurers will monitor patients' lengths of stay to ensure that the patients are discharged quickly. If an insurer determines that the patient has received all the appropriate tests and treatments, the insurer will not authorize additional care and will refuse to pay for additional days.

Covered Lives—individuals included in an insurance plan.

Direct Service Delivery Plan—a plan used by HMOs where the HMO pays the provider in advance and the provider agrees to provide certain services.

Disease Management—a plan often used for chronic, long-term illnesses. The physician, or provider, is given a mandated, systematic, population-based approach that defines the patient diagnosis or problem and the specific intervention(s) to take with all patients who meet this definition.

Fee for Service—when the provider is reimbursed a specific amount of money, reasonable and customary charges, for each service and/or product that is provided. A discounted fee for service reimburses the provider for the service and/or product but with a discount, either a fixed amount or a percentage, as specified in the payer–provider contract, subtracted from the fee.

Gag Rules—providers need protection for due process in their relationship with payers because payers may expect that providers remain quiet about the incentives payers give providers.

Gatekeeper—a primary care physician or nurse practitioner who determines whether care is necessary and, if so, makes the decision whether the patient should be referred to a specialist. In an HMO, when consumers need care they must first see a gatekeeper. The advantage to the patient is that there is no charge to see the gatekeeper, and no insurance paperwork is necessary for reimbursement. In addition, there is no charge for specialty care, as long as the gatekeeper makes the referral and the contract specifies that specialty care is available.

Health Maintenance Organizations (HMOs)—an insurance plan where the plan pays the provider in advance. The purchaser (an employer or an individual) pays a monthly fee to the HMO. The HMO agrees to provide healthcare services specified in the contract for no additional costs to the employer or the individual. The consumer sees a gatekeeper who determines what care the consumer needs.

Managed Care—any method of healthcare delivery that is designed to cut costs yet provide needed services.

Payer Mix—the percentage of different payers (i.e., Medicare, Blue Cross, self-pay) who paid for services to a healthcare organization over a year.

Performance-Based Reimbursement— data collected on patient outcomes—length of stay, readmission rates, adverse reactions, deaths, etc.—within a healthcare organization (provider performance). Payers use this evaluation before contracting with providers for healthcare services.

Preferred Provider Organizations (PPOs)—an example of a service benefit plan. It consists of a group of providers—such as physicians and hospitals—who have agreed to provide services at lower than usual rates to enrollees. The PPO acts as the intermediary between providers and consumers. The PPO pays prearranged fees for services provided. The enrollee incentive is to use the providers in the plan and not have to pay for many of the services provided. If an enrollee chooses to go to a physician not included in the PPO, the PPO only pays part—or none—of the fee, with the enrollee having to pay the remainder.

Practice Patterns—where physicians are under scrutiny about their practice. Data are collected on such things as length of stay and individual physician data is compared with other physician data.

Preadmission Certification—the insurer approves care in advance. If this is required, and certification is not obtained, the insurer can refuse to pay for the care.

Preferred Provider Organizations (PPOs)—an example of a service benefit plan that consists of a group of providers, such as physicians and hospitals, who have agreed to provide services at lower than usual rates to enrollees. The PPO acts as the intermediary between providers and consumers. The PPO pays prearranged fees for services provided. The enrollee incentive is to use the providers in the plan and not have to pay for many of the services provided. If an enrollee chooses to go to a physician not included in the PPO, the PPO pays only part—or none—of the fee, and the enrollee has to pay the remainder.

Prospective Payment— the payer determines the cost of care before the care is given. The provider is then told how much will be paid to give the care.

Provider Protection—legislation aimed at either limiting incentives offered to providers or revealing the incentives to patients.

Retrospective Payment—indemnity insurance where payment occurs after the care is given.

Service Benefit Plan—plans that directly pay providers after negotiating and specifying the prices paid for each healthcare service. In service benefit plans, the patient pays part of the costs through deductibles and coinsurance.

Underwriting—when an insurance company acts as an administrator of the pool of money collected from all its members and pays the defined illness care coverage to a provider when the consumer receives healthcare services.

Value-Based Reimbursement—when providers are reimbursed based on achieving positive patient outcomes (providing what patients value). In this new value-based environment, providers are not reimbursed for never events, for not following designated protocols of care within the required and specified time, or for having patients who need to be readmitted to the hospital in less than a month. The better the hospital's performance, the higher the value-based incentive payment.

Volume-Based Reimbursement—when payment to providers is based on the volume of patients who receive care.

Withholds—when an HMO, or payer, holds part of the physician or hospital income until the end of the year and pays it back to the physician or hospital based on performance.

References

American Hospital Association. (2011, September). *Hospitals and care systems of the future*. Retrieved from http://www.aha.org/about/org/hospitals-care-systems-future.shtml

Bernreuter, M. (2001). Spotlight on … the American Board of Nursing Specialties: Nursing's gold standard. *JONA's Healthcare Law, Ethics, and Regulation, 3*(1), 5–7.

Finkelman, A. (2001). *Managed care: A nursing perspective*. Upper Saddle River, NJ: Prentice Hall.

Institute of Medicine. *The future of nursing: Leading change, advancing health—report recommendations*. Retrieved from http://www.iom.edu/~/media/Files/Report%20Files/2010/The-Future-of-Nursing/Future%20of%20Nursing%20 2010%20Recommendations.pdf

Kovner, C., & Lusk, E. (2012). Introduction: How can we afford to die? *Nursing Economic$, 30*(3), 125–126.

Longest, B., Rakich, J., & Darr, K. (2000). *Managing health services organizations and systems* (4th ed.). Baltimore, MD: Health Professions Press.

Mitty, E. (1998). *Handbook for directors of nursing in long-term care*. Albany, NY: Delmar.

National Council of State Boards of Nursing. (n.d.). *About NCSBN*. Retrieved from https://www.ncsbn.org/about.htm

Storfjell, J., Omoike, O., & Ohlson, S. (2008). The balancing act: Patient care time versus cost. *Journal of Nursing Administration, 38*(5), 244–249.

Trautman, D. (2011, April). Healthcare reform 1 year later. *Nursing Management*, 26–31.

Microeconomics in the Hospital Firm: Competition, Regulation, the Profit Motive, and Patient Care

Mary Anne Schultz, PhD, MBA, MSN, RN

OBJECTIVES

- Provide a broad view of the economics involved in the hospital environment that includes competition, regulation, and patient care.
- Understand the impact of regulation in the U.S. healthcare system and costs associated with it.
- Demonstrate the impact of electronic medical records and how this affects the healthcare industry.

Since the introduction of a *prospective payment system (PPS)* for health care 25 years ago, hospital services have become increasingly driven by the market forces of price and quality. Rooted in a tradition of caring, hospitals were once seen as places where people could be healed and have their physical needs met—all through the professionalism and trust of healthcare providers. This was the hospital's *mission*. Today, hospitals are businesses, big and small, where patient care is but one service and patients are no longer the only constituent. The processes are now high technology, caring, curing in some cases, research based, and financially driven, serving a number of stakeholders such as physicians, investors, patients and families, and employees such as nurses, to name a few.

Balancing the goals of the players and supporting the many purposes of a hospital require identification of the pressures shaping its operation. Chiefly, these are (1) *competition*, (2) *regulation*, (3) the *profit motive*, and (4) quality patient care. This chapter examines these key forces from the standpoint of theory and practices in both *microeconomics* and cost accounting. Health care once derived its processes almost solely from mission, but now a hospital's *margin* is first because without a (*profit*) margin the organization, like all businesses, ceases to exist, and hence there is no mission. This chapter in no way provides a comprehensive survey of these interrelated forces but instead offers an explanatory primer, with examples, for a hospital's economic and business behavior. An overview of the disciplines of both microeconomics and cost accounting is provided to acquaint the reader with what is probably an entirely new way of thinking (and talking) about the institution called a hospital. This way, the profession, through the *nurse managers* and other nurse administrators, communicates with key nonprovider hospital decision makers, such as the chief executive officer or chief financial officer, with the same language and thus on a level playing field.

Microeconomics, Cost Accounting, and Nursing

This section addresses the question, "What is microeconomics (and, in turn, cost accounting) and what has it to do with nursing?" *Economics*, the study of how society allocates scarce resources, can be divided into two categories, macroeconomics and microeconomics. *Macroeconomics* (the prefix *macro* meaning large) is the study of the market system on a large scale. Macroeconomics considers the aggregate performance of *all* markets (so, the performance or outcomes of *all* companies or firms in *all* industries) and gives us indices or measures (indicators) of a nation's economy such as stock prices, interest rates, jobless claims, and housing starts. For purposes of this chapter, macroeconomics might serve as a context within which we describe the typical hospital (hospital *firm*) behavior with respect to (1) revenue optimization, (2) expense reduction, and (3) production of patient outcomes at an acceptable (not maximal) level of quality. *Microeconomics*, the study of individual consumers in relationship to their markets, is concerned with the choices made by smaller economic units such as consumers or individual (hospital) firms. A key topic in this chapter, microeconomics gives us concepts such as profit, profit maximization, price strategy, and nonprice competition to consider.

Cost accounting is an element of financial management that generates information about the *costs* of an organization and its components. As such, it is a subset of accounting in general and encompasses the development and provision of a wide range of financial management that is useful to managers in their organizational roles. Keep in mind that the goal in generating this information is to provide a basis for decision making. A quintessential question in our field is this: What should the nurse-to-patient ratio be and on what basis is this decided? The field of cost accounting, borrowing from *financial accounting* (information generated by firms largely for external purposes, e.g., the Internal Revenue Service) while encompassing *managerial accounting* (information generated by firms for their own internal use), affords us tools to address the tough staffing questions such as break-even analysis, profitability analysis, make versus buy decision making, marginal cost calculations, and cost–quality trade-off analysis. The relationship of the accounting disciplines is depicted in **Exhibit 11–1**. It is the considered opinion of the author that these domains, economics and accounting, were once considered mutually exclusive from the field of nursing. Only as the number of nurses undertaking formal study of these quantitative disciplines, such as in Master of Business Administration (MBA) or Master of Public Health (MPH) programs, increased did our field place itself on equal footing with lay administrators at the top of the hospital hierarchy.

The nurse at the top of the administrative hierarchy, the nurse executive, may have trained with advanced preparation in all three disciplines discussed here, microeconomics, cost accounting, and nursing. The American Organization of Nurse Executives (2005) published its view of the core competencies that the nurse executive should have. Among these are analyses of supply and demand data, analysis of financial statements, articulation of business models based on economics, strategic and business planning, and the development of future business skill sets in leadership team members, all of which are listed under the Business Skills subsection of the document. This is brought to the attention of the reader to dramatize how important it is for current and future nurse leaders to maintain their own skill set in business and financial matters and to massage this process with key leaders in their organizations such as nurse managers. The deployment of nurse resources at the unit level could quite possibly be the most important decision made in hospital care because it is through the provision of quality nursing care that quality patient outcomes are realized.

Today, baccalaureate nursing schools traditionally require one course in leadership, often at the senior level. This course may not include financial content. Some schools are beginning to offer a separate course in nursing management that does address lower level financial decision making, for example, the use of budgeting and marketing tools for nurse managers on the unit level. All, or nearly all, baccalaureate programs offer a course in health systems that analyzes healthcare organizations on the macro level, but the core quantitative courses and tools needed to place nursing on equal footing with lay decision makers reside in MBA or MPH programs and only some Master of Science in Nursing (MS or MSN) programs, including the new DNP programs (doctorate in nursing practice), in which the volume and type of financial preparation for these future leaders vary.

This does not mean that every baccalaureate or higher prepared nurse must be a manager per se. It also does not mean that the nurse administrator must be a junior chief financial officer. Rather, a nurse executive must possess the financial knowledge necessary to make system-focused decisions that integrate the clinical and business aspects of health care (Lemire, 2000).

Exhibit 11–1   Relationship of the Accounting Disciplines

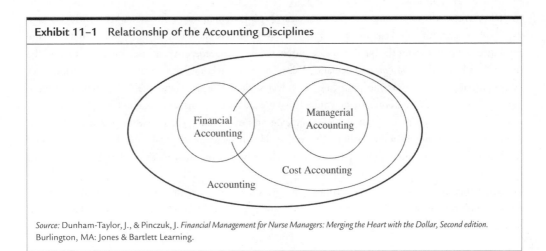

Source: Dunham-Taylor, J., & Pinczuk, J. *Financial Management for Nurse Managers: Merging the Heart with the Dollar, Second edition.* Burlington, MA: Jones & Bartlett Learning.

Nursing administration, one form of advanced practice (Harris, Huber, Jones, Manojlovich, & Reineck, 2006), is an at-risk specialty given numerous reports of dropping enrollment in graduate nursing administration programs (Herrin, Jones, Krepper, Sherman, & Reineck, 2006); a perceived lack of attractiveness of nursing administration as a viable graduate program choice (Rudan, 2002); widespread nurse executive burnout (Rollins, 2008); and the dire situation of the aging nurse faculty workforce (Berlin & Sechrist, 2002). Without this vital specialty, nursing could lose its scientific basis for practice, nurse managers at the unit level might lose recently acquired gains in real autonomy and decision making, and, most of all, research done by nurses on the effectiveness of their measures will continue to be invisible in healthcare quality, health services research, health policy, and health care finance initiatives (Lang, 2003). This discussion is an appeal to the reader regarding the uniqueness of the nursing administration specialty as well as the special challenges afforded the profession if our critical mass of economic and systems thinkers continues to deteriorate.

Competition

Theory of the firm, the theory of *supply and demand*, explains and predicts price, quantity of products, and the likelihood of survival of firms in a competitive industry. Before the PPS was introduced into the healthcare market, hospital firms operated on a *cost-plus basis*, billing insurers for the total consumption of resources by an individual patient. After 1983, hospitals were switched to a *diagnosis-related group (DRG)* basis for reimbursement, receiving compensation for what a typical patient within a medical diagnosis and selected other medical conditions would consume. This departure from the cost-plus reimbursement scheme ended the era of price competition in health care, and hospitals began to compete on a nonprice, or quality, basis, which is when patient outcomes magnified in importance.

For centuries, the relationship of the demand for a product or service to its supply has been thought to be largely the result of the intervening variable of price. In the fictional "market for widgets," supply of a product consistently meets the demand for it, given a set of assumptions about the market for *widgets*. This theory, theory of the firm, explains a lot about the way the world works pending the strength of these assumptions: a large numbers of buyers and sellers, perfect information about the product, absence of barriers to entry and exit as a business entity in the industry, and homogeneity of the product. Note that a full description of all four assumptions as they pertain to markets for health care is beyond the scope of this text, yet a focus on two of the assumptions—a large number of healthcare buyers and sellers and the existence of good information—is key.

In health care, the four assumptions are less clearly visible than in the fictitious market for widgets for a variety of reasons. Among them are the fact that relatively little is known to the *buyer* of hospital care (the insurance company) about the quality of care purchased from the *seller* (in our case, the hospital), and the demand for hospital care is a *derived* demand. This is to say that it comes from health insurance companies as the intermediary between hospital care providers such as hospitals and the individual consumer–patient. When health care entered the competitive arena, decision makers became highly sensitized to the customary business practices of restricting *expenses* and maximizing revenue while producing a service of measurable quality whenever possible. (Note that the language "an acceptable level of quality" should not be confused with something time-honored verbalized by nursing such as "the highest possible level of quality.")

The change from a system loosely concerned with quality of care, through the professionalism and trust of providers, to a system that prices services strategically while competing on quality has resulted in a cost-conscious era unlike that ever seen before. It is widely recognized that as hospitals compete to provide services, they attempt to (1) optimize profit through pricing strategies, (2) reduce expenses through decisions about personnel and equipment, and (3) achieve reimbursable patient outcomes by satisfying recipients of care through both high-technology and caring approaches. This means that hospitals seek to strike a vital balance between cost reduction and quality of care to adapt successfully to external competitive threats to their survival. For example, the ratio of nurses or *operating expenses* to patient days is a resource input that may influence the output of the system in the provision of quality care.

Better care provision (a result of wise resource allocation) may result in better patient outcomes (output) that results in better reimbursement and is alleged to be a benefit of an openly competitive, deregulated hospital market. Hospitals that can demonstrate higher quality of care, or even adequacy of care, will win higher reimbursement, or bids, for reimbursement plans, more patients, and better-qualified care providers. Over time, "good" hospitals will survive because they have established a pattern of good outcomes. The higher the hospital's performance or improvement, the higher the value-based incentive payments.

Additional evidence that this theory, theory of the firm, which explains a lot of how the world works, explains at least some things about how the world of hospital care works can be found through such organizations as HealthGrades, a leading independent healthcare ranking company (see www.healthgrades .com), and *U.S. News and World Report*'s ranking system (see http://health.usnews.com/sections/health/ best-hospitals). Both report such measures as risk-adjusted mortality rates and complication rates as patient-population-specific measures of comparative quality.

Also, hospitals can be designated as Magnet hospitals by the American Nurses Credentialing Center (ANCC; see www.nursecredentialing.org/Magnet/ProgramOverview.aspx), which means they meet process and structural criteria validated by a site visit from the ANCC. Only those hospitals known to be a good place to practice nursing are ranked as such, and the term originally meant that the hospital "attracted" nurses and patients.

The inner workings of these organizations cited in the previous two paragraphs and detailed descriptions of their methodologies, too complex to be reported here, can be found at their respective websites. Also, a primer on what risk-adjusted mortality rates means, as an overall general measure of quality or at least adequacy of any one hospital, is discussed in a later section. In summary, the importance of these hospital ranking systems, or stamps of approval as the public might see them, is this: The information about the quality of the product or service of a hospital is accurate enough to be used for comparison ratings used by payers as well as by others interested in these data. Hence, the information qualifies as perfect information (not to be taken literally).

What microeconomic theory states regarding the eventual number of hospital firms within an industry under long-run equilibrium (hospitals that rival or compete over a long time) is this: Those hospital firms with better products or services will survive, but those with inferior products and services will not. This is the result of the achievement of quality held by payers and consumers, which, in part, drives the industry's (derived) demand. Unfortunately, relatively little is known about the tenets of competition in health care. More will be known as variations in the quality of patient outcomes based on reimbursement in hospitals become available in the future. So, the usefulness of this theory for the explanation and prediction of future activities in health care remains challenged. This is not to say that "Supply and demand—it just doesn't work in health care!" is an emotionally charged statement devoid of reason. It is, instead, appropriate to say that predictive power of the theory in health care is limited more than its explanatory power interpreting the how and why of a hospital firm's behavior. Stated another way, all hospitals seek to maximize patient outcomes/reimbursement and thus maximize performance ratings.

In the world of competitive hospital management, decision makers continually forecast, or second guess, what their rivals will do when they introduce such novelties as courting new profitable patient populations or programs such as breast centers, cancer centers, symptom-management clinics, and addiction rehabilitation. In short, hospitals must innovate with new programs, new patient populations, or quality initiatives to survive and better achieve the continuum of care in the value-based environment. New sources of (perfect or symmetric) information on hospital care continually become available in both print and electronic media, so decision makers must be savvy regarding patient outcome comparisons. Just as automobiles are rated for gas consumption and airlines for on-time arrivals, payers and consumers contract for hospital care based on price and quality through managed care negotiations.

Regulation and Managed Care

The soaring cost of health care has been one of the most pressing domestic issues for decades. Politicians and pundits speak of how changes in laws could affect this crisis, sometimes provoking a discussion of socialized medicine and cross-country comparison of U.S. versus "other" healthcare expenditures and outcomes. With no clear answer to this type of healthcare ill emerging soon, most would agree that although our healthcare system is among the most market oriented (competitively driven) in the world, it remains *the* most heavily regulated sector of the U.S. economy (Conover, 2004). This author states that the costs of regulation are the benefits we would derive with alternative uses of those resources. After reviewing the literature on 47 different kinds of healthcare regulations, it was estimated that the net burden of health services regulation on society was $169.1 billion annually. For the novice in economic thinking, let's examine what some of the costs of regulation are said to be. In lay terms, it is the sum total of all expenditures by federal or state regulators that oversee, inspect, supervise, monitor, or award privileges to healthcare providers such as physicians, nurses, and hospitals. In just a quick survey of hospital and nursing regulation costs alone, consider these:

- The Centers for Medicare and Medicaid Services (CMS) utilization reviews of appropriateness
- Office of Safety and Health Administration (OSHA) inspection of workplace safety
- The National Labor Relations Board monitoring of nurse unions
- National Council of State Boards of Nursing licensing exam requirements
- Every state board of nursing, medicine, pharmacy, respiratory therapy, and physical therapy
- American Association of Colleges of Nursing and National League for Nursing accreditation of nursing schools
- National Practitioner Data Bank housing information on practitioners
- Limitations on medical resident or registered nurse (RN) working hours
- Fraud and abuse protections

Each one of these organizations or protections has staff, overhead, a place of business to run, and extensive reporting requirements to yet another governmental or quasi-governmental organization. The author makes a convincing case that if health care were deregulated, the cost savings from this could realize gains in health promotion and prevention.

Although in our discussion of rivalry and what hospital firms must do to survive, indeed thrive, a convincing case is made about the benefits of the competitive, or market-driven, environment for hospital care, this is not diametrically opposed to regulatory efforts. This needs to be said because, in essence, a highly competitive market-driven industry is a bit like the polar opposite of one that is highly or completely regulated as is the case in countries with a national single-payer health system. In short, the market for hospitals is not what is known as "purely competitive" as is the market for widgets; far from it.

It holds, instead, a complicated mixture of free-market principles, huge regulatory demands, a demand for sick-care services that is derived and not direct, and the most complicated reimbursement scheme known in modern times in any industry.

Managed care, a concept and term invented by Alain Enthoven (1986), was originally intended to reduce healthcare costs to society through the restriction of resource allocation and improve the overall health of individuals. Now it is a generic term for healthcare payment systems that attempt to control costs through utilization monitoring; health maintenance organizations and preferred provider organizations are examples. In the old cost-plus world, physicians as clinicians (not clinicians and businesspersons) had free unrestricted aim over treatment plans and resource allocation for their patients. This system, focused on physicians and, arguably, hospitals, involved a complete arbitrariness to clinical decision making, and if science (as in evidence-based medicine) was involved, all the better. Imagine a world where the faith and trust in the physician as provider were sacrosanct. Depending on the age of the reader, probably you cannot imagine it, even in your wildest dreams. Also beyond the imagination for some, there was a time that insurance companies paid for resources used without much, if any, review processes for appropriateness of treatment.

Managed care, now considered an economic success and a social nightmare, has in fact reduced healthcare costs to society by tying clinical decisions to economic ones that previously were mutually exclusive. In these arrangements, a hospital or group of doctors agrees to provide services in exchange for third-party payment. Managed care networks make available to their members only those providers authorized by the plan. Often, this designation is geographically derived, thereby restricting individuals' choices to go to what they see as the "best" orthopedic or cancer care hospital or doctor if unavailable locally. It is worth mentioning that individuals still have free choice (lots of it)—if they are willing to get out their checkbook! This statement is a positivist (or factual) one amid the rhetoric of concerns from individual patients and physicians about how things used to be or ought to be. The way things "ought to" or "used to" be was inflationary, and there isn't an informed health consumer around who doesn't know this.

In managed care, the provider (physician, nurse in advanced practice, or hospital) provides covered services at a discounted rate in exchange for a steady revenue stream. If the novice reading this wonders why providers would "settle for less" by receiving a discounted rate, consider the alternative. Providers would have an uncertain revenue stream that challenges their abilities to cover the basic costs of doing business (reduces *uncertainty*) plus there are few, if any, alterative ways of conducting business, generally speaking. Stated another way, consider what is known as *the first rule of finance*: A dollar today is worth more than a dollar tomorrow as a result of the time value or opportunity cost of money. That is, any entity that gains revenue in a timely manner not only can retire debt (an asset) but invest; hence, the time value of money is realized. Remember that fee-for-service medicine has all but disappeared, taking with it the old model of the solo-practice physician, and patients who pay out of pocket are rare.

Under a per diem rate agreement, the managed care plan pays the hospital a fixed rate for each day of care, when in fact nurses are in a particularly strategic position to observe that costs per diem to the institution can be (very) variable for one patient stay. Consider the surgical patient who consumes relatively few resources on the morning of admission for a procedure that afternoon. Once the patient enters the operating room, costs to the institution soar steeply and remain high as the patient travels to the postanesthesia recovery room, not to mention more if intensive care is involved. For a monthly fee, the hospital must provide the specified services to the third-party payer's enrollees such as this patient. Under this arrangement, the hospital is ensured money in a relatively timely fashion (based on the average consumption of patients within that diagnosis-related group and other clinical factors) and the patient–consumer knows he or she will be covered for surgeries that are preapproved.

The overall aim of managed care is to make the patient a better healthcare customer, evaluating whether she or he is getting what she or he is paying for (assuming the individual pays health insurance premiums, which most do). Also, the burden of prevention and wellness increases in importance for the patient, and, presumably, physicians and advanced practice nurses share in this responsibility by virtue of recent changes in medical and nursing education. In this system, the patient has less control over selection of the doctor or hospital and may be responsible for higher deductibles and copayments as well as penalties for services done outside the network.

From a positive (or factual) point of view, the real cost savings to the healthcare system and society at large is through reduction and *elimination of unnecessary* services, tests, and procedures and time delays through the authorization process where untold numbers of individuals drop off, or attrition out of, the care-seeking process. It needs to be said that to the extent that costs are held down by reduction in *necessary* services, tests, procedures, and premature hospital discharge, there are, in fact, real detriments to patients and to society. Many healthcare professionals and consumers are now claiming that the term *managed care* translates to "discounted care," but adhering to the intent of this chapter, the positive or factual view of healthcare business operations, the author looks disparagingly upon this rhetorical and editorial change.

Profit Motive and Patient Care

Amid the rhetoric and hysteria regarding hospitals and profit, not enough is said about why a hospital exists. A hospital exists to satisfy the needs of its various stakeholders. Among these are physicians, nurses, and other employees; patients and their families; consumers; researchers; schools of medicine and nursing; and the community at large, to name a few. Although many agree that today's hospital exists for the provision of sick care, this is not to say there are no other compelling reasons for it to subsist. It is a business entity and, as such, it responds to many demands from the players, or stakeholders. Among these demands are the volume and morbidity of patients, requests from physicians and nurses in advanced practice for necessary equipment and efficient flow of patients, concerns from patients and families about inefficient or substandard care, training opportunities for students of medicine and nursing, and an outright appeal for more nurses from basically anyone! The profit motive drives all of these.

In an influential book in its time, *The Profit Motive and Patient Care* (Gray, 1991), the author made the previously unexplored claim that two unique accountability factors exist in health care that do not exist in other organizations: the vulnerability of the consumer (patient) being served, and the absence of payers at the point of service. He goes on to state:

> In many different ways the profit motive—on the part of organizational providers of health care, suppliers of their capital, physicians, employers who provide benefits for their employees, and organizations that administer health benefits plans and monitor the performance of health care providers—has come to shape the behavior of all parties. An ethos that emphasizes trust, community service, professional autonomy, and devotion to interests of individual patients is being replaced with undisguised self interest, commercialization, competition, and the management of care by third parties. . . . These shifts will shape how providers and purchasers of service respond to the two great accountability problems. (p. xi)

A cursory reading through these remarks prompts one to believe there is a lament here—perhaps about "the way things *ought* to be." Yet on closer examination, it appears that Gray, instead, is making logical positivist (factual) remarks. His explanation of whom the important players (stakeholders) are and how they are motivated to perform has far-reaching implications for the overall philosophical *and* business approaches that healthcare providers, such as nurses, might take. His was among the first credible writings to shake the foundations of why a hospital exists as well as to articulate the important forces shaping the behavior of the stakeholders.

In this section, it is necessary to debunk some myths still prevailing in certain sections of our society, sometimes even among healthcare providers (some of whom should know better!):

Myth 1: We are a nonprofit entity; we don't have profit.
Myth 2: We are here to provide the highest possible quality of care.

These are among the most important misconceptions forwarded by many stakeholders, among them nurses. Replacing what might be our wishes (myths) with factual statements helps us understand the pervasive economic forces shaping our work and provides resolve for nursing research aims and hypotheses.

Getting the Word Profit Back

The first myth—that of no profit—has hung around for decades. First, it is important to clarify our terminology. As to profit status, hospitals are now classified as either investor owned (IO), formerly known as "for-profit," or not-for-profit (NFP), formerly known as "nonprofit." All hospitals have profit, *and* each of them chases profit as fast and furiously as the next, period. They may differ on many other factors, chiefly *how* they approach profit optimization as well as descriptive characteristics such as public versus private ownership, urban versus rural, small-margin versus large-margin, safety-net versus non-safety-net, high-mortality versus low-mortality, and teaching versus nonteaching, to name some. A number of these factors may, in fact, covary with profit status. For example, major teaching hospitals tend to be NFP hospitals and nearly all IO hospitals are private, but it is thought that the variable of profit status, and possibly outcomes, is the prime mover of organizational behavior.

Profit, loosely defined as the excess of revenues over expenses, is as necessary to hospitals, irrespective of profit status, as oxygen is to the living system. Almost no hospital could survive without it because it could not remain liquid or solvent. Without it, a hospital eventually goes out of business just like any other entity, leaving services unprovided and employees out of jobs. Profitability, as a construct, is measured by these variables: total margin ratio, operating *profit margin*, nonoperating gain ratio, and return on equity. As you continue reading the next section on the cost inputs for varying levels of quality, keep in mind that costs to the hospital (what is expensed on the hospital's income statement) relative to revenue (money given to the hospital in lieu of care provided) are nearly synonymous with profitability, at least in the short run.

Finally, an accounting note about the differences in IO versus NFP hospitals. In lay terms, the key differences between these two sets of hospitals on the matter of profit goes like this: All that matters is where you put it, what you call it, and what you do about it! Restating this old joke another way, the dollar line item of profit is found on the income statement of general funds for NFPs versus the profit and loss statement for the corporation; profit is called "profit" in the IO world versus a "positive fund balance" in the NFP one; and the IO distributes profit (after taxes) at year's end to the shareholders, whereas the NFPs cycle profits back into facility maintenance or expansion after paying no taxes. This partly whimsical look at what the terms mean (and do *not* mean) causes this author to conclude "I want the word *profit* back!" given that although there is a cost–quality trade-off (see next section), there is *not necessarily* a cost–profit trade-off.

Quality of Care: At What Level? At What Cost?

In this chapter's discussion of competition, it was stated that a hospital is *not* in the business of providing the best care money can buy but that a hospital *is* in the business of providing quality of care at a certain acceptable level where reimbursement is received. It is time to examine why.

Measurement of the costs of providing care quality, long a perplexing problem, is a function of the cost of providing quality *and* the costs of failing to do so.

Lowering quality also has costs to the organization. Besides reimbursement losses, this lowers the quality of care for patients. This can bring about more detrimental effects for patients to deal with, including death, and the organizational reimbursement and reputation suffer; and remember, reputation *is* an asset. So, as lowering quality occurs, this erodes the hospital's competitive position and thus longer-term viability.

This cost–quality trade-off explains the behavior of firms in every competitive industry, including the hospital firm in health care. Although seemingly abstract constructs, hospital decision makers use this paradigm as freely as a living system uses carbohydrate for fuel in the cell.

In conclusion, what can be said about the profit motive and patient care? Profit, as an incentive, is here to stay. *Profit* is not a dirty word. Further, cost–quality trade-offs drive operational (day-to-day) decisions in all organizations in a competitive industry. Also, cost shifts (costs to the hospital, or expenses) might be borne by the individual, or perhaps the employer, if the individual is discharged prematurely and too sick to resume employment. Revenues would shift from one governmental organization such as CMS to another if they could. And dramatically changing one variable, such as RN staffing, necessitates significant changes in another, such as expenses for other personnel—a topic that will prove essential to our national debate about hospital staffing.

Quality Patient Care

The discussion of profit motive demonstrated how a hospital comes to provide not the best care money can buy but instead an acceptable level of quality. The acceptable level of quality is driven by its cost. Next, to compete on a quality of care basis, the hospital must report *measurable* aspects of quality of care—patient outcomes (presumably at an acceptable level)—to various governmental (state health departments and federal agencies) and nongovernmental organizations, such as the Joint Commission. Through processes such as these, the information about the quality of care in one facility is said to be *perfect information*, a cornerstone of a competitive industry. The information can also be characterized as *symmetric* in that both the buyer (the insurer) and the seller (the providers) have access to it.

The old quality assurance model, now nearly extinct, was limited in at least two ways: Quality cannot be *ensured*, and the information, or knowledge, was *asymmetric*, known to the seller (a provider hospital) but not necessarily to the buyer. Therefore, under this old model, it was practically impossible for hospitals to modify their care provision processes in a competitive way because they had no information about the performance of their rival hospitals.

Given the preponderance of information-reporting requirements, it is assumed that hospitals have numerous opportunities for improvement—assuming that these many reporting requirements translate to internal care-improvement processes. Next, through the movement now known as *transparency* (symmetric knowledge), hospitals can bid competitively to purchasers, boasting superior quality outcomes. A third quintessentially important thing this information preponderance gives us is the *incentive* for public programs (e.g., Medicare) and private insurers to reward and reimburse quality of care and efficiency.

This incentive program has the overall goal of making hospitals miss reimbursement when they err with never events.

It is essential to note that the *quality and availability of the information* to both buyers and sellers make hospital nonprice competition possible.

Information on Quality and the Risk-Adjustment Process

A time-honored claim that hospitals and other providers have made regarding quality measures in general is that their patient populations contain more *risk* factors than others, hence the appearance of "not looking good" to the state or inspection agency. Granted, patient populations from hospital to hospital (or even from doctor to doctor) likely always differ on factors other than the care provided, but, arguably, meaningful points of comparison have been devised by clinical and biostatistical experts within many agencies.

One such agency is California's Office of Statewide Health Planning and Development (OSHPD). California was among the first states to develop a database of risk-adjusted quality measures, and the California Hospital Outcome Project reported to the public for the first time in 1995 and has continuously updated and improved its risk-adjustment processes ever since. The project worked first with a common and costly condition, acute myocardial infarction, by reporting risk-adjusted mortality; discharge abstracts served as the basis for data collection for more than 400 hospitals representative of more than 68,000 patients.

Biostatisticians know that databases this large do, indeed, allow for meaningful points of comparison across hospitals for reasons to be explained in advanced texts of statistics and econometrics. Generally speaking, risk-adjusted measures of quality of care, such as acute myocardial infarction mortality, are in fact useful tools for the comparison of hospitals on the quality of care provided, but imperfectly so. In the California hospital project, the mortality measure was defined as the observed number of deaths from acute myocardial infarction divided by the number of qualifying persons admitted with this primary diagnosis multiplied by the statewide rate. The risk-adjustment process is described in detail in workbooks provided to all by the state (again, the information is symmetric; Office of Statewide Health Planning and Development [OSHPD], 1996a, 1996b). By making the process known to all, agencies such as this assert they have satisfactorily responded to providers' claim about disparate findings based on (unmeasured) risk factors. In fact, on a yearly basis as the press releases come out about new editions of the data, the project offers the opportunity for hospital providers to respond in writing about why their facility "looked worse than expected" in the measures. This way, the project measures are refined yearly in part on the basis of the responses of participating hospitals. Since inception of this project, the agency has made available other outcome measures, all risk adjusted, that are reflective of common and costly conditions. These include complication rates of cervical and thoracic diskectomy, maternal admissions, hip fractures, and community-acquired pneumonia.

Earlier, this chapter expresses the thought that for our profession to be seated at the table of quality initiatives in the context of the hospital business entity, we need expert knowledge of the economic and quality measures being discussed. Further, societal decision makers and gatekeepers, such as the OSHPD and CMS, would benefit from nursing representation to make the hospital measures, now used for reimbursement, meaningful. Fortunately, through the years, as nursing acquired a critical mass of administratively prepared nurses, it has become common for nurse executives from hospitals and/or representatives of our professional societies to be invited to such tables where the decisions are made. Because this was not always the case, it could be considered progress of the profession through acquisition of the same knowledge *and* the same financial language spoken by lay administrators that made this possible. Also look at CMS data.

Healthcare Policy: The Staffing Ratios Debate

The relationship between nurse staffing and patient safety is reasonably well established, especially when patient outcomes such as medical-surgical mortality rates (Aiken, Smith, & Lake, 1994), acute myocardial infarction mortality rates (Schultz, van Servellen, Litwin, McLaughlin, & Uman, 1997), community-acquired pneumonia mortality rates (Schultz, 2008), failure to rescue (Needleman, Buerhaus, Mattke, Stewart, & Zelevinsky, 2002), and shorter lengths of stay (Lang, Hodge, Olson, Romano, & Kravitz, 2004), to name a few, are considered. How patients fare has long been thought to be to the result of the number of professional nurse staff available as well as their preparation, visibility, and experience. Additional organizational variables known to be important are leadership style of the nurse manager, the overall quality of leadership in the institution, whether staffing and other operational decisions are decentralized, physician satisfaction with nursing care, and the nature of the information system used for patient care. Research on hospital characteristics and their relationships to patient outcomes has broadened to include additional variables important in the complex relationships of people and technology relative to quality. For instance, positive cultures are less expensive and achieve better outcomes. It is the opinion of the author that as these associations are identified and contextualized clearer policy implications can be investigated.

Mandated minimum nurse-to-patient staffing ratios were legislated in California in 1999 and implemented January 1, 2004. Also being considered is the importance of having patient classification system data to support the appropriate RN staff requirements. Some of the impetus for the movement toward mandating nurse staffing ratios through governmental and scientific imperatives comes from the challenging conclusions offered by the Institute of Medicine's (2002) report *To Err Is Human*. This report shook both the scientific and lay communities with its most memorable finding: Between 44,000 and 98,000 deaths occur each year as a result of medical errors. There is hardly a scientific journal that focuses on these types of organizational studies that does not report the influence of nurse staffing, often in the form of RN hours per patient day or RN to all staff hours.

The beginner in politics and policy might ask, "Isn't this a no-brainer? More nurses equals better patient care, right?" Only a fool would disagree, and certainly, more nurses sound as good as motherhood and apple pie! But so, too, do more police in a neighborhood and fewer pupils per teacher in schools. The following subsections provide the novice nurse–politician some food for thought on the potential implications, or consequences, of such legislation in the context of the (1) operation of a hospital within a community or (2) market for hospitals as a whole. The implications can be summarized in four parts: hospital operations including closure, feasibility and the nursing shortage, political opportunity costs, and costs to society. The implications, economic consequences of legislation addressing what staffing *should be* (*normative economics*), are couched in *positive economics*, or *what is*, factually.

Hospital Operations and Closure

As mentioned previously, the healthcare workforce accounts for at least 50% of a hospital's costs (Kazahaya, 2005). Most of this is nursing personnel costs. Starting with the assumption that some hospitals staff significantly better than the minimum staffing ratios suggest while some staff significantly lower as a baseline, there is a variance around the regulated minimum ratio (also known as "the floor" ratio). Hospitals staffing well below this floor ratio will experience a rapid rise in operating expenses and lost reimbursement and a subsequent drop in operating profit margin. This endangers the hospital's *liquidity* (ability to meet short-term obligations) and *solvency* (ability to meet maturing obligations as they become due). Hospitals staffing well above the floor ratio have an incentive to drop nurse staffing levels depending on the cutoff point of where reimbursement is negatively affected as well as the ultimate response of their rivals, that is, whether neighboring hospitals can afford to remain in business after enactment of this law. Finally, hospitals staffing at about the mandated level may experience no significant change in their financial and, subsequently, business activities, so their staffing may continue as is.

Consider other hospital operations that are disrupted as a consequence of what many nurses thought was a great idea. As reported in *Medical News Report* (2004):

- Elective procedures have been postponed, canceled, or moved to a nearby facility.
- Community hospitals have a more difficult time transferring patients to tertiary care facilities because beds cannot always be staffed.
- Emergency room (ER) wait times have increased.
- ERs have increasingly switched (or requested to switch) to diversion status.
- Night shifts are nearly impossible to staff.
- There is a huge shift to contract (agency or registry) nursing staff, causing a significant rise in expenses, often tens of millions of (unforeseen) dollars in a year.
- The regulations make the hospital increasingly vulnerable to lawsuits, especially on the occasion when staffing is less than required.
- When the regulations allow for "licensed" nurses in the equation, RN unions block the effort to fill a void with licensed practical nurse hours, thereby inflating union-to-union conflict.

Evidence supporting the view that this mandate was too costly for hospitals to continue operating is seen in the number of hospitals that closed in the years during implementation phase-in of the California law. Twenty hospitals closed (9 in 2003, 8 in 2004, 3 in 2006; OSHPD, 2006), citing factors on the revenue side of the profitability equation (drop in inpatient revenue and utilization issues). The costs to hospitals of the mandate cannot be underestimated. It is important to note that many forces, both internal and external, cause a business to close and that many of these factors, when they occur simultaneously, push the firm close to the "edge," or more specifically, to the margin. Usually, a hospital firm that closes had both failing business (patient care processes) *and* economic activities (on both revenue and expenditure sides) in the preceding years that ultimately caused its demise. To date, no one empirical effort has isolated the impact of such a law on a hospital's propensity to close due to the complexity of the issues.

Recall from the discussion of profit that when expenses rise in one category, pressure is exerted in the hospital system (or any business) to (1) reduce expenses in another category, (2) make up the expensed activity with an increase in revenue, or (3) both. To formulate a guiding principle on hospital profit-maximizing behavior, Needleman (2008) suggests these questions to consider:

- How much would it cost to increase nurse staffing?
- Would these costs be offset by cost savings from better reimbursement, reduced LOS, and fewer complications?
- Would the hospital realize these cost savings, or, because of how the hospital is paid, would these savings be captured by payers?
- Can the hospital attract additional profitable patients on the basis of its nurse staffing?
- Are there cost savings other than those achieved via better patient care that might also be realized if nurse staffing is increased?

So, it should be clear that changing a regulation on the most significant personnel expenditure a hospital budget contains, RN hours, has far-reaching consequences for both hospital business and economic activities. This subsection looks at the core organizational dynamics of a single hospital, which is a very limited aspect of the staffing ratios laws. Even looking at these activities in all hospitals in a state or the nation offers only a partial view of the consequences of mandated ratios as described here. Read on to see how a hospital's behavior cannot be viewed in such a microcosm because of its essential bond to the other subcategories, such as the sporadic nursing shortage.

Feasibility and the Sporadic Nursing Shortage

In the past, hospitals, lawmakers, providers, consumers, and society as a whole were increasingly concerned about the international nursing shortage and its subsequent impact on the quality of care. After implementation of California's safe-staffing law, RN hours per patient day on medical-surgical units rose significantly, perhaps by as much as 21% (Donaldson et al., 2005). Yet the nursing shortage, predicted to be a deficit of 400,000 RNs by 2020 (Buerhaus, Needleman, Mattke, & Stewart, 2002), continued to beg the question of where the nursing hours came from. Over decades, it was a long-standing principle of hospital staffing to "borrow" nurse hours from unit to unit to (1) satisfy short-term patient care demands, for example, a number of new admissions arriving at the same time as intensive care unit transfers, and (2) satisfy regulatory and reporting requirements. Patient care demands may have been met, whereas regulatory and reporting requirements almost certainly were.

Many obstacles hinder compliance with mandated staffing requirements. Consider these real-world examples from *Medical News Report* (2004):

- Hospitals may start a shift in compliance but not end that shift in compliance.
- Hospitals may start and end a shift in compliance, but the middle of the shift is in question.
- Nurse recruitment efforts have been accelerated but often are not associated with the desired result of satisfactory staffing.
- California's law requires nurses to be on standby to cover breaks for bedside nurses, which is a requirement that is practically impossible to meet.
- Penalties exist for noncompliance.
- Nurses increasingly report not taking their breaks, given the lack of coverage while they are to be gone.
- Hospitals could be held *criminally* liable for adverse outcomes in the context of staffing that is less than required by mandate, even in view of evidence of the intent to comply.

These remarks point to regional shortages within one hospital carrying yet another set of concerns for patient safety. Chiefly, these concerns are costs associated with noncompliance, nurse recruitment (especially as nurses from outside the country are involved), and legal defense. Also, there were no accompanying changes in the revenue side of the hospitals' profit equation. The examples offered in this subsection highlight merely a few of the difficulties hospitals are having with the mandate. Additional issues include workplace safety, nurse injuries, nurse dissatisfaction, turnover, and propensity to stay in current positions. This subsection, not a comprehensive review for all issues related to a hospital's nurse pipeline, emphasizes some of the more immediate feasibility issues posed by such regulations. And this does not take into account how this will affect reimbursement.

Political Opportunity Costs for Nursing

Highly publicized political wars have taken place, most notably in California and New York, over the staffing ratios debate. Both states had nurse unions that were successful in getting legislation sponsored that evolved into statewide acute care hospital staffing mandates, but at what political cost? California's

12-year battle (California Nurses Association, n.d.) spanned the reign of two governors, and New York's campaign (Gerardi, 2006) was similarly protracted, both being punctuated by statewide town hall meetings, numerous "call to action" alerts to other professional societies, consumption of resources of nursing associations of all types, and bad press labeling nurses as unyielding and self-serving. In California, such ill will attracted national attention when Governor Arnold Schwarzenegger summarily dismissed both the nurse union's leadership and membership *as well as* nurses in general by calling nurses "a special interest group" that is just angry because "I kick their butt" (Marinucci, 2004).

These campaigns occurred just as the state of the research was judged *not* to categorically support the thesis of better care provision through more RNs in each case. In fact, the research results are mixed (Burnes Bolton et al., 2007), reporting that although a clear and consistent rise in nurse staffing did exist post regulation in California, it was not accompanied by a commensurate rise in quality as measured by significantly fewer falls or pressure ulcers. In a study reported by Mark and Harless (2007), a superior distribution of outcomes (mortality and LOS) with a *lower* level of RN staffing was found. In sum, the evidence points to the prevailing conclusion that there is a strong, but not yet totally conclusive, case for an impact of nurse staffing on mortality (Needleman & Buerhaus, 2003) and other adverse outcomes. This is not unlike the teachers union advocating for better teacher-to-student ratios, having to defend the national outcry (and *some* empiricism) that we are a nation of people who lack necessary reading, writing, and critical thinking skills.

If you believe, as some do, that science drives policy and legislation—and that's a leap—you have now identified a gap between just what we recommend on the matter of staffing mandates (the normative economic view) and a recommendation accompanied by a cogent economic rationale (the positive economic position) and plan. Stated another way, consider the words of Keepnews (2007):

> Ongoing research on the impact of nurse staffing regulation can yield important information that can guide continued staffing policy efforts. Understanding the impact of such efforts should include evaluating the outcomes of recent legislation in Oregon and Illinois as well as continued examination of staffing ratios in California. Successful efforts will need to transcend traditional boundaries between researchers, policy analysts, advocates, and organizations. (p. 236)

Costs to Society

Social policy is the domain that aims to improve human welfare and to meet human needs for education, health, housing, and social security. It is that part of public policy that has to do with social issues; among them is health. There was a time when *health* was considered the absence of disease. Couple this limited definition of health with the Hippocratic admonition "to do no harm" to identify what the public expects from a hospital: to emerge from the experience with an improved state of health or, at a minimum, to avoid increased morbidity *as a result of* seeking hospital care. Although it is touted as a modern concept, we would do well to remember that the Hippocratic admonition regarding harm emerged centuries ago (Hippocrates, n.d./2004). Previously, it was noted that, at a minimum, quality care is identified as the absence of adversity or the absence of adverse events.

The costs to society of this adversity are understudied or underreported in modern health services research. The costs to society include, but are not limited to, the alternative use of hospital resources in a community (e.g., feeding the poor, housing the homeless), consumption of a tax basis (in the case of NFP hospitals) for same, the costs of ill health for individuals and employers such as the opportunity cost of lost time and productivity at work, unreimbursed expenses related to caring for the underinsured or the uninsured, as well as the alternative use of people and technology resources in other employment.

This subsection briefly lists some questions for further study in the context of the costs to society of mandated staffing ratios with respect to the latter two factors—the function and purpose of safety-net hospitals and the opportunity realized in the operation of a hospital in a community context.

Safety-Net Hospitals

Defined as hospitals disproportionately serving vulnerable, including financially vulnerable, populations, *safety-net hospitals* also experienced a sustained significant rise in nurse hours after enactment of safe staffing ratios. To assume that a higher nurse-to-patient ratio affects the financial structure of hospitals the same way across the board is folly. Safety-net hospitals are at-risk institutions, by definition. They have consistently been financially vulnerable organizations when viewed from the revenue side of the profit equation. With large numbers of underinsured or uninsured patients, they have no position from which to compete on price and may not have the resources to compete on the basis of quality. It would stand to reason that although they budget for *bad debt expense*, this line item varies considerably because it is volume dependent and sensitive to changes in the macroeconomic condition. In short, when the region of its location "has a bad year," this institution, among all institutions there, has an even worse one! It is close to impossible for such a hospital to court more attractive (paying) patients not only because of geography but because of poor internal economic conditions, including liquidity crises.

A study done by Conway and associates (2008) reported that nurse staffing ratios in California hospitals were relatively unchanged from 1993 to 1999, and then showed a sharp significant increase in 2004, the year of the ratios implementation. The study reported that hospitals more likely to be below the minimum had high Medicaid/uninsured patient populations and were government owned, nonteaching, urban, and located in more competitive markets. Most of these hospitals were considered part of the safety net that "catches" uninsured and underinsured patient populations, which, presumably, have poorer health outcomes as a baseline. Also, these hospitals are thought to be extraordinarily sensitive to governmental mandates on staffing, with safety-net hospitals reporting significantly fewer professional staff relative to patients in the years after the Balanced Budget Act of 1997 (Lindrooth, Bazzoli, Needleman, & Hasnain-Wynia, 2006).

Having just stated that the competitive position of these hospitals is weak to begin with (they are less able to compete on the basis of price or quality), it stands to reason that they run a high risk of closure, particularly in view of the fact that the mandate obliges them to spend more on nurse staffing. With this loss of flexibility to vary nursing skill mix come inefficient allocation of scarce resources and an inability to make trade-offs in other hospital services. The subsequent drop in operating profit margin (and perhaps other measures of profitability) could easily cause negative consequences for patients such as premature discharge, recidivism, and higher complication rates. With the Medicare pay-for-performance structure, it is easy to see the handwriting on the wall for such environments, with closure looming in the future.

Nowhere more apparently is the strain felt than in the ER of a safety-net hospital. Long a point of entry for the financially strapped patient, the ER at hospitals such as the Los Angeles Memorial Hospital (Inglewood, California) found it necessary to divert patients to a neighboring hospital, Centinela Freeman, of the same Centinela Freeman Health Care System. Memorial's ER was the 10th to close in Los Angeles County in the 2001–2006 period. Memorial Hospital had lost $30 million in that time frame, and the hospital's executive said the closure was necessary to help the system save money (Quinones, 2006). Meanwhile, Centinela Freeman's ER saw a majority of nonurgent cases, approximately 60% of the total clientele, which begs the societal questions: Where should those patients have gone for more cost-effective care to begin with? Where will they go now and in the future? Why did the hospital's leadership not redirect its activities given the staggering loss of $30 million over 5 years?

As providers, especially safety-net hospital providers, struggle with these enmeshed issues of geographic limitations, a tangible floor in revenue, and dropping profit margins in light of rising bad debt expenses, it is no wonder that the hospital executive has an eye on cash flow relative to debt (cash-flow-to-debt ratio) because it is *the* prime predictor of hospital closure. Once again, without a margin there is no mission, despite outcries from community leaders in Inglewood and elsewhere that health care is a right. Is it? If yes, who pays for it?

A Hospital Firm Within a Community Context

Recall that in the subsections on hospital operations and the nursing shortage, a number of questions were raised relevant to reducing or delaying services (diversion to neighboring ERs), the potential for a hospital to realize other cost savings as RN hours rise (better reimbursement, some *economies of scale*, perhaps, with nursing duties in common with nonlicensed personnel), and the costs to the hospital of recruiting and retaining nurses—all of which are accentuated in a regulatory climate in which RN ratios are mandated. Here are some questions posed by the author when considering the impact of such a *government intervention* on small-margin hospitals. Bear in mind that small-margin hospitals include those considered safety-net hospitals or those classified as rural.

- Will there be a drop in the employees' *total compensation package*, say, a reduction in health benefits or a rise in premium prices, in an effort to offset the rise in operating expenditures?
- As the line item for RN hours increases, what happens to the expenditures for nonprofessional nurses and ancillary nursing personnel?
- As these nonprofessional nurse budgets get trimmed, will it be necessary to start outsourcing programs in preparation for layoffs?
- As resources become more constrained, what is the subsequent impact on measurable levels of quality? On reimbursement?
- What is the effect of the change in levels of quality on managed care contract negotiations? In short, will the insurer continue to send covered lives to a facility thought or known to be substandard?
- As measurable levels of quality are affected, what is the impact of this on the hospital's creditworthiness?
- As the hospital's creditworthiness is adversely affected, how compromised is the hospital in borrowing, even in the short term, to meet economic obligations such as employee wages and other compensatory line items? How will a hospital's payment to its suppliers be affected?
- If the hospital does, in fact, close, what is the impact of this event on the unemployment rate in the surrounding community, especially if the hospital is the largest employer around?
- If the hospital closes, what are the costs to society of airlifting or otherwise transporting the most critical of cases to the appropriate environment of care?

As decision makers in small-margin hospitals, including the nurse executive, wrestle with these tough questions, it remains in the mind's eye of the observer whether the charge "well, it's a hospital that *should* have closed anyway" is defensible. This discussion does not provide an answer to such normative queries. Instead, the measures (or variables) necessary to construct an individual answer are offered from the logical positivist (factual) economic view.

In concluding this discussion of one of the most challenging healthcare policy questions of modern times, mandated nurse staffing ratios, I remind you to remember some guiding principles from positive economics, that is, costs shift, revenues shift, and this will *always* be the case. Costs and revenues shift both within and outside the hospital firm. As in the case of borrowing nurse hours from unit to unit to "look good" or claim compliance with such mandates, what is the subsequent impact on patient care on the unit from which the borrowing occurred? As each hospital chases profit as fast and furiously as the next or neighboring competitor, how long will it continue to play the shell game of shifting ER patients from one safety-net hospital to another or allowing premature discharge? This last causes recidivism that results in no reimbursement if patients are readmitted within a month for the same problem. Finally, as far as costs to society are concerned, how is the health of a region or the nation affected by the loss of hospitals that fail seemingly from the economic or quality point of view?

The Business Case: Electronic Medical Record Systems in Hospitals

Although information systems, including the electronic medical record (EMR), are considered essential to the quality and efficiency of our healthcare system as a whole, the high cost of these systems is prohibitive in successful widespread implementation, especially in hospitals. Vital to daily operations, these systems bring many benefits such as safety, accessibility, retrievability, and convenience. They are a major organizational investment, especially with respect to start-up costs (the initial one-time expenses). This section discusses some costs, some benefits, the relationship of these costs and benefits, and the elements of a successful business case for a hospital's EMR system. As done previously, this section offers reader some measures (variables) to consider when idealizing that healthcare systems, especially hospitals, *ought* to have a computerized record-keeping and decision-support system.

Clinical information systems that computerize documentation of physicians, nurses, and other care providers, now nearly 20 years old, hold the promise of numerous benefits—for the healthcare system or hospital, for the patient, and for the health of the nation. Among them are patient safety, accessibility, legibility, process-adherence evidence, data-mining capabilities (Manjoney, 2004), retrievability, convenience, and a reduction in indirect care time. The downside is that privacy issues, costs including upgrades, data transfer inaacuracies, implementation problems, etc. occur. Like the previous section on legislative mandates for professional nurse staffing, the desirability of successful EMR implementation (accompanied by ongoing maintenance and subsequent upgrades) ensure that the integrity of the system is intact. This could be considered a no-brainer in that more time could be devoted to bedside care and patient outcomes such as fewer medication errors and increased patient satisfaction would occur. However, this is more complex due to ongoing maintenance and subsequent upgrades (including staff time and additional expense) that ensure the integrity of the system.

Costs for the Hospital

The major costs in acquiring an EMR system include the costs of hardware, software, networking, maintenance, installation, and training as well as opportunity costs (Agrawal, 2002). Direct costs such as training are expensed on the hospital's income statement, and big-ticket items such as the hardware and contracted software are listed as assets on the balance sheet and depreciated over their useful life. This is a way of spreading out the tremendous cost outlay over time. This is also a way to pair these economic activities with the business or strategic plans the organization might have to determine an asset's future benefits. For example, an EMR system is known to be associated with increasing patient satisfaction and reductions in risk-adjusted mortality or complication rates. It is possible that these improved patient outcomes could be leveraged in a hospital's managed care contract negotiations with insurers.

This matching of economic and business activities begins the process of identifying the benefits of the technology relative to its costs.

Other direct costs are for hardware, software, training time, and salary and support fees. Indirect costs, those expenses associated with ongoing operational costs, include software maintenance and support fees, salaries for support staff, fees related to space and utilities (Nahm, Vaydia, Ho, Scharf, & Seagull, 2007), and the expenses of safety/security measures. Note that all costs mentioned thus far are borne by the health care-providing institution, in this case, the hospital. The next section, however, discusses that the benefits are shared by more than just this one entity.

Benefits for the Hospital and Patients

Implementation of a system has both tangible and intangible benefits, further complicating a discussion of the dynamics of benefits and costs. Some tangible benefits are concrete measurable gains derived directly from the EMR system, further expanded in the next paragrph. The intangible, or hard-to-quantify, benefits are such things as patient and user satisfaction and safety, increased compliance with federal or state regulations, decreased staff turnover, future leverage derived from the same, and hospital reputation.

Other difficult-to-calculate benefits include reduced resource use (partially from reduced LOS), improved quality through convenient access to information at the point of care, enhanced data capture, enhanced business management, and improved legal compliance with subsequent reduction in claims. In an econometric model making the business case for EMR implementation, Kaiser Permanente justified the costs for an inpatient EMR system through such benefits as increased RN and medical records efficiency; decreased RN overtime; reduced lab expenses, chart review time, and physical therapy wait time along with reduced inappropriate admissions, avoidable days, ER diverts, forms expenses and medical records supplies; fewer adverse drug events; and redeployment of space (Garrido, Raymond, Jamieson, Liang, & Wiesenthal, 2004). On the revenue side, improved coding accuracy for Medicare risk was mentioned.

Here is where we see a shared-benefit situation. In the case of adverse drug events, the hospital realizes as much as a 2.2-day reduced LOS for those events associated with injury. The patient is spared the inconvenience of the same amount of time plus the reduced opportunity cost of further morbidity from hospital-acquired conditions and, presumably, a shortened recuperation time with subsequent earlier return to work or productivity. At this point, the patient, the family, and the employer begin to share the benefits that resulted from costs incurred by only the hospital in the business case model. Yet if this is in keeping with a hospital or healthcare organization's mission (as is certainly the case for Kaiser Permanente), the business model is said to be a successful one.

Many different ways of calculating the hospital's return on investment (ROI), the benefits in relation to costs, exist. (See **Exhibit 11–2**.) Among these are *net present value* (NPV), payback analysis, and

---

Exhibit 11–2 Definitions

Cost-to-benefit analysis compares the cost of program goals that are being considered to the cost of implementing the proposed venture's benefits. If the benefits are greater than the cost, you have a positive cost benefit. A cost-benefit example can be found in Trepanier and colleagues (2012).

Return on investment (ROI) simply calculates the bottom line from your investments in the assets used for the investment, for example, positive ROI of 6% on the investment. Examples of ROI can be found in Pine and Tart (2007).

Break-even analysis identifies the cost and number of units that must be sold at a minimum to recover the fixed costs. This is defined further in Chapters 12 and 16.

break-even analysis. In each of these, many other influences must be assessed simultaneously, making the ROI analysis, by definition, very complicated. Among these are inflation, deflation, changes in business and strategic goals, shifts in healthcare management methods, and changes in Medicare reimbursement rates. Well beyond the scope of this text, econometric models identifying the multiple simultaneous influences on a successful analysis of this sort yield a partial solution for justifying the enormous outlay of costs for such information technology projects as EMR. Executive administration would do well to cost-out both sides of the analysis in the short, intermediate, and long terms.

Conventional wisdom leaves little doubt about the ability of information technology to improve clinical outcomes, but equally compelling evidence of the positive financial return of the same has yet to be established. Because the trend in reimbursement mechanisms continues to move toward outcomes achieved, technology may prove to be beneficial. However, equally compelling is pay for performance limiting reimbursements, the downturn in the U.S. economy, and security issues and other unexpected negative side effects of technology. Large purchases may continue not to be good business decisions. This means that there are currently inadequate incentives for hospitals to act on this important aspect of the hospital infrastructure, especially when many of the benefits are difficult to quantify and forecast, not to mention government intervention. This also means that as incentive programs to reward early adoption of technology or other innovations and quality of care are realized, they will act as a catalyst for the implementation of large-scale EMR projects in hospitals everywhere.

Kaiser's Business Case

In the account of a successful business case for a large-scale multihospital adoption of electronic medical records, Garrido and associates (2004) describe how Kaiser Permanente is investing $3 billion over 10 years to enhance the quality of care for its members. This is a marketing effort so that providers will continue to use Kaiser as the HMO of choice for employees. Kaiser Permanente HealthConnect is an EMR system for both inpatient and outpatient information management. The authors identified 36 categories of quantifiable benefits that contribute to a positive cash flow within 8.5 years. However, this business case is contingent upon other simultaneous factors, some of which are assumptions: leadership commitment, timely implementation, partnership with labor, coding compliance, and workflow redesign.

To be phased in over 3 years, theirs is a system that integrates the clinical record with appointments, registration, and billing. It is a system that includes workflow procedures, charting tools, and decision-support rules that will be shared by all Kaiser Permanente regions in 37 hospitals and 533 medical offices. To calculate NPV (net present value), two time lags were accounted for. The first was the implementation lag, the time between installation, training, and actual use. The second was the benefit realization lag, accounting for benefits such as malpractice liability reductions that may not manifest until years after full use is realized.

Net cash flow, the difference between the quantifiable benefits of the system and its costs of implementation and support, was projected for part way through the eighth year of phase-in. More than $2 billion realized cash flow is anticipated from the $1 billion investment over the investment horizon. Projected payback of the system within its 10-year life confirms the potential for it to generate long-term return on investment. Process improvements enabled by the project affect LOS, a key driver of savings where approximately 35% of net benefits are identified. Other significant areas of savings include lower transcription costs, timely manner of changes in care delivery (e.g., processing of physician orders), 30–50% reduction in medical record supplies and non–payroll expenses, and reduction in off-site medical record storage.

The difficult-to-quantify benefits include the adoption of care management protocols and best practices known to improve health outcomes. Again, entities other than the one outlaying the expenses—the hospital—are the patients and their families who benefit from streamlined care delivery and more efficient and informed admission and discharge processes. Although the strategic benefits from these enhancements are significant, the value attributed to them is difficult to measure. These, along with quality improvement, patient safety, continuity of care, and patient centeredness, are all part of Kaiser Permanente's strategic plan, so the business case can account for goals within those plans being met. Kaiser anticipates this system will be associated with higher nurse satisfaction, reduced burnout, and subsequent decreased turnover—so much so that intermediate and longer-term nurse recruitment expenses could be reduced. Another yet-to-be-quantified benefit will likely be a related reduction in registry nurse expenses as well as reductions in new nurse orientation, education time, and expense. Finally, a societal benefit is the rich flow of information for clinical, epidemiologic, and health services research. The data could be used for benchmarking, identification of best practices, and clinical outcome studies. There may be unidentified surprises as they continue along this path.

In conclusion, healthcare information systems play a central role in both the quality of care and daily operations (Nahm et al., 2007). They are extraordinarily expensive, even when the potential benefits are considered. Recall some of the lessons learned in this chapter's discussion of profit seeking: Costs shift, revenues shift, and this will *always* be the case. Costs and revenues shift both within and outside the hospital firm, as do costs and benefits, as shown. This is the factual view for any big-ticket item that a hospital might consider (such as substantially increasing professional nurse staffing or EMR implementation). This chapter does not provide an answer to normative queries on whether an EMR system *should be* implemented. Instead, the measures (or variables) necessary to construct an individual answer are offered from the logical positivist (factual) economic view.

As each healthcare organization addresses the issue of widespread implementation of an EMR, it will be increasingly important for decision makers to evaluate the nuances of their own business cases. Given that many factors obscure the construction of a clear business case for EMR, hospitals are forced to consider the *avoidance of an expense* (e.g., future litigation costs, less reimbursement if pay-for-performance mandates are not met) as parallel with *actual expense reduction* (including less reimbursement, if that has already occurred), especially in the short term. Similarly, they are forced to identify benefits that are realized by the hospital as well as those gained by the individual patient, his or her employer, or society as a whole. The propensity of a hospital to invest this way will likely be enhanced by the changing CMS rules on nonreimbursement for selected hospital complications. Forcing a hospital to pay for its own mistakes, such as certain hospital-acquired infections, raises the question of what type of electronic system it will take to capture the processes associated with these adverse outcomes for purposes of both quality improvement and revenue sustainability.

Summary

Hospitals, wrote Lewis Thomas (1983) in *The Youngest Science*, are "held together, glued together, enabled to function . . . by the nurses" (pp. 66–67). This chapter offers background information on the nature of competition and why it is important in the market for hospital care. In the discussion of profit motive and patient care, the reader was asked to join in debunking some myths about why a hospital exists to fulfill its purpose—to satisfy the needs of various stakeholders such as employees, the community at large, as well as patients and providers such as physicians and nurses. The regulatory arena was addressed last in the context of the hospital system as a dynamic microcosm of activity affected, sometimes dramatically, by legislative and societal mandates such as safe staffing laws. All of this reflects the complexity of the system.

Some of this monetary analysis is, in fact, a brand new way of thinking for those who have not studied formally in the fields of economics, accounting, or finance. It is hoped that, through this examination of what it takes for a hospital firm to survive competitive circumstances, future cohorts of nurses can preserve the only sustained hospital foundation—the practice of professional nursing. As stated by Buerhaus and associates (2002), "Nursing matters greatly in the hospitals' ability to provide quality of care and prevent avoidable adverse outcomes" (p. 130). The prevention of avoidable adversity is going to contribute most significantly to the survival of hospital firms through the coming years.

Most of the statements on hospital conditions and the business activities therein are from the domain of positive economics ("what is" or "what exists"), leaving the reader to draw his or her conclusions in the normative economic ("what *should* be") field of endeavor. Nursing's history, of course, has been to embrace the *mission* of caring, often with less investment in the *impact* of the ideals such as safe staffing on the hospital's *margin*. The chapter-opening quote, "No margin, no mission" (quoted in Langley, 1998), focused discussion on the consequences of nursing's advocacy. This is to say that without a sustainable *margin* of profit, a hospital, like all businesses, fails to provide service, employ personnel, pay its suppliers, or fulfill its *mission*.

Discussion Questions

1. Support or refute the statement "Well, supply and demand . . . it just doesn't work in health care!"
2. Discuss how margin and mission are related in the hospital environment, or aren't they?
3. Frame arguments for or against the policy of mandated minimum staffing ratios in the positive versus normative economic dichotomy.
4. Are hospitals competing on the basis of price, quality, or both? Explain.
5. Is hospital care overly regulated? Why or why not?
6. What is healthcare regulation and what are some of its costs?
7. Why is the provision of sick care (hospital) services said to be a *derived* demand?
8. Should there be minimum safe staffing ratios—from the standpoint of the patient? Why or why not?
9. Should there be minimum safe staffing ratios—from the standpoint of the hospital? Why or why not?
10. Should there be minimum safe staffing ratios—from the standpoint of the profession? Why or why not?
11. From an economic perspective describe the cost of regulation in the healthcare environment.
12. What is your definition of profit?

Glossary of Terms

American Nurses Credentialing Center—the world's largest and most influential nurse credentialing organization and a subsidiary of the American Nurses Association. American Nurses Credentialing Center is best known for promoting excellence in practice through its Magnet Recognition Program and Pathways to Excellence Program.

Asymmetric Knowledge—a state or condition in which buyers and sellers of a product or service have significantly different sets of information.

Bad Debt Expense—accounts receivable that will likely remain uncollectible and will be written off. It is a line item for which the hospital budgets.

Buyer—one who purchases healthcare services, often the health insurance company.

Competition—effort of two or more parties to gain the business of a third by offering preferably favorable terms.

Cost—dollar value of inputs used in the production of goods and services (output). Types of costs are variously termed and defined. These include direct, indirect, medical, nonmedical, future, intangibles, fixed, variable, marginal, and opportunity. Not to be confused with *expenses;* it is a broader term.

Cost Accounting—an element of financial management that generates information about the costs of an organization and its components. A subset of accounting, in general. Encompasses the development and provision of a wide range of financial information useful to managers in their roles.

Diagnosis-Related Groups (DRGs)—Medicare initiated payment to hospitals on this basis beginning in 1984. The prices for the groups are updated yearly by Medicare to reflect changes in reimbursement protocols.

Economics—study of how a society allocates scarce resources and goods.

Economies of Scale—also known as "returns to scale," it is the degree to which the cost of providing a good or service falls as quantity (measured by patient days) increases because fixed costs are shared by the larger volume of units.

Expense—a more exact concept than *cost*; the exact dollar amount a firm spends on a unit of production. Divided into two major types on a hospital's income statement, there are operating expenses (direct line items for the cost of inputs) and nonoperating expenses (less directly assigned costs, e.g., overhead).

Financial Accounting—system that records historical financial information and provides summary reports to individuals outside of the organization of what financial events have occurred and what the financial impact of those events has been.

Firm—the company, the hospital.

Government Intervention—actions on the part of government that affect economic activity, resource allocation, and especially free choice on the purchase of products or services.

Healthcare Economics—economics concerned with issues related to scarcity in the allocation of health and healthcare service provision.

Incentive—reward to an organization or individual for a behavior. Differs from *motive*, which is a psychological term describing an inner state.

Liquidity—ability of a firm to meet its short-term financial obligations, that is, pay bills, as they become due.

Macroeconomics—a branch of economics concerned with how human behavior affects outcomes in highly aggregated markets, such as the markets for labor or consumer products. In the healthcare context, the behavior of all hospital firms.

Managed Care—a system that manages healthcare delivery with the aim of controlling costs. Typically reliant on a physician or nurse in advanced practice, the clinical activity is paired with the economic activity that is thought to reduce frivolous expenses and moral hazard.

Managerial Accounting—the process of identifying, analyzing, interpreting, and communicating financial information so that an organization can pursue its goals. Differs from financial accounting in that it is an internal process, whereas financial accounting focuses on reporting financial activity to an outside source.

Margin—the point at which one more unit of input no longer yields one more unit of output—it yields less.

Microeconomics—a branch of economics concerned with the behavior of individuals and a (hospital) firm. The activities of individuals and businesses with regard to the allocation of resources and the production and distribution of goods and services.

Mission—a healthcare organization's raison d'être; why it says it exists.

Motive—internal psychological state of arousal propelling a person (or organization) to approach a goal.

Net Present Value (NPV)—future stream of benefits and costs converted into equivalent values today. Today's value of an investment's future net cash flow minus the initial investment.

Normative Economics—judgments about "what ought to be" in economic matters. By definition, they cannot be proved false because they are based on assessments, but they can (and should) be supported by facts or positive economics to be most useful.

Nurse Manager—supervisory nurse who has complete operational and financial authority for a unit or units on a 24/7 basis; her or his practice is said to be decentralized.

Operating Expenses—line-item entries on the income statement traceable to a hospital's day-to-day business, for example, salaries and bad debt expense. These are different from nonoperating expenses, such as insurance and maintenance of equipment.

Perfect Information—a state of complete knowledge about the product of a firm and possibly the actions of other players in it. Not to be taken literally, it is the basis for the purchase of a certain volume of products at a particular price.

Positive Economics—study of "what is" in economic relationships.

Profit—excess of revenue over expenses.

Profit Margin—excess of revenue over expenses divided by total revenue. An index of the amount of profit generated by each dollar of revenue.

Prospective Payment System—introduced by the federal government in 1983, a system by which Medicare reimburses hospitals at a predetermined rate, largely based on discharge medical diagnoses, for its patients. Aimed at influencing hospital behavior through financial incentives that encourage more cost-efficient care, the hospital receives a flat-rate reimbursement for a diagnosis-related group into which each patient falls based on clinical information such as age, gender, and comorbidities for a medical diagnosis, irrespective of actual consumption of services.

Regulation—form of government intervention designed to shape the behavior of an economic entity—organizations or individuals. Healthcare providers such as physicians, nurses, and hospitals are said to be highly regulated, referring to such things as approval by boards of medicine or nursing and licensure by states.

Risk—state of uncertainty containing possible adversity or undesired outcomes. If quantifiable, this expectation of loss is said to carry a certain probability.

Seller—economic agents who are accountable for the production and sale of healthcare services, for example, the hospital.

Solvency—ability of a firm to meet its maturing obligations as they become due.

Symmetric Knowledge—knowledge about a hospital's performance (patient outcomes) possessed by both the healthcare buyer and seller.

Total Compensation Package—sum total of an employee's payment for services rendered including salary and benefits.

Uncertainty—lack of certainty, either subjective or objective. It differs from risk in that it cannot be easily quantified.

Widget—an abstract unit of production.

References

Agrawal, A. (2002). Return of investment analysis for a computer-based patient record in the outpatient clinical setting. *Journal of the Association for Academic Minority Physicians, 13*(3), 61–65.

Aiken, L., Smith, H., & Lake, E. (1994). Lower Medicare mortality among a set of hospitals known for good nursing care. *Medical Care, 32*, 771–787.

American Organization of Nurse Executives. (2005). *The AONE Nurse Executive Competencies.* Retrieved from www .aone.org/resources/leadership%20tools/PDFs/AONE_NEC.pdf

Berlin, L., & Sechrist, K. (2002). The shortage of doctorally-prepared nurse faculty: A dire situation. *Nursing Outlook, 50*, 50–56.

Buerhaus, P., Needleman, J., Mattke, S., & Stewart, M. (2002). Strengthening hospital nursing. *Health Affairs, 21*, 123–132.

Burnes Bolton, L., Aydin, C., Donaldson, N., Brown, D., Sandhu, M., Fridman, M., et al. (2007). Mandated nurse staffing ratios in California: A comparison of staffing and nursing-sensitive outcomes pre- and postregulation. *Policy, Politics & Nursing Practice, 8*, 238–250.

California Nurses Association. (n.d.). *CNA's 12-year campaign for safe RN staffing ratios.* Retrieved from http://www .nationalnursesunited.org/page/-/files/pdf/ratios/12yr-fight-0104.pdf

Conover, C. (2004, October 4). Health care regulation: A $169 billion hidden tax. *Policy Analysis, 527.* Retrieved from http://www.cato.org/pubs/pas/pa527.pdf

Conway, P., Tamara Konetzka, R., Zhu, J., Volpp, K., & Sochalski, J. (2008). Nurse staffing ratios: Trends and policy implications for hospitalists and the safety net. *Journal of Hospital Medicine (Online), 3*, 193–199.

Donaldson, N., Bolton, L., Aydin, C., Brown, D., Elashoff, J., & Sandhu, M. (2005). Impact of California's licensed nurse–patient ratios on unit-level nurse staffing and patient outcomes. *Policy, Politics & Nursing Practice, 6*, 198–210.

Enthoven, A. (1986). Managed competition in health care and the unfinished agenda. *Health Care Financing Review, Annual Supplement, 8*, 105–119.

Garrido, T., Raymond, B., Jamieson, L., Liang, L., & Wiesenthal, A. (2004). Making the business case for hospital information systems—a Kaiser Permanente investment decision. *Journal of Healthcare Finance, 31*(2), 16–25.

Gerardi, T. (2006). Staffing ratios in New York: A decade of debate. *Policy, Politics & Nursing Practice, 7*, 8–10.

Gray, B. (1991). *The profit motive and patient care: The changing accountability of doctors and hospitals.* Cambridge, MA: Harvard University Press.

Harris, K., Huber, D., Jones, R., Manojlovich, M., & Reineck, C. (2006). Future nursing administration graduate curricula, Part 1. *Journal of Nursing Administration, 36*, 435–440.

Herrin, D., Jones, K., Krepper, R., Sherman, R., & Reineck, C. (2006). Future nursing administration graduate curricula, Part 2: Foundation and Strategies. *Journal of Nursing Administration, 36*, 498–505.

Hippocrates. (n.d./2004). Book 1, Section 2. (F. Adams, Trans.). In *Of the epidemics* (p. 5). Kessinger Publishing.

Institute of Medicine. (2002). *To err is human: Building a safer health system*. Washington, DC: National Academy Press.

Kazahaya, G. (2005). Harnessing technology to redesign labor cost management reports. *Healthcare Financial Management, 59*(4), 94–100.

Keepnews, D. (2007). Evaluating nurse staffing regulation. *Policy, Politics & Nursing Practice, 8*, 236–237.

Lang, N. (2003). Reflections on quality health care. *Nursing Administration Quarterly, 27*, 266–272.

Lang, T., Hodge, M., Olson, V., Romano, P., & Kravitz, R. (2004). Nurse–patient ratios: A systematic review on the effects of nurse staffing on patient, nurse, employee, and hospital outcomes. *Journal of Nursing Administration, 34*, 326–337.

Langley, M. (1998, January 7). Nuns' zeal for profits shapes hospital chain, wins Wall Street fans. *Wall Street Journal*, pp. A1, A11.

Lemire, J. (2000). Redesigning financial management education for the nursing administration graduate student. *Journal of Nursing Administration, 30*, 199–205.

Lindrooth, R., Bazzoli, G., Needleman, J., & Hasnain-Wynia, R. (2006). The effect of changes in hospital reimbursement on nurse staffing decisions at safety net and nonsafety net hospitals. *Health Services Research, 41*, 701–720.

Manjoney, R. (2004). Clinical information systems market—an insider's view. *Journal of Critical Care, 19*, 215–220.

Marinucci, C. (2004, December 8). At tribute for women, Schwarzenegger angers nurses. *San Francisco Chronicle*, p. A1.

Mark, B., & Harless, D. (2007). Nurse staffing, mortality, and length of stay in for-profit and not-for-profit hospitals. *Inquiry, 44*, 167–186.

Medical News Report. (2004, February). New nurse-to-patient ratios present challenges in California. Retrieved from http://www.nursingworld.org/MainMenuCategories/Policy-Advocacy/State/Legislative-Agenda-Reports/State-StaffingPlansRatios

Nahm, E., Vaydia, V., Ho, D., Scharf, B., & Seagull, J. (2007). Outcomes assessment of clinical information system implementation: A practical guide. *Nursing Outlook, 55*, 282–288.

Needleman, J. (2008). Is what's good for the patient good for the hospital? Aligning incentives and the business case for nursing. *Policy, Politics & Nursing Practice, 9*, 80–87.

Needleman, J., & Buerhaus, P. (2003). Nurse staffing and patient safety: Current knowledge and implications for action. *International Journal for Quality in Health Care, 15*, 275–277.

Needleman, J., Buerhaus, P., Mattke, S., Stewart, M., & Zelevinsky, K. (2002). Nurse-staffing levels and the quality of care in hospitals. *New England Journal of Medicine, 346*, 1715–1722.

Office of Statewide Health Planning and Development. (1996a). *Study overview and results summary*. Sacramento, CA: Author.

Office of Statewide Health Planning and Development. (1996b). *Technical appendix*. Sacramento, CA: Author.

Office of Statewide Health Planning and Development. (2006). *Hospital closures in California*. Retrieved from www.calhealth.org

Pine, R., & Tart, K. (2007, January–February). Return on investment: Benefits and challenges of a baccalaureate nurse residency program. *Nursing Economic$, 25*(1), 13–19, 39.

Quinones, S. (2006, September 22). Closure of Memorial ER is protested. *Los Angeles Times*, p. B4.

Rollins, G. (2008). CNO burnout. *Hospitals & Health Networks, 82*(4), 30–34.

Rudan, V. (2002). Where have all the nursing administration students gone? Issues and solutions. *Journal of Nursing Administration, 32*, 185–188.

Schultz, M. (2008, July). *The association of hospital structural and financial characteristics to mortality from community-acquired pneumonia*. Paper presented at the Congress on Nursing Research of Sigma Theta Tau International, Singapore.

Schultz, M., van Servellen, G., Litwin, M., McLaughlin, E., & Uman, G. (1997). Can hospital structural and financial characteristics explain the variations in hospital mortality caused by acute myocardial infarction? *Applied Nursing Research, 12*, 210–214.

Thomas, L. (1983). *The youngest science: Notes of a medicine-watcher*. New York, NY: Penguin.

Trepanier, S., Early, S., Ulrich, B., & Cherry, B. (2012, July–August). New graduate nurse residency program: A cost-benefit analysis based on turnover and contract labor usage. *Nursing Economic$, 30*(4), 207–214.

Budget Principles

Part V provides the "bread and butter" information on budgeting. It is important that nurse managers, as well as other nurse administrators, have this basic knowledge.

Chapter 12 provides basic budget principles and terminology and gives an explanation of the break-even budget strategy. Then, Chapter 13 adds to the budgeting knowledge base to show a nurse manager how to both evaluate and develop a nursing expense budget. Certain principles should be followed when developing a budget, including figuring nonproductive time, to be sure enough staff are budgeted.

Another very important budget responsibility for nurse managers, and other nurse administrators, is evaluation of budget variances. These are explored in Chapter 14. Some budget variances are less critical or occur because of circumstances already anticipated, such as staff training during the installation of a new clinical documentation system. But some variances can indicate serious problems nurse managers can fix—including charges that should not have occurred in that cost center. Variances can provide clues as to money that can be saved. Although tracking variances is presented as an activity to do monthly, the nurse manager needs to perform certain activities on a daily basis to achieve maximum budget savings. Although a number of nurse managers still do not have this kind of budget responsibility, especially in Veterans Administration facilities or long-term care freestanding facilities, we recommend that such a process be consistently used in all settings.

Chapter 15 discusses important budget responsibilities that have resulted since prospective payment was implemented. Here the nurse manager/administrator, along with the rest of the administrative group, needs to examine actual reimbursements received and compare them with the actual costs of services provided. This is best accomplished as an interdisciplinary activity that reflects all actual costs. Nurse managers can affect certain costs, while other costs need to be handled by other departments or by the executive group. Examining reimbursement/cost ratios ensures that the facility is not spending more to provide service than the reimbursement amount received.

CHAPTER 12

Budgeting

R. Penny Marquette, DBA, Janne Dunham-Taylor, PhD, RN, and Joseph Z. Pinczuk, MHA

OBJECTIVES

- Provide basic budget principles and terminology.
- Provide examples of how the budget is put together.
- Identify the interface between the nurse manager, information services, and the finance department.
- Explain the basic cost concepts.
- Identify certain costs and their behavior.
- Discuss the composition and differences between an operating budget and a capital budget.

Introduction

There are nurse managers who are not privy to budget information, but most nurse managers are both privy to budget information (at least in their area of authority) and responsible for budgets. Although the extent to which nurse managers are involved in the budget process varies by healthcare organization, most nurse managers find themselves being involved with budget preparation, holding spending to within budget limits, dealing with differences between the budget and actual performance (called *budget variances*), and identifying budget errors.

For most nurse managers, budget information and activities are involved with *spending*. Having r*evenue* information is not as common. On the revenue side, nurse managers may know the breakdown between private pay, Medicare/Medicaid, and paying/nonpaying patients. In some systems, the actual reimbursement amount is shared with the nurse manager. Finally, the nurse manager is often involved with the entire area of case management, which involves daily issues of determining whether an insurance plan will pay for services provided. Nurse managers must understand the vital link between the amount of money received from all insurance carriers (including Medicare and Medicaid) and the critical role of charting, which supports the billing documents.

Budgets and Patient Care

Budget responsibility offers an opportunity for the nurse manager to be an advocate for patients. As the level of management closest to the services delivered to patients, a nurse manager with a firm grip on relevant budget information influences patient care, ensuring that the patient receives the best and safest services possible.

All managers are most effective when they are able to make sound decisions and defend those decisions with others in the organization. This is equally true for the nurse manager who needs the *skills and the vocabulary* to determine what financial information is available, acquire that information, and interpret its impact on patient care. Unfortunately, the nurse manager often must ferret out the data he or she needs to do this job. Data are often badly organized or even hidden from line managers.

Data Systems

Computer systems are becoming the norm in large healthcare organizations. By *system*, we mean integrated computer programs that can interface with one another.[1] For example, in an ideal situation, a nurse manager faced with staffing a unit for the coming week has access to selected data from the finance department, the human resources department, and the nursing department. With data from these sources, the nurse manager knows how much money is available in the budget for the unit, the salaries of cost center personnel, which employees have already worked this month, who has vacation scheduled, and so on. If the patient classification system is also interfaced, the nurse manager additionally has a description of the patients needing care and the anticipated hours of care needed for each patient. With this information, the nurse manager can evaluate whether the present staffing is adequate, too high, or too low to meet patient needs.

Presently, there are computer programs that do all of these tasks in isolation. The problem has been that the programs cannot "talk to each other." They are isolated programs, not computer systems. Although the information may be available, it is not easily retrieved and involves collecting data from many sources.

Charts of Accounts

Within the finance department, the provision of easy, orderly access to extensive cost information requires an organizing device. That device is called a *chart of accounts*. Most charts of accounts consist of two parts. The first is a listing of all units of the organization for which cost information should be gathered. In health care, this might include laundry, rehabilitation therapy, infection control, housekeeping, operating room, X-ray, home health, physical therapy, separate nursing units, food service, finance, and others. The second part is a list of those elements of cost that occur in those *cost centers*. These elements of cost include such items as salaries, various fringe benefits, legal fees, pharmaceuticals, building supplies, grounds repair, equipment repair, oxygen, medical supplies, linen replacement, uniforms, copying, advertising, postage, and so on. Some expenses occur in only one unit of the organization, but most occur in several places. By properly organizing the chart of accounts, we can compare similar costs across different units and even compare costs of similar units across different healthcare institutions.

The typical format of a chart of accounts is a decimal system where a number representing the cost or revenue center of the organization appears before the decimal and the element of cost appears after. When such charts are first designed, the numbers are not consecutive. Gaps are left in the numbering so that new departments and new types of costs can be inserted in places where they best belong. For example, you would want to keep all kinds of salaries close together on the chart to help you find them quickly. (Unfortunately, the longer the list, the more likely it is that you will run out of room in logical order and begin adding items to the end of the list.)

A brief example that uses the chart of accounts recommended by the American Hospital Association (AHA) may be helpful. Assume an outpatient clinic has three departments: Respiratory Care, Laboratory, and Rehabilitation Services. The chart of accounts might appear as shown in **Exhibit 12–1**. With these data,

Exhibit 12–1 Chart of Accounts for the Outpatient Clinic

Account Name (organizational unit)	Department Charge Numbers (elements of cost)	
6170 Respiratory Care	.000	Salaries Supervisors
7091 Rehabilitation Services	.010	Salaries - RNs
7010 Laboratory	.020	Salaries - LPNs
	.030	Salaries – Aides
	.160	FICA (Social Security)
	.340	In-Service Training
	.360	Pharmaceuticals
	.420	Oxygen
	.430	Solutions
	.440	Medical Supplies
	.441	Billable Supplies
	.450	General Supplies
	.480	Instruments
	.490	Microfilming
	.491	Minor Equipment

Exhibit 12–2 Cost Comparisons Using a Chart of Accounts			
	Account Name (organizational unit)		
	6170	7091	
Department Charge Numbers (elements of cost)	Respiratory Care	Rehabilitation Services	7010 Laboratory
.000 Salaries - Supervisors			
.010 Salaries - RNs			
.020 Salaries - LPNs			
.030 Salaries - Aides			
.160 FICA (Social Security)			
.340 In-Service Training			
.360 Pharmaceuticals			
.420 Oxygen			
.430 Solutions			
.440 Medical Supplies			
.441 Billable Supplies			
.480 Instruments			
.490 Microfilming			
.491 Minor Equipment			

we have an account numbered 6170.480 to collect the costs for instruments purchased by the Respiratory Care department. Account number 7091.480 collects the same costs for Rehabilitation Services.

Comparisons of costs by department can be facilitated by organizing data as shown in **Exhibit 12–2**. Data from the individual cells in this chart represent specific cost elements within specific healthcare units. These costs form the basis for many of the analytical financial tools used to measure healthcare entity performance.[2] In addition to the advantage of being able to compare costs across departments within a single institution, using a standardized chart of accounts allows healthcare entities to compare themselves with similar institutions in their own communities and elsewhere in the country.

Nursing: A Big Budget Item

Nursing department costs often comprise 25% to 30% of the healthcare organization's budget. Because the nursing budget is so large, it often becomes the subject of close scrutiny. This makes it all the more important for nurse managers to have information available to respond quickly and effectively to such scrutiny with documented facts. Some questions to consider are the following:

- Do I have enough information about the nursing personnel? Data the nurse manager might want quickly at hand include starting dates; salaries and salary ranges, including ceilings for different classifications of personnel; sick, vacation, and personal time off available and already taken; hours worked each week; shift(s) worked; and overtime paid.
- Do I have adequate information about the patient population served? Do I have a good handle on the type and severity of illness, length of stay or visit, satisfaction level, and method of payment?
- How productive are the personnel in my assigned area? How can I demonstrate the level of productivity that exists? Could this level of productivity be improved?

- What changes could be made to reduce costs?
- How do selected cost changes affect the quality of service delivered?
- Is my organization and/or my area of responsibility financially viable?

Integrity

As with all aspects of health care, integrity is an essential component of the financial function. In the budget process, the nurse manager is faced with a choice: Does one ask for what is needed or "pad" the budget request, assuming it will be cut later? Padding does *not* include reasonable slack. Things never go perfectly as planned. Leaving some slack in the budget is reasonable and prudent. Padding, on the other hand, involves asking for more than you know you will need.

Remember first that your reputation is at stake. Once you have a reputation for padding your budget, every request you make will be examined with a fine-tooth comb. Your numbers will be assumed not to be accurate. On the other hand, if you develop a reputation for prudence and accuracy, that reputation, once established, will support your requests in future years. The authors—representing nursing and finance— unanimously recommend that you choose to be truthful. Crying wolf eventually is recognized. An honest relationship between those involved is always preferable for everyone concerned, including the patient.

Interfacing with the Finance Department

As they deal with their cost center budgets, most nurse managers find themselves forced to interface with their finance department. We say *forced* because there exists an army of reasons why these encounters are generally stressful. Part of our goal in this text is to make those interactions work more smoothly.

Although budgeting and financial terms are used throughout business, government, and nonprofit organizations, this terminology is not tightly standardized. Terms that mean one thing in a factory mean something at least slightly different in a healthcare setting. To make matters worse, terminology is not standardized across all hospitals (or any healthcare facility) and is certainly not standardized across different healthcare environments. For example, a nurse manager who has worked at one hospital and then moves to another or who moves from a hospital to home care will discover differences in terminology and budget forms.

Finally, the financial people in the healthcare organization are likely to come from nonhealthcare business backgrounds. By looking at terminology from both a nursing and an accounting/finance perspective, the nurse manager will learn the links needed to communicate more effectively and maximize mutual understanding of terminology, concepts, and issues when working with financial personnel.

We have one more important instruction before we begin to examine the budgeting process and the dictionary of budgeting terminology. When you seem to be at an impasse when working with your financial people, skip the frustration stage and move on to *defining your terms*. Assume that you may be using a term differently. Once you understand the underlying concepts, you can simply ask, "How are you defining fixed cost? What are you including?" This approach can quickly move you beyond the stage where the finance person is looking at you as though you are an idiot, and you are getting ready to smack him or her with your unit's budget!

The Budget Process

To be most effective, budgeting should be an integrated function within the organization, and all departments should participate. Then, the nurse manager will be an integral part of the organizational whole.

Start with the Strategic Plan

The strategic plan outlines the programs and services to be provided for the upcoming year, including priorities and new opportunities to be pursued. Unfortunately, this process of strategic planning often does *not* include all the managers who need to understand the budget process. The nurse manager may not understand the goals of the organization, may not have seen the strategic plan, or may not have been involved in setting those priorities that specifically deal with the nurse manager's areas of responsibility. When this happens, the resultant budget is not as accurate as it might be. For example, those developing the budget may not know that a surgeon has changed an operating technique, turning an inpatient length of stay into an outpatient procedure. This change (becoming increasingly common with microsurgical techniques) affects multiple levels of the budget, including most nursing costs. A few years ago, this type of procedural change occurred with gallbladder surgery. If finance department personnel are unaware of such changes, both the revenue budget and the spending budget may end the year with major differences (called *variances*) between budget and actual.

Strategic plans need to take into account new surgical/medical/diagnostic advances that can require a different staff mix. For example, in long-term care, staff mix formerly included registered nurse coverage for 8 hours a day with 24-hour coverage being provided by licensed practical nurses/certified nurse aides. Now, with the increased complexity of the patient population, the staff mix has changed to 24-hour registered nurse coverage and increased numbers of licensed staff.

Another factor to consider if third-party reimbursement (including Medicare and Medicaid) is using the per diem payment method is that you must know what is included and excluded in the per diem. For example, if per diem includes all medications and the patient is placed on Lovenox bid at $80 to $90 an injection, the budget is affected.

Generally, there are separate budgets for each organizational unit. Units are defined as either *cost centers* or *profit centers*. Profit centers have direct patient billing. These include the operating room, X-ray, laboratory, and outpatient. Cost centers do not bill patients directly; instead, they support the profit centers. Some cost centers have little direct relation to patient care. Payroll, custodial, purchasing, and senior management are examples of such cost centers. Other cost centers do support patient care but do not bill patients directly for their services. These include most nursing services, food service, and medical records.

Cost centers may be identified by their physical location (a floor) or by their function (all cardiology-related costs). Nurse managers are usually responsible for at least one cost center budget. As the manager's organizational responsibilities grow, so does the number of budgets for which the manager is responsible. When nurse managers move to a different organization, even at a similar healthcare entity, it is important that they inspect the new budget, line by line, to get an accurate picture of how the budget is constructed. A line item may reflect salaries and benefits at one institution; salaries alone in another; and salaries, benefits, and overtime at a third.

The Finance Department

Often, the budget process begins with the finance department. This process begins at a specified time, perhaps 6 months before the new fiscal year.[3] The finance department generates a budget for next year based on actual spending during the current year. Major differences between the current budget and actual spending are investigated, and anticipated cost changes are factored in for such items as employee raises, supply and pharmaceutical cost increases, and the general rate of inflation. The system should include input from the nurse manager. For example, the nurse manager's cost center might be experiencing full census when the current budget reflects 80% occupancy. If changes have occurred, the nurse manager must provide changes to finance department personnel.

Although budget figures are generally *annual* estimates divided by 12 (or 13), costs do not flow evenly through the year, and nurse managers should be prepared to explain short-term variations. For example, a clinic may anticipate an increased demand for immunizations in August before school starts in the fall, an orthopedic cost center may anticipate more fractures during ski season, or a psychiatric cost center may have a decreased census during the convention of the American Psychological Association because most of the admitting psychiatrists attend this meeting. Only front-line managers understand these variations, which is another reason why nurse managers should help prepare the budget.

The value of those working *for* the nurse manager should also not be underestimated. This point in the budget cycle is a good time to talk with unit employees about budget issues. Staff can suggest how to provide patient care in a more cost-effective manner while still achieving quality standards. It is also very helpful if administrators *from all departments* can meet and discuss changing circumstances and spending priorities.

Each Unit Submits a Budget to Help Achieve the Strategic Plan

The budget process starts at the top with the strategic plan, but once that is set it moves back to the trenches and the budget is generally built from the bottom up. As each unit submits the costs (and/or anticipated revenue if in the operating room or in a revenue-producing cost center) associated with achieving its portion of the mission, the *finance* or *cost and budget* department aggregates these costs into an overall, entity-wide budget. Clearly, the nurse manager must know what strategic goals are expected of the unit to determine the associated costs.

The Nurse Executive

Once the nurse manager has reviewed the next year's budget and provided feedback on changes, the budget is often sent to the nurse executive for further review. To negotiate successfully with the nurse executive, the nurse manager needs to consider the broader scope of responsibility that the nurse executive holds. The nurse manager can consider what role the nurse executive holds in the organization's strategic plan and how his or her unit can help fulfill that role.

Developing Budget Numbers

Most budgets are based on the prior year's budget, actual performance, or a combination of the two. It is typical for entities (whether business, government, or nonprofit) to simply take last year's plans, adjust for obvious errors in estimate, add on a little for inflation, and continue on. Called a *line-item budget*, this budgeting program clearly does not start with the strategic plan! Nevertheless, it is simple, and it is the most common approach to budgeting.

There is an opportunity here. If something has changed in the environment, this type of budgeting process allows the nurse manager to take the initiative and seek additional funding when the underlying circumstances have changed. For example, if the strategic plan of the hospital has changed to focus on patients with higher levels of acuity, the opportunity exists to argue effectively for a higher proportion of registered nurses or nurse practitioners. Unfortunately (or fortunately, if you are the one in hiding), activities are often funded long after they fail to support the strategic mission of the organization.

During the Year

Throughout the year the nurse manager must compare the budget (the plan) with actual results. The quality of reporting that supports this work varies from organization to organization. In the best case scenario, the nurse manager receives regular reports on a pay-period-by-pay-period basis, month-by-month basis, and a year-to-date basis. The year-to-date numbers represent actual and budgeted numbers for the portion of the fiscal year that has passed. For example, if the budget year begins in January and it is now April, the budget report will include the actual and budget numbers for April, along with the actual and budget numbers for the 4-month period that includes January through April. These year-to-date figures help smooth out minor fluctuations and help the nurse manager see whether the unit is on target. Additionally, year-to-date numbers also *highlight growing differences between budget and actual numbers that require immediate attention.*

Variance Reporting

In a well-run system, each unit receives a regular monthly report showing the actual activity, the budgeted activity, and the difference between the two, called the *budget variance.* This report enables the nurse manager to focus on those areas where things are not going according to plan.

End of the Budget Year

As the end of the fiscal year approaches, the finance department often asks that purchases for the last month of the fiscal year be completed early in the month so that finance can more accurately reflect yearly expenditures by the end of the fiscal year. In fact, as the end of the budget period approaches, nurse managers are sometimes faced with the unusual problem of wanting to spend more money.

Starting 6 months before the end of the fiscal year, nurse managers should begin examining their budgets (including grant budgets) to evaluate their remaining funds. The disposition of unspent funds varies from organization to organization and grant to grant. In the worst case scenario, unspent funds are returned to the administration *and* the following year's allocation is reduced by the same amount. (This is another place where budget "padding" can come back to haunt you.) In the next least attractive situation, the unspent funds are returned to the administration and you are commended for your careful control over organizational resources. In the best case scenario, you are allowed to retain (or roll over) all or a portion of your remaining funds.[4] It is the nurse manager's job to know how unspent funds are handled at the end of the fiscal year and to plan accordingly.

Like our advice on honesty in the budget process, it is best to avoid spending money on things you really do not need. On the other hand, if you have needed new patient beds for 2 years and this year you have money left over, it would be a shame to lose it because you failed to plan ahead.

Fixed and Flexible Budgets

A *fixed budget* predicts a certain level of costs, ignoring the level of activity that occurs.[5] In reality, the cost of nursing services varies greatly with census and acuity. Because the fixed budget is not too useful when activity is shifting, many organizations prepare a *flexible budget.* The flexible budget has different levels of cost based on levels of activity. The nurse manager may plan a flexible budget to cover different scenarios, for example, a 100% census versus a census of 95%.[6]

Some health care systems have computer programs that automatically prepare flexible budgets. Sometimes, however, this is still a manual activity for the nurse manager. But a note of warning: Even when a computer program takes over the number crunching, the nurse manager should evaluate the assumptions underlying which costs change and which stay constant. A flexible budget provides guidance in anticipating cost increases when volume increases in terms of either census and/or acuity.

Optimistic, Pessimistic, or Realistic Budget Estimates

Another approach that many organizations take is to have each manager prepare his or her budget at two or more levels: optimistic (census or department activity levels are very high), pessimistic (census or department activity levels are very low), and realistic (department or activity levels stay the same as the previous year). First, this approach forces managers to consider which costs and services are absolutely essential: What can't the unit do without? Second, it forces the manager to consider the most attractive expansion of costs and services: What would you do if you were rolling in money? Even though these budgets may never be used, the thought process involved in their preparation helps the manager deal with changing realities.

Midyear Budget Adjustments

Cash receipts are often less than the amount expected, necessitating midyear budget cuts.[7] It is best if the nurse manager has a plan for this possibility, rather than being forced to do budget cuts at the last minute.

Everyone Brings Something to the Table

Different groups in the organization have unique information crucial to the overall effectiveness of the budget. Nurses often do not know what *revenues* were generated last year (which the finance department does know), whereas finance personnel do not understand the myriad problems encountered in taking care of patients (which nursing personnel do know). The most accurate budget predictions are achieved when people from all departments contribute the unique information they have.

Measuring and Adjusting for Inflation

Accountants and finance people adjust for inflation using a *price index*. The price index you are most likely familiar with is the *Consumer Price Index (CPI)*, which measures "the increase (or decrease) in the cost of living for an urban family of four" (U.S. Department of Labor Bureau of Labor Statistics). There are other price indices, including the *Wholesale Price Index*, which measures price changes in individual industries and sectors of the economy, including a *market basket* of goods and services in health care.

All price indices are in the form of the to/from ratio:

> Prices in the period we are going "to"
> Prices in the period we are coming "from"

To illustrate all price indices, let's look at the way the CPI is developed. First, a panel of experts (usually economists) decides what items an average urban family of four spends its money on: food, housing, clothing, education, medical costs, entertainment, and so on. For the moment, assume that those are the only items on the list. The panel must now decide how to define one unit of food or one unit of housing. These decisions can be pretty arbitrary *as long as they remain consistent from year to year*. That consistency, however, is actually impossible. How do you compare a unit of entertainment in 1945 with a unit of entertainment in 2009? Most of the things we do for entertainment in the twenty-first century did not exist at the end of World War II. The panel is simply left to do the best it can.

Generally, the finance department personnel indicate expected levels of inflation for different kinds of equipment, supplies, and pharmaceuticals. They get this information from the market basket index. If contracts for equipment and supplies change, it is important that the correct cost of these items be reflected in the budget.

Basic Cost Concepts: How Costs Are Defined

Cost accounting is an industrial invention. It comes from an environment where things are manufactured. Even today, cost accounting is not heavily applied to businesses that are service entities and provide services instead of goods.

Imagine a business that manufactures surgical carts. They have certain requirements: a building, insurance, electricity, equipment, materials to make the cart (legs, wheels, shelves, handles, glue, sandpaper, paint), labor to take those materials and shape them into a cart, and, finally, labor to oversee the process and do the paperwork (accounting, payroll, insurance, and taxes). We will go back to this simple example as we "cross-walk" nursing terminology for costs with accounting/finance terminology for costs and try to identify the places where misunderstandings are most likely to occur.

In manufacturing, there are three types of costs: direct materials, direct labor, and overhead. *Direct materials* are those large enough to be identified with a specific product. In the example of the surgical cart, the legs, the wheels, the shelves, and the handles all classify as direct materials. For a patient who comes into the hospital for the surgical insertion of a pacemaker, the pacemaker itself is clearly a direct material.

Indirect materials, on the other hand, are materials that cannot be associated with a specific product in a *cost-effective manner*. These costs may or may not relate directly to the product, but it would be so time-consuming and expensive, there would be no overall benefit. *Indirect materials are part of overhead*. In the example of the surgical cart, indirect materials include items like glue, sandpaper, and paint. For the surgical patient, indirect materials include things like antiseptic swabbing in the operating room, surgical gloves, and surgical masks.[8]

Direct labor is the labor that actually turns direct materials (also called *raw materials*) into a finished product. In our surgical cart example, direct labor is the person who puts the cart together. In our hospital environment, floor nurses are direct labor. The physician who inserts the pacemaker is direct labor.

Indirect labor encompasses those persons who do not actually turn direct materials into a finished product. In the industrial example, indirect labor includes the foreman, the person who runs the raw materials storeroom, the accountant, the custodian, the payroll clerk, and others. In our hospital, indirect labor includes all these people, plus the housekeeper, the dietitian, the medical records clerk, and many others. *Indirect labor is part of overhead.*

Overhead is composed of two things, of which you already know—indirect materials and indirect labor. These, however, are a tiny portion of overhead. The main overhead costs are often called the "costs to get ready to manufacture." In our surgical cart example, these costs include the building, insurance, electricity, and equipment. In our hospital example, overhead includes all these costs plus many others: insurance billing, kitchen staff, dietitians, medical records, accounting, billing, payroll, finance, and management.

Basic Cost Concepts: How Costs Behave

The definitions of types of costs (direct materials, direct labor, and overhead) interact with two important concepts of how costs behave: *fixed costs* and *variable costs*. Because healthcare environments are different from manufacturing environments, this is an area where misunderstandings can easily occur, and one where the nurse manager can play a role in educating finance and accounting personnel about the unique aspects of healthcare environments.

Fixed Costs

Fixed costs are those that stay the same regardless of the level of activity. The first example of fixed costs is those costs that would exist even if the organization were shut down. In a manufacturing environment, that would include such things as rent, insurance, taxes, depreciation on (the consumption of) buildings and equipment (although perhaps at a lower or higher rate than if the equipment and buildings were in use), a minimal level of utilities, and so on. Also, fixed are those costs that stay the same whether the organization manufactures 1 surgical cart or 10,000. Many overhead costs fall into this category (manufacturing supervisors, accounting, billing, payroll, finance, and top-level management).

From a nursing administration perspective, fixed costs (including minimum staffing requirements) are the minimum costs that are always paid regardless of the volume of activity.[9] Regardless of patient activity, whether it is measured by patient visits, patient acuity, or patient minutes, hours, or days, certain costs are always present. Examples include a cost center or department secretary working the day shift regardless of patient volume, telephone service, electricity, heating and cooling, staff development, quality assurance, dietary personnel, financial personnel, administration, infection control, and other cost center supplies that do not fluctuate with volume.

There is a subtle difference between the nursing concept of fixed costs and the manufacturing concept. As a profit-focused entity, a business would not consider the cost center secretary a fixed cost (he or she can be laid off), and staff development is certainly not fixed and can be delayed or skipped entirely. Perhaps most important, the concept of minimum staffing is alien to a finance or accounting person from a manufacturing background. In a healthcare environment where most financial managers come from a business background, the need to understand the *business* concept of *costs* is increasingly important. If finance department personnel tell you what your fixed costs are, have them explain how they have defined these costs. Generally, the nurse manager or nurse executive will need to educate finance department personnel about minimum staffing. You should be prepared to explain the concept of minimum staffing and present examples of actual minimum staffing requirements for your unit(s).

Variable Costs

Variable costs are those that change depending on the level of volume. In a manufacturing environment it is a simple concept—the more surgical carts we make, the more costs we have. *All direct materials tend to be variable costs.* In manufacturing, *direct labor* may also be a variable cost because unneeded workers can be sent home (manufacturing has no concept of minimum staffing). Notice, also, that some elements of overhead are variable, including indirect materials, quantity of utilities used, and the amount of depreciation on buildings and equipment. In a healthcare environment, volume is a more complex concept. Volume includes not only the census numbers but also patient acuity, patient minutes/hours/days, and patient visits. Variable costs occur *in addition* to fixed costs to yield the organization's total cost:

$$\textit{Total costs} = \textit{Fixed costs} + \textit{Variable costs}$$

Staffing, beyond the minimum, is a variable cost based on the variable patient census. Other typical variable costs are forms used on a per-patient basis, medical and surgical supplies, and both linen and food costs. Although it is important to know these definitions, particularly when planning your budget, be aware that depending on the sophistication of your finance department's software, they may be unable to split out fixed and variable costs with a useful degree of accuracy.

Mixed Costs

Most costs are neither purely fixed nor purely variable. They are what we call *mixed costs*. Utilities are a good example. Even if an organization shuts down, it still needs a minimum level of electricity to light the yard and heat the building in the winter. That level of utilities is a fixed cost. If the organization is up and running, however, it needs more electricity to run the equipment, for lights, and for higher levels of heat or air conditioning. So, electricity is actually a mixed cost—part fixed and part variable. Staffing provides a similar example. There may be minimum levels of staffing (fixed cost), but as the census moves upward or the average patient acuity increases, the staffing level rises as well.

In general, we do not attempt to split most costs into their fixed and variable components. Rather, we tend to classify them as either fixed or variable and ignore the area of overlap. In a healthcare environment, you may be best served by considering minimum staffing as a fixed cost and other staffing as a variable cost. Remember that you may need to explain this unique aspect of healthcare costing to your finance department.

Exhibit 12–3 illustrates the relationship between fixed and variable costs over a *relevant range*.[10] The horizontal axis in Exhibit 12–3 represents activity level.

In our business, that could be the number of surgical carts made, whereas in a nursing unit it could be the number of patients or patient days. The vertical axis represents *total* cost. The horizontal line *above the axis* represents fixed costs, staying the same regardless of the level of activity. The slanting vertical line represents the variable costs, increasing as the volume increases. The dotted line shows that at a census of 20 patients, this unit would have an average annual cost of $X dollars. Notice that at shutdown, there would still be costs. Even with a volume of zero, the fixed costs remain.

Exhibit 12–3 not only illustrates the relationship between the different kinds of costs, but it is also a flexible budget. This one diagram (Exhibit 12–3) can provide budget numbers, including both fixed and variable costs, for census levels from 0 to 30 patients on a unit. Similar diagrams, or charts that move these numbers into columns for ease of use, can be prepared for many kinds of individual costs and for the overall costs of an organization. The important thing is to remember the names of the costs, the way they behave, and the manner in which they are put together.

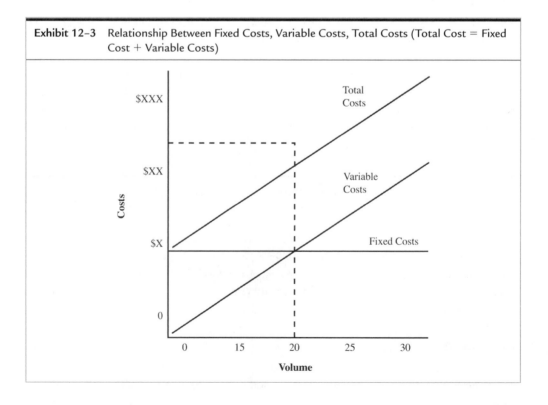

Exhibit 12–3 Relationship Between Fixed Costs, Variable Costs, Total Costs (Total Cost = Fixed Cost + Variable Costs)

Break-Even Analysis

To stay in operation, the *minimum* long-run goal of any organization must be to at least *break even*. When one breaks even, the costs of operations exactly equal the revenues. There is no profit and no loss. More revenues result in a profit, and fewer revenues (or more costs) result in a loss. When an entity operates below the break-even point, it must borrow or dip into savings from earlier periods when profits were made. Clearly, these are short-term solutions, and when they are exhausted the entity will be forced to close.

Breakeven can be shown graphically and calculated mathematically. Both the visual and the mathematical approaches are based on the definitions of costs. Remember that there are two kinds of costs: fixed costs and variable costs. By adding a revenue line to Exhibit 12–3, we create **Exhibit 12–4**, a graphical representation of breakeven. In Exhibit 12–4, the *fixed cost line* has been eliminated to simplify the diagram. It has been replaced with a shaded area. Notice again that the *variable* costs begin to rise from the base of fixed costs—costs that continue even when activity drops to zero. The new element in Exhibit 12–4 is the revenue line. The revenue line begins at zero—*no activity, no billing*. Thereafter, it climbs at a steady rate toward the upper right corner of the graph. The slope of the revenue line (the rate at which it climbs) is dependent on the rate of billing—bigger bills, steeper climb. Using the same measures on the horizontal and vertical axis as we used in Exhibit 12–3, our revenue slope would be based on the total revenue as it related to the average census or patient day. That is a crude measure, and there are many other measures that could be used. Nevertheless, at best, the break-even chart is a tool that will give you a rough idea of the activity level needed to remain solvent.

Remember, the more detailed your cost analysis is, the better this tool will work for you. A break-even analysis for a procedure will be more accurate than a break-even analysis for a unit or department. Similarly, a break-even analysis for a unit or department will be more accurate than a break-even analysis for an entire healthcare institution. Unfortunately, at some point, the break-even point for the organization as a whole becomes the issue in question.

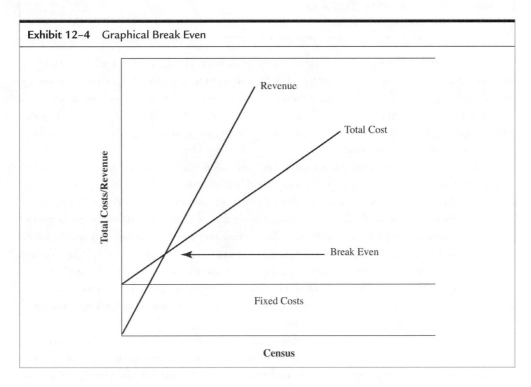

Exhibit 12–4   Graphical Break Even

Mathematically, break even is calculated using the formula that follows. It indicates that one breaks even when the revenues equal the expenses. Because both revenues and variable costs are a function of activity level, in this case patient days, *we must know both the average cost and the average revenues as we add patients to the census.* Given that, breakeven occurs when revenues per patient day equal fixed costs plus variable costs per patient day. The question we want to answer is this: *How many patients do we need in house, on average, to break even?* What is the break-even census?

> *Breakeven occurs when*
> *Revenues/Patient day × Census = Fixed costs + Variable costs/Patient day × Census*

Assume the following data:

Revenue per patient day	$ 2,000
Variable cost per patient day	$ 110
Fixed costs per year	$ 1,000,000

> *Revenues/Patient day × Census = Fixed costs + Variable costs/Patient day × Census*
> *$2,000 × Census = $1,000,000 + $110 × Census (2,000 − 110) × Census = $1,000,000*
> *Census = $1,000,000 ÷ 1,890*
> *Census = 529 per year*

You can verify your answer:

> *Revenues/Patient day × Census = Fixed costs + Variable costs/Patient day × Census*
> *$2,000 × 529 = $1,000,000 + $110 × 529*
> *$1,058,000 = $1,000,000 + $58,190*

Your answer may not be exact. First, these are estimated numbers. You cannot be certain that your fixed costs will be $1,000,000, or that your average daily patient revenue will be $2,000, or that your average daily variable cost will be $110. What the break-even analysis has given you is a rough estimate. If, as you move into the year, you find that your estimates of revenues or costs are badly off target, or you find that your average census is only 475, you can go back to the drawing board and change the underlying realities or face a very bleak financial situation.

Similarly, *if your variable revenues do not exceed your variable costs, you can never break even.* If, in this example, the revenues per patient day had been $2,000 but the variable costs per patient day had been $2,001, no amount of activity will result in a break-even situation. You will lose $1 per patient day, and the harder you work, the farther in a hole you will find yourself. This understanding of the fact that variable revenues must exceed variable costs leads to an alternative way to think about the break-even calculation. This is not a change in either the concept or the calculation. It is simply an approach that avoids the manipulation of an algebraic equation and is easier for some people to remember.

Start with your fixed costs. They exist *whether or not* there are patients in the beds. To cover your fixed costs, you must make more revenue on the patients than you have costs caused by the patients. This "extra" revenue can then be used to cover your fixed costs.

Next, think about the revenues and the variable costs. These elements change with activity. In essence, if there were no patient in the bed, neither the revenue nor the variable cost exists. So, a patient, in a bed, creates both a variable revenue and a variable cost. The term for the difference between these two is *contribution margin*. Contribution margin is the amount available to *contribute* toward covering fixed costs. When you have just enough contribution margin to cover fixed costs, you arrive at breakeven:

$$Break\ even = \frac{Fixed\ costs}{Revenues\ /\ patient\ day - variable\ costs\ /\ patient\ day \times census}$$

$$Break\ even = \frac{\$1,000,000}{\$2,000 - \$110}$$

$$Break\ even = \frac{\$1,000,000}{1,890} = 529\ patients\ per\ year$$

If one approach to calculating breakeven works, so will the other. Perhaps the most important concept of breakeven is the understanding that some costs and most revenues are a function of activity. Some costs, however (perhaps most costs in a typical small healthcare institution), are fixed and continue even after the shutdown point. When you consider actions that will improve profitability or reduce a loss situation, you must clearly identify which elements of cost and revenue you can best affect to improve profitability.

Alternate Ways to Organize the Budget

Thus far, we have been using a line-item budget. Line-item budgets are organized first by a cost center and then by the line items the cost center spends its money on. Line items include such items as salaries, supplies, telephone, linen, and copies.[11]

Another approach to organizing the budget is called a *program, performance, product-line, or community-benefit budget*. This budget is organized not around a department or unit but around a purpose. For example, a program budget might be organized around a product line in kidney care. The budget could include the transplant program, dialysis costs, outpatient care, and so forth. A program budget for cardiology might include cost center budgets for the operating room, recovery room, coronary intensive care, cardiac step-down, and cardiac rehabilitation services.

Although program budgets are conceptually appealing, they are not common. They are difficult to build, difficult to coordinate, and difficult to use as cost-control mechanisms. Perhaps the best way to get a picture of the overall cost of a program budget is to compile the program budget after the line-item budgets are complete. A program budget for cardiology might include 100% of the costs associated with coronary intensive care, cardiac step-down, and cardiac rehabilitation services, along with some percentage of the costs for the operating and recovery rooms.

Unfortunately, patients do not always fall cleanly within a product line. For example, when a cardiac patient requires kidney dialysis, it is unlikely the cost will be picked up. Remember that budgeting is always an estimate; you never have perfect data. When building a program budget, it is important not to miss the less obvious costs associated with such things as counseling cardiac patients and members of their families, training or ongoing education of staff, and recruitment and retention of staff.[12]

The purpose of a community-benefit budget is to identify specific costs allocated to meet social responsibilities in the community. These items include services for the poor and educational or outreach programs that enhance people's health in the community.

Capital Budgeting Versus Operational Budgeting

Budgets can be divided into two major divisions: the *operating budget* and the *capital budget*. Most nurse managers primarily work with the operating budget, which has been the focus of this chapter thus far. Operating budgets cover the day-to-day costs of a unit, including such things as wages for regular and temporary workers, medical and office supplies, equipment rental, repair and maintenance, travel and education, and dues and subscriptions. Like all budgets, operating budgets represent the "best guess" for costs over a coming period.

The *capital budget*, on the other hand, covers the purchase of land, buildings, and long-lived (at least 2 years) equipment.[13] The capital budget is developed separately from the operating budget and is often funded through separate sources such as capital campaigns, designated internal savings, and grants. Nurse managers are most often involved in capital budgeting when they request expensive, long-lived equipment for their units. In most organizations, financial rationale must support the request for an item from the capital budget. The following are the most obvious reasons for purchasing long-lived equipment:

1. A necessary item is broken and must be replaced.
2. A newer, better piece of equipment exists that will provide better patient service or equivalent patient service at a lower cost.
3. A new piece of equipment exists that will provide new patient services and help to generate new revenues.

The process of providing a rationale for capital spending is called *capital budgeting*. There are two fundamental differences in the way capital budgeting is approached in business (which may be your finance director's background) and in health care. First, from a *business* point of view, the underlying concept behind capital budgeting is that if the future revenues or the future cost savings from a new project or a new piece of equipment exceed the cost, this purchase will increase the overall profitability of the organization. From a *healthcare* point of view, on the other hand, most capital purchases are based on the requirements of quality patient care. Second, in *business,* if a project is deemed to be profitable, the funds to undertake that project will likely be borrowed if they are not available internally. In *health care*, on the other hand, funds are generally limited and capital projects will compete against each other for available capital funding.

An operating room nurse manager requesting a new autoclave or a new computer system is often faced with a set of forms from the finance department asking for a justification for the expenditure of capital funds. **Exhibit 12–5** through **Exhibit 12–7** are adaptations of the forms suggested by the AHA.

Sometimes when requesting capital funds it is necessary to give further explanation about why such funds are necessary. One possible format is given in Exhibit 12–6. Assuming that the department has more than one capital request, the set of requests will be summarized on a capital requests worksheet similar to the one shown in Exhibit 12–7.

The trick to completing these forms is to ask yourself why you need the new equipment. Focus first on patient care needs, and then on cost and/or revenue considerations. Remember to look at the big picture. Failure to fix equipment or failure to acquire new equipment that is faster, more accurate, and/or less invasive may result in patients choosing to go elsewhere for a wide range of associated services and thus a loss in revenue for the organization. If a piece of equipment is broken but the patient continues to come for patient services, there are often patient care issues (including possible negative patient outcomes), personnel costs associated with doing without that piece of equipment, and decreased revenues.

When you prepare your request, keep detailed copies of your notes and calculations *whether or not there is room for that amount of detail on the forms and whether or not it is requested.* Remember to

- Make your calculations explicit.
- Label everything.
- Show every intermediate calculation.
- Recopy when you are done and keep your notes where you can pull them up to justify your numbers.

Exhibit 12–5   Request for Capital Equipment or Services

1. Department _____   Date of request _____
2. Equipment or service requested _____
3. Name of primary requestor _____
4. Type of request:
   - ○ Required by regulation or accreditation   ○ Replacement of existing service
   - ○ Expansion of existing service   ○ Addition of new service
5. Department priority: Priority number _____ out of _____ requests.
   _____
6. Brief description of general specifications (including major components) and possible vendors.
   _____
7. Brief description of use and capability.
   _____
8. List by name and/or job classification the hospital staff who will operate the requested equipment.
   _____

TENTATIVE cost information:

Number of units _____   Personnel cost/year _____
Cost per unit _____   Lease or buy recommended _____
Total equipment cost _____   Estimated useful life _____
Installation cost _____   Supply cost/year _____
Transportation cost _____   Maintenance cost/year _____

9. Optional comments. Describe the present system used to accomplish the same or similar function, why the present system is not adequate, and what other departments and areas will be affected or will support the project. Additional sheets can be used when necessary.

_____   _____
Signature of person completing form   Date

Exhibit 12–6   Problem and Solution Statement

Requesting department _____   Date of request _____
Project title _____   Accountable manager _____
_____

PROBLEM STATEMENT

1. Description of the problem:

2. Which medical and hospital staff have helped define the problem?

SOLUTION STATEMENT

3. Briefly describe the proposed solution to the problem:

4. How will the proposed project resolve the problem?

5. What alternative solutions are available, and why were they rejected?

6. What are the standard uses associated with the project?

_____   _____
Signature of person completing form   Date

Exhibit 12-7   Capital Request Worksheet

Department Priority Number	Title of request and brief description	Requested month of purchase	Required by law or JCAHO*			Quantity	Unit Cost	Estimated Acquisition Cost	For Administrative Use	Referral to Medical Equipment Committee
			Check Appropriate Box						Check Information Needed for Review**	
			Replacement	Expansion	New					
									□ R □ P-S □ N □ I □ C □ E □ F	
									□ R □ P-S □ N □ I □ C □ E □ F	

* If JCAHO standard is the reason for acquisition, complete the Needs Assessment section.
** Letters stand for R = Request Form, P-S = Problem and Solution Statement, N = Need Assessment, I = Impact Assessment, C = Clinical Assessment, E = Equipment Assessment, F = Financial Assessment

Finally, remember to be *specific about your assumptions*. Your work as nurse manager will most likely be reviewed first by the nurse executive, who will set priorities over the full range of nursing services. If the nurse manager requests additional information or clarification, the quality of your notes will be critical in supporting your request.

Generally, you can round your costs and savings to the nearest dollar. Remember that these are estimates, and pennies are not generally accurate or helpful. Larger organizations may have you round everything to the nearest hundred dollars.

Budgeting Revenues

Throughout this chapter, we have focused on budgeting for cost control. Most nurse managers work with costs, not revenues. Nevertheless, when you budget revenues, or set your own prices, there are additional things that you should know.

Revenues Versus Cash Flows

First, it is important to understand the difference between revenues and cash flows. *Revenues* are charges made to patients or other clients. When these charges are made, the healthcare organization believes that it is has earned the payment and that it has a reasonable chance of receiving the money. Accounting (and finance) records a revenue when it is earned, *not* when the cash is received. When the revenue is earned, the accounting department bills the patient (or the insurance company) and records both the fact that the revenue is earned and the fact that the patient is obligated to pay. This step of recording the revenue is called *recognizing a revenue*.

An example may help to clarify the situation. Think of a department store at Christmas. December is a department store's biggest month of the year in terms of both sales (revenue) and expenses (various kinds of costs). *Yet very little money changes hands in December*. Most of the money associated with the Christmas season changes hands in January and February as people pay their charge account bills and the department store pays for the merchandise it purchased for the holidays. Accountants call this *accrual accounting*—revenues are recorded when a sale is made and the seller has done the work, not when the cash is received. Similarly, most expenses are recorded when the organization has an *obligation* to pay, not when the cash changes hands.

Money (cash) is different from revenue. In healthcare settings, money is received long after the revenue is recorded (recognized). Although some procedures involve direct payment from patients, money generally arrives when the insurance company or Medicare or Medicaid pays the bill. To complicate matters further, when accountants and finance people talk about receiving money, they often say that they *realized* a revenue. To *realize a revenue* is to receive the cash. This situation is not helped by the fact that even accountants and finance people occasionally get these terms backward! For this reason when someone talks to you about revenues, it is often useful to clarify exactly what they mean.

If a healthcare organization has a very low population of indigent patients, the difference between revenues and cash flows may be very small. Even in this case, however, the *timing difference* between when services are given and revenues are earned (recognized) and the payment date when revenues are received in cash (realized) may cause difficulties for the organization.

Nurses play a vital role in moving revenues from recognized to realized by charting. Every third-party payer relies on the accuracy and detail of the patient's chart to validate payment. Until the charts are "clean," payment will be withheld. Poor paperwork can be a bottleneck that chokes off cash flow to the entire organization.

When a nurse manager enters any healthcare environment for the first time, whether that environment is a hospital, home health care, long-term care, ambulatory center, or other, it is important to learn how patient billing works and to develop an understanding of the time lag between submitting patient charges and receiving private insurance or government reimbursement (Dunham-Taylor & Pinczuk, 2006).

Predicting (Budgeting) Revenues

Operating at a profit requires both revenues and costs to be carefully controlled. We attempt to control costs through careful budgeting. We attempt to manage revenues through careful price setting and by packaging a set of services that patients want to buy and insurance companies will pay for. Revenues are predicted in the same manner as expenses. First, you examine each major revenue source for the past 2 to 5 years and project the historical trend forward to next year. Next, carefully examine each revenue to decide whether it will behave differently next year than it did in the past. Finally, add any new "revenue streams" coming on line from new goods and services.

Pricing to Cover Your Costs

Pricing is done in several aspects. Beds and physical therapy services, for example, are priced on a per patient per day or per patient per hour basis. On the other hand, procedures such as surgeries and laboratory tests are priced on a per event basis. Last, goods such as pharmaceutical supplies and prostheses are priced on a per unit basis. Regardless of the good or service we are pricing, in the long run prices must cover all costs—direct labor, direct materials, and overhead. Thus, to set long-run prices, you must have a good idea of what your costs are. Prices are not based solely on costs, but *on average, costs will define the lower bound of pricing.*

For each individually priced good or service, you must try to identify the cost of all the direct materials, direct labor, and overhead associated with providing that good or service and add them together to arrive at the cost—the *lower bound* of the price for that item. Some of these costs are reasonably easy to estimate. Others require enormous estimations. For the examples that follow, let's assume we have a good estimate of our average census for the coming year. We are estimating an average census of 500 patients per day, or 182,500 patient days during the year:

$$500 \text{ patients per day} \times 365 \text{ days per year} = 182,500 \text{ patients per year}$$

Direct Materials and Direct Labor

Careful cost budgeting can provide you with reasonably accurate cost figures for direct materials and direct labor. Direct nursing labor is generally applied, or added to the cost of a patient day, based on average census figures or patient classification system data. If we use only the patient census as an example to arrive at a cost per day per patient for direct care nursing services, we would estimate our total direct care nursing salaries, wages, and benefits for the year and then divide by 182,500 to arrive at a direct labor cost per day. Assume that the labor cost for direct nursing on one unit is $175,000 per year. The nursing cost to be added to each patient's daily bill is then $0.96.[14]

$$\frac{\$175,000 \text{ labor cost}}{182,500 \text{ patient days}} = \$0.96 \text{ labor cost per patient day}$$

Developing the estimated cost for direct nursing services is a complex problem that involves concepts of minimum staffing, staff mix (i.e., registered nurses vs. licensed practical nurses vs. nurse aides and full time vs. part time), and other elements such as shift differential.

Direct materials are easier to budget—the pacemaker is billed to the patient who receives it. Again, the cost of the pacemaker (or the bedside wash kit or the prosthesis) is the minimum charge for that item.

Overhead

Overhead is far more difficult to evaluate and is the reason that pricing is an art, not a science. Let's start with the easiest parts of overhead—indirect labor and indirect materials. Let's assume your *total* costs are calculated as *annual* costs, so you have an idea of the total cost for these items for the year. They can be calculated with some degree of accuracy for indirect labor, and indirect materials can be based on last year's costs. However, even if we knew total costs with absolute accuracy (which we rarely do), we still need to know how to *allocate those costs to billable elements of patient care.*

For example, if you know that a group of supervisory salaries cost $150,000 a year, how do you allocate that cost to patient billings to ensure that the cost is recovered? The unfortunate answer is that you can never be absolutely sure. You can, however, make a very good guess. For example, to spread the supervisory cost we might use our best estimate of patient days. Because we are estimating an average census of 500 patients per day during a 365-day year, we would spread our $150,000 salary cost over 182,500 patient days. Accordingly, we will *attach* $0.83 for this class of supervisory salaries to each patient's daily bill for room and board.

> Step 1: 500 patients per day × 365 days per year = 182,500 patient days per year
> Step 2: $150,000 in supervisory costs ÷ 182,500 patient days = $0.8222 per patient day. Let's round to $0.83 per patient day.

If we are exactly correct in our census estimate, we *distribute* or *allocate* $151,475, and we will recover this cost from our patients and their insurance companies.

$$182,500 \text{ patient days} \times \$0.83 \text{ per patient day} = \$151,475$$

If our census falls short, we will have *underapplied* this class of overhead. For example, if our census only averages 490, we will apply only $148,446. If we actually spent the $150,000 we anticipated, we have failed to recover $1,554 in supervisory salaries from our patients.

> Step 1: 490 patients per day × 365 days per year = 178,850 patient days per year
> Step 2: 178,850 patients days × $0.83 per patient = $152,990 recovered from patient billings

Alternatively, if our census is larger than anticipated—for example, 505 patients per day—we will have *overapplied* our supervisory salaries by $2,990. In other words, we will have realized an additional $2,990 more than anticipated.

When doing this type of budgeting, vary your assumptions and see what happens. Called *sensitivity analysis*, this exercise allows you to check the outcome if your assumptions are wrong (and they always are). In this example, for instance, will you recover the entire $150,000 if your census is 497 instead of 500? How about 495? By testing several alternatives, you can pick a minimum price that provides a reasonable degree of comfort in terms of recovering your costs.

Indirect labor is, perhaps, the easiest example we can provide, although other indirect costs such as linen costs, utilities, and patient meals can be budgeted in a similar manner. Notice that although linens and meals are direct costs in the sense that they directly touch each patient's time in the hospital, they are treated as indirect costs because it is not efficient to allocate them on a per patient basis. Linens and meals are like the paint on our surgical carts. Although not truly overhead (like the utilities and supervisory salaries), they are more easily and cost-effectively handled as indirect materials.

For such items as surgical supplies, we move beyond a per patient allocation and try to associate each kind of supply with the type of procedure that uses that item. We estimate the number of procedures, the quantity of supplies, the total supply costs, and then divide to arrive at a cost per procedure.

Allocating Long-Lived Assets

The hardest item to allocate is the "using up" of buildings and equipment. Land, buildings, and equipment are most commonly called *fixed assets, fixed tangible assets,* or *plant, property, and equipment.* These are long-lived assets (more than 2 years), and their cost is spread over the asset's useful life. The name of this cost is *depreciation* or *amortization.*[15]

In some cases, it might be possible to allocate the cost of a machine directly to patient care. For example, if you knew that a piece of surgical equipment would last through 200 surgical procedures and then be scrapped as no longer reliable, you could divide the cost of the equipment by 200 and *apply* the result to the cost of each surgical procedure. If we can do this, this element of depreciation is treated as a direct cost (one that can be directly associated with a specific element of patient care). Unfortunately, it is rare that equipment can be treated in this manner, and it is virtually impossible to do it with a building. Here we need to make some very *big assumptions.*

Assume we build a $20 million building. We need to recover that cost by charging patients for the building. The question becomes how much to charge per patient per day. If we are lucky, we financed part of the building with grants or a capital giving campaign. Nevertheless, when the building is "used up," we will have to replace it and we cannot be certain that grants and donations will be available when the time comes to do that. Prudence dictates that we try to add the full $20 million cost of the building to patient charges over the building's useful life.

First, we need to estimate the useful life of the building. Assume it is 40 years.[16] Then, we need to estimate the volume of activity that will go through that building each year for the next 40 years. Let's stay with our estimate of 500 patients per day. Remember, that was 182,500 patient days per year. In 40 years, that is 7.3 million patient days. That is $2.74 per patient per day to recover the cost of the building over its 40-year life.

> Step 1: 500 patients per day × 365 days per year = 182,500 patient days per year
> Step 2: 182,500 patient days per year × 40 years = 7,300,000 patient days over 40 years
> Step 3: $20,000,000 building ÷ 7,300,000 patient days = $2.74 per patient day

Equipment is handled in the same way, but because its life is shorter than a building's, our estimate of useful life is better. Remember, however, that in a high-tech environment like a hospital most depreciation is not caused by physical deterioration but by obsolescence. Our equipment might last 5 years, but if someone comes out with a new piece of equipment that performs the procedure with far less stress to the patient, we'll probably want to replace that equipment long before its 5-year life expires.

Land is not depreciated because it lasts "forever." It is placed on the list of assets and there it remains until you sell it.

What Did We Forget?

Doubtless, you have noticed that we have only scratched the surface. Even when we talk about spreading the cost of buildings and equipment, we are ignoring such items as repairs and maintenance. Hopefully, you never find yourself at the "top of the budgeting food chain" until you have had years of experience in health care—years to learn the ropes, budget a unit, budget a clinic, budget overall nursing services—and before you are the person responsible for budgeting an entire entity and possibly setting its prices. But, in the meantime, you may have input into price setting, and some of the same ideas that matter in setting prices help you understand the ways in which costs behave.

Notes

1. *Interface* can have many different meanings. At a minimum, it implies the sharing of data. It can also mean that when one system is changed, all related systems are also updated.

2. One such tool is ratio analysis, which compares one financial or performance element to another (for example, nursing cost per patient day or in-service training cost per dollar of registered nurse salaries). Another is a management technique called benchmarking, where entities can compare their costs for an activity to the same costs for other, similar units.

3. In some organizations, the fiscal year is divided into 13 months to reflect equal time periods, each 4 weeks in duration. This has some advantages over a 12-month fiscal year where the number of days per month varies. With 13 identical 28-day "months," it is easier for a nurse manager to compare staffing costs in February (when the census was up) with July (when the census was down). The combination of fiscal and calendar years can be confusing. Often in health care, different calendar and fiscal years are used. Usually, the budget period coincides with other financial reporting devices such as managerial reports, balance sheets, and profit-and-loss statements. It is not uncommon, however, to have federal government grants where the fiscal year (and thus the year for grant application, funding reports, and spending deadlines) corresponds with the federal government's fiscal year of October 1 through September 30.

4. Even when it is policy to allow a rollover of unspent funds, it is common for these funds to be "swept up" by the administration in years when financial results are poor.

5. A fixed budget can be compared with planning the cost of a wedding while ignoring the number of invited guests. Of course, a fixed budget is appropriate for some things. The bride's bouquet, for example, costs the same amount whether the wedding has 50 or 500 guests. Similarly, in a nursing unit with a nurse manager, the nurse manager's salary is the same whether the census is 50% or 100%. Most costs, however, vary with volume.

6. A flexible budget is sometimes called a variable budget, but this term is not generally used by finance and accounting people. Accordingly, we suggest that the term *flexible budget* be used to describe a budget where costs vary according to volume (level of activity) or acuity.

7. Shortfalls can be caused by changes in the census, problems with insurance reimbursement, lower-than-anticipated receipts from Medicaid and/or Medicare, or budget shifting, where one unit loses funds to compensate for overspending in others.

8. Historically, because health care enjoyed "cost-plus" billing, health care was far more willing to treat small costs as direct costs. If a cost could be identified with a patient or procedure, the hospital could bill the insurance company and receive reimbursement. Health care treated everything from aspirin to surgical trays as direct costs. With diagnosis-related groups and capitation, the rationale for that type of detailed record-keeping has changed.

9. It is important to note that the definition of a cost as fixed or variable would change if, for example, a cost center or an entire institution were closed!

10. All financial figures, including cost estimates, rely on the concept of relevant range: the range of activity over which your estimates (particularly estimates of fixed costs) remain reasonable. If, in our manufacturing example, we needed to go to a second or third shift, almost all our fixed cost estimates (particularly indirect labor) change. In a healthcare environment, there is a census or acuity level at which the underlying assumptions of the budget process change. One needs to watch for that point to avoid outcomes that are very different from what was planned.

11. The term *appropriations budget* is used by all governmental agencies, including governmental healthcare entities such as Veterans Administration hospitals. The "appropriation" (short-hand for an "appropriations budget") has been passed by a governmental, legislative body and represents a legal permission to spend money on specified items. Appropriations budgets are unique in that they are often very detailed in terms of line items. In a private healthcare institution, the ability to switch money from one line item to another line item (e.g., from full-time salaries to part-time salaries) lies within the organization. With an appropriations budget, on the other hand, the organization may have to petition the legislative body to move money from one budget category to another. The second major difference in governmental budgets is that they almost always recapture unspent funds at the end of each budget period.

12. Another term often heard is *zero-based budgeting*. With zero-based budgeting, the manager theoretically begins the budget cycle not with last year's budget but with a blank piece of paper. Every cost is then created and justified, building the new budget from scratch. Although some variations of zero-based budgeting are used for small units and projects, zero-based budgeting is simply too time consuming and costly to be used routinely. Where you do find true zero-based budgeting is during the creation of totally new programs and services. A hybrid of zero-based budgeting and program budgeting exists when programs are regularly reevaluated to determine whether or not they should continue. This type

of analysis, called a sunset review, is a practical addition to the line-item budget and its tendency is to always assume that last year's programs will simply continue with a slight increase in cost.

13. Because heavy record-keeping costs are associated with equipment, most organizations set a lower limit on the dollar amount of purchases to be called, and accounted for, as "equipment." This threshold amount may be $500 or $5,000. The larger the organization, the higher the threshold is likely to be. When long-lived equipment with a cost below this threshold is purchased, it is treated as "minor equipment supplies" and expensed. Businesses handle low-value equipment in much the same way, generally using the term *small tools*. Thus, surgical scissors, which may last 5 years but cost only $250, will probably be included as minor equipment supplies in the operating budget.

14. With the increased incidence in 23-hour observation patients, we may want an hourly cost. To figure the hourly cost, divide the daily figure by the 24 hours in each day to also get a usable figure for direct nursing cost per hour.

15. Technically, this cost should be called *depreciation* when an asset is owned and *amortization* when the asset is leased. In practice, however, both words may be used interchangeably.

16. There are published lists of estimates for the useful lives of long-lived assets, such as from the AHA and the American Institute of Certified Public Accountants. Ultimately, the best estimates depend on years of experience in a single environment (e.g., health care).

Discussion Questions

1. What challenge do nurse managers face when dealing with financial data that will help them to make sound decisions and defend that decision with others in the organization?
2. What difficulties exist for nurse managers who must accumulate data from different computer systems?
3. Because the nursing department costs are a large part of the overall budget, what information (documented facts) should the nurse manager be able to retrieve quickly and effectively to respond when the budget is scrutinized by administration?
4. Why is it important for the nurse manager to provide a reasonable and fair operation budget?
5. What challenge does the nurse manager face when interacting with nonhealthcare personnel who have only a business background?
6. Why do hospitals have a strategic plan, and why is it important that the nurse manager understands this plan and the goals for the healthcare organization?
7. Although budget figures are generally annual estimates divided by 12 (or 13), costs will not flow evenly through the year. Why and how should nurse managers be prepared to explain short-term variations?
8. How should a nurse manager prepare to handle minimum staffing requirement costs in the budget process in case this is challenged?
9. Besides a department budget approach, what other alternatives are available in a budgeting process?

Glossary of Terms

Breakeven—when one breaks even, the costs of operations exactly equal the revenues. There is no profit and no loss.

Budget Variance—the difference between the projected budget and the actual budget.

Capital Budget—covers the purchase of land, buildings, and long-lived (at least 2 years) equipment.

Cost Center—does not bill patients directly; instead, support the profit centers.

Depreciation or Amortization—the hardest item to allocate is the "using up" of buildings and equipment. Land, buildings, and equipment are most commonly called *fixed assets, fixed tangible assets*, or *plant, property, and equipment*. These are long-lived assets (more than 2 years), and their cost is spread over the asset's useful life. The name of this cost is depreciation or amortization.

Direct Labor—the labor that actually turns direct materials into a finished product.

Direct Materials—materials large enough to be identified with a specific product.

Fixed Budget—predicts a certain level of costs, ignoring the level of activity that occurs.

Fixed Costs—costs that stay the same regardless of the level of activity.

Flexible Budget—different levels of cost based on levels of activity.

Indirect Labor—those persons who do not actually turn direct materials into a finished product. Indirect labor is part of overhead.

Indirect Materials—materials that cannot be associated with a specific product in a cost-effective manner. Indirect materials are part of overhead.

Line-Item Budget—simply takes last year's plans, adjusts for obvious errors in the estimate, adds a little for inflation, and continues on.

Mixed Costs—most costs are neither purely fixed nor purely variable. They are what we call *mixed costs*. Utilities are a good example.

Operating Budgets—cover the day-to-day costs of a unit, including such things as wages for regular and temporary workers, medical and office supplies, equipment rental, repair and maintenance, travel and education, and dues and subscriptions. Like all budgets, operating budgets represent the "best guess" for costs over a coming period.

Overhead—composed of indirect materials, indirect labor, and the "costs to get ready to manufacture," such as the building, insurance, electricity, and equipment.

Profit Center—bills patients directly.

Program, Performance, Product-Line, or Community-Benefit Budget—a budget not organized around a department or unit but around a purpose. For example, a program budget might be organized around a product line in kidney care. The purpose of a *community-benefit budget* is to identify specific costs allocated to meet social responsibilities in the community.

Realize a Revenue—to realize a revenue is to receive the cash payment from the client.

Recognizing a Revenue—when charges are made to patients, the healthcare organization believes that it has earned the payment and that it has a reasonable chance of receiving the money. Accounting (and finance) records a revenue when it is earned, *not* when the cash is received. When the revenue is earned, the accounting department bills the patient (or the insurance company) and records both the fact that the revenue is earned and the fact that the patient is obligated to pay.

Revenues—charges made to patients or other clients.

Variable Costs—those costs that change depending on the level of volume.

Reference

Dunham-Taylor, J., & Pinczuk, J. (2006). *Health care financial management for nurse managers: Applications from hospitals, long-term care, home care, and ambulatory care.* Sudbury, MA: Jones and Bartlett.

Budget Development and Evaluation

Janne Dunham-Taylor, PhD, RN, and Joseph Z. Pinczuk, MHA

OBJECTIVES

- Show how to both evaluate and develop a nursing expense budget.
- Illustrate how to develop a budget, including figuring nonproductive time, to insure that enough staff is provided.
- Examine what role the nurse manager should take when creating a standard definition of nursing workload needs with the finance department.

Introduction

Budget responsibilities usually include an evaluation of the adequacy of the budget and, at times, the development of a new budget. Budget evaluation is an important activity because a cost center budget may not have been *totally* evaluated for years. A piecemeal evaluation to add raises or cut the budget may have occurred but is not sufficient in the overall budget evaluation process. What has been appropriate for the last 10 years is not necessarily what is needed presently. This chapter is designed to help the nurse administrator determine whether the overall budget is appropriate and adequate to meet present patient needs.

Budget evaluation needs to occur on both a monthly and a yearly basis. The *monthly evaluation* is concerned with looking at the past month's (or, better yet, the present month's, if available) expenditures to determine whether budget variances are appropriate.

The *annual evaluation* is more in-depth and provides the nurse manager and nurse executive with data that either demonstrate the budget is appropriate and does not need to be changed or that the budget should be specifically altered to better meet current program needs. This in-depth evaluation process is also appropriate when there is sufficient patient population or volume changes to warrant a budget reevaluation and possible midyear budget adjustments. In this longer process, question everything:

- Are budget line items appropriate amounts for the patient population being served? Go through line by line and evaluate each category.
- Are we spending less than the reimbursement amount to provide the specified services? Have we lost any reimbursement because of nursing care issues? What will need to be changed to meet the changing reimbursement requirements?
- Are there more efficient ways—staffing, facilities, other resources—to better meet patient needs? For instance, if everyone is working straight 8-hour or 12-hour shifts, chances are the staffing is too heavy for certain times and may be too lean for other times. Or with facilities, would a better physical setup help save staff time? With resources, is there a computerized documentation system in place that helps save staff, especially registered nurse (RN), time?
- Is the staffing plan effective?
- Can staff productivity be improved?
- Is the staff mix appropriate for the patient population served?
- How could the leadership be improved? (If there are leadership problems, these need to be fixed because they cost a lot of money.)
- Are there unresolved organizational systems process issues that are costing money unnecessarily for the organization? Are there organizational systems that could be streamlined?
- Are there new safety measures, regulatory guidelines, or accreditation standards that affect the budget?
- Does the new budget reflect cost inflation or anticipated raises?
- Are there new innovations or quality improvement strategies that have budget implications?
- What would increase patient—and patient family—satisfaction? Would these measures affect the budget?
- What would improve staff satisfaction and turnover?
- How will Medicare and Medicaid reimbursements, or other reimbursement discounts, affect the budget?

Start a dialogue about these questions with all nursing staff, physicians, other disciplines, and patients and their families. You can obtain invaluable input and find other approaches that better serve patient needs. Include the nurse executive in this process. The nurse manager must always have an accurate picture of the entire organization, understanding how unit issues fit with this larger picture. Many issues need broader organizational involvement. In fact, some issues necessitate the executive team or board action—the nurse executive will be more involved at this level. However, many issues, both on the unit and interdepartmentally, can be fixed by the nurse manager or by the nurse manager working with other department directors.

We would be remiss here not to emphasize the importance of nurse executive expectations of the nurse manager. These expectations are critical to overall organizational success. In the budget evaluation process, the nurse executive should expect monthly variance reports and annual evaluations of each cost center budget from the nurse manager. The reports should include recommendations and rationales for any budget changes needed for each cost center.

The budget calculations presented in this chapter have additional uses. These data provide objective evidence to determine and compare staff workloads, to measure outcomes, and to provide quality or research data. In addition, these data could be compared with benchmark data from other organizations.

Budget Terminology

Full-Time Equivalent

Before evaluating a budget, it is necessary to introduce some additional budget terms that were not introduced earlier. First, the term *full-time equivalent* (*FTE*) is used in all healthcare organizations. A nurse manager is responsible for a specified number of FTEs. An FTE is a unit of measurement that represents one person who works a full-time position. In other words, a person working 40 hours a week works 2,080 hours a year.[1]

> *1 FTE = 40 hours a week × 52 weeks a year = 2,080 hours a year*

However, more than one person can fill one FTE. Part-time employees work less than one FTE. To figure out hours worked, let's consider that an employee works 0.8 FTE. How many hours per week does this person work? Using the following equation, we can calculate that this employee works 32 hours per week. See **Exhibit 13–1** for a listing of different FTE hours.

> *0.8 FTE × 40 hours per week = 32 hours per week*

Exhibit 13–1   FTE Hours

FTEs	Hours per Week*	Hours per Year*
.1	4	208
.2	8	416
.3	12	624
.4	16	832
.5	20	1,040
.6	24	1,248
.7	28	1,456
.8	32	1,664
.9	36	1,872
1.0	40	2,080

*Based on an 8-hour day—this would need to be changed for a 7.5-hour day.

A nurse manager responsible for 50 FTEs most likely has 70 to 80 persons reporting directly to him or her. This includes both full-time and part-time staff. An industry standard is that *a nurse manager is most effective if responsible for fewer than 50 FTEs.* When responsible for more than 50 FTEs, there are too many people on direct report, and the nurse manager will not be as effective. More legal and patient safety issues begin to occur when a nurse manager is responsible for too many FTEs.

Unit of Service

Unit of service is used by healthcare organizations to measure specific services a patient uses within a specific time frame (i.e., patient minutes, hours, days, visits, births, treatments, operations, or other patient encounters). *Patient days* are the number of inpatients present at midnight. One patient day is given for each day the patient is present on an inpatient unit. Sometimes terms are used such as *average daily census*. Average daily census may also be the average number of emergency department/home visits or outpatient treatments for a month or a year.

The patient day is used to determine the *length of stay* (*LOS*) or the average length of stay (ALOS). This averages individual patients' lengths of stay within a cost center or facility for a month or a year. Patient days are also used to determine the *occupancy rate*. If a long-term care unit has 50 beds and 40 are filled, a percentage is determined for the number of beds actually filled. So, the long-term care unit would have an occupancy rate of 80% (40 filled beds ÷ 50 bed capacity = 0.8, or 80%).

Nursing Workload

Using the various units of service specified here causes a problem in that all patients do not require the same amount of nursing care. For instance, one treatment could take a half hour, whereas another could take 2 hours. Or one patient requires intensive care, whereas another needs only the step-down unit. Or a home care nurse could drive 30 miles to make a visit, whereas other visits require only a 5-mile drive. Therefore, further unit-of-service specification is needed to accurately reflect *nursing workload*, or the volume of work performed by nurse caregivers.

One way to better specify units of service for **nursing workload** is to use *nursing hours per patient day* (*NHPPD*) or *hours per patient day* (*HPPD*). NHPPD gives the number of nurse staff hours needed to provide care to an inpatient in 24 hours. NHPPD and HPPD are produced by patient classification systems.[2] NHPPD and HPPD most often have the same meaning; however, at times the definition is different.[3] For instance, if a healthcare organization uses a patient classification system to measure NHPPD, finance may use HPPD using only patient census data. In this case, the two terms are different and have different measurement. As discussed previously, this is an example where it is important to find out the definition/measurement of either the term NHPPD or HPPD. Because there is not a standardized definition for either term, be sure to clarify definitions.

Another similar term is the *relative value unit* (*RVU*), used by reimbursement systems. On an inpatient unit, the RVU represents the complexity of a procedure.

The NHPPD, when used as a patient acuity factor in a patient classification system, is produced from descriptors about a patient. In this process, the nurse supplies the descriptors about the patient, the descriptors are entered or scanned into the computer, and the patient classification system assigns weights for each descriptor. Then, the weight total is given. This weight total places the patient into one of several levels of nursing care needed on a 24-hour basis. Once the level of care is determined, the patient classification system can supply actual nursing care hours (NHPPD) needed that day.

All levels of direct nursing care staff—RNs, licensed practical nurses (LPNs)/licensed vocational nurses, and nursing unlicensed personnel such as technicians, assistants, aides—are included in the NHPPD. There is no standard for which specific nursing personnel are included in the NHPPD figure.[4] For example, the direct care nursing staff might include RNs and nursing assistants on one unit and have RNs, LPNs, and nursing assistants on another unit. In some hospitals, the nurse manager is included. In other organizations, the nurse manager is not included or is included only if giving direct care.

Several issues need to be considered when using acuity data. First, the NHPPD is *not* standardized between patient classification systems. Thus, there are differences in the hours of care for the same type of patient when using different patient classification systems (Shullanberger, 2000):

> Cockerill et al.'s (1993) comparison study of four widely used nursing workload measurement tools (including GRASP) demonstrated that with different workload measurement tools there were significant clinical and statistical differences in estimated hours of (nursing) care. Discrepancies of up to 30% were noted in the costs associated with caring for exactly the same patients. (p. 132)

Second, even within the *same* patient classification system, the NHPPD *measurements* are not always standardized. In the factor evaluation classification systems, the nurse executive can choose the base hours of care given. At one hospital it might be 5.5 NHPPD, whereas at another the nurse executive might choose 6.0 NHPPD. Most likely this number will be higher for a tertiary care hospital or medical center and lower for a smaller, less acute general hospital that sends the more acute patients to the tertiary center. The classification system then uses this base number to compute the hours of care needed for most nursing care areas within that hospital. The acuity number is higher for a critical care area and lower for a rehabilitation floor—all determined by the patient classification database.

Third, it is very important that *reliability* (would two nurses rate the same patient in the same way?) and *validity* (does the tool actually measure the appropriate activities that nurses are doing?) have been regularly evaluated for the patient classification system. The first thing to examine is whether the patient classification system has actual reliability and validity established. Some internal patient classification systems do not have reliability and validity established at all—and they may not take into account significant nursing staff time spent on such things as admissions, discharges, and transfers. They also may not include such functions as an IV team.

The second issue with reliability and validity occurs *within* the healthcare organization. Reliability needs to be evaluated regularly by having a nurse from a different unit rate the patient already rated by unit staff. Evaluation of validity is also necessary annually. For example, the classification system may say that nursing hours for orthopedic patients are 6.0 NHPPD. If the unit is long and narrow with supplies at one end of the unit and charts in another area not as accessible for certain patient rooms, nursing staff may need slightly more than 6.0 hours to complete the care for certain orthopedic patients. Perhaps the system does not take into account that psychiatric nurses spend a lot of time teaching families as part of the RN role. In this case, these nurses might be spending more hours of care with their assigned patients than the patient classification system reflects.

Fourth, *acuity data*, if available, should be used *instead of census figures* because census figures do not account for the acuity of the patient. If acuity data are not available, one could benchmark with like units.

There is another reason the NHPPD would more closely reflect actual nursing care hours than census data. Census data are gathered at *midnight*. Patients admitted and discharged within the same day may not be reflected by the midnight census at all. The patient classification system generally collects data around 11 AM and may be done on a per-shift basis. It is more likely to pick up short-stay patients as well as admissions, discharges, and transfers.

On the census issue, the American Nurses Association (2008) supports not using census data:

> [O]ne size (or formula) does not fit all. In fact, staffing is most appropriate and meaningful when it is predicated on a measure of unit intensity that takes into consideration the aggregate population of patients and the associated roles and responsibilities of nursing staff. Such a unit of measure must be operationalized to take into consideration the totality of the patients for whom care is being provided. It must not be predicated on a simple quantification of the needs of the "average" patients but must also include the "outliers." (p. 5)

Overhead

You may see a column named "overhead" on your budget sheets. Overhead items are indirect costs. *Overhead* includes benefits such as health insurance and Social Security, depreciation on buildings or equipment, and nonproductive time (although sometimes this is mixed in with the labor budget figures). Overhead usually includes departments not giving direct care such as administration, housekeeping, maintenance, finance, medical records, and human resources. Overhead can be computed in several ways: Administration costs may be divided by the census and billed to each inpatient unit in a hospital, housekeeping and utility costs can be computed by square footage, and linen computed by the pounds of linen used. Finance traditionally will use the same step-down allocation for overhead as filed with the Medicare and Medicaid cost reports.

In most cases, overhead figures on the budget sheet are neither determined nor much affected by a nurse manager's efforts to save costs. Occasionally, such as with pounds of linen, the nurse manager could encourage staff to use linen more expeditiously and thus save on this cost. The overhead figures generally are the responsibility of the executive team and determined by the finance department. However, the nurse manager should know how the overhead is determined, especially when the nurse manager is checking the budget for accuracy or building a budget from scratch.

Product Lines

Healthcare organizations may use a term, *product line* or *service line*, that represents total services for a particular group of patients or similar patient diagnoses. For example, typical product lines may be cardiology, oncology, burns, or women's health. The product line can represent operating room, inpatient, ambulatory, long-term care, and home care services for that product line and sometimes can serve as a "profit center" within the accounting system. Usually, when using product lines, there are administrators—including nursing—assigned to each line.

Patients often need treatment in more than one product line. This causes problems, for example, when a patient is admitted into the orthopedic product line for knee surgery but also has diabetes, emphysema, and cardiac arrhythmia. So, treatment includes aspects not actually defined, nor costed out, by the product line.

Loss Leaders

There may be services that a healthcare organization considers a *loss leader*. These services do not make money—in fact, they lose money—but benefit the organization by bringing patients to the organization for services or gain potential patients because patients see that hospital personnel are friendly, helpful people. Loss leaders can include such services as the emergency department and women's health programs.

Another unit that often loses money but remains in general-service hospitals is the pediatric unit. This establishes the full-service designation for the hospital even though the department loses money. It also can help the community if there are no other pediatric inpatient units in the community. Minimum staffing is the issue here—there are so few patients that *minimum staffing* (needing two staff members on at all times) actually *overstaffs* the unit. To deal with this issue some hospitals have adopted strategies where additional patients are diverted to this unit (i.e., short-stay patients, ill children of employees, day care patients), or hospitals even station pediatric outpatient services there.

Vertical Integration

In *vertical integration*, a hospital might want to add long-term care beds or home care services to increase profits but have additional options to save costs. For instance, it is cheaper to quickly move a postoperative patient into a skilled nursing facility unit—a less expensive option than holding the patient on an inpatient unit for an additional day or days. Or the hospital might start a health maintenance organization or preferred provider organization. It could even buy a medical supply company. All these additions are related services that expand the service options of the hospital.

Annual Evaluation of the Cost Center Budget: Building a Nursing Expense Budget

Now we will evaluate a nursing expense budget. As we go through this process, we introduce additional budget terminology. Most often, the nurse manager is given an established cost center budget. Yet changes continue to occur (e.g., the patient population changes, the acuity rises, a different staff mix is needed, the location or environment changes, or new reimbursement regulations occur). How does a nurse manager evaluate whether this historical budget accurately reflects current needs?

One way the nurse manager can determine whether the budget is adequate is to build a unit budget from scratch. This provides objective data that can then be used for the evaluation process. Too often, a nurse manager tells the nurse executive, or finance personnel, that budget changes need to be made "for quality reasons" or "the patients are more acute" or "to meet accreditation standards." It is certainly important to meet accreditation or quality standards. And the acuity may have actually increased. However, the nurse manager is more effective when he or she backs up this statement with objective data, when the objective data are available. Building a budget from scratch provides objective data that then can be compared with the actual budget.

The nurse manager and nurse executive may need to either propose different budget amounts that more accurately reflect the services rendered or, within the same budget amount, reallocate how the money is used to better provide the needed services. When a change can be documented with objective evidence, it usually has the best chance of being supported by the nursing executive, the finance executive, and the executive team.

A hospital example is given here. However, examples in long-term care, home care, and ambulatory care can be found in Dunham-Taylor and Pinczuk (2006). Using the hospital example in this chapter, each step is defined in detail in the following sections, with the total process reflected in **Exhibit 13–2**.

Exhibit 13–2   Building a Budget from Scratch by Calculating Direct Care FTEs

Step 1:   Average NHPPD × Patient Census/Year or # of Visits/Year = Average NHPPD/Year.
Step 2:   Average NHPPD/Year ÷ 2,080 Hours = Total Nursing Direct Care FTEs.
Step 3:   Figure nonproductive hours per FTE or get this figure from Human Resources.
Step 4:   2,080 Hours ÷ ____ Nonproductive Hours per FTE = ____ Productive Hours per FTE.

(continues)

Exhibit 13–2   Building a Budget from Scratch by Calculating Direct Care FTEs (*continued*)

Step 5:   2,080 Hours ÷ _____ Productive Hours per FTE = _____ Actual FTEs.
(This step figures how many actual FTEs are needed to cover both productive and nonproductive time for each FTE.)

Step 6:   Take Total Nursing Direct Care FTEs determined in Step 2, and multiply times Actual FTEs determined in Step 5.
(Total Nursing Direct Care FTEs × Actual FTEs = Total Nursing Direct Care FTEs including both productive and nonproductive time.)

Step 7:   Determine the percentage of each nursing staff category to give direct care (staff mix). Then multiply the percentage of each nursing staff category × the total Actual FTEs determined in Step 6, to calculate how many FTEs are needed for each nursing staff category.

Step 8:   Determine the cost of the nursing staff by actually putting in salary [or salary and benefit] amount for each nursing staff category. Total this amount for the total direct care cost for the division.

Step 9:   Determine the percentage of staff that will be appropriate by shift. Divide the number of FTEs needed for each nursing staff category calculated in Step 7 by the percentage of staff needed by shift to determine FTEs in each nursing staff category by shift.

Step 10:   Determine the part-time versus full-time ratio. Divide the FTEs determined in Step 9 by the part-time or full-time ratio. Then adjust the ratios to accurately reflect staffing needs.

Historical Data Sources of Services Rendered

To build a budget from scratch, one needs to collect available historical patient data. Some possible hospital data sources include historical census data (patient days) or visits per year; other volume indicators not on the census such as observation patients; and the NHPPD or HPPD. Admissions, discharges, and transfers may already be included in patient classification hours of care data, but, if not, these activities take additional nursing staff time; the NHPPD or HPPD that can be obtained from patient classification data, hopefully document this.

Patient classification data are most helpful and most accurate if reliability and validity have been established. If there is no patient classification system, or if the system does not have reliability and validity, the nurse administrator may have to use census data. If so, it still can be helpful to establish acuity levels for certain groups of patients by benchmarking with like units. The medical records department may have the most accurate data about short-stay or observation patients. Other sources may include the literature or an actual measurement of the amount of time it takes a nurse to perform certain tasks.

Available historical data are totally inaccurate if major changes occur that the data do not reflect. For example, perhaps a physician who is a large admitter is retiring and no one is taking his or her place. A nurse manager would then need to use data that would exclude that physician's patients. Or as technology developments occur—such as what happened with knee surgery—it might be possible to do a less invasive procedure that will change the data because the patient stay statistics will now be much lower. In this case, the nurse manager would need to find out how many patients came in the previous year for this surgery, find out the care hours they required, and correct the data to reflect this new development.

Let's walk through this evaluation exercise with an actual example of a nurse manager creating a budget. You are the nurse manager of 4W, an orthopedic division. The orthopedic unit nurse manager figures the average NHPPD for the year is 6.6 (**Exhibit 13–3**). This means the direct care nursing staff gives an average of 6.6 hours of care in 24 hours to each patient on the orthopedic unit. This figure needs to be compared with the average hours of care for the previous year. If the figures are similar, the current staffing level might be adequate. However, if the average figure is 6.4, the current staffing level might be inadequate.

Exhibit 13–3 Determining the Average NHPPD for the Previous Year	
Month	**NHPPD**
January	6.7
February	6.5
March	6.8
April	6.5
May	6.5
June	6.4
July	6.6
August	6.7
September	6.8
October	7.0
November	6.5
December	6.4
Average for Year	**6.6**

Source: Dunham-Taylor, J., & Pinczuk, J. *Financial Management for Nurse Managers: Merging the Heart with the Dollar, Second edition.* Burlington, MA: Jones & Bartlett Learning.

The NHPPD figure can be further broken down into the individual classifications of nurse direct caregivers (i.e., RNs give 3.4 hours of nursing care, LPNs provide 2 hours of care, and the nursing aides give 1.6 hours of care within 24 hours). The patient classification system specifies such information with established staffing ratios for the orthopedic unit.

Calculating Direct Care FTEs

Once appropriate historical data have been collected, the nurse manager can begin the calculations to build the cost center budget. First, take the nursing hours worked in 24 hours and multiply by the patient census or number of visits:

Average NHPPD × Patient census or number of visits = Direct care FTEs

If patient classification system data are not available, the nurse manager could actually compute direct nursing care hours worked by employee classification for the past year. Or the nurse manager might want to develop some data: *n* patients who had 0.5-hour visits this past year and *n* patients who required an hour-long visit this past year. In long-term care, the minimum data set could be used.

Now let's go back to the example of the 4W nurse manager. The census data for 4W shows 6,800 patient days on 4W last year—or an average of 18 to 19 patients each day.[4]

6,800 ÷ 365 = 18.63 patient days
This means there was an average of 18 to 19 patients on 4W each day.

Historically, there is a patient classification system that is reliable and valid on 4W. The acuity data from the patient classification system indicate that

- 50% of the patients are at Level 3 receiving 8.0 NHPPD
- 30% of the patients are at Level 2 receiving 6.0 NHPPD
- 20% of the patients are at Level 1 receiving 4.0 NHPPD

Going back to the previous equation, to determine the nursing hours worked in 24 hours the 4W nurse manager uses the patient classification system to determine the NHPPD or direct care nursing hours worked in 24 hours. The nurse manager computes the NHPPD as follows (*remember that to multiply 50%, it becomes 0.50 in the equation*):

$$
\begin{aligned}
&\text{50\% Level 3 patients @ 8 hours/day*} &= \text{4.0 NHPPD } (0.5 \times 8 = 4.00) \\
&\text{30\% Level 2 patients @ 6 hours/day*} &= \text{1.8 NHPPD } (0.3 \times 6 = 1.80) \\
+ \quad &\text{20\% Level 1 patients @ 4 hours/day*} &= \text{0.8 NHPPD } (0.2 \times 4 = 0.80) \\
\hline
& &\text{6.6 NHPPD}
\end{aligned}
$$

*For 24 hours.

So, you, as the 4W manager, have determined that the average NHPPD for 4W is 6.6. Now you are ready to finish the equation:

$$6.6 \text{ NHPPD} \times 6{,}800 \text{ patient days/year} = 44{,}880 \text{ NHPPD/year}$$

Continuing with this example, you are ready to compute the direct nursing care FTEs for 4W. You remember that an FTE represents 2,080 hours/year. Now you are ready for another equation:

$$\text{NHPPD/year} \div 1 \text{ FTE} = \text{Total nursing direct care FTEs}$$
$$44{,}880 \text{ NHPPD/year} \div 2{,}080 \text{ hours} = 21.58 \text{ nursing direct care FTEs}$$

Therefore, 21.58 FTEs are needed to give direct nursing care for the 6,800 patient days the previous year. There is a major flaw here. Do you see what it is?

Productive and Nonproductive Time

The 21.58 FTEs include *productive* time or actual time worked. This means the budgeted FTEs do not cover anyone taking a holiday, going on vacation, or getting sick. The 4W nurse manager knows that employees receive paid time for 8 holidays a year, 10 vacation days a year, and 10 sick days a year.[5] (Another term used in some organizations is *paid time off*, or *PTO*, which combines sick and vacation time. If actually sick for more than a specified time, such as 4 days, the PTO time reverts to additional sick time.) In addition, staff are given time off to attend two staff development days, so this needs to be included in the 4W nurse manager's budget projection. The term for this is *nonproductive time* or time where an employee is paid but is not actually working.

Usually, the human resources department can give a nurse manager a nonproductive time figure. This figure is often for the entire organization. However, it is possible that this figure is not totally accurate for 4W. For example, if the 4W nurse manager has been an effective administrator and the retention rate is high, the 4W staff members receive more vacation time than the organizational average. In this case, the 4W nonproductive time average will be higher than the human resources department number.

For this 4W example, let's say that the human resources department does not have a figure for nonproductive time and, to simplify the equation, that all the direct care nursing staff have the same number of nonproductive days. To calculate the direct nursing staff nonproductive time, the 4W manager uses the following calculation:

	2 weeks of vacation	*= 80 hours/year*
	10 sick days	*= 80 hours/year*
	8 holidays	*= 64 hours/year*
+	*2 education days*	*= 16 hours/year*
		240 hours/year total nonproductive time

Thus, each 4W staff member has 240 hours a year of possible nonproductive time.[6]

Even though every employee does not always take all this time in 1 year, it is better to figure this total into the equation—unless at the end of employment unused nonproductive time is not paid back to the employee. Then, one could use the average number of nonproductive hours taken per year by employees. Even then one has to be careful: If someone has a lot of sick time accrued and suddenly has surgery or an extensive illness, he or she will use much more than the average number of hours for that year. This is another factor that the human resources department will consider with its nonproductive figure: the average number of sick days taken by all employees for the year.

Because each FTE represents 2,080 hours a year but part of these hours (240 hours in the 4W example) is nonproductive time, the next step you need to compute is how many actual FTEs are needed, taking the nonproductive time into consideration. One way of calculating this is as follows:

2,080 hours (1 FTE) − 240 nonproductive hours per FTE = 1,840 productive hours per FTE

This means that of 2,080 hours paid to a full-time employee each year, on 4W direct care staff will actually work only 1,840 hours annually.

Next, you need to divide one FTE by 1,840 productive hours to determine the actual number of FTEs needed for the year:

2,080 hours ÷ 1,840 productive hours = 1.13 actual FTEs
(2,080 hours = 1 FTE)

This shows that for every 2,080 patient care hours, it is necessary to actually have 1.13 FTEs. One can translate the 1.13 figure into percentages—100% of the FTE (1 FTE) plus 13% of another FTE.

Usually, nonproductive costs are included in the division budget. This may include a factor for funeral leave or other such benefits where staff members are actually paid for nonworked days.

Benefits

Other benefits such as social security, healthcare insurance, and worker's compensation are not included here because these cost extra money but do not affect actual work hours. Such benefits—and sometimes sick and vacation time are included with these figures—may be 20% to 25% additional cost for a full-time employee. Such benefit costs may be included in a cost center budget or may be included in a different cost center such as a special human resources budget. Once again, there is not a standard for benefit costs and what cost center to put them in.

$$\textit{\$40,000} \times \textit{1.25} = \textit{\$50,000}$$
$$\textit{(1.25} = \textit{125\%)}$$

Both nonproductive time and benefits can be expensive for the organization to provide. For example, for an RN making $40,000 a year, if 25% of the salary is needed for benefits, in addition to the actual salary, the organization is actually paying $50,000 for each full-time RN. This means that an additional $10,000 a year is spent for the benefits for this RN. Thus, if writing a proposal for a new RN position, the nurse administrator needs to take into account that the actual cost for a new RN is $50,000—even though the actual budget statement shows only $40,000. The remaining $10,000 for benefits will be reflected in another cost center budget—most likely, human resources.

In the 4W example, the 240 nonproductive hours for the RN making $40,000 a year actually costs $4,615.20 a year.

$$\textit{\$40,000/year RN salary} \div \textit{2,080 hours/year} = \textit{\$19.23/hour}$$
$$\textit{240 hours/year nonproductive time} \times \textit{\$19.23/hour} = \textit{\$4,615.20}$$

Other Personnel Cost Factors

Other personnel costs factors that need to be considered before having actual personnel costs are holiday pay, shift differential, charge differential, overtime, on-call pay, cost of staff temporarily transferred to this cost center, as-needed staff used including sitters, funeral leave, jury duty, orientation, or education costs, tuition reimbursement—if not already included in the cost center budget—and other costs such as differentials for having a Bachelor of Science in Nursing degree, for specialty or other certification, and for a specialty area such as critical care or operating room. Tuition reimbursement is another cost, although this often is allocated to the human resources cost center.

A common practice in times of nursing or other interdisciplinary shortages is to pay extra to the staff experiencing a shortage. For example, one decides to pay a critical care differential. The message given to other nurses is that they are not as valued as a critical care nurse. Also, once a differential is started, the personnel involved will be very upset if this is ever taken away. Once a shortage is resolved, it can be tempting for administrators to dispense with the extra pay. *Nurse administrators should really think carefully about the implications if additional pay is given to a specific group based on a shortage.* Quick fixes usually do not work and may end up being permanent.

Direct Care Staff FTEs Needed

As the 4W nurse manager, you know that the budgeted direct care FTEs (*direct staff*) must include both productive and nonproductive time. To compute actual direct care staffing FTE needs for 4W, you need to multiply the productive FTEs by 1.13 FTE, which takes into account the nonproductive time. This figure, 24.4 FTEs, takes into account both productive and nonproductive hours of staff.

> *21.58 FTEs × 1.13 FTE = 24.39, or 24.4 direct care nursing staff FTEs needed on 4W*
> *(40 hours/week = 1 FTE based on an 8-hour day)*

Determine the Staff Mix

Now another issue confronts the 4W nurse manager: What direct care staff mix is appropriate for 4W? The term *staff mix* is a marketing term that specifies what kind of direct care staff will provide optimum care within the available budget dollars. Because this is a medical-surgical division with a 6.6 average NHPPD, there is a need for an appropriate RN ratio.

When making staff mix decisions, start with the patient care requirements. In the 4W example, the patients are acute, postsurgical, orthopedic patients, and therefore a higher ratio of RNs is preferable. Other things to consider include nursing delivery system practices as well as structure and organizational issues. For instance:

- What is the division size?
- How are assignments made?
- What is the layout of the nursing division?
- Are there delivery system practices such as unit staff accompanying patients to X-ray, an IV nurse, or other off-unit responsibilities?
- What is the nursing department structure?
- Are additional support staff available, such as an orthopedic technician or a float pool? (Sometimes the orthopedic technician is on another budget, i.e., an operating room cost center budget.) If so, these people need to be included in the staffing for the appropriate number of hours worked on 4W. Benchmarking data on staffing for other orthopedic units might be helpful as well.

In our example, as the 4W nurse manager, you choose to have a staff mix of 70% RNs and 30% nursing assistants. Thus, for the 24.4 FTEs of direct care nursing staff needed on 4W, the nurse manager determines that 17.1 FTEs will be RN staff. We continue to use this figure in this example. Fralic (2000) advocates creating a staffing plan based on a slightly lower number, such as 7.3 NHPPD or 7.4 NHPPD if the actual NHPPD was 7.5, to give some additional flexibility to the nurse manager. Then, if the average NHPPD suddenly goes above 7.5, a staff member could be added on a shift without going over budget. In addition, this strategy could save money if fewer staff were actually needed on a shift.

> *24.4 FTEs direct care nursing staff × 0.70 RN staff = 17.1 RN FTEs*

The remaining FTEs will be used for nursing assistants.

> *24.4 FTEs direct care nursing staff − 17.1 RN FTEs = 7.3 nursing assistant FTEs*
> *OR (It is always best to double-check your figures.)*
> *24.4 × 0.3 = 7.32 or 7.3 (The 0.3 is from 30% nursing assistant staff mix.*
> *It is always best to round to the nearest tenth.)*

Indirect Nursing Staff

In the preceding section, the direct care nursing staff requirements were computed. Now we determine the *indirect* FTE requirements. Here, the nurse administrator decides what *indirect staff* members are necessary for optimal functioning of a cost center. Still using 4W as an example, you know that two unit secretaries are needed for each day and evening shift. (Staff work 8-hour shifts on 4W.) To compute the unit secretary FTEs, how many FTEs are needed to fill a 7-day-a-week position? If the unit secretaries work 8-hour shifts, then

> *8 hours × 7 days/week = 56 hours/week*
> *56 hours/week ÷ 40 hours/week = 1.4 FTEs per shift*
> *(40 hours/week = 1 FTE based on an 8-hour day)*

To cover both day and evening shifts, you need 2.8 unit secretary FTEs.

As previously noted in the section titled "Direct Care Staff FTEs Needed," the 2.8 FTEs only reflect productive time worked. If there is a mechanism to replace the unit secretaries while they take vacation or sick time, such as a hospital-wide pool, costs for the nonproductive time could be charged to 4W when someone from this pool is actually used on 4W.

Another option to cover the nonproductive time is to hire part-time unit secretaries who are willing to work extra shifts when the other unit secretaries are sick or on vacation. A budgeted amount reflecting up to 0.4 additional unit secretary FTEs would be added to the budget to cover this additional time worked.

> *2.8 productive unit secretary FTEs × 1.13 productive and nonproductive time = 3.2 unit secretary FTEs*
> *(3.2 unit secretary FTEs 2.8 productive unit secretary FTEs = 0.4 unit secretary FTE nonproductive time)*

Another choice that can be made is not to replace the unit secretaries when nonproductive time is taken. This presents a problem because the division may have no unit secretary 13% of the time. This can be costly because the other RNs and nursing assistants will have to do the unit secretary duties—answer the phone, do the required paperwork, greet visitors—in addition to their regular duties. This can mean that expensive RN time is spent completing clerical functions. This is a waste of licensed staff time. Perhaps a better option is to specially train certain nurse aides, who are paid at a slightly higher level, to also complete the unit secretary work.

Occasionally, the unit secretary hours are considered under direct care hours. The advantage to putting the unit secretary in the direct care hours is that when the census is low the nurse manager could replace the unit secretary with a caregiver. The disadvantage of this is that the unit clerk could be counted into the NHPPD as a direct caregiver, thus decreasing caregiver hours. We recommend the unit secretary not be considered in direct care hours.

In considering indirect nursing personnel, the nurse manager FTE needs to be included. Going back to the 4W example, you have responsibility only for 4W, so one FTE would be allocated to the nurse manager position. An industry standard currently is that when the nurse manager takes sick or vacation time, no additional FTEs are allocated to cover this time. Often, the assistant nurse manager/charge nurse covers the unit.

There are additional indirect nursing costs for the division. Indirect unit personnel costs might include staff development, clinical specialist time, and/or assistant nurse manager time, if not included in the direct care staffing. Often, staff development and/or clinical specialist time are found on other cost center budgets.

Total Cost Center FTEs

Continuing with the 4W example, as the nurse manager, you have now figured the total FTEs for the cost center personnel budget:

	1.0	*Nurse manager FTE*
	17.1	*RN FTEs*
	7.3	*Nursing assistant FTEs*
+	3.2	*Unit secretary FTEs*
	28.6	*Total FTEs for 4W*

Dividing FTEs into Shifts

You now need to determine the percentage of FTEs on each shift. As a general rule of thumb, because the patients are more acute, staff are more evenly distributed across shifts. Using 8-hour shifts on a general care division, the industry standard is that most direct care nursing staff are allocated to the day shift (40–45%) with a bit less for the evening shift (35–40%) and the fewest for the night shift (20–35%). A lot of this is determined by the actual patient population needs on the unit. Using 12-hour shifts, the industry standard is that most direct care nursing staff are scheduled for days (50–60%) with the rest of the staff working the night shift. There is no absolute industry standard for shift allocations. This distribution relies on the judgment of the nursing staff and nursing administration.

On 4W, you determine that there will be 40% of the direct care nursing staff working day shift, 35% on the evening shift, and 25% on the night shift. This decision was made because the majority of medications happen on days and evenings, and most surgical procedures are scheduled on days. Also, days and evenings experience the most admissions and discharges. Now you can determine the FTE distribution for each shift:

	RN	NA
Day Shift		
17.1 RN FTEs × 0.40 = 6.84, or 6.8 RN FTEs	6.8	
7.3 RN FTEs × 0.40 = 2.92, or 2.9 NA FTEs		2.9
Evening Shift		
17.1 RN FTEs × 0.35 = 5.98, or 6 RN FTEs	6.0	
7.3 RN FTEs × 0.35 = 2.55, or 2.6 NA FTEs		2.6
Night Shift		
17.1 RN FTEs × 0.25 = 4.27, or 4.3 RN FTEs	4.3	
7.3 RN FTEs × 0.25 = 1.82, or 1.8 NA FTEs	+	1.8
	17.1	7.3

To check your figures, add them together. They should total 17.1 RN FTEs and 7.3 nursing assistant FTEs.

Determine Part-Time Versus Full-Time Ratio

After determining the FTE distribution by shift, you have another decision to make: *What percentage of staff should be part time versus full time?* You need to make a thoughtful decision here because too many part-time staff means a lack of continuity on the division. On the other hand, if there are too many full-time staff, it will be impossible to cover weekends with adequate staffing. Ideally, a ratio of about 60% full-time personnel and 40% part-time personnel, or 65% full-time and 35% part-time, is preferred. It allows for some flexibility in staffing yet achieves continuity.

Going back to the 4W example, you decide to use the 60:40 ratio and figure the FTEs for both classifications of nursing personnel, checking the figures:

	RN	NA
Day Shift		
6.8 RN FTEs × 0.60 = 4.08, or 4.1 full-time RN FTEs	4.1	
6.8 RN FTEs × 0.40 = 2.72, or 2.7 part-time RN FTEs	2.7	
2.9 NA FTEs × 0.60 = 1.74, or 1.7 full-time NA FTEs		1.7
2.9 NA FTEs × 0.40 = 1.16, or 1.2 part-time NA FTEs		1.2
Evening Shift		
6.0 RN FTEs × 0.60 = 3.6, full-time RN FTEs	3.6	
6.0 RN FTEs × 0.40 = 2.4, part-time RN FTEs	2.4	
2.6 NA FTEs × 0.60 = 1.56, or 1.6 full-time NA FTEs		1.6
2.6 NA FTEs × 0.40 = 1.04, or 1 part-time NA FTEs		1.0
Night Shift		
4.3 RN FTEs × 0.60 = 2.58, or 2.6 full-time RN FTEs	2.6	
4.3 RN FTEs × 0.40 = 1.72, or 1.7 part-time RN FTEs	1.7	
1.8 NA FTEs × 0.60 = 1.08, or 1.1 full-time NA FTEs		1.1
1.8 NA FTEs × 0.40 = 0.72, or 0.7 part-time NA FTEs	+	0.7
Total	17.1	7.3
(NA = nursing assistant)		

Now another challenge emerges as you compute the full-time calculation. Several of the full-time FTE numbers are a fraction. A full-time person fills 1 FTE, not a fraction of an FTE. So, you must change several calculations. This first occurs on the day shift with both the RN FTEs and the nursing assistant FTEs. There are 4.1 full-time RN FTEs and 2.7 part-time RN FTEs. Here it is best to take the leftover 0.1 full-time RN FTE and add it to the part-time RN FTEs. There are 1.7 full-time nursing assistant FTEs—you can either have 1 or 2 full-time nursing assistants. In these cases, you must think of the implications. You could decide to have 2 FTEs be full time, with a resulting 0.9 FTE for part-time nursing assistants on days. Alternately, you could choose to have 1 full-time nursing assistant and 1.9 part-time nursing assistant FTEs.

There is no right answer to this dilemma: You must consider the implications of each. There probably will be less continuity with the second option, but it offers more flexibility with scheduling. The authors, however, would choose to go with the first option because of availability of personnel. It can be very difficult to find nursing assistants who want to work part time. Because the nursing assistant salaries are lower than other nursing personnel, they would prefer to have a full-time job with benefits.

Looking at the RN FTEs on the evening shift, the same problem occurs. Here there are 3.6 full-time RN FTEs. So, you must choose between three or four full-time RNs. In this case it may be best to choose to have four full-time RNs rather than three because if the RNs have every other weekend off, there will be two full-time RNs on every weekend. When one RN goes on vacation or is sick, there will still be continuity with another full-time RN available. So, you will plan to have four full-time evening RN FTEs and two part-time evening RN FTEs, which totals six evening RN FTEs.

As you change the budget figures, keep an ongoing tally of the changes as you add or subtract FTEs. In the end, the tally should add to zero. In the following 4W example, you change the FTE designations as follows and keep a tally:

Had	*Change To*	*Day Shift*	*Tally*	
			RN	*NA*
4.1 to	*4 full-time RN FTEs*	*[4.1 − 4 = 10.1]*	*+0.1*	
2.7 to	*2.8 part-time RN FTEs*	*[2.7 − 2.8 = −0.1]*	*−0.1*	
1.7 to	*2 full-time NA FTEs*	*etc.*		*−0.3*
1.2 to	*0.9 part-time NA FTEs*			*+0.3*
		Evening Shift		
3.6 to	*4 full-time RN FTEs*		*−0.4*	
2.4 to	*2 part-time RN FTEs*		*+0.4*	
1.6 to	*2 full-time NA FTEs*			*−0.4*
1.0 to	*0.6 part-time NA FTEs*			*+0.4*
		Night Shift		
2.6 to	*3 full-time RN FTEs*		*−0.4*	
1.7 to	*1.3 part-time RN FTEs*		*+0.4*	
1.1 to	*1 full-time NA FTE*			*−0.1*
0.7 to	*0.8 part-time NA FTEs*			*+0.1*
17.1 RN FTEs and 7.3 NA FTEs, or 24.4 Total FTEs			*0*	*0*
(NA = nursing assistant)				

Once again, you can double-check the numbers. The part-time and full-time numbers should add up to the total FTE number for that position classification; the total direct care staff FTEs should still add up to 24.4.

The last action of the nurse manager, if using these numbers to actually staff the division, is to determine the number of actual part-time staff to hire. Using the 4W example, there are 2.8 RN part-time FTEs on day shift. To staff for weekends, it is probably best to have at least four employees in part-time positions—two for each weekend if everyone gets every other weekend off. So, you could choose to make a couple positions 0.7 or 0.8 FTEs and two positions for less time. One option is to have two 0.8 FTE positions and two 0.6 FTE positions. Gear this decision by part-time staff availability and preferences. And be flexible and change the FTE designations if new staff members prefer different numbers of work hours. The main goal is to stay within the 17.1 RN FTEs and the 7.3 nursing assistant FTEs.

There is no industry standard here. The FTE part-time designations are a result of personal preference, availability of potential employees, and good judgment. For example, if you had 2.6 part-time FTEs for a shift, you would not want all the part-time employees to be 0.4 FTEs only working 2 days each week. Continuity would really be an issue if this were the case. On the other hand, if you have only 0.8 part-time FTEs for a shift, it might be preferable to have two different people hired to allow more flexibility in staffing.

Calculate Nursing Care Hours Needed per Day

Now that we have figured productive and nonproductive time, let's go back to the 44,880 NHPPD given the previous year. Assuming that the average number remains the same for this current year, we can divide the 44,880 NHPPD by 365 days to determine the actual number of nursing care hours needed each day, or 122.96 hours.[7] In the box provided one can see that on the day shift the nurse manager should have 34 RN hours and 15 nursing assistant hours; on evenings 30 RN hours and 13 nursing assistant hours; and on nights 22 RN hours and 9 nursing assistant hours. Full-time and part-time staff scheduled to work each shift should add up to these numbers. (All final numbers have been rounded to an even hour.)

4W Nursing Care Hours Needed per Day
44,880 NHPPD / 365 days = 122.96 nursing care hours needed each day
Skill Mix
122.96 hours × 0.7 RN = 86 RN hours needed over 24 hours
122.96 hours × 0.3 NA = 37 NA hours needed over 24 hours
Shifts
86 RN hours × 0.40 day shift = 34 day shift RN hours
37 NA hours × 0.40 day shift = 15 day shift NA hours
86 RN hours × 0.35 day shift = 30 evening shift RN hours
37 NA hours × 0.35 day shift = 13 evening shift NA hours
86 RN hours × 0.25 day shift = 22 night shift RN hours
37 NA hours × 0.25 day shift = 9 night shift NA hours
(NA = nursing assistant)

If 4W has a staffing plan, you could evaluate the staffing plan by comparing it with these numbers of staff per shift. In other words, when 4W has 18 to 19 patients with an average acuity of 6.6 NHPPD (these were the averages for 4W the previous year), the staffing plan should agree with the hours per shift designated previously.

Figure Actual Personnel Costs

To calculate actual personnel costs, the nurse administrator needs either actual salary costs of the personnel or average salaries for different personnel categories (i.e., nurse manager, RNs, LPNs, nursing assistants, nursing technicians, and ward clerks). Usually, this information can be provided by the department or by finance personnel. If available, use actual salaries and computer software programs or finance department programs to generate these data. Additional costs such as shift differential, charge pay, on-call pay, and other costs discussed earlier in this chapter may need to be included in this equation.

Other factors affecting personnel costs on a unit are such functions as an IV team, escort service, sitter, or orderly. Often, these services are located within the centralized overall nursing department budget under a different cost center than the unit center. In some systems, when these services are used by a cost

Exhibit 13–4	Calculate Actual Personnel Salary Dollars				
1.0	Nurse Manager FTE (average Nurse Manager salary)	× $36.00/hour	× 2,080 hours*	=	$74,880.00
17.1	RN FTEs (average RN salary)	× $26.00/hour	× 2,080 hours*	=	$924,768.00
7.3	NA FTEs (average NA salary)	× $12.00/hour	× 2,080 hours*	=	$182,208.00
3.2	Unit Secretary FTEs \(average Unit secretary salary)	× $10.00/hour	× 2,080 hours*	=	$66,560.00
Total Salary Dollars Needed					**$1,248,416.00**

*2,080 hours/year = 1 FTE

(Note: This calculation does not include additional benefits, differential, or bonus dollars.)

center, the employee costs for that shift or service are billed to that cost center. If such functions exist and are regularly used on a unit, these costs would need to be added to the unit personnel costs. The same is true when regularly using replacement staff from another cost center.

Thus, in the 4W example, as the nurse manager, you could calculate the actual salary costs as illustrated in **Exhibit 13–4**. In this example, no other unit personnel have been identified. If such personnel exist and are necessary for the appropriate functioning of the unit, it would be important to include them in this budget.

There will probably be additional costs to figure into this equation. For instance, perhaps shift differential is paid for both the evening and night shifts, holiday time is paid when employees actually work holidays, and on-call pay is given. Pay raises or premiums are other possible costs. If per diem or traveling staff will be used, they should be added to the budget.

Overtime—often meaning staff are paid time and a half (1.5)—is another factor. You would assume that some overtime will be used. The industry standard is that overtime should not exceed 2%. The nurse manager could look at what was actually used the year before and determine whether this amount was reasonable under the circumstances. For example, if one nurse is on sick leave and two others leave their positions, accruing additional overtime could be a reasonable way to staff the unit to deal with this temporary situation. However, if overtime is consistently used by all the nurses to chart, other solutions may be necessary. Perhaps the workloads or skill mix needs to be adjusted. Maybe a computerized charting system would really save RN time. Maybe the nurse manager leadership needs to be examined because there is so much turnover on the unit. If additional money is paid for other reasons, be sure to add them to the budget if they seem realistic and reasonable.

The nurse manager may or may not have to include fringe benefits into these costs. Fringe benefits include health insurance, Social Security payments, and other benefits. At times, these costs are shown on the nurse manager's cost center budget, but often they are not and instead appear on the human resources budget. These are significant costs—20% to 25%—so the executive team always needs to include this expense when determining labor expenses.

Information Systems Technology

It is best to do budget calculations, as well as staff scheduling, using a computer program. Some programs can schedule staff based on patient classification data, give staffing and variance reports, and compare what was actually spent with what was budgeted. Many staffing programs can be linked with budget and payroll data. It is ideal to have all this information integrated together.

If such programs are unavailable, the next step is to ask personnel in the finance department whether they are using an existing program that could compute these data. Another option is to use an existing spreadsheet software program. Dunham-Taylor and Pinczuk (2006) provide examples of spreadsheet systems.

Minimum Staffing

When evaluating the budget, you must understand another concept: *minimum staffing*. When the patient volume reaches a certain low level of service, it becomes a liability because more staff must be present than are actually needed to take care of the existing patients. This is because there are minimum staffing issues. Minimum staffing is a fixed cost. Remember that *fixed costs* are those costs that stay the same regardless of the level of activity.

To figure minimum staffing let's begin with an inpatient example. For an inpatient cost center staying open every day of the year, the industry standard is that two personnel are available to care for patients regardless of the number of patients. Minimum staffing for an inpatient cost center is pictured in **Exhibit 13–5**. Note that it is best not to include unit secretary time in the minimum staffing or fixed cost section of the budget because this allows for more budget flexibility for the nurse manager.

You may need to determine the actual salary dollars involved for your cost center. See **Exhibit 13–6**, assuming an average salary amount per staff classification. Often, the human resource department or finance department personnel have determined the average salary for each personnel category. Although

---

Exhibit 13–5   Inpatient Unit Direct Care Minimum Staffing for 24 Hours

Day Shift	Evening Shift	Night Shift
8 hours = 1 RN	8 hours = 1 RN	8 hours = 1 RN
8 hours = 1 Aide/Tech/LPN/RN	8 hours = 1 Aide/Tech/LPN/RN	8 hours = 1 Aide/Tech/LPN/RN
16 hours	**16 hours**	**16 hours**

Add the hours from each shift:

16 hours + 16 hours + 16 hours = 48 hours/day

Exhibit 13–6   Inpatient Unit Direct Care Minimum Staffing Cost/Day

Day Shift	Evening Shift	Night Shift
(8 hours = RN–Amy) @ $28/hour* = $224/day*	(8 hours = 1 RN–Bill) @ $26/hour* = $208/day*	(8 hours = 1 RN–Carol) @ $27/hour* = $216/day*
(8 hours = 1 NA–Robert) @ $12/hour* = $96/day*	(8 hours = 1 NA–Sue) @ $12/hour* = $96/day*	(8 hours = 1 NA–Tom) @ $12/hour* = $96/day*

Add the salary rate from each staff member:

$224 + $208 + $216 + $96 + $96 + $96 = $936/day* (minimum staffing cost per day)

$936/day × 365 days = $341,640/year*

*Benefits and shift differential not included.

NA = nurse aide.

this salary amount could be used to determine the fixed cost of minimum staffing, it may not be as accurate. For instance, if most staff RNs in a cost center have been there for many years, most may be at the top of the salary range. The human resources average staff RN salary figure may be lower. So, it would be preferable to use the actual salaries rather than the human resources figure in this example.

So far, our minimum staffing example has included only the actual direct care nursing staff. Minimum staffing on an inpatient cost center also includes the nurse manager and other consistent cost center/department employees such as the cost center secretaries. To determine the fixed cost per day for the nurse manager, let's assume that the nurse manager is responsible for one cost center. Because the daily cost is based on 7 days in the week, the actual daily rate for the nurse manager would be the nurse manager's hourly salary multiplied by 5.7 hours a day (a fixed cost per day).

> *Nurse Manager*
> *40 hours/week ÷ 7 days/week = 5.7 hours/day*
> *5.7 hours/day × $36/hour = $205.20/day*

If a cost center secretary is always present on the inpatient cost center for a 12-hour shift, this would be added to minimum staffing. In this case, the hourly rate of the cost center secretary is multiplied by 12 hours per day.

> *Unit Secretary*
> *12 hours/days × $10/hour = $120.00/day*

Thus, the minimum staffing actually costs $1,261.20 per day or $460,338.00 per year (**Exhibit 13–7**). So, actually looking at the staffing budget for that unit, $460,338.00 would be a fixed cost.

The financial personnel may determine the fixed costs within the nursing cost center budget differently. Usually, they understand neither what minimum staffing is nor how to measure it. If the finance staff tell you what your fixed costs are, be sure to have them define how they have determined these costs. Usually, the nurse manager or nurse executive will need to educate finance department personnel about minimum staffing. The nurse manager/executive should both explain and show financial personnel actual minimum staff examples.

Exhibit 13–7   Total Inpatient Unit Direct Care Minimum Staffing Cost/Day

Direct care staff = $936.00/day*

Nurse manager = $205.20/day*

Unit secretary = $120.00/day*

Total = $1,261.20/day*

$1,261.20/day × 365 days = $460,338.00/year*

*Benefits and shift differential not included.

After determining the *fixed* cost of staffing—minimum staffing—the rest of the staffing budget is then variable staffing costs. See **Exhibit 13–8** (minimum staffing and variable staffing) to see how this might actually look for a unit. *Variable costs* are those costs that change (vary) depending on the level of activity or volume. So, staffing over and above the minimum staffing is a variable cost. Variable costs occur in addition to fixed costs. Thus, the staffing needed above and beyond minimum staffing would increase or decrease as the patient volume increases or decreases. The volume determining the staffing would be related to the number of patient minutes/hours/days, patient acuity, or patient visits.

If a nurse manager were asked to prepare a *flexible, or variable, budget* giving alternative plans for different levels of spending, the nurse manager would have to figure both minimum staffing and variable staffing at different volume levels. Dunham-Taylor and Pinczuk (2006) provide an example of a flexible budget presented as an Excel spreadsheet.

Systems differ when using a flexible, or variable, budget. In some systems, this just means that there are two or more levels of spending (several fixed budgets at various occupancy levels) determined for different volumes of patients. In some systems, variable budgets change as the volume of patients and the acuity of patients change. For example, this budget could vary as the patient population changes throughout the day. A nurse manager in such a system could see what budget amount was available for the upcoming shift

---

Exhibit 13–8 Fixed (Minimum Staffing) and Variable Staffing

(Average HPPD = 6.5)

Patients		Days			Evenings			Nights		
		RN	LPN	NA	RN	LPN	NA	RN	LPN	NA
25	Variable Direct Caregivers	4	2	1	3	2	1	2	1	1
20		3	2	1	2	2	1	2	1	1
14		2	1	1	2	0	1	1	1	1
		1	1	1	1	1	1	1	1	1
9		1	0	1	1	0	1	1	0	1
8	Fixed Direct Caregivers / Minimum Staffing									
7										
1		1	0	1	1	0	1	1	0	1

RN = registered nurse
LPN = licensed practical nurse
NA = nurse aide
UC = unit clerk

based on the current patient population. If there is a variable budget, the nurse manager must discuss how finance department personnel determined the gradations in the variable budget.

As the budget changes, it is important for the nurse manager to decrease variable costs in relation to the decrease in volume. When the census or acuity falls below the minimum staffing pattern, the nurse manager and nurse executive might consider closing/consolidating cost centers or assigning patients in a manner that maintains a census on several cost centers that cover the fixed costs of minimum staffing.

Equipment and Supply Costs

The nurse manager also needs to examine equipment and supply costs. These costs often include such items as education, travel, standard office and medical supplies not used by specific patients, telephone costs, equipment lease/rentals, equipment repair, uniform allowance, books, and consulting charges.

Once again it is important to look at the historical data. If these data were accurate and reflected what is anticipated for another year, there is no need to change the data. However, most often the costs in these categories existed for years and may not be totally accurate for present patient needs. Past experience can be helpful when looking at these data. If nurse managers have been regularly going over budget variances each month, it is often quite obvious that certain budget categories are insufficient to cover supply costs for the present group of patients, whereas other budget categories may not be used as much or at all. It is important to make sure that supplies are expensed to the proper line item to reflect adequate expenditures. If these expenditures are accurate, they may need to be adjusted each year to better reflect actual use. If they remain accurate, the nurse manager may not need to do much with these data.

In addition to the historical data, the nurse manager must anticipate what might change for the coming budget year. Will the unit purchase new equipment that requires a change in supplies? Are physician practice patterns changing? Are there anticipated inflationary costs to consider?

For the evaluation process, the nurse manager needs to consider all changes that have occurred, or are expected to occur, on the unit that might result in more or less being spent in equipment and supply costs. The nurse manager needs to provide additional documentation as to why the amounts need to be changed in certain budget categories. For example, if the cost center is treating a different kind of patient, the nurse manager might need to provide the number of such patients anticipated for the next year and document typical supply needs required. Additionally, the nurse manager should specify any equipment and supplies that might be used less frequently.

Determining Variance Between Historical and Newly Figured Budgets

Now that an accurate budget has been completed, it is time for the nurse manager to compare these data with the current historical budget. Do they agree? If so, you can proceed with the budget planning process, knowing that the data are accurate. However, if there is a discrepancy—or variance—between both budgets, you need to do some additional work. The first step is to discuss this issue with the nurse executive or with your supervisor if you do not directly report to the nurse executive.

By having computed the budget from scratch, you have objective data to use when defining the problem and suggesting solutions. It gives you actual objective data; finance department personnel are more likely to listen when presented with such data. It is easy to argue that additional staffing is needed for "squishy" reasons, such as this is needed to improve quality or to meet accreditation requirements. However, having *objective evidence* provides better documentation of actual patient needs, and the executive team will be more likely to hear it. After all, the nurse manager best understands and represents actual patient needs. Patients benefit—and the nurse manager has more success—when actual numbers can be presented to verify patient needs.

If the patient acuity/volume is higher, this provides actual data that verify additional staffing needs. Perhaps if the patient volume is higher, the nurse manager can suggest a different staff mix to better meet the needs of these patients. The nurse manager may propose opening a swing unit, available at times of peak census, or possibly the problem is that more staff are needed because nonproductive time was not taken into account.

If the patient volume has decreased within a cost center, other strategies can be considered. First, current staffing levels may need to be decreased. However, current staffing levels can be decreased only to the minimum staffing level. If below the minimum staffing level, other strategies could be to increase the patient volume on the cost center such as by merging cost centers; alternately, the nurse manager could close the cost center and send the patients to a similar cost center not at full patient capacity. This action is complicated by other issues such as medical patients with infections not being preferable patients to divert to a surgical unit or labor and delivery area and by staff cross-training issues.

Be creative in thinking through the most appropriate strategy. Things do not need to be done the same way! After thinking through such issues and discussing them with the nurse executive, it may be necessary for you to write a thoughtful proposal or business plan clearly defining the problem as well as discussing one or more potential solutions.

Other Ways Actual Cost Data Can Be Used

Cost data can be used in additional ways:

- **Assignment comparability:** If these concrete cost data are available, when a staff member questions having a heavier load than other staff, the nurse manager can actually compare the acuity levels for assigned patients. These data can also be used for staff evaluation. If one staff member can safely care for a higher volume of patients, this staff member might deserve additional merit pay. Or a staff member might need to be mentored and/or counseled as to how to safely care for a higher volume of patients.
- **Intraunit comparability:** Using our 4W example, the nurse executive or nurse managers on similar cost centers within this healthcare organization could compare staffing, skill mix, and budget information. For example, two medical cost centers with similar acuity ratings could be compared (**Exhibit 13–9**). Here 6E and Tower have fairly similar NHPPD. However, Tower has a higher

Exhibit 13–9	Personnel Budget Sheet				
		General Hospital Personnel Budget **FY 20XX**			
Medical *Cost Centers*	*NHPPD*	*Days*	*Direct* *FTEs*	*Indirect FTEs*	*Total* *FTEs*
4W	6.6	6,800	24.3	3.8	28.1
6E	5.8	6,200	22.2	3.8	26.0
6.2	6.2	7,300	30.4	3.8	34.2

number of patient days, whereas 6E has fewer patient days. Each unit could be costed out to determine whether there was comparable staffing on each of these units.

- **Benchmarking:** The cost data can also be used to compare with other similar services across the country using available benchmarking data such as the Premier or VHA data for hospitals. Premier or VHA can give extensive data on skill mix, labor costs, overtime used, and wages paid certain types of employees and can even provide the nurse manager a vehicle to network with peers from similar units nationally. When using such data, it is important to make sure you are not comparing apples and oranges—you may believe you are comparing like categories yet may not be. For example, skill mix for a pediatric unit is totally different from the skill mix on a critical care unit. It is important to get definitions of what is actually included for that category. To do this, we recommend that you contact a person at the facility to verify like activities.

- **Skill mix issues:** Skill mix could be an issue. One could compare skill mix on similar units or with benchmarking data. The acuity could dictate the skill mix (i.e., an intensive care unit with higher acuity is generally staffed with a higher RN ratio than a general care unit is). So, it would be important to make sure that the units you are benchmarking are actually serving the same degree of patient acuity.

- **Full-time/part-time ratios:** The ratio of full-time staff to part-time staff must also be evaluated. It is possible that there are constant staffing problems on weekends because the ratio of full-time staff is too high. Or, if a lot of part-time staff work 1 to 3 days a week, it may become impossible to keep all staff informed as to changes and continuity of care can be challenged. The cost data can provide helpful information to determine whether the part-time-to-full-time ratio is appropriate.

- **Establishing a staffing plan or flexible staffing model:** Another strategy for nurse managers is to establish ideal staffing levels—a staffing plan—for different volumes of patients when there are wide variations in patient acuity and/or numbers of patients served. When the volume is low, perhaps part-time staff or specific full-time staff work fewer hours, or staff are floated to other cost centers. If volume is high, this is reversed. Part-time staff work more hours, full-time staff earn overtime, a float pool is available to supply additional staff, or additional agency staff are hired. It is always best to carefully plan various strategies that can be implemented when a certain volume of patients is present. Additional staff training is needed when staff are expected to work at different clinical sites. Planning for several scenarios ahead of actual happenings can help to eliminate stress for both staff and administrators and maintain a continuity in quality of care. If staffing needs change, this staffing plan can be used as a flexible staffing model where a computer system—or the staffing personnel—automatically sets appropriate numbers of staff at the designated staff mix.

Thus, an annual evaluation of the budget can be helpful not only to determine that the allocated budget dollars are appropriate but for other staffing and supply/equipment issues as well.

Notes

1. Occasionally, in certain geographic areas, employees are paid for 7.5 hours rather than 8 hours for a day's work. In this case, the workweek is not 40 hours but 37.5 hours; the year is 1950 hours, not 2080 hours. If this is the case in your facility, use 1950 hours rather than 2080 hours.
2. Not all patient classification systems produce NHPPD or HPPD data. Prototype systems usually do not, whereas other task-based or care interaction models usually do.
3. In this chapter, NHPPD is used, but HPPD could be substituted.
4. Make sure the census data include all short-stay patients.

5. In some systems, different categories of employees may have a different number of vacation days.
6. This assumes that all part-time and full-time employees receive sick, vacation, or other nonproductive time. If part-time employees do not receive nonproductive benefits, include only their productive time. If employees do not use all their nonproductive time, we recommend that you still compute the full amount because this could possibly be used in the future.
7. This assumes that the census and acuity remain at the average level determined by last year's figures. If you know other information that would change these numbers, use those figures. Increases or decreases in census or acuity need to follow a staffing plan based on these numbers.

Discussion Questions

1. Nurse managers have many responsibilities when it comes to the development of the budget. What issues would be considered most important for the nurse manager in this process? Who should be involved?
2. This chapter deals with specific units of service for nursing workload requirements. What role should the nurse manager play and how should the manager interact with the finance department for a standard definition for measurement?
3. How should a nurse manager use a patient classification system to justify NHPPD measurements for various units for budget purposes that would be understood by the finance department? How would nursing prove that the patient classification system is consistent in measuring the patient acuity for the various patient areas?
4. Generally, the finance department provides the overhead allocations for the nursing units. If your department is considered a revenue department for budgeting purposes, why is it important for you to know how overhead expenses are allocated to your unit?
5. As a nurse manager, you have to set up a new patient service budget. What sources of information do you need to build that budget?
6. Why is it important to have a patient acuity classification system to calculate minimum staffing needs?

Glossary of Terms

Average Daily Census—average number of inpatients present at midnight for a month or a year. May also be the average number of emergency department/home visits or outpatient treatments for a month or a year.
Direct Staff—staff that give direct care to patients.
Fixed Costs—costs that stay the same regardless of the level of activity. In staffing, minimum staffing is the fixed cost.
Flexible, or Variable, Budget—alternative plans for different levels of spending.
Full-Time Equivalent (FTE)—unit of measurement that represents a person or people working 40 hours a week and 2080 hours a year. One person who works a full-time position is one FTE, whereas part-time employees work less than one FTE.
Hours per Patient Day (HPPD)—the number of nursing staff hours needed to provide care to an inpatient in 24 hours. NHPPD and HPPD most often have the same meaning; however, at times the definition is different. For instance, a healthcare organization uses a patient classification system to measure actual hours of care needed (NHPPD), whereas finance may use HPPD using only patient census data. In this case, the two terms are different and have a different measurement. This is an example where it is important to find out the definition/measurement of either the term NHPPD or HPPD. Because there is not a standardized definition for either term, be sure to clarify definitions.
Indirect Staff—those employees (including the nurse manager) who do not give direct care to patients.
Length of Stay—an individual patient's duration of staying within a cost center or facility for a month or a year. The number of patient days one patient is in the facility.
Loss Leaders—services that do not make money—in fact lose money—but benefit the organization by bringing patients to the organization for services or gain potential patients because patients see that hospital personnel are friendly, helpful people. Loss leaders can include such services as the emergency department and women's health programs.
Minimum Staffing—needing at least two staff members on duty at all times to staff a unit.
Nonproductive Time—time where an employee is paid but is not working, such as holidays, sick time, vacation time, and/or paid time off (PTO).

Nursing Hours per Patient Day (NHPPD)—the number of nursing staff hours needed to provide care to an inpatient in 24 hours. NHPPD and HPPD most often have the same meaning; however, at times the definition is different. For instance, a healthcare organization uses a patient classification system to measure actual hours of care needed (NHPPD), whereas finance may use HPPD using only patient census data. In this case, the two terms are different and have a different measurement. This is an example where it is important to find out the definition/measurement of either the term NHPPD or HPPD. Because there is not a standardized definition for either term, be sure to clarify definitions.

Nursing Workload—the volume of work performed by nursing caregivers. One way to better specify units of service for nursing workload is to use NHPPD or HPPD.

Occupancy Rate—Patient days are used to determine the occupancy rate. If a long-term care unit has 50 beds and 40 are filled, a percentage is determined for the number of beds actually filled. So, the long-term care unit would have an occupancy rate of 80% (40 filled beds ÷ 50-bed capacity = 0.8, or 80%).

Overhead—indirect costs, including benefits such as health insurance and Social Security, depreciation on buildings or equipment, and nonproductive time (although sometimes this is mixed in with the labor budget figures). Overhead usually includes departments not giving direct care such as administration, housekeeping, maintenance, finance, medical records, and human resources. Overhead can be computed in several ways: Administration costs may be divided by the census and billed to each inpatient unit in a hospital, housekeeping and utility costs can be computed by square footage, and linen by the pounds of linen used. Finance traditionally uses the same step-down allocation for overhead as filed with the Medicare and Medicaid cost reports.

Patient Days—number of inpatients present at midnight. One patient day is given for each day the patient is present on an inpatient unit.

Product Line (Service Line)—total services for a particular group of patients or similar patient diagnoses. For example, typical product lines may be cardiology, oncology, burns, or women's health.

Productive Time—actual time worked.

Relative Value Unit (RVU)—term used by reimbursement systems. On an inpatient unit, the relative value unit represents the complexity of a procedure.

Staff Mix—marketing term that specifies what kind of direct care staff will provide care.

Unit of Service—used by healthcare organizations to measure specific services a patient uses within a specific time frame, that is, minutes, hours, days, visits, births, treatments, operations, or other patient encounters.

Variable Costs—those costs that change (vary) depending on the level of activity or volume. In staffing, variable costs are those that are over and above minimum staffing.

Vertical Integration—a hospital might want to add long-term care beds or home care services to increase profits to have additional options to save costs. For instance, it is cheaper to quickly move a postoperative patient into a skilled nursing facility—a less expensive option than holding the patient on an inpatient unit for an additional day or days.

References

American Nurses Association. (2008). *Principles for nurse staffing with annotated bibliography*. Kansas City, MO: Author.

Dunham-Taylor, J., & Pinczuk, J. (2006). *Health care financial management for nurse managers: Applications from hospitals, long-term care, home care, and ambulatory care*. Sudbury, MA: Jones and Bartlett.

Fralic, M. (Ed.). (2000). *Staffing management and methods: Tools and techniques for nursing leaders*. Chicago, IL: AHA Press.

Shullanberger, G. (2000, May–June). Nurse staffing decisions: An integrative review of the literature. *Nursing Economic$, 18*(3), 124–148.

Budget Variances

Norma Tomlinson, MSN, RN, NE-BC, FACHE

OBJECTIVES

- Recognize the value of budget variance analysis as a tool for managers and staff to control costs.
- Define and apply unit of service as the denominator in budget analysis.
- Explain the difference between revenue charges and actual dollars received for care provided.
- Analyze the impact of unbudgeted overtime, contract labor, or orientation hours on the salary budget.
- Identify the source of increased supply usage or errors in the periodic inventory expense report.
- Understand the impact of benefit expense and how it is related to man-hours worked.

Introduction

Budgets are usually created several months before the beginning of the fiscal year. Annual budgets are based on assumptions about the types and volumes of patients that will be cared for over the coming year and the resources required to provide that care. The difference between the budget and actual performance is the *budget variance*. Well-researched and analyzed budget variance becomes a powerful tool in controlling cost while ensuring safe, effective care.

A nursing unit or department is a *cost center*. Data comparing budgeted dollars to actual dollars are usually provided on a monthly basis by the finance department for each cost center. It normally shows data for the month and year-to-date (YTD). It is important, therefore, to be aware of the beginning of your fiscal year. If your fiscal year begins with January and it is now February, the data for January and YTD are the same because both include only 1 month's data (January). If your fiscal year begins July 1 and ends June 30, in February the YTD will include 7 months of data (July through January).

The *cost center report* compares the actual costs with the budgeted amount. Often, these reports show the percentage of the difference, or variance, between what was budgeted and what actually was spent. If it does not, you can calculate the percentage of variance by taking the difference between the actual and the budget and then divide that number by the budget. For instance, using **Exhibit 14–1**, multiplying the difference between the budget and actual by 100 gives you the percentage of variance. Therefore, the actual budget amount was 25% greater than the budgeted amount.

Often, an operational report shows the data for the prior year for the same time frame to give you an additional perspective to gauge whether you are doing better or worse than the same time last year.

Types of Variance

The statistics, or types of variance, discussed here include the volume or units of service, revenue, man-hours, information about salary expense, benefit expense, and nonsalary expense.

Expense Budget

In an expense budget, units of service for inpatient cost centers are often broken into patient days for patients admitted and observation hours when the patient time on the unit was short enough that it did not qualify to become an admission. *It is important to capture all of your unit activity.*

If your report does not delineate these two types of patient days, it is very important to determine whether the statistics include both. The man-hours to care for a patient in observation status can actually

---

Exhibit 14–1   Comparing Budgeted Amount with Actual Amount Used

Budget = $200

Actual = $250

$200 (budget) − $250 (actual) = − $50 variance

The difference between the budgeted amount and the actual amount is $50.

$50 (variance) ÷ ($200 (budget) = 0.25

0.25 × 100 = 25 percent (To get the percentage, one multiplies this amount by 100.)

Therefore the actual amount was 25 percent greater than the budgeted amount.

be more time intensive per day because admission and discharge activities have to be done within the same day (23-hour patient) or the next day. If the unit experiences many outpatient or observation days and these are not included in the statistic for patient days, your data are skewed. It can appear that your hours of care per patient day as well as other costs are very high when benchmarked against other comparable nursing units that count all activity (see **Exhibit 14–2**).

If you are responsible for a unit that does not keep patients 24 hours per day, your volume statistic will be different. For example, if you are responsible for an operating room, an endoscopy suite, or a postanesthesia care unit, your volume statistic will be patients or procedures. It is very important to understand which is being counted because a single patient may have several procedures done during the same visit.

- In obstetrics, the volume statistic may be patient days, both mother and baby, or it may be births. In obstetrics, the volume of outpatient tests must be captured as well. That volume can involve a significant number of man-hours.
- In the emergency department, the usual volume statistic measured is the number of visits. However, in these days of overcrowding, when patients can be held in the emergency department waiting for beds for more than a day, it is important to capture those hours beyond the time that the patient could have been admitted to an inpatient bed.
- Long-term care normally counts patient days.
- Some home care organizations weight visits for productivity based on greater weight for opening or reopening a case because of the extensive documentation required to meet regulatory requirements.

It is very helpful when operational reports also provide data about full-time equivalents (FTEs), average hourly rate, and a breakdown of data per unit of service. When looking at the data, you need to understand the meaning of parentheses. In the examples provided in this chapter, negative variances (bracketed data) for *statistics* and *revenue* are favorable. Negative variances (data in parentheses) on *expenses* are unfavorable.

In Exhibit 14–2, actual volume for patient days for both the month (735) and year (3,662) is higher than that budgeted (655 for the month and 3,354 YTD) and higher than what was experienced in the prior year (3,356). The actual observation days (15) for the month were higher (by 1) than the budgeted days (14) but lower (by 1) than the same month last year (16). Year-to-date the observation days are right on target for what was budgeted (68) but lower than last year (75). When combined, the total units, or total patient days, for both the month (750) and YTD (3,730) are higher than what was budgeted (669 for the month and 3,422 YTD) and what was experienced in the prior year (681 for the month and 3,431 YTD). The positive (higher) volume variance of 12.1% for the month and 9.0% YTD becomes very important later when analyzing the resources used to care for that volume of patients.

Exhibit 14–2   Example of a Monthly Report of Statistics for a Surgical Nursing Unit

| Department Operations Report for the period ending 11/30/200_ Main 7 | | | | | | | | | |
| MONTH | | | | | YTD* | | | | |
Actual	Budget	Var%	Prior	Statistic	Actual	Budget	Var%	Prior
735	655	(12.2)%	665	Unit Patient Days	3,662	3,354	(9.2)%	3,356
15	14	(7.1)%	16	Observation Days	68	68	0.0%	75
750	669	(12.1)%	681	Total Units	3,730	3,422	(9.0)%	3,431

*YTD = Year-to-Date

Revenue Budget

Revenue is as important to monitor as expense. Looking at a revenue and expense budget, managers might believe their department is generating a very high profit margin, *even when it really is not. Reported revenue* reflects *charges* generated for the month and YTD by the department, *not actual dollars received for that care.*

In areas with a high population of Medicaid, self-pay, and managed care as the source of payment, the percentage of charges captured can be less than 50%. By multiplying the total revenue by the percentage of charges captured, you can identify the approximate amount of collectible revenue that will result from the care provided and billed. Subtracting the total expenses, which are actual dollars expended, usually does not leave a high profit margin, if any.

> *Total revenue × Percentage of captured charges = Approximate collectible revenue*
> *Approximate collectible revenue − Actual expenses = Net revenue*

For example, the annual revenue budget for Main 7 is $4,119,257. That is the total amount of expected charges to be generated by Main 7 for the year. The budgeted annual expense is $1,816,255. Net revenue is those dollars remaining after expenses are subtracted from revenue. If the hospital received 100% of charges, the net revenue is

> *$4,119,257 − $1,816,255 = $2,303,002*

However, if the true capture of charges is 50%, half of $4,119,257, or $2,059,628.50, is all that will be collected. The net revenue then becomes

> *$2,059,628.50 − $1,816,255 = $243,373.501*
>
>   *$4,119,257*   *Annual revenue (from expected charges)*
> *−$1,816,255*   *Budgeted annual expense*
>   *$2,303,002*   *Total revenue (from expected charges)*
>
> *When charges were actually 50% of what had been anticipated:*
> *$4,119,257 × 0.50 =*   *$2,059,628.50*   *Actual revenue*
>   *−$1,816,255.00*   *Budgeted annual expense*
>   *$243,373.50*   *Net revenue*

That leaves a *small* margin for unexpected additional costs such as greater overtime dollars required or the unanticipated cost of new safety devices.

Before becoming depressed, keep in mind that other departments such as Pharmacy, Laboratory, Radiology, and Surgery normally show much higher positive revenues for the same patients. Those departments would not see higher profits if those patients were not receiving care on your unit.

Just as volume is reported for both inpatient and outpatient, the corresponding revenue is reported in the same manner (**Exhibit 14–3**). In the example shown in Exhibit 14–3, just as with volume, actual inpatient revenue is higher for the month ($355,501) and YTD ($1,794,790) than that budgeted ($318,724 for the month and $1,632,062 YTD). It is also higher than that experienced in the prior year ($286,985 for the month and $1,488,463 YTD). Outpatient revenues for both the month ($5,469) and YTD

Exhibit 14–3	Example of a Monthly Report of Statistics for a Revenue Budget								
Department Revenue Report for the period ending 11/30/20XX Main 7									
MONTH					YTD				
Actual	**Budget**	**Var%**	**Prior**	**Statistic**	**Actual**	**Budget**	**Var%**	**Prior**	
(355,501)	(318,724)	(11.5)%	(286,985)	Inpatient Revenue	(1,794,790)	(1,632,062)	(10.0)%	(1,488,463)	
(5,469)	(5,860)	6.7%	(4,436)	Outpatient Revenue	(23,482)	(28,464)	17.5%	(26,991)	
(360,970)	(324,584)	(11.2)%	(291,421)	Total Revenue	(1,818,272)	(1,660,526)	(9.5)%	(1,515,454)	

($23,482) are less than the budgeted amounts ($5,860 for the month and $28,464 YTD) and less than that experienced in the prior year ($4,436 for the month and $26,991 YTD).

Outpatient or observation charges are usually not reimbursed at a very high rate. Therefore, the shift to higher inpatient charges when the patient stays long enough to convert to an inpatient stay, and experiences less outpatient charges, is positive.

Total revenues for both the month ($360,970) and YTD ($1,818,272) are greater than the budgeted amounts ($324,584 for the month and $1,660,526 YTD) and more than that experienced in the prior year ($291,421 for the month and $1,515,454 YTD). So, this reflects the same pattern (increased amounts) as the volumes.

Man-Hours Budget

Because staffing is usually the most expensive resource in the provision of care, the amount and type of man-hours expensed to a nursing unit is very critical. The monthly operations report usually does not break down the man-hours by job classification such as registered nurse (RN), licensed practical nurse (LPN), nursing assistant, and unit clerk. That information is normally provided in biweekly reports that show individual employee hours and/or man-hours or FTEs by job classification (**Exhibit 14–4**).

Although biweekly reports may not correspond to the exact days, or the month, covered by the operations report, they provide good data to monitor if your mix of staff corresponds to that budgeted. Man-hours are usually broken down into contract, productive, paid time off (PTO), overtime, education, orientation, and other.

Contract labor is usually the most expensive man-hours. Contract staff can be through local agencies or the more expensive "travelers" who are agency personnel assigned for several weeks or months at a time and usually live in local temporary housing. Although they may provide for better continuity of care than local agency staff, their costs include at a minimum hourly rate, rent, food, travel, and car rental.

Productive man-hours are those hours where employed staff members provide care for patients. In the case of direct caregivers such as RNs, LPNs, and patient care technicians, it is the time they are assigned on the nursing unit actually providing hands-on care to patients. For indirect caregivers such as unit clerks, it includes the time they spend on the nursing unit providing their specific indirect services.

Nonproductive man-hours include PTO, such as vacation, holidays, jury duty, sick time, and any other time off where the employee is paid by the organization but does not actually work during that paid time. It is an employee benefit. PTO may be expensed (charged) to the cost center at the time that it is earned or at the time that it is taken.

The time at which PTO is expensed is important to know when analyzing the unit costs for the month. If it is expensed to your department *at the time it is earned*, you will see it charged as an expense against your department based on the hours worked during that month. In this case, it goes into a "bank" that the employee draws against when it is taken. Your department is not charged for it again when the employee

Exhibit 14–4   Example of a Biweekly FTE Report

Pay Period xx	1/13/XX–1/26/XX				
Name	Classification	Productive FTE	Nonproductive FTE	Overtime FTE	Total FTE
T. Moore	Manager	1.0	0	0	1.0
Subtotal	**Manager**	**1.0**	**0**	**0**	**1.0**
A. Todd	Charge RN	1.0	0	0.1	1.1
S. Shaw	Charge RN	1.0	0	0	1.0
Subtotal	**Charge RN**	**2.0**	**0**	**0.1**	**2.1**
R. Barry	RN	1.0	0	0.2	1.2
J. Brown	RN	0.45	0.45	0	0.9
C. Collins	RN	0.9	0	0	0.9
R. Dix	RN	0.9	0.1	0	1.0
E. Fisher	RN	0.6	0	0	0.6
J. Robinson	RN	0.9	0	0	0.9
R. Smith	RN	0.45	0.45	0	0.9
Subtotal	**RN**	**5.2**	**1.0**	**0.2**	**6.4**
J. Edwards	LPN	0.9	0	0	0.9
R. Falls	LPN	0	0.9	0	0.9
E. George	LPN	0.9	0	0	0.9
T. Hall	LPN	0.6	0.3	0	0.9
Subtotal	**LPN**	**2.4**	**1.2**	**0**	**3.6**
J. Adams	PCT	0.9	0	0	0.9
N. Coates	PCT	0.6	0	0	0.6
T. East	PCT	0.9	0	0	0.9
Subtotal	**PCT**	**2.4**	**0**	**0**	**2.4**
A. Thomas	Unit Clerk	1.0	0	0	1.0
S. Vender	Unit Clerk	1.0	0	0	1.0
Subtotal	**Unit Clerk**	**2.0**	**0**	**0**	**2.0**
TOTAL		**15.0**	**2.2**	**0.3**	**17.5**

Note: These are fictitious names.

takes the time off because it was already expensed to you once. You will see it in the detail of what was paid to the employee on your biweekly report.

However, those dollars are not added to the total on your monthly report. If you need to replace the employee to cover the man-hours required to care for the volume of patients, you will be charged only for the hours worked by the replacement employee. If, on the other hand, PTO is charged to your budget *only when taken* by the employee, you will see it included in the total on the monthly report. If, because of volume, you had to replace the employee to cover the man-hours required to care for the volume of patients, you will be charged for that employee's hours, as well.

In most organizations, PTO is earned based on the hours worked. If you use part-time staff members more than their allocated FTE, they will earn PTO on those hours, as well. That will increase the nonproductive time and dollars expensed to your department.

Overtime is that time worked over 40 hours in a week if on a 40-hour workweek. It can include, at the discretion of the organization, hours worked over a scheduled 8-, 10-, or 12-hour shift *even if less than 40 hours are worked in a week*. It can also include time designated as overtime at the discretion of the organization, such as any hours called in and hours worked when on-call. Although discretionary overtime pay can be a positive retention tool, it is also an added expense. It is important to know what the policy is in your organization regarding the designation of overtime.

On-call pay is a minimal hourly rate paid to staff who are not at work but who have committed to be available to work on short notice. It is important to know whether in your organization on-call pay hours stop when the individual is called into work. Some organizations stop on-call pay at the time the employee clocks into work. In this case, if employees clock out before the end of their time on-call, the on-call pay picks up again when they clock out. Some organizations continue to pay the on-call pay in addition to any hours worked while on-call.

Education and orientation hours are those spent learning and meeting the competencies required for the employee's position. With implementation of electronic medical records and new regulatory rules, many hours of mandatory education are being added to the cost of staffing to ensure that all employees are educated about the changes.

In **Exhibit 14–5**, the data demonstrate a large increase in contract labor that has been utilized both for the month (344 hours) and YTD (1,840 hours). Year-to-date in the prior year shows only 284 hours of contract labor was used for the month.

Note the following:

- The budget of 1,575 hours YTD shows that the shortage of employed nursing staff was recognized and plans were made to use agency staff. However, because of the volume of patients and the shortage of regular employed staff, 16.8% additional contract hours were used in addition to what had been budgeted.
- Productive hours were higher than budgeted for the month (5,759) and YTD (28,469) as well.
- PTO was over by 7.2% for the month but 1.0% lower than budgeted YTD.
- Overtime was less than budgeted.

Exhibit 14–5   Example of a Monthly Report of Man-hours for a Surgical Nursing Unit

Department Man-hours Report for the period ending 11/30/20XX Main 7

MONTH					YTD*			
Actual	Budget	Var%	Prior	STATISTIC	Actual	Budget	Var%	Prior
344	315	(9.2)%	258	MAN-HOURS CONTRACT	1,840	1,575	(16.8)%	284
5,759	5,267	(9.3)%	5,291	MAN-HOURS PRODUCTIVE	28,469	26,893	(5.9)%	26,860
611	570	(7.2)%	573	MAN-HOURS PTO	2,883	2,912	1.0%	2,988
192	270	28.9%	363	MAN-HOURS OVERTIME	1,117	1,380	19.1%	1,627
764	750	(1.9)%	667	MAN-HOURS ED/ ORIENT/ETC	3,392	3,825	11.3%	3,933
7,670	7,172	(6.9)%	7,152	TOTAL MAN-HOURS	37,701	36,585	(3.1)%	35,692
44.86	41.95	(6.9)%	41.83	TOTAL FTES	43.24	41.96	(3.1)%	40.94

*YTD = Year-to-date

- Education/orientation hours and other hours such as on-call were over for the month but under YTD.
- The total man-hours for the month were 6.9% greater than that budgeted for the month.
- The man-hours were 3.1% greater than budgeted YTD.
- The FTEs are based on conversion of the man-hours worked into FTEs (2,080 hours per year = 1.0 FTE).

Salary Budget

Salaries are normally the largest expense for a cost center. Salaries are broken down into the same categories as man-hours. The percentage of variance in salaries not only reflects the number of man-hours used to care for a particular volume of patients, but it also reflects the mix of staff providing that care, such as RN, LPN, nursing assistant or patient care technician, and unit clerk. Salaries for the department usually include the unit manager. If nursing education is decentralized, it may include a nursing educator for the unit. If the unit has a clinical nurse specialist, that salary may be charged to the unit, as well.

In **Exhibit 14–6**, productive salaries are higher for the month ($85,670) than budgeted ($76,243), with the variance percentage being 12.4% over budget for the month. The same is true YTD ($424,059 actual against a budget of $381,320 and 11.2% over budget).

Note the following in this example:

- PTO salary is 20% higher for the month ($9,125 actual against a budget of $7,601) and 11.3% higher YTD ($43,208 actual against a budget of $38,826), reflecting the additional PTO earned for the hours worked above budget.
- Overtime is under budget by 32.1% for the month ($4,547 actual against a budget of $6,701). YTD overtime is under budget by 34.9% ($22,283 against a budget of $34,237).
- The ratio difference between the variance percentage of contracted man-hours-to-budget for the month of 9.2% in Exhibit 14–5 is very different from the variance percentage of contracted salary-to-budget for the month of 109.7% in Exhibit 14–6. This reflects the extremely high cost

Exhibit 14–6 Example of a Monthly Report of Salaries for a Surgical Nursing Unit

Department Salary Report for the period ending 11/30/200_ Main 7

| | MONTH | | | | | YTD | | |
Actual	Budget	Var%	Prior	SALARY EXPENSE	Actual	Budget	Var%	Prior
85,670	76,243	(12.4)%	80,107	SALARIES PRODUCTIVE	424,059	381,320	(11.2)%	399,027
9,125	7,601	(20)%	8,567	PTO	43,208	38,826	(11.3)%	42,621
4,547	6,701	32.1%	9,611	SALARIES OVERTIME	22,283	34,237	34.9%	42,610
18,319	8,734	(109.7)%	13,939	CONTRACT SALARIES	95,318	43,670	(118.3)%	15,357
900	2,070	56.5%	251	SALARY/LUMP - SUM/ RETENT	1,982	5,988	66.9%	3,251
8,279	9,184	9.9%	7,119	ED/ORIENT/ ON-CALL/ETC	39,699	46,838	15.2%	48,424
126,840	110,533	(14.8)%	119,594	TOTAL SALARY EXPENSE	626,549	550,879	(13.7)%	551,290

of contracted labor. This is explored further in this chapter when variance analysis and variance reporting are discussed.

- The salary–lump sum/retention is 56.5% below budget for the month ($900 actual against a budget of $2,070) and 66.9% under budget YTD ($1,982 against a budget of $5,988). This could reflect less use of this benefit by the staff in filled positions, or it could reflect open positions.
- Education, orientation, and on-call costs are under budget for the month by 9.9% ($8,279 against a budget of $9,184) and under budget YTD by 15.2% ($39,699 against a budget of $46,838). This could reflect less orientation and/or less regular staff able to use the education dollars budgeted for the unit.

The percentages of the total salary expense line compared with the total units line (in Exhibit 14–2) can provide a big-picture view to determine whether your use of staff is in line with the volume of patients cared for during the month and YTD. In this case for the month, Main 7 was 12.1% above budget on volume of patients (from Exhibit 14–2), whereas salary expense was 14.8% greater than budget. YTD Main 7 was 9% above the budget for volume of patients but 13.7% over budget for salary expense.

When budgeting for the year, you should calculate each expense line based on one unit of service. This budget often is based on the cost per unit of service for the same expense line item from the previous year, plus information about changes that would affect that item. For example:

> If last year the total cost of productive salaries was $941,757 to care for 8,488 patient days, the cost per patient day was $941,757 divided by 8,488 = $110.95 per patient day.

If this year it is anticipated that salaries will increase 3% and that staffing mix and hours of care per patient day will remain the same, the expectation is that the productive salary per patient day will be 3% higher than last year or $110.95 × 1.03 = $114.28 per patient day. This becomes an indicator to use each month as you evaluate your costs. In this specific instance:

$110,533 budgeted salary expense for the month ÷ 669 budgeted units for the month =
  $165.22 budgeted per patient day (from Exhibit 14–2)
$126,840 actual salary expense for the month ÷ 750 actual units for the month =
  $169.12 actual expense per patient day (from Exhibit 14–2)
$165.22 budgeted per patient day − $169.12 actual expense per patient day = −$3.90
The negative number means it actually costs $3.90 more per patient day than had been budgeted for the month.

The same can be done YTD:

$550,879 budgeted salary expense YTD ÷ 3,422 budgeted units YTD = $160.98 budgeted per patient day
$626,549 actual salary expense YTD ÷ 3,730 actual units YTD = $167.98 actual expense per patient day
$160.98 budgeted per patient day − $167.98 actual expense per patient day = −$7.00
So, it actually costs $7.00 more per patient day than had been budgeted YTD.

This shows that so far this year it has cost an additional $7.00 per patient day for salary above what was budgeted to care for patients on Main 7. However, during the current month the $7.00 has been reduced to an average of $3.90 per patient day. Although not back to the budgeted salary expense, the salary expense to care for patients on Main 7 is improving from that experienced in previous months.

Benefit Expense

Benefit expense includes retirement, group health, flex benefits, and Federal Insurance Contributions Act, or FICA (**Exhibit 14–7**). Group health is the employers' portion of the cost for health insurance that can include dental, vision, life insurance, and disability. Flex benefits can be called many things, including special benefits such as dollars returned to employees who maintain specified health habits and physical parameters as an incentive to reduce health insurance costs. FICA is the law that covers Social Security and Medicare. The employer is responsible to pay half of the bill for the employee, and it is charged to your department. Keep in mind that because FICA is based on earned income, if your salary budget is over or under budget, FICA will be over or under budget as well.

Nonsalary Expenses

Nonsalary expenses can include, but are not limited to, purchased professional services, patient nonchargeable supplies, instruments, implants, intravenous solutions, drugs, medical supplies, food service, department supplies, forms and paper, minor equipment, freight, maintenance contracts, repairs, equipment rental, dues and memberships, certification and recertification, books and publications, and travel.

Purchased professional services can include fees paid to physicians contracted to provide services. This could include fees for medical director administrative services such as those paid to the medical head of a psychiatric department. It can also cover fees paid to other professionals who are not employees but who provide services where the hospital both submits charges and receives the reimbursement. An example is for a contracted group of psychologists who provide services to patients where the hospital bills for those services and keeps the revenue. There can also be purchased professional services paid to a physician specialty in short supply that does not receive adequate reimbursement for the services they provide. If these services are critical to the operation of the hospital, the hospital can, using fair market value to ensure compliance with legal parameters, provide a level of compensation in addition to what that specialty collects for billed services. Frequently, anesthesiologists are compensated in this manner in addition to what they bill and collect. This charge is usually budgeted under the anesthesia cost center.

Exhibit 14–7   Example of a Monthly Report of Benefits for a Surgical Nursing Unit

Department Benefits Report for the period ending 11/30/20XX Main 7									
MONTH						YTD			
Actual	Budget	Var%	Prior	Benefit Expense	Actual	Budget	Var%	Prior
4,104	2,674	(53.5)%	3,011	**Retirement**	18,655	13,535	(37.8)%	15,212
10,342	11,533	10.3%	14,112	**Group Health**	51,174	58,551	12.6%	65,960
1,297	1,022	(26.9)%	1,007	**Flex Benefits**	6,977	5,172	(34.9)%	5,092
6,778	5,800	(16.9)%	6,325	**FICA/Taxes**	32,078	29,353	(9.3)%	32,099
22,521	21,029	(7.1)%	24,455	**Total Benefits**	108,884	106,611	(2.1)%	118,363

Patient nonchargeable supplies include items that are necessary to care for the patient but cannot be charged directly to the patient, such as admission kits and syringes. It is important to know which supplies can be charged to the patient and which cannot. Usually, chargeable items have stickers or bar codes indicating they can be charged to the patient.

The instrument expense can be very large in an operating room based on the cost of reusable instruments that wear out and require replacement on a regular basis. This would not be the case on a medical-surgical unit.

Implants can be a very large expense for items in the operating room such as joints for total knee and hip replacements or for the cost of cardiac stents in a cardiac catheterization lab.

Intravenous solutions may be expensed to the department or may be expensed to the pharmacy. Usually, intravenous solutions without medications added are expensed directly to the nursing units. Intravenous solutions with medications added are usually expensed to the pharmacy.

Drugs are usually charged to the nursing unit only when patient charges have not been made and when floor stock is used. The same occurs with medical supplies.

Be very aware of the expense your unit incurs for lost charges. That is, if patient chargeable items such as drugs or supplies like catheterization kits are not charged to the patient, when the drug or kit is replaced, it is charged to the unit. If the staff are not careful about entering charges for patient chargeable supplies, expensive and unnecessary costs occur. More and more organizations have invested in drug and supply vending equipment that requires patient data to be entered before the door can be opened to get the drug or supply. This results in automatic charging of the item and provides automatic data to ensure inventory replacement to maintain par levels in the drug and supply vending machines.

Food service is not patient meals but includes those items that are stocked on the nursing unit for patient use in addition to meals. This includes such items as sodas, crackers, sandwiches, and fruit. This is an item to watch carefully. If your kitchen is very easily accessed, visitors may be consuming food for patients. Although staff are usually aware that the food is for patients, staff may consume these items as well. If you have special celebrations on your unit and have the dietary department provide the food, the cost of the food will be expensed to this subaccount.

Department supplies include office supplies such as ink cartridges for the printers, pens, and pencils. It also includes hand soap, paper towels, and other items that are necessary to care for patients but are not used specifically on a patient.

Forms and paper can be a significant expense. If still using paper documentation in departments such as obstetrics and gynecology, there may be use of copyrighted nursing documentation forms from an outside vendor. Preprinted physician orders and clinical pathways need to be updated as evidence-based practice changes. When policies change, the forms documenting the activity affected by those policies must be changed to match the new policies. Old printed forms may be wasted, or the organization may choose to wait months while stockpiles of the old forms are used before implementing the new policies. At the same time, the setup and printing of new forms can be a significant cost. Most organizations are moving to electronic medical records, reducing the expense of forms.

Minor equipment includes equipment that costs less than the level set by the organization to capitalize the equipment. It can include items such as ophthalmoscopes, video equipment, sphygmomanometers, and chairs. It is important to know when budgeting whether the items you anticipate replacing or purchasing fall into minor equipment or capital purchases. It is not unusual to find that an item with a cost close to the line between minor equipment and capital that was put into the capital budget ends up costing less than anticipated. If it falls below the line for capital, it goes into the minor equipment subaccount even though not budgeted for it.

Dues and memberships include those that are paid for by the organization. An example is payment for the manager of an operating room to belong to the local, state, and/or national Association of periOperative Registered Nurses.

Books and publications include textbooks and journals specific to the nursing care provided on the specific unit. Computer-based learning programs and computerized reference websites may also be included in this category.

Travel is a nonsalary expense that can vary widely. This line item covers all expenses incurred when staff travel to educational programs and includes airfare, car rental, hotel, and food. It also includes reimbursement for mileage when staff travel between locations on the job such as to attend a meeting at another hospital within a system. In home care, this can be a very expensive line item because staff members drive between patients' homes. It is very important in home care to teach staff to set up their route for patient visits on a given day based not only on services tied to specific times, such as drawing fasting blood sugars, but also on the proximity of patient homes. Unnecessary mileage can be cut and staff productivity raised by shortening the time spent driving between patients.

Other expense is a line item (subaccount) that should be used as little as possible and only when the item does not fit the description of any other subaccount. Most nonsalary expenses will fit into one of the other line items and should have been budgeted accordingly. Expense charges to your department should be reviewed for accuracy. If a charge that was budgeted in one subaccount is charged to another subaccount, it is important to recognize and put the item into the correct subaccount. Otherwise, one subaccount may appear under budget whereas another appears over budget. Also be sure that all charges to your department belong to your department. Many people enter charges to your department and errors can easily happen. By identifying and reporting errors, credits are made and should be noted on the report the following month. Keep track of this month-to-month when reviewing your reports to ensure that credits have been posted properly.

Freight may or may not be a line item that is allocated to the nursing unit. Freight charges can be minimized with appropriate planning. The operating room, for example, may have high freight costs if needs are not well anticipated. Overnight charges for implants or supplies significantly increase the cost of freight. Some organizations expense freight directly to the nursing unit that special orders or uses an item. Some allocate freight charges according to a predetermined percentage of total charges to specific nursing units. Others keep freight charges as a single item in the purchasing department budget and charge it accordingly. Ask how freight charges are handled in your organization so that you will know how to respond to the data.

Exhibit 14–8 shows the following:

- No purchased professional services were budgeted or used by Main 7 during the month. However, YTD $250 was actually charged to this subaccount in a previous month, although no money was budgeted for this purpose.
- The patient nonchargeable subaccount was over for the month by 160.9%. The actual YTD expense was $30,934 against a budget of $11,858. YTD this subaccount was over by 52.4%. The actual expense was $92,458 against a budget of $60,656.
- The subaccount for drugs was 100% positive for the month because no expenses were charged to the subaccount and $32 was budgeted. The same is true for YTD with no expenses charged to the subaccount, but $165 was budgeted.
- Food service was over budget for the month by 23.4%. Actual expense was $975 against a budget of $790. YTD food service was over budget by 21.8%. Actual expense was $5,252, although $4,313 was budgeted.

Exhibit 14–8   Example of a Monthly Report of Non-salary Expense for a Surgical Nursing Unit

Department Non-salary Expense Report for the period ending 11/30/200_ Main 7

MONTH					YTD			
Actual	Budget	Var%	Prior	Non-salary Expense	Actual	Budget	Var%	Prior
0	0	0.0%	0	Purchase Professional	250	0	0.0%	0
30,934	11,858	(160.9)%	14,338	Patient Nonchargeable	92,458	60,656	(52.4)%	59,995
0	32	(100.0)%	0	Drugs	0	165	100.0%	0
975	790	(23.4)%	1,068	Food Service	5,252	4,313	(21.8)%	4,736
0	68	100.0%	0	Medical Supplies	0	349	100.0%	0
2,038	1,866	(9.2)%	2,472	Department Supplies	9,668	9,546	(1.3)%	6,429
197	245	19.6%	264	Forms and Paper	1,024	1,254	18.3%	1,204
959	1,134	15.4%	47	Minor Equipment	5,148	5,670	9.2%	1,529
0	216	100.0%	0	Equipment Rental	0	1,080	100.0%	0
0	1	100.0%	0	Dues & Membership	0	5	100.0%	0
136	46	(195.7)%	0	Books & Publications	225	46	(389.1)%	40
228	207	(10.1)%	470	Travel	567	1,058	46.4%	1,325
0	82	100.0%	0	Other Expenses	0	410	100.0%	37
35,467	16,545	(114.4)%	18,659	Total Non-salary Expense	114,592	84,552	(35.5)%	75,295

- Medical supplies, like drugs, were 100% positive for the month. No expenses were charged against the account, although $68 was budgeted. YTD medical supplies were also 100% positive. No expenses were charged to the account, but $349 was budgeted.
- Department supplies were over budget for the month by 9.2%. The actual expense for the month was $2,038 against a budget of $1,866. YTD department supplies are 1.3% over budget with an actual expense of $9,668 against a budget of $9,546.
- Forms and paper were under budget for the month by 19.6%. The actual expense was $197 against a budget of $245. YTD forms and paper were under budget by 18.3%. Actual expense was $1,024 against a budget of $1,254.
- Minor equipment was under budget for the month by 15.4%. The actual expense for the month was $959 against a budget of $1,134. YTD minor equipment was under budget by 9.2% with actual expense of $5,148 against a budget of $5,670.
- Equipment rental was 100% positive for the month with no expenses charged against a budget of $216. YTD was also 100% positive with no expense charged against a budget of $1,080.
- Dues and memberships was 100% positive for the month with no expense charged to a budget of $1. YTD the budget is also 100% positive with no expense against a budget of $5.
- Books and publications was 195.7% over budget for the month because of the expense of $136 against a budget of $46. YTD books and publications was 389.1% over budget with the expense of $225 against a budget of $46.
- Travel was over budget by 10.1% for the month because of the expense of $228 against a budget of $207. YTD travel was under budget by 46.4% with the actual expense of $567 against a budget of $1,058.
- Other expenses were 100% positive for the month with no expense charged against a budget of $82. YTD other expenses were also 100% positive with no expense charged against a budget of $410.

Exhibit 14–9 Total Monthly Salary and Non-salary Expenses for a Surgical Nursing Unit

| | | | | Total Department Expense Report for the period ending 11/30/20XX Main 7 | | | | |
| | MONTH | | | | | YTD | | | |
Actual	Budget	Var%	Prior	Total Expense	Actual	Budget	Var%	Prior
126,840	110,533	(14.8)%	119,594	Total Salary Expense	626,549	550,879	(13.7)%	551,290
22,521	21,029	(7.1)%	24,455	Total Benefits	108,884	106,611	(2.1)%	118,363
35,467	16,545	(114.4)%	18,659	Total Non-salary Expense	114,592	84,552	(35.5)%	75,295
184,828	148,107	(24.8)%	162,708	Total Expenses	850,025	742,042	(14.6)%	744,948

The total of salary (Exhibit 14–6), benefit (Exhibit 14–7), and nonsalary (Exhibit 14–8) expenses is listed below the expense budgets in **Exhibit 14–9**.

Note in review of the subaccounts under Nonsalary Expense that one line item, patient noncharge-ables, accounts for almost all of the budget overage both for the month and YTD. As with the total salary expense line, to get the big picture of nonsalary expense, the total nonsalary expense line should be compared with the total units line for both the month and YTD. In this case, Main 7 was 12.1% (Exhibit 14–2) over budget because of the volume of patients for the month. Total nonsalary expense was up 114.4% for the month. YTD Main 7 was 9% above the budget for volume of patients and 35.5% above budget for total nonsalary expense. This sounds terrible! However, before coming to this conclusion, further analysis is needed.

The *budgeted* nonsalary expense per unit of service is the total budgeted nonsalary expense for the month ($16,545) divided by the budgeted total units for the month (669 from Exhibit 14–2) = $24.73 per patient day. The *actual* total nonsalary expense YTD ($35,467) divided by the actual total units YTD (750 from Exhibit 14–2) = $47.29 per patient day. The difference between the budgeted nonsalary expense per unit for the month ($24.73) and the actual ($47.29) is $22.56.

> $16,545 (budgeted total nonsalary expense for the month)
> ÷ 669 (budgeted total units for the month)
> = $24.73 per patient day
> $35,467 (actual total nonsalary expense for the month)
> ÷ 750 (actual total units for the month)
> = $47.29 per patient day
> $24.73 (per patient day) − $47.29 (per patient day)
> = −$22.56 per patient day
> So, the nonsalary expense is significantly over at $22.56 per day more than what was budgeted.

This is quite a significant overage and requires appropriate analysis. The budgeted nonsalary expense YTD ($84,552) divided by the budgeted YTD total units (3,422) = $24.71. The actual total nonsalary expense YTD ($114,592) divided by the actual total units YTD (3,730) = $30.72 per patient day. The difference between the budgeted nonsalary expense per unit YTD ($24.71) and the actual YTD ($30.72) = $6.01 per patient day.

$84,552 budgeted nonsalary expense YTD
    ÷ 3,422 budgeted YTD total units
    = $24.71 per patient day
$114,592 actual total nonsalary expense YTD
    ÷ 3,730 actual total units YTD
    = $30.72 per patient day
$24.71 per patient day − $30.72 per patient day
    = −$6.01 per patient day

This tells us that the $22.56 nonsalary budget problem for the month is atypical because YTD the overage per patient day is $6.01. Although not as significant as the problem for the month, it still requires understanding and a plan for correction if at all possible.

Variance Analysis

Variance analysis includes finding all the pieces of the puzzle, putting them together, and understanding what the data are telling you about your operations. The pieces of the puzzle include all the various reports you are sent by, or can find online from, the finance, materials management, and human resources departments, as well as unit-specific reports of daily or weekly activity that you create and track. These reports are uniquely named by the organization but include specific types of information. From finance you should receive a monthly *distribution register*. This lists accounts payable payments made for your department. This can include items charged to your department by personnel in your department as well as from personnel in other departments. For instance, supplies required to repair broken equipment on your unit may be charged to your department by facilities management.

It is important to communicate effectively with support departments so that there are no surprises on this report. It will also save you time when preparing your *variance report* if you have made note during the month of special charges that will appear on your department's report. An *accounts payable accrued but not invoiced report* identifies items received on a purchase order but not yet invoiced. An example is dollars you anticipate to be billed for traveler agency staff used during the month. Why not just wait until the bill arrives next month and explain it then? The reason is that you want to link expenses as closely as possible to what happened during the time frame that your variance report covers, which is this particular month. If you know that during the month you will be using 160 hours of traveler agency RN staff because of increased patient volume and open RN staff positions, you want the expense for that to show in the month where it happened. If you wait until the bill comes the following month and the volume is down during the following month, or you have filled the positions and are not using agency staff during the following month, it is much harder to reconcile and explain the expenses that appear to belong in that following month. It is better to tell finance to accrue for the services you estimate will be used during the current month. When the actual bill arrives, it will be applied against what was accrued and already be explained.

A *revenue and usage report* identifies charges by financial class and charge code. Financial class tells us whether the patients were Medicare, Medicaid, private insurance, or self-pay. Charge code tells us how many charges were made for specific services. In the case of a surgical unit, there should be charges for admitted patient days and observation patient days. In surgery, there will be charges for the initial minimum time for using an operating room.

Additional charges under a different code will show for additional increments of time beyond the basic charge. It is important to review this to see that it matches the activity in your department. If on a surgical nursing unit you know that you had 15 observation days but no charges show for those days, you will want to follow up to determine why those charges did not get posted. These become lost charges unless caught before the patient bill is completed and sent out by finance. It is important to find out from your finance department how many days post patient discharge late charges can be added so that the charges are not lost. Lost charges can be minimized if the daily department log is reviewed on a daily basis and reconciled.

The *daily department log* is an excellent tool to ensure that input errors are rectified before a patient's bill is completed. By reviewing this log, you can tell whether a patient in obstetrics and gynecology was charged for 10 deliveries instead of 1. Likewise, if you review the daily department log against the log showing births, there is an opportunity to identify lost charges for a delivery that occurred in the last 24 hours that does not appear on the daily department log. The charges can then be input within a time frame that allows for capture.

The *period inventory expense report* lists expenses from materials management. This is an important report to review to determine both whether supplies are being used effectively and whether your unit was charged appropriately for what was ordered. If you note an increase in the number of intravenous catheters being used per patient day, you will want to investigate. Do you have a bad lot of intravenous catheters, resulting in multiple attempts by staff to start intravenous lines? Did the hospital just change to a new safety intravenous catheter and the staff is in a learning curve? Did you order a certain number of boxes of intravenous catheters and get charged for that number of cases of intravenous catheters rather than boxes? Unless someone is checking this report, the problem would go unnoticed. By noting and investigating, you not only explain the variance but prevent it from continuing. If it is a bad lot, material management may be able to get free replacements. If it is a change in product and a learning curve, select staff members may need reeducation. If it is a charge for cases rather than boxes and it is reported, you will receive a credit for it the following month, bringing your YTD into line.

Payroll reports are biweekly reports that reflect hours by type being paid to each employee. These should reflect the hours worked by staff and should match the daily staffing plan actually worked. Regular hours, overtime hours, shift differential, education hours, and PTO should be listed for each employee. Any special pay-by-type should appear as well. This could be added pay for being a preceptor for new employees or other unique special-pay categories. If you use an automated system for clocking in and out, you may receive individual employee reports from that system that allow you to make manual corrections prior to payroll being cut. Review of these data can identify whether staff did not clock in or out appropriate to the hours the worked-unit-staffing plan reflects. It can also identify other errors that can be corrected to accurately reflect staff worked or productive time. Recognize that biweekly reports do not exactly match to the hours worked, and charged, to a department during a given month.

For instance, as shown in **Exhibit 14–10**, if your workweek is Sunday through Saturday and the month begins on Monday of the second week of a pay period, that pay period will include 8 days from the previous month as well as the first 6 days of the current month. The 7th through the 20th will make up the next biweekly report. If it is a 30-day month, the 21st through the 4th of the following month will make up the next biweekly report.

How then can you compare these reports with the hours and dollars charged to your department for the month? You can't. The important work is to ensure that the hours and dollars charged to your department each pay period are accurate. Finance accrues expenses for the days that have not been covered in the

Exhibit 14-10	Calendar for Sample Month					
Sun	**Mon**	**Tues**	**Wed**	**Thurs**	**Fri**	**Sat**
31	1	2	3	4	5	6
7	8	9	10	11	12	13
14	15	16	17	18	19	20
21	22	23	24	25	26	27
28	29	30	1	2	3	4

current month and reverses them the next month. The important information to know is how the hours and dollars charged to your department for the full month compare with budget. If you are watching the biweekly reports closely, you will not have many surprises.

Unit productivity reports are important to watch as well. Many organizations use national productivity products that compare the productivity of hospital departments with those in comparable hospitals throughout the country. It is crucial to ensure that the specific operations of your department are specified when building the base of organizations for comparison. If your surgical unit cares for orthopedic patients, be sure to identify the type (orthopedics) to determine your comparison group. That is, if your unit cares for patients post joint replacement and post spine surgery, the base of hospital nursing departments you are being compared with should care for the same type of patients. If they care for some post joint replacement, general surgery patients and no spine surgery patients, the comparison may not be valid. You may have some unique differences that need to be added to the equation to have a valid comparison. For example, if your department includes a decentralized nurse educator, add it to the equation. The comparison groups may not have that position in their departments. Also determine whether the productivity tool includes all man-hours or whether education and orientation hours are excluded. Once you have validated that your comparison groups are comparable, this becomes a very helpful tool for benchmarking.

National comparative productivity tools normally report data in quartiles of productivity. The budget should reflect the FTEs the hospital expects to be achieved for the quartile of productivity. For example, the FTEs budgeted for Main 7 are set for the 50th percentile of productivity compared with other comparative hospital units throughout the country. The staffing patterns scheduled should reflect that required to meet the productivity levels budgeted. One of the benefits of using a national productivity tool is that you have the ability to contact staff at other hospitals in your comparison group to network for ideas to improve productivity.

Turning to **Exhibit 14–11**, let's examine productivity measurement. Note the following:

- The volume corresponds to the actual patient days identified for the month for Main 7 in Exhibit 14–2.
- The paid FTEs of 44.86 for the month and 43.24 for YTD correspond to Exhibit **14**–5. Productive man-hours include man-hours contract (344) + man-hours productive (5,759) + man-hours overtime (192) = Total productive man-hours (6,295).
- *Mid* stands for the comparative midpoint of productive hours per unit of service for the 50th percentile for comparative hospitals, derived from the national productivity tool.
- The actual productive hours per unit of service for the month were total productive man-hours (6,295) ÷ Total volume (750) = 8.393. This is lower than the national midpoint.

Exhibit 14–11   Example of a Monthly Comparison of Actual Productivity Performance to Comparative Midpoints for Actual Volumes Report

					Main 7 Productivity						
Name	Vol	Paid FTE Month	Paid FTE YTD	Mid	Actual Month	Actual YTD	Ed/Or % YTD	FTE Month	FTE YTD	Prod Index Month	Prod Index YTD
Main 7	750	44.86	43.24	8.791	8.393	8.425	9%	(2.2)	(1.9)	104.7	104.3

- The actual productive hours per unit of service YTD were 8.425, also below the national comparative goal of 8.791 hours per unit of service.
- The 9% for education/orientation hours and earned PTO hours has been extrapolated from those identified as productive because these hours are not direct patient care hours.
- The next column reflects FTE variance from the comparative midpoint for the month is (2.2). This means that 2.2 fewer FTEs were utilized to provide direct patient care based on the units of service than the goal for the month.
- The next column reflects FTE variance from the comparative midpoint YTD is (1.9). This means that 1.9 fewer FTEs have been used to provide direct patient care based on units of service than expected YTD.
- The productivity index for the month shows that the staff worked at a productivity level of 104.7% compared with similar hospitals and 104.3% YTD. The productivity index is calculated by dividing the national midpoint (8.791) by the actual productivity for the month (8.393) = 104.7%.

From a financial standpoint this is a very positive level of productivity both for the month and YTD. Review of patient satisfaction data and other quality data for the unit will reflect whether this level of productivity is positive from a quality standpoint, as well.

If you do not use a national productivity tool to compare your department with others, compare your monthly productivity with your budget by determining your budgeted and actual hours of care per patient day:

1. Subtract from the total man-hours those hours that are not used for direct patient care. This includes PTO, education, and orientation.
2. Then, divide the man-hour number by the total budgeted units of service.

What follows is an example comparing actual with budget. This example uses the information for the month from Exhibit 14–2 and Exhibit 14–5.

Use your productivity data to understand your variance. If your productivity was less than budgeted for the month, determine the reason. Did you have many staff in orientation but did not get their hours posted to the education subaccount? This would result in education hours being allocated to productive hours. Did you have many days with volumes that forced staffing to minimum levels? An example is an oncology unit with a census of only four patients for 5 days. For patient safety it is still required that two staff members be present on each shift, thereby resulting in a much higher number of hours of care per patient day than required for care of oncology patients. Understanding these data helps you not only to create the variance report for the month, but also helps you and your staff identify areas to explore for changes to improve productivity while ensuring quality of care.

> Budgeted hours for PTO (570) + Budgeted hours for education/orientation
>   (750) = 1,320
> Total budgeted man-hours for the month is 7,172 − 1,320 (PTO/education/orientation)
>   = 5,852 (direct patient care hours for the month)

The total budgeted units of service for the month are 669 patient days. Divide the total budgeted direct patient care hours (5,852) by the total budgeted units of service (669) to calculate 8.75 budgeted hours of care per patient day. Compare budgeted hours of care per patient day with actual hours of care per patient day.

> Actual hours for PTO (611) + Actual hours for education/orientation (764) = 1,375

Total actual man-hours for the month is

> 7,670 − 1,375 (PTO/education/orientation) = 6,295 (direct patient care hours for the month)

The total units of service for the month are 750 patient days. Divide the total direct patient care hours (6,295) by the total units of service (750) to calculate 8.39 hours of care per patient day. Then, subtract the actual hours of care per patient day from the budgeted hours of care per patient day:

> 8.75 − 8.39 = 0.36

This is fewer hours of care per patient day than budgeted, so it becomes a positive variance.

Variance Report

The variance report is a summary of the major exceptions to the budget that are experienced during a given time frame and an explanation of why the exceptions occurred. Most organizations expect these reports on a monthly basis. This important report identifies opportunities to understand and control the exceptions, or variances, to the budget. It is important not only for the manager to understand but also for the manager to help staff understand and become a part in controlling costs. Managers can use the monthly variance data to involve staff in identifying and planning the activities needed to make midstream corrections.

To focus on the items of most importance, only those variances that are large are noted in the report. You need to know what level of variance is expected to be included in your report. For purposes of this chapter, a variance of at least 10% for statistics and man-hours and at least 10% and greater than $1,000 for the month for each line item reflecting dollars is included in the report. YTD information is only referenced to note overall trends for those variances reported on for the month. As a rule, review of the "total" line under each large category such as "total salary expense" or "total nonsalary expense" gives you an idea as to the significance of that area's impact on the budget. Line-by-line review points to specific areas for focused analysis.

Statistics

Refer to Exhibit 14–2. The actual volume of inpatient days for the month (735) was 12.2% above the budget (655), with the total patient days (750) 12.1% above the budgeted total patient days (669). You will use these data in your report to explain variance based on volume. In review of YTD data, actual inpatient days are above budget by 9.2% with YTD total units up 9.0%. In analysis it is determined that the addition of a new orthopedic surgeon has increased the volume of surgeries, whereas the other surgeons are experiencing the number of surgeries expected from them. However, because the new surgeon started practicing at the hospital only 3 months before and has been increasing volume each month, this trend should be noted with a plan to ensure adequate staffing anticipating additional volume throughout the remainder of the fiscal year.

Revenue

Revenue, in ratio to the volume statistics, is also above budget. This information is also used to explain variance for overages in specific line items that are related to the volume and subsequent revenue. Referring to Exhibit 14–3, the total inpatient revenue for the month of $355,501 is higher than the budgeted inpatient revenue of $318,724. Budgeted charges for Main 7 inpatient days can be determined by dividing the budgeted dollars ($318,724) by the budgeted volume (669) = $476.42. The same can be done for observation day charges. Budgeted charges for observations days are $5,860 ÷ 14 = $418.57. Admitted patient days are paid at a higher rate than observation days. Therefore, the higher volume in admitted patient days, and one less observation day than budgeted, results in positive revenue for the month of 11.2%, or actual ($360,970) − budget ($324,584) = $36,386. YTD revenue is up 9.5% from budget, or actual ($1,818,272) − budget ($1,660,526) = $157,746. There is a positive variance in revenue both for the month and YTD based on volume.

Man-Hours

Analysis of man-hours without analysis of salary expense information can be deceiving. In the example in Exhibit 14–5, the only variance significant enough to report is overtime, which is down 28.9%. That appears very positive. Overtime hours for the month were down by 78 hours from those budgeted (budget 270 − actual 192 = 78). Contracted man-hours were over only 9.2%, not enough to be reported. Contracted hours were over by 29 hours (actual 344 − budget 315 = 29). Productive man-hours were over only 9.3%, or 492 hours (actual 5,759 − budget 5,267 = 492). PTO was over only 7.2%, or 41 hours (actual 611 − budget 570 = 41). Education and orientation hours were above budget by only 1.9%, or 14 hours (actual 764 − budget 750 = 14). The total man-hours were up only 6.9%, reflecting 498 hours (actual 7,670 − budget 7,172 = 498). The total volume was up by 12.1%. The trend YTD is similar with total man-hours above budget by only 3.1%, whereas total units are above budget by 9%. This looks very positive, but is it?

Salary Expense

This begins the line items to review for reporting purposes on the monthly variance report. Referring to Exhibit 14–6, dollars do not correlate in the same ratio to man-hour statistics (Exhibit 14–5). Productive man-hours for the month were up by only 9.3%. The dollars represented by those man-hours were up 12.4%, or $9,427 (actual $85,670 − budget $76,243 = $9,427). PTO man-hours were up by only 7.2%. The dollars reflecting those man-hours were up 20.0%, or $1,524 (actual $9,125 − budget $7,601 = $1,524). The salary–lump sum retention was under by 56.5%, which sounds positive and very significant. In reality, it amounts positively to only $1,170 (budget $2,070 − actual $900 = $1,170). Education/

orientation/on-call was also under budget. That positive variance of 9.9% reflects only $905 (budget $9,184 − actual $8,279 = $905).

Now compare the contract man-hour coverage, which was 9.2% and too small to report, with the contract salary variance of 109.7%. This significantly reflects the high cost of contract labor. The 29 hours over budget for contract labor resulted in a negative variance of $9,585 (actual $18,319 − budget $8,734 = $9,585). Added together, the positive and negative variances in salary expense result in a negative total salary expense variance of 14.8%, or $16,307 for the month. This is far worse than the negative 6.9% of total man-hours.

To fully understand the variance in salary expense, it should be analyzed by dollars per unit of service. Refer back to the calculations made earlier in the section titled "Salary Budget"; the actual salary expense per patient day was $3.90 more per patient day than what was budgeted. In analysis you note that you have three full-time RN positions and two part-time LPN positions vacant. The good news is that you have hired three full-time RNs who will begin orientation in 2 weeks. Also, because you have involved staff in understanding the negative impact that those open positions have on overtime, part-time RN staff have been wonderful picking up additional hours, thus keeping overtime down. The mix in staffing has changed, resulting in RNs covering some of the hours of care per patient day that should have been covered by LPN staff. Contracts are coming to an end for two of the traveler contracted RNs who have been covering open positions, and they will not be renewed. Given the expectation of continued higher volume of patients than budgeted, it will be important to fill the open part-time LPN positions to get the mix of staff back to that budgeted.

Discussions were held with the nurse recruiter to find two part-time LPNs. Although the recruiter currently had no part-time candidates, she had one full-time LPN candidate who has experience on a surgical nursing unit. Given the continued high volume and the fact that one LPN currently on staff is in school and wishes to work most weekends to be off for weekday classes, based on staff discussions you determine you could cover the schedule using a full-time LPN. You have scheduled the full-time LPN candidate for an interview. When this plan is fully implemented, the salary expense per unit of service should get back in line with the budget.

A review of total salary expense YTD is similar to that for the month. YTD total salary expense is over 13.7%, or $75,670 ($626,549 − $550,879 = $75,670). An ongoing review of YTD after implementation of the changes being made will be important. Although by the end of the fiscal year, you may not be able to get salary expense per unit of service to meet that budgeted, it should improve significantly from that currently experienced.

Benefit Expense

Although benefits are an expense borne by the department, managers have little control over them. Retirement, group health, and flex benefits are based on choices made by employees. Analysis of benefit expense is useful for future budgeting purposes and to note the impact that it has on the department as a whole.

In Exhibit 14–7, the total benefit expense line shows that overall this category has little negative impact on the budget for the month. The variance to budget is a negative 7.1%, reflecting a negative dollar impact of only $1,492 (actual $22,521 − budget $21,029 = $1,492). Although retirement and group health meet the reporting requirement for a line item by being over or under budget by at least 10% and $1,000, there is normally not an expectation that these will be covered in the variance analysis. Retirement is over budget by 53.5%, reflecting $1,430 (actual $4,104 − budget $2,674 = $1,430). Group health is under budget by 10.3%, reflecting $1,191 (budget $11,533 − $10,342 = $1,191). Flex benefit dollars, although 26.9% over budget, amount to only $275 (actual $1,297 − budget $1,022 = $275). FICA taxes hospital portion, although over budget by 16.9%, reflects an overage of only $978. This overage is the result of the increase in patient volume and the subsequent increase in taxed dollars paid to staff. The budgeted benefits per unit of service are actually below budget. This is calculated as for other unit of service categories or line items:

> *Budgeted benefits for the month ($21,029) ÷ Budgeted volume (669)*
> *= $31.43/unit of service*
> *Actual benefits for the month ($22,521) ÷ Actual volume (750)*
> *= $30.03/unit of service*
> *So, the actual cost per unit of service was down:*
> *($31.43 − $30.03 = $1.40) $1.40 per unit of service*

A quick review of total benefit expense YTD shows that YTD the negative impact of benefits to help absorb the additional hours used to cover the added patient days has been only 2.1%, or $2,273 (actual $108,884 − budget $106,611 = $2,273).

Nonsalary Expense Analysis

In Exhibit 14–8, patient nonchargeables are over by 160.9% for the month, reflecting an overage of $19,076 (actual $30,934 − budget $11,858 = $19,076). What is the difference per unit of service?

The budget called for $17.72 per unit of service determined by dividing the budgeted dollars ($11,858) by the budgeted volume (669) = $17.72.

Actual for the month was $41.25 per unit of service:

> *Actual dollars $30,934 ÷ Actual volume 750 = $41.25*

This major difference creates a good point to test whether the budget was logical based on prior year data. In review it is found that for the same month prior year there was $21.05 per unit of service (prior year month actual dollars $14,338 ÷ prior year month actual volume 681 = $21.05).

To get an even better perspective, you go to the prior year YTD data and do the math:

- The prior year YTD actual dollars spent on patient nonchargeables was $59,995.
- Divide this by the prior year YTD actual volume of 3,431 patient days and you find that the prior year YTD average cost per unit of service for patient nonchargeables was $17.49.
- The budgeted cost per unit of service of $17.72 was somewhat aggressive considering the usual increase in cost of goods from one year to the next and considering the prior year average YTD was $17.49, or 23 cents more than that budgeted for the current year. However, it was known when budgeting that the hospital had engaged a new buying group that committed to reducing the cost of supplies as well as a plan to introduce an automated supply cabinet system.

Looking at recent months (not shown in this chapter), you determine that although the cost had been slightly higher than that budgeted, it was never over the prior year average of $21.03 per unit of service. You know that during the month of November your department converted to an automated supply cabinet system that required switching out many patient nonchargeable items. The last inventory expense report from materials management itemized all the supplies added but none of those removed. A phone call to the director in materials management finds that the credits, which should amount to $17,547 for those patient nonchargeables removed, were not placed in time to be reflected in the November reports.

He assures you that the credits will show in December, bringing the cost for patient nonchargeables back in line with the budget.

Using this new information, you determine what the actual budget should have been if the credits had been placed.

> *Actual for the month ($30,934) − Credits that should have been applied ($17,547) = $13,387*

Therefore, the actual cost per unit of service was

> *Revised actual ($13,387) ÷ Actual volume (750) = $17.85*

Although this is higher than budgeted, all the changes with the new buying group have not been put into place. Therefore, the total decrease in the cost of goods has not been realized.

There are no other line items that meet the requirements for variance reporting. Armed with the information that you have, you are now ready to complete your monthly variance report for your cost center, Main 7. This will be done in an Excel spreadsheet (**Exhibit 14–12**).

Summary

The annual budget is based on assumptions based on experiences from the previous year and what is expected to occur in a given department or cost center during the coming fiscal year. The difference between the budget and what happens is called the *variance*. When you compare the budget to what actually occurred each month and YTD and analyze the variance, you have powerful data to understand what is happening on your unit. Given the multiple departments that can charge items to a given cost center, it also allows for review and accountability to ensure that items are charged correctly or credited in a timely manner. This also maintains the integrity of the data for future budgeting purposes.

Budget variance analysis that uses a line-item-by-line-item approach to determine cost per unit of service puts the information into an understandable context. It reflects the impact of volume and staff mix changes, new technology changes, and other variables experienced throughout the year. Translating and sharing that information with unit staff allows for planning and implementation of measures to creatively manage fiscal resources required for excellence in patient care.

Discussion Questions

1. Why is it important for a nurse manager to understand variance reporting? How does this reporting become a valuable tool?
2. In an inpatient unit, why is it important to determine which statistics are being captured and included to reflect your unit activities?
3. What challenges are present in capturing statistics for the emergency department?
4. What mistake must a nurse manager not make when reviewing the revenue report for his or her department or unit?
5. Because staffing is usually the most expensive resource in the provision of care, what reports would provide you valuable information for this expense?
6. Contract labor is usually the most expensive man-hours. Why?
7. In your man-hour analysis, why is it important to keep track of education and orientation hours?
8. The monthly distribution register for your department should be carefully monitored. Why?
9. You are reviewing a monthly budget where the pay period included both the previous month and the present month you are reviewing. What does a nurse manager do about this issue? What is the financial department personnel's role in this situation?

Exhibit 14-12   Monthly Variance Report

Month and Year: **2-Nov**

Unit #: 7   Unit Name: Main 7   Reported by: N. J. Tomlinson

Account #	Description	Budget	Actual	Variance	Variance %	Explanation
1	Salaries Productive	$76,243	$85,670	$(9,427)	–12%	Total Volume over budget by 12.1% (actual 750 – budget 669 = 81). New surgeon providing higher volume.
4	PTO	$7,601	$9,125	$(1,524)	–20%	Additional PTO earned based on additional hours worked mostly by part time staff to cover volume and 3 FT RN & 2 PT LPN open positions.
9	Salaries Overtime	$6,701	$4,547	$2,154	32%	OT hours under budget by 28.9% (budget 270 – actual 192 = 78). OT salaries under budget based on 3 FT RN & 2 PT LPN positions being covered by contract labor, relief staff and PT staff increasing man-hours.
10	Contract Salaries	$8,734	$18,319	$(9,585)	–110%	Using contract labor due to open positions and volume over 12.1%. Salaries/unit of service are over $3.90 due to use of contract staff. Have filled 3 FT RN positions to start in 2 weeks. Will not renew agency contracts.
	Total Salary Expense	$126,840	$110,533	$16,307	–15%	Productivity is 104.7% for the month & 104.3% YTD. YTD actual salary/unit of service is $7 more than budgeted. However, during the month that has been reduced to an overage of $3.90/unit of service. With filling positions and eliminating contract staff, this should return to budgeted levels.
26	Patient Nonchargeables	$11,858	$30,934	$(19,076)	–161%	Volume up 12.1%. Credits for $17,547 for automated supply cabinet conversion not credited during month. Will be credited next month. With credits, cost/unit of service would have been $17.85. While not on budget, all changes with new buying group not completed.
	Total Non-salary Expense	$35,467	$16,545	$18,659	–114%	With credits the actual cost/unit of service is $17.85 against a budget of $17.72. This should be achieved with use of automated supply cabinet conversion and changes with new buying group.

Glossary of Terms

Benefit Expense—includes retirement, group health, flex benefits, and FICA.

Nonproductive Man-Hours—include paid time off (PTO). PTO includes vacation, holidays, jury duty, sick time, and any other time off.

Payroll Reports—biweekly reports that reflect hours by type being paid to each employee.

Productive Man-Hours—hours where employed staff members provide care for patients.

Reported Revenue—reflects charges generated for the month and year-to-date by the department, not actual dollars received for that care.

Revenue and Usage Report—identifies charges by financial class and charge code.

Variance Analysis—includes finding all the pieces of the puzzle, which include the various reports that you are sent by the finance, materials management, and human resources departments.

Variance Report—summary of the major exceptions to the budget that are experienced during a given time frame and an explanation of why the exceptions occurred.

Comparing Reimbursements with Cost of Services Provided

Patricia M. Vanhook, PhD, MSN, RN, FNP-BC

OBJECTIVES

- Determine areas within the nurse manager's control that influence profitability.
- Recognize whether a service is profitable.

Note to the Reader

1. This process is most effective when completed as a collaborative interdepartmental effort.
2. The information in this section only provides an example. You need to find out current information when actually following these procedures. It is also important to reevaluate the data as conditions/reimbursement/costs change.

Introduction

One very important question the nurse manager needs to answer is *whether the overall unit expense budget falls within the reimbursement amount.* The evaluation activity described in this chapter helps the nurse manager to recognize whether a service line is profitable and determine areas within the nurse manager's control that influence profitability. To accomplish this, the nurse manager needs to have a clear understanding of the different mechanisms of cost accounting used to reflect both services and reimbursement. This chapter explains and provides examples of cost and reimbursement for acute care, hospital outpatient, ambulatory surgery, skilled care, and home health. It is imperative the nurse manager is well versed on this topic to understand and to respond appropriately to cost and reimbursement questions generated from the departmental operations reports produced by finance.

Reimbursement

Over the past 20 years, hospitals, healthcare agencies, and primary care providers have moved from a retrospective cost reimbursement system to a prospective payment system (PPS) where the payer determines the cost of care before the care is given. Under prospective payment, the agency is paid a set fee regardless of the amount of resources used to provide the service. This type of payment system creates some financial risk for the agency and keeps costs under control for the insurer, while also providing financial rewards for services provided at a lower cost. If the agency can deliver services under cost and under the prospective payment reimbursement fee, the difference equates to profit for the agency. However, if services cost more than the reimbursement amount, it results in a monetary loss. Therefore, prospective payment was an attempt to control rising healthcare costs through improved efficiency within the healthcare agency.

In prospective payment, rates are negotiated between the provider and the insurer under a contractual agreement for a year. Reimbursement rates may be for all services offered or for one specific service area, called a "carve-out," such as laboratory. Within the healthcare setting, financial administration under a *capitation* system requires critical financial management and knowledge of the payers.

This has been compounded by the change from a volume-based reimbursement system to a value-based reimbursement system "focused on outcomes, population health management and a patient-centered, coordinated care-delivery approach" (Health Research and Educational Trust, 2013, p. 4). In this new environment, reimbursement can be lost when certain specified care is not received, when never events occur, and when patients are readmitted within 30 days of discharge. *Nurse managers have a key role in avoiding this lost reimbursement.* Organizational performance on quality measures is used from year to year to determine reimbursement amounts that can be lowered when quality is not achieved.

Thus, it is important that the nurse administrator understands the various healthcare payers to appreciate the diversity of billing and reimbursement methods. The two types of payers for healthcare services are public and private. Federal and state are public payers and include Medicare and Medicaid. The insured and uninsured are considered private payers, which are various insurance plans, indemnity insurance, and self-pay.

Reimbursement Sources

For those aged 65 years and older, Medicare is the primary payer for acute care hospitalizations. The home health or skilled care manager will also note a higher percentage of patients covered by Medicare and Medicaid referred to their services because these patient populations continue to be the highest users of acute, skilled, and home health care. Why is this important? It means the government sets the trend for reimbursement for other payers. The nurse administrator must understand the drivers of payment and how this affects the overall revenue for the unit and for the healthcare organization.

Why do differences in reimbursement exist? *Different payers use different strategies for payment of claims.* Therefore, a healthcare agency's reimbursement varies according to negotiated contracts and standard fees from Medicare or other insurers. Insurance companies and managed care organizations negotiate reimbursement with healthcare entities that provide services for their patients. Contracts are established, generally for a year, and are renegotiated by the executive management team at contract end.

This payment pattern is further complicated because the mechanisms of reimbursement vary between acute care, long-term care, skilled nursing, and home health. Payment to the hospital and a long-term care facility is determined by the reimbursement structure the payer uses. It is important to note skilled care may be performed in a long-term care facility and is reimbursed by Medicare for the first 120 days. The residents' care is then reimbursed predominantly by Medicaid and a few private payers.

Different reimbursement mechanisms for services provided may be based on a per diem (specified daily) rate from private insurance carriers, a negotiated fee from managed care (HMO) or PPOs, a prospective payment by assigned diagnosis-related groups (DRGs) or resource utilization groups (RUGs) from Medicare, or the patient who is classified as self-pay. Therefore, *payment is not standardized and varies by the type of reimbursement structure.* The payment amount can differ within these structures as well. For instance, a different negotiated discount could be given to one PPO versus another PPO. The nurse manager can obtain from the finance or billing department a breakdown of payer categories and reimbursement amounts for the patients served.

The largest hospital payer, Medicare, reimburses by an assigned DRG code or an assigned RUG, with a fixed dollar amount for all services provided during the hospital or skilled care stay. Therefore, knowledge of patient and payer mix is essential to understand the variation in reimbursement. Again, the nurse manager should know this information. In addition, the Centers for Medicare and Medicaid Services (CMS) does a "market basket analysis,"[1] and reimbursement is adjusted annually based on the inflation of prices of goods and services incurred by the facility.

The concept of RUGs is that there are conditions that require similar resources and services and therefore reimbursement can be calculated based on the resources used by the skilled nursing facility patient. Routine services such as room, board, administrative services, nursing care, and therapy services are the components of the RUG that are summed to determine the reimbursement.

Reimbursement for home health varies by service. Each payer has fee schedules for the various visits as well as fee schedules for durable medical equipment and for respiratory and infusion therapy services. Under home health care, the prospective payment reimbursement is determined by the standardized assessment tool, Outcome and Assessment Information Set (OASIS), or negotiated fees from private insurance and HMOs. OASIS is mandated by Medicare. *Under prospective payment, neither intensity of services nor supplies can be applied as additional charges.* Instead, the agency must try to maintain costs within the reimbursement schedule.

Medicare established a PPS, called ambulatory patient category (APC), for hospital outpatients. A relative weight is given to each procedure, and payment is determined by multiplying the relative weight by average costs of similar services within that weight.

Costs

As *costs* are examined, it can be helpful to compare the costing of hospital care with that of manufacturing. Consider the patient as the process of manufacturing a car. The patient progresses through stages beginning with admission to discharge, much as a car begins with a frame and is complete at the end of the assembly line. The patient discharge is the outcome of the hospital stay. This is not to say each and every patient receives the same services or that each and every disease process is the same. The nurse manager uses this thought process to identify all areas involved with the patient, including administration, registration, laboratory, radiology, diagnostics, pharmacy, dietary, housekeeping, maintenance, materials management, physician, building and utilities, and nursing with each contributing to the cost of the hospital, skilled care, or long-term care stay.

Hospital cost determination mirrors other businesses and industries with the exception that hospitals have high fixed costs (administration, depreciation, utilities, maintenance, etc.) and must attempt to cover these costs by increasing inpatient volume, adding services, using stringent contract management, and investing in capital to attract more business. Costs are calculated as direct or indirect, and fixed or variable. *The nurse manager should consider him- or herself as both the chief executive officer and chief financial officer of his or her nursing unit or department and develop a good understanding of costs and revenue.* This chapter presents how to determine nursing unit costs and manage the budget.

Hospital outpatient service payments, under the APC, were based on historical average costs. Here, relative payment weights were assigned by calculating the APC median cost of a midlevel cardiovascular clinic visit (that was found to be the most common outpatient service) and assigned a numerical value of 1.0. The assignment of each APC group relative payment rate was determined by dividing the median cost of each APC by the median cost for the midlevel cardiovascular visit.

There are two significant items the nurse manager must understand from this discussion. First, comparison of relative relationship of one APC to another, by knowing the median payment weight is 1.0 and understanding the reimbursement will be less or greater, is based on the variation from 1.0. Second, the hospital is reimbursed separately for each APC billed. Therefore, a patient may have radiological and endoscopy procedures on the same day, with each procedure reimbursed independently.

The concept of RUGs is that there are conditions that require similar resources and services and therefore costs can be calculated based on the resources used by the skilled nursing facility patient. Direct and indirect costs include routine services such as room, board, administrative services, nursing care, and therapy services that are the components of the RUG.

Home health cost determination varies somewhat from inpatient services. The home health agency manager considers different types of visit costs that are provided by a service line that includes nursing care, therapy services, and nursing assistance. The average cost per visit is calculated, much the same as acute care, by applying direct and indirect costs, and allocating for special fees such as accreditation services and other intermittent expected fees. The costs are averaged for the Medicare Cost Report and charges are set at an amount greater than the costs to recoup costs from high level care patients and to provide an established level for contract negotiations for private carriers that ensure costs are reimbursed.

Clarifying the Cost Issue

Defining Costs, Charges, and Payments

It is a common fallacy that the terms *cost* and *charges* can be used interchangeably. *Costs* and *charges* are not interchangeable terms, and the nurse manager needs to understand the difference. *Costs* are determined by the organization's financial accounting system, which takes into account actual costs of supplies, manpower, facility, and administration for services provided. *Charges* are determined by the allocation of costs to the revenue-producing centers and then are used to project an amount needed to recover all the costs. Finally, *payment* is the amount the healthcare agency actually receives for the services provided. All payers pay differing amounts for the same service depending on the type of payer and the contractual agreement between the agency and the insurer.

Projection of reimbursement is calculated by a payment-to-cost ratio that indicates the percentage of costs that are covered by reimbursement. Healthcare organizations use the private-payer reimbursement as a cushion to offset the reimbursement from Medicare and Medicaid because it does not cover the full cost of the services provided. As less is received from all sources, it becomes harder to stay solvent.

The manager must remember that each private payer negotiates fees contractually with the healthcare agency, and payment *may or may not* cover costs. **Exhibit 15–1** demonstrates a fictional example of charge, payment, and cost of a hospitalization. The hospital calculated the costs of care to be $7,250 and determined the charge to be $9,500 to capture any extended costs that may occur as well as to recoup losses that may be experienced from Medicare and Medicaid reimbursement. Contract negotiations between the

Exhibit 15–1 Comparison of Cost to Charge and Payment*

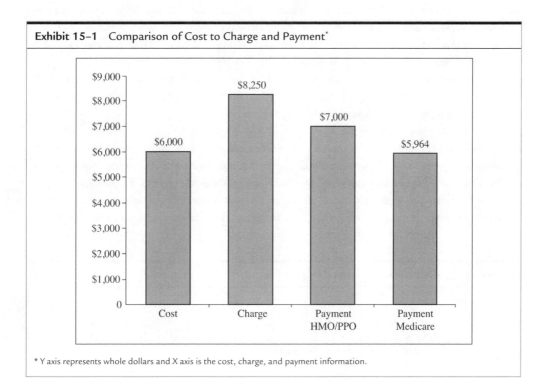

* Y axis represents whole dollars and X axis is the cost, charge, and payment information.

hospital and the HMO and PPO agreed on the reimbursement for the hospitalization to be $8,250. The last column represents the prospective payment from Medicare, which equals approximately 99.4% of the actual costs incurred.

Cost of Service Versus Reimbursement

What if more money is being spent on providing the service than is brought in by the reimbursement? In this case, the executive team needs to determine an effective way to either provide the service and cut the overall budget, decide to take a loss on the service, or stop providing the service. It is possible that we cannot answer this question because we do not know how much a service costs and the actual revenue amount that is realized. This section provides some helpful suggestions that can lead us to finding some answers.

The key financial question is, *Are we spending less than the reimbursement amount to provide the specified service?* A *yes* answer is desired. However, if the answer is that we are spending more than the reimbursement amount, or worse, that we do not know, *immediate action* needs to be taken by the entire management group—including the nurse manager.

Calculating the answer to this question is complicated because most often many cost centers—that is, nursing, pharmacy, laboratory, dietary, medical records, therapies—have been involved in providing the service. So, to answer this question the interdisciplinary team needs to figure all the actual costs expended to provide the specified service. This activity is sometimes called *costing a service*. This costing exercise should take place for all major services provided within the healthcare organization. Let's break this down into priority levels for the nurse manager. The first issue is determining cost.

Cost Determination Methods

Four distinct methods of cost determination are used in health care today (Udpa, 2001). The first method is the *cost-to-charge ratio (CCR)*. Medicare specified this method be used to report annual costs. Thus, most healthcare organizations today use this ratio as the primary source of all hospital costs and cost accounting information (Magnus & Smith, 2000). This report, called the *Medicare Cost Report*, is used by the CMS to calculate and update reimbursement rates. Nationwide data are available as public information from the Healthcare Cost Report Information System, or HCRIS, (at www.cms.gov.) and healthcare agencies use this information to benchmark their costs and performance.

The information contained in the *Medicare Cost Report* includes CCRs for inpatient, outpatient, departments, and functions such as medical education, utilization data, and financial statement data. The report is required for all Medicare-certified hospitals, skilled nursing facilities, home health agencies, and renal facilities. The ratio is determined by dividing the costs by the charges. **Exhibit 15–2** demonstrates the CCR calculation. A ratio under 1.0 (equal costs and charges) is positive and indicates that the organization is making money on the service. A ratio over 1.0 indicates the organization is experiencing

---

Exhibit 15–2   Calculation of Cost-to-Charge Ratio

Cost ÷ charge = cost-to-charge ratio

Examples:
1. If costs are $50 and charges are $100:
   $50 ÷ $100 = 0.5 cost-to-charge ratio (in the black)
2. If costs are $100 and charges are $50:
   $100 ÷ $50 = 2.0 cost-to-charge ratio (in the red)

a loss—the costs are more than the charges (expected reimbursement). In the first example, the service is making money. In the second example, the service is losing money.

Using the CCR, it is assumed that reimbursement (revenue) reflects the intensity of care, and therefore indirect costs (overhead) are assigned accordingly. This method of cost determination does not allow for a full assessment of the true revenue production of a service because all service areas are considered profitable if the healthcare agency as a whole is profitable. In addition, this means that the higher the revenue generation, the higher the proportional allocation of overhead regardless of actual resource utilization. The nurse manager should be aware that CCR could lead to misrepresentation of cost when evaluating the profitability of a service.

The second method of cost accounting is *volume-based measures*, which is much like it sounds. Here, the indirect costs are assigned according to the volume (which may be visits, admissions, nursing hours per patient day) or machine hours (in radiology and the laboratory). A typical example of this measure is demonstrated (**Exhibit 15–3**) when the patient volume increases by 15% on a nursing unit and the nursing hours remain the same. The allocation of indirect cost is increased by 15%. Nursing hours did not increase to accommodate an increase of patient volume, yet the department is allocated higher overhead. It is difficult for the nurse manager to demonstrate increased productivity under this method of cost assignment. The nurse manager must understand the method of allocation of indirect costs to explain variation.

The third approach to cost allocation is the *per diem approach*. This approach accumulates the indirect costs, divides by the number of patient days to determine per diem costs, and allocates the indirect cost equally to all the nursing units. This method considers all patients the same regardless of intensity of care. In a facility that cares for various types of patients, such as intensive care and obstetrics, this method of costing may also distort departmental costs. For example, in 1 month a 10-bed cardiovascular intensive care unit has 100% occupancy and the 30-bed obstetric unit occupancy rate is 55%. The indirect costs are distributed equally to the units when the per diem method of cost allocation is used. This means the departmental operations reports for the obstetric unit and the cardiovascular intensive care unit have the same dollar amount for indirect expenses even though the obstetric unit had fewer patient days.

The last method, *balanced scorecard and activity-based costing*, became a part of the industry in the 1980s but quickly lost favor because of the resources required to initiate and maintain this process (Easier Than ABC, 2003). Over time, the advancement of healthcare management software technology has allowed health care to use activity-based costing (ABC) as a means of identifying true patient costs. This method of costing is more closely aligned with the true costs of caring for the patient (Ross, 2004; Udpa, 2001; Young, 2007). Activity-based costing methodology also resembles performance improvement methods as processes and outcomes are evaluated. The complexity of "procedures and tests involved, the intensity of nursing care, the duration of an activity, and the intricacies of operative and postoperative care" identify

---

Exhibit 15–3   Volume-Based Cost Calculation

For an average daily census of 18:

- Budgeted direct cost (salaries and benefits) for average daily census of 18 = $18,331
- Budgeted indirect costs (professional fees, depreciation, and utilities) for nursing unit for average daily census of 18 = $5,781

For an average daily census of 21:

- Average unit census per day for month $X = 21$
- Actual direct costs for census of 21 = $18,331
- Actual indirect costs for nursing unit for census of 21 = $6,648

the true costs (Udpa, 2001, p. 36). In this method, all areas and processes of patient interaction are identified and costs are allocated to the activity center.

The balanced scorecard adds the quality dimension to cost and reimbursement data. For instance, cost drivers outside the system, such as patient satisfaction, can be measured and reflected in the overall scorecard. In this example, by combining these tools the nurse manager has an excellent overview of the financial aspects from cost, reimbursement, and quality perspectives.

Exhibit 15–4 is an example of a balanced scorecard used by a hospital nurse manager to assess the unit performance against budget and revenue. This type of detail can be obtained from the finance department in a scorecard format if the agency uses this method of analysis. If the agency does not use a scorecard, the nurse manager can create one using information obtained from finance and spreadsheet software. In the example given here, the unit is under budget on expense and over budget on revenue, an excellent position. To truly determine whether the unit is financially sound, the manager needs to *clarify whether the revenue information is what was billed or whether it was the actual amount received.* The nurse manager must remember it is not possible to obtain this information in a timely manner because of delays in both billing and receiving the actual payment from payers.

The following studies have used the activity-based costing method through the hospital cost accounting system to both assess costs and to improve performance and patient care. Lester, Bosch, Kaufman, Halpern, and Gazelle (2001) determined the actual inpatient costs of a patient undergoing endovascular abdominal aortic aneurysm repair. In their study, the direct costs were allocated to the individual units and the indirect costs were spread evenly among all departments. Time studies were performed, and supply costs for each department were monitored. Surgery and radiology comprised 62% of the cost, with nursing contributing 22%, anesthesia 12%, and 4% attributed to an "other" category. The nursing costs reported in the study were allocated to the nursing unit on which the patient received postoperative care. Although nursing costs were noted to contribute only a quarter of the costs, the surgical nursing costs were not separated from the total cost of the operative suite. By combining all nursing costs, it is assumed the total nursing costs would have represented a larger percentage than was presented in the study. However, the nursing costs, whether combined or separate, would continue to demonstrate a lesser percentage when compared with all other costs.

Popp and associates (2002) studied the cost of craniotomies to identify factors that affect the profitability of this procedure. The cost allocation method used was from a cost accounting system that used relative value units (RVUs) to assign actual costs. The method to determine the RVU is based on the principle used by Medicare to reimburse ambulatory and physician costs. By assigning RVUs to tasks, the costs were allocated to different cost centers, which included surgery, radiology, laboratory, pharmacy, anesthesia, physical therapy, rehabilitation, and room and board (nursing). Their findings also supported the research of Lester and coworkers (2001) by identifying 80% of costs for a craniotomy that were allocated into four major areas: operating room, room and board, pharmacy, and anesthesiology. In this study, room and board (nursing) contributed approximately 33% to the overall costs. From the two studies presented, the nurse manager can begin to recognize that although total nursing personnel costs are the highest cost center of a hospital, *the individual nursing unit contributes a quarter to a third of the overall cost of care for a hospitalized patient.*

Nurse Manager's Role in Cost Control

The nurse manager usually has access to information that assists with identification of overall agency costs. Cost drivers that increase healthcare costs include salaries and wages, bad debt expense, depreciation and

Exhibit 15–4   Performance Indicators

a.

St. Mercy Hospital
Somewhere USA

Year:	FY 200_
VP:	Nancy Nurse
Director:	Perry Person
Dept:	Medical

PERFORMANCE INDICATORS	NOV GOAL	JUL	AUG	SEP	OCT	NOV	DEC	JAN	FEB	MAR	APR	MAY	JUN	YTD TOT	YTD GOAL	FY04 GOAL
GROWTH																
Total Inpatient Unit	364	401	308	371	364	365								1,809	1,791	4,263
Total Inpatient Unit LYSM	322	361	346	383	377	322								1,789	1,789	4,370
Total Outpatient Unit	29	21	57	28	49	39								194	186	425
Total Outpatient Unit LYSM	47	28	25	37	42	47								179	179	386
Total Unit	393	422	365	399	413	404								2,003	1,977	4,688
Total Unit LYSM	369	389	371	420	419	369								1,968	1,968	4,756
COST																
Total IP Revenue per IP Unit	$506.13	$497.16	$491.94	$494.79	$494.65	$499.62								$495.78	$506.13	$506.13
Total OP Revenue per OP Unit	$324.59	$168.90	$388.28	$344.11	$377.10	$392.21								$356.12	$324.59	$324.58
Total Revenue per Unit	$492.73	$480.83	$475.75	$484.22	$480.71	$489.25								$482.25	$489.05	$489.67
Salary Expense per Unit	$157.61	$182.54	$169.73	$163.36	$158.81	$152.51								$165.44	$158.15	$159.32
Supply Expense per Unit	$9.56	$8.93	$8.46	$8.89	$8.35	$7.65								$8.42	$9.37	$9.16
Non-Salary Expense per Unit	$27.52	$25.50	$32.62	$26.09	$25.76	$25.32								$26.93	$27.50	$27.38
Total Expense per Unit	$185.13	$208.04	$202.35	$189.45	$184.57	$177.83								$192.37	$185.65	$186.70
Gross Margin per Unit	$307.60	$272.79	$273.40	$294.76	$296.14	$311.43								$289.88	$303.40	$302.97
PEOPLE																
Productive Manhour per Unit	8.1767	9.2633	10.3583	9.1105	8.7301	8.9210								9.2534	8.1746	8.1756
Total Manhours per Unit	8.9135	10.0061	10.8079	9.8303	9.4000	9.6263								9.9156	8.9114	8.9124
Overtime Hours	62	91	15	101	133	14								354	314	745
Overtime % of Productive Hours	1.94%	2.34%	0.40%	2.78%	3.68%	0.38%								1.91%	1.94%	1.94%
Total FTEs	19.88	23.97	22.39	23.01	21.98	22.75								22.82	20.26	20.09
Avg Hourly Rate	$17.91	$20.63	$16.12	$16.69	$16.90	$15.84								$17.21	$17.97	$18.10
Contract Labor Costs	$2,431	$19,168	$468	$32										$19,668	$12,000	$28,705
Contract Labor Hours	44	488	102	17	1									607	217	520
Contract FTE Equivalent	0.25	2.77	0.58	0.10	0.00									0.70	0.25	0.25
VARIANCE																
Productive Manhour Variance		459	797	373	229	301								2,159		
Total Manhour Variance		462	692	366	201	288								2,010		
Productive FTE Variance		2.61	4.52	2.19	1.30	1.76								2.48		
Total FTE Variance		2.62	3.93	2.15	1.14	1.69								2.31		
Productive Salary Variance		$9,469.74	$12,842.59	$6,225.65	$3,870.07	$4,770.04								$37,154.12		
Total Salary Variance		$9,522.00	$11,153.20	$6,112.97	$3,403.53	$4,568.63								$34,583.98		

(continues)

Exhibit 15–4   Performance Indicators (*continued*)

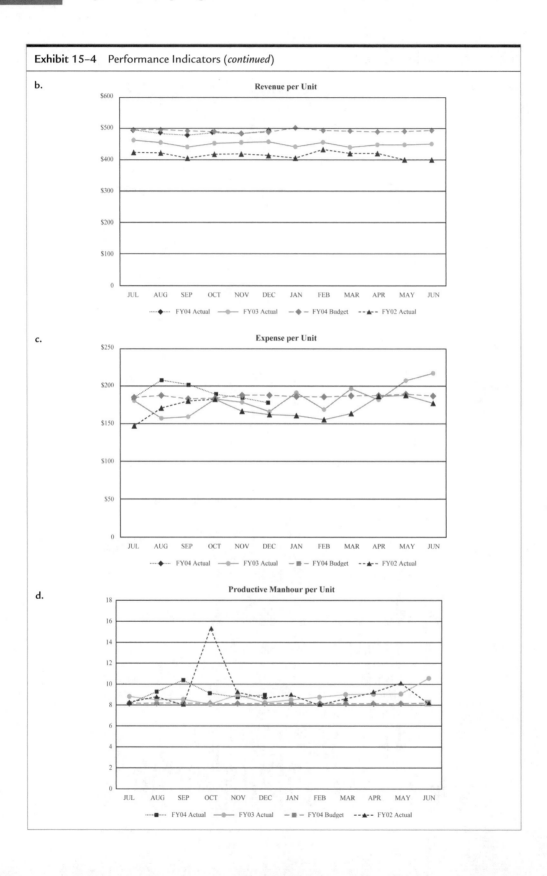

interest, supplies, and direct fringe benefits (an example is given in **Exhibit 15–5**). Understanding the relationship of these drivers to the total operating revenue provides guidance for the nurse manager, who can identify cost areas within his or her control. In this example, the median cost per hospital discharge was $5,619 (Nursing Leadership Academy, 2003). **Exhibit 15–6** demonstrates the contribution of each cost component to the overall total cost for one hospitalization episode.

Kane and Siegrist (2002) reported aggregated cost data for inpatient and outpatient care. *Nursing comprised 33% of the cost for outpatient and approximately 50% of the inpatient cost.* In 2002, salaries of healthcare workers increased by 6.1% as a result of workforce shortage (Carpenter, 2003). However, reimbursement rates did not increase to accommodate this increase in cost of providing care. Kane and Siegrist (2002) noted that small increases in nursing costs have a tremendous impact on the overall cost of hospitalization. The manager must be aware of this impact and plan the budget to accommodate annual performance evaluation raises.

Is the nurse manager able to control bad debt, depreciation, interest, or liability insurance? Of course not. Areas of cost the nurse manager cannot control need to be understood but are not the nurse manager's responsibility. Instead, the executive team must be concerned with these costs. Utilities, equipment expense, maintenance, and administrative costs are fixed costs that do not change as volume changes. (Of course, if the administrative team decides to take actions that decrease costs in these areas, the fixed cost amounts can change.) During the budget period, the manager may be responsible for projecting these costs, or they may be supplied from the finance department. Whether the manager is given this

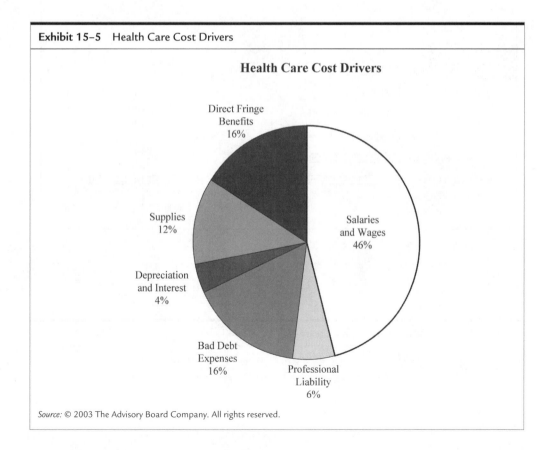

Exhibit 15–5   Health Care Cost Drivers

Health Care Cost Drivers

Direct Fringe Benefits 16%

Supplies 12%

Salaries and Wages 46%

Depreciation and Interest 4%

Bad Debt Expenses 16%

Professional Liability 6%

responsibility or the fixed costs are supplied by the finance department, the manager must ensure allocations are made for unusual seasonal or billing issues that may increase or decrease the expense that has been noted by historical data.

For example, fees associated with accreditation may occur only once every 2 to 3 years, and the cost of this service may be distributed among the nursing units under professional services. Another example is the expense of rental equipment such as specialty beds. The nurse manager is aware of increased use during the winter months because of the increase of ventilator patients. The astute manager, being a clinician, will not only ensure this information is supplied to finance during the budgeting processes but also will be able to provide sound rationale for the requested increased allocation.

Costs within the realm of nursing administrative control are variable costs. These costs vary in direct relationship to volume. Examples of variable costs include nursing hours, patient care supplies, pharmaceuticals, laboratory, and dietary services. Variable costs per patient day are calculated by dividing the patient days for the month into the total variable expense. Knowledge of the costs per patient day assists the nurse manager to improve control of the variation and be fiscally astute. **Exhibit 15–7** demonstrates how the nurse manager can calculate the variable (controllable) costs per patient day.

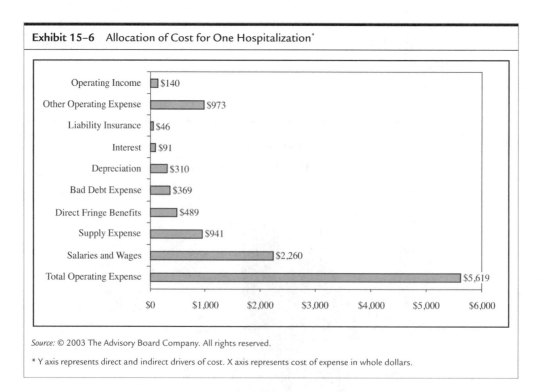

Exhibit 15–6 Allocation of Cost for One Hospitalization*

Source: © 2003 The Advisory Board Company. All rights reserved.

* Y axis represents direct and indirect drivers of cost. X axis represents cost of expense in whole dollars.

Exhibit 15–7 Calculation of Variable Costs

Cost per unit of service equals total variable expense divided by patient days.

($450,000 variable expense ÷ 500 patient days = $900 per patient day)

Managing Expenses with a Cost Accounting System

Under prospective payment it is crucial for the healthcare agency to know the exact costs of care to make responsible and accurate management decisions. The cost of care on a nursing unit may be tracked through a financial cost accounting software system. Cost accounting software was developed after the implementation of prospective payment in the 1980s and has continued to be refined into a useful management tool (Durham, 2000). However, as Durham (2000) reported, less than 30% of healthcare agencies use cost accounting software because of the constant updates necessary to ensure that information is current. The new manager should determine whether the agency uses this technology as a means of financial assessment. If this information is available to you, your job is to diligently manage expenses.

Exhibit 15–8 is a fictitious example of a surgical services report generated from a cost accounting system. The report is for DRG 209, which is "major joint/limb reattachment," and includes hip replacement and fractures that use orthopedic hardware. This summary provides information regarding the number of orthopedic hip surgical cases, cost per case, and hospital charge per case for the operating room for supply items. Note this report does not include personnel costs because the nurse manager only requested supplies to evaluate this area for cost-saving opportunities. For healthcare agencies with this type of software, the nurse manager can request a report customized to the unit and patient population.

Exhibit 15–8   Cases/Cost/Charge Summary for DRG 209 Surgical Services

Metrics	Cases	Cost/Case	Charge/Case
Perspective Clinical Summary			
Anesthesia supplies	464	12	63
Anti-embolism hose/devices	359	96	184
Cath lab/angio supplies	1	124	234
Dialysis supplies	1	35	64
GI/Endo supplies	2	60	335
Implants ortho hardware	501	2,620	7,606
Med/surg supplies	522	2,332	9,840
Orthopedic soft goods	212	109	180
Ostomy supplies	39	6	11
Pacemaker/pacing supplies	2	57	130
Pulmonary/endo supplies	1	8	23
Respiratory supplies	494	35	190
Suction supplies	458	35	190
Urological supplies	440	24	45
TOTAL		**5,553**	**19,095**

Departmental Operations Report

What if you begin work as a new manager at an agency that does not have a cost accounting system? How do you determine the cost of care on your unit? The most efficient process is to determine the average daily census and review the departmental operations report from finance. **Exhibit 15–9** is part of a departmental operations expense report for November 20XX from nursing unit 5 North.

How do you, the new manager, analyze this information? This is shown in **Exhibit 15–10**. The actual and budgeted average daily census can be calculated by dividing the actual or budget expenses total amount by the actual or budget per unit amount. The actual average daily census (this might also be called the average patient volume per day) was 12.7, whereas the budget had projected an average daily census of 16.7 patients. Although the total expenses were 18% less than budgeted (−18% variance that was favorable), the cost per individual patient was higher by 7.8% (7.8% variance that was unfavorable). The contributors of these variances may be linked to employee costs, supply costs, and how overhead is allocated to the department. The manager would need to investigate each possible contributing factor to identify opportunities to reduce expenses or to explain the variation that may in fact be to the result of a higher patient acuity requiring increased nursing staff to provide safe, good quality care.

Now, what if you do not have an operations report? Unfortunately, in many healthcare organizations costing does not take place at this level of detail. A usual mode of practice is to examine the overall bottom line for the organization or to examine costing of a major service, represented by a product line or group of designated cost centers (i.e., cardiology or women's health). Here, the total reimbursement is compared with the total expenditures. In this case, if there is an overexpenditure for one group of patients or services, there needs to be a savings accrued by another group of patients or services because the overall goal is that the bottom line is "in the black" (**Exhibit 15–11**).

The problem with this method is that the *organization may not be aware that one service is losing money and another service is saving money*. Using the hospital example, one DRG may be delivered over cost (losing money), whereas another DRG is costing less than the DRG (profit). So, in a time when the reimbursements are not what were anticipated, services may be asked to cut equally, yet services for one DRG have been efficient, whereas another has not. The nurse manager, working with the nurse executive, can

---

Exhibit 15–9   Departmental Operations Expense Report

Nov 20XX 5 North	Actual	Budget	Variance	Variance %	Favorable/Unfavorable
Expenses Total	87,121	106,305	−19,184	−18	F
Per unit	229.27	212.61	16.66	7.8	U

Exhibit 15–10   Calculation of Average Daily Census from Departmental Expense Report

Actual Expenses Total ÷ Actual Expenses Per Unit ÷ 30 (days in the month)
   = Actual Average Daily Census
      $87,121 ÷ $229.27 ÷ 30 = 12.7 Actual Average Daily Census

Budget Expenses ÷ Budget Expenses Per Unit ÷ 30 (days in the month)
   = Budgeted Average Total Daily Census
      $106,305 ÷ $212.61 ÷ 30 = 16.66 Budgeted Average Daily Census

Exhibit 15–11	Comparison of Revenue and Costs of Two Strategic Service Units				
Strategic Service Unit	Revenue (actual)	Departmental Cost (actual)	Variance	Variance %	Favorable/ Unfavorable
Cardiology	$706,313	$650,980	$55,333	8.5%	F
Women's Health	$325,987	$309,687	−$16,299	5%	U

use these data as an argument as to why cuts should not apply to the unit or units coming in under costs. The following DRG examples are used to further explain actual costs and reimbursement.

DRG Costing Examples

Let's examine a hospital DRG to determine whether we are spending more or less than the reimbursement amount to provide the specified service. You are a hospital nurse manager/director/nurse executive responsible for an orthopedic cost center. A typical service provided on this cost center is DRG 209: Major Joint/ Limb Reattachment Procedure, Low Extremities—No Complications (for Total Hip Replacement) and the Medicare reimbursement for this DRG is $9,269. Do you actually know how much you are expending to provide that DRG?

In this particular DRG, there is a further complication: The costs of the prosthesis and direct supplies needed to do the total hip replacement may expend more than 50% of the reimbursement dollars. So, the amount of money left to provide all other services this patient requires from admission to discharge must be low enough to stay within approximately 50% ($4,600) of the reimbursement amount. The question then is whether the service provided to a patient utilizing DRG 209 is less than $4,600. Or, in providing that service, is the service cost above that amount? If the latter is true, the organization is losing money on each patient having a total hip replacement. ***With profit margins as tight as they currently are in health care, it is very important that the nurse manager—as well as the executive team—know actual costs of the services provided.***

Using the total hip replacement example, figuring out costs is further complicated because the reimbursement amount includes services and supplies delivered from several cost centers (i.e., operating room, laboratory, pharmacy, radiology, physical therapy, and the orthopedic inpatient unit). So, if the orthopedic nurse manager is working on the cost of this DRG, other cost center managers need to provide their departmental costs of service assigned to each hip replacement patient to calculate the total DRG cost. (Interdepartmental collaboration is very important. This is a good example that portrays the importance of department managers working together effectively.)

As a nurse manager figures nursing costs on the orthopedic inpatient unit, she or he will need to figure out the cost of the nursing care provided as well as the cost of materials and supplies, pharmaceuticals, and other expenses incurred while on this unit. If the nurse manager takes a typical patient and works out costs incurred with that patient, this can provide a basis for determining costs associated with the DRG. When examining nursing time spent with the patient, if there is a patient classification system in place, this can be used. If this is not available, there is a way to cost out the direct and indirect nursing time spent for this patient. (An example can be found in Finkler, Jones, and Kovner, 2013.)

The following provides a specific patient example to demonstrate a case scenario for a patient admitted for a total hip replacement.

Jill Anderson is a 78-year-old woman with severe degenerative arthritis of the right hip. She has been evaluated by the orthopedic surgeon, who recommends a total hip replacement. Ms. Anderson agrees to the surgery and is scheduled for the procedure 1 week from the office visit. **Exhibit 15–12** is a representation of the hospital costs incurred for a 3-day length of stay for a total hip replacement (DRG 209).

Exhibit 15–12   Costs for DRG 209 Total Hip Replacement

Day	Med surg	OR	Pharmacy	Pharmacy IV	Implants	Pathology	Lab	Supplies	Blood	Physical Therapy	TOTAL
1 (Adm)	480	2,800	253	120	4,600	54	380	217	175	0	9,079
2	480		384				32			175	1,071
3	480		64				21			126	691
4 (D/C)			22	42			32				96
Total	1,440	2,800	723	162	4,600	54	465	217	175	301	10,937

As the manager can see, the cost of providing this service is greater than the reimbursement by $1,668 ($10,937 actual cost – $9,269 reimbursement = $1,668 actual loss), and an average case load of 500 total hips for the year would cost the hospital $834,000.

How can this procedure be profitable for the hospital? First, the interdisciplinary team must work aggressively to transfer the patient to another level of care, such as skilled care, as soon as medically indicated. The hospital also generates additional revenue from the other services the orthopedic surgeon orders for the patient, such as the surgical procedure, outpatient radiology studies, outpatient physical therapy, and referrals to a skilled nursing unit housed within the facility. By standardization of the hip prosthesis being used, the hospital can negotiate a contract with a supplier to be the vendor of choice and thereby decrease costs. Also, the hospital may opt to purchase a prosthesis that costs less money. In addition, the volume of patients can be an important factor. We know that excellent patient satisfaction leads to the patient using the facility as his or her hospital of choice. As the manager can see, many global issues are reviewed by management in deciding to provide a service line.

Now, let's take the same patient admitted to the skilled nursing unit. As you recall, the skilled units are reimbursed by RUGs consisting of the costs for administration, room and board, nursing service, and therapy services. The length of stay on the skilled unit for Ms. Anderson is 11 days.

Ms. Anderson's RUG category is "ultra high" because her admission assessment indicated her need for nursing care, physical therapy, and occupational therapy (U.S. General Accounting Office, 2002). In the ultra high category, therapy must demonstrate Ms. Anderson received a total of 720 minutes of services in 7 days (Medicare SNF-PPS Indices, 2003). The reimbursement and cost for the ultra high category is noted in **Exhibit 15–13**. As you can see, the skilled care facility is losing $800 per day of care and services provided to Ms. Anderson. In addition, as her therapy and nursing care requirements decrease as she improves, the reimbursement also decreases. After her 7-day assessment, the reimbursement for her care decreases to $296.15 per day.

How does a healthcare agency afford to care for patients like Ms. Anderson? Van der Walde and Lindstrom (2003) report that freestanding skilled nursing facilities have fewer Medicare and more private pay patients, whereas a skilled nursing facility in an acute care facility admits a higher percentage of Medicare patients. As their report indicates, the freestanding skilled nursing facilities are profitable, whereas skilled nursing facilities in an acute care setting are not profitable. Many hospitals have closed their skilled nursing facilities because of the continued financial drain on the agency.

The next two examples demonstrate costs and reimbursement for a home health and same-day surgery patient. It is probable that ACA will change the available days, but this scenario presents a way to approach

Exhibit 15–13	RUG III Reimbursement for Ultra High Level of Care			
Category	Nursing Care	OT, PT, Speech	Room, Board, and Administration	Total Rate per Day
Ultra high*	$142.32	$186.01	$55.88	$384.21
Actual costs	$444.03	$574.30	$165.77	$1,184.10
Difference	−$301.71	−$388.29	−$109.89	−$799.89

* Difference in RUG rates obtained from http://www.cms.gov/providers/snfps/snfpps_rates.asp. Actual costs calculated from historical data from a skilled nursing facility.

the costing exercise for home health. As you recall, home health came under prospective payment in October 2000, and outpatient surgery also began to be reimbursed by APCs in 2000. The following case scenario is provided to explain the method used for a scenario about home care.

Mr. Harold James is a 78-year-old diabetic, hypertensive, African American with new onset atrial fibrillation who has survived a right hemispheric stroke (DRG 14). His deficits include left hemiparesis and speech difficulties, and he is discharged from a skilled nursing facility to home with a home health referral. Home health skilled nursing care includes medication management for diabetes and anticoagulation in addition to medication education. The following additional services will be used: physical therapy three times a week, speech therapy twice a week, and certified nursing assistant visits three times a week. As Mr. James continues to improve, the certified nursing assistant visits will be discontinued and occupational therapy will begin services three times a week. Medicare covers 60 days of home health service, and a total of 66 home visits will be made during the 60-day period (www.cms.gov/).

Because home health for this patient is primarily labor intensive, the manager can predict the cost of care by calculating the salaries and benefits for each team member, adding supplies and overhead, multiplying by number of visits, and finally multiplying this number by two (average hours spent in the home by each caregiver). **Exhibit 15–14** demonstrates this calculation.

Under prospective payment, our patient reimbursement is $6,098. Because the total cost for Mr. James is $6,428.80, the agency will lose $330.80 for this patient (i.e., $6,428.80 total cost – $6,098 reimbursement = $330.80). For this reason, many home health agencies have limited the complex cases they enroll in their service (van der Walde & Choi, 2003b).

In the present scenario, the home health manager is also faced with the issue of the short-term home health admission. For example, a new diabetic may be ordered to receive home health visits for teaching. The visits are limited to three. The cost of admitting the patient to the service is $200 due to the time and intensity of the assessment as well as completion of OASIS. Our previous calculation indicates the cost of the two remaining visits (plus supplies of $25) is $155.10. The payer reimburses only $90 for each visit ($270 total), and the agency again loses $85.10. Although the manager may believe this is a small amount, over time the agency will not be self-sustaining as a result of losses from complex patients and short-term admissions. Therefore, the home health manager must be creative and identify areas of savings such as decreasing supply costs that are not reimbursable and set budget expenditures based on historical data that provide insight into payer reimbursements, as well as the types of patients admitted to the agency.

The same-day surgery patient, under prospective payment, receives services reimbursed by APC codes. These are based on RVUs, which are a measure of time and resources that are bundled into hundreds of assigned categories (van der Walde & Choi, 2002). Many outpatient services have benefited from the APC process of reimbursement, more so from the private payers than Medicare. **Exhibit 15–15** shows

Exhibit 15–14   Projection of Home Health Care Costs for 60 Days of Care

Salary/hr × benefits (20%) + supplies + overhead × no. visits × average time/visit =costs

RN costs	= ($18.79/hr × 0.2)	+ $37.45	+ $30	× 12	× 2	=	$2,160.00
PT costs	= ($19.50 × 0.2)	+ $0	+ $30	× 16	× 2	=	$1,708.80
CNA costs	= ($8.50 × 0.2)	+ $20.00	+ $30	× 16	× 2	=	$1,926.40
OT costs	= ($19.00 × 0.2)	+ $0	+ $30	× 6	× 2	=	$633.60
Total costs	=						$6,428.80

CNA, certified nursing assistant; OT, occupational therapy; PT, physical therapy; RN, registered nurse.

Exhibit 15–15   Same Day Surgery Cost and Reimbursement for Laparoscopic Cholecystectomy

51.23 Laparoscopic cholecystectomy	Charge code units (RVU)	Charges	Actual payment	Total Direct Costs	Total Indirect Costs	Total Cost
Private Insurance						
1662 Anesthesia	9	$1,658		$240	$77	$317
1665 Same day surgery	29	$4,514		$1,140	$927	$2067
1710 Central supply	6	$264		$131	$34	$165
1715 Pharmacy	12	$352		$96	$21	$117
1720 Pathology	1	$175		$12	$9	$21
1722 Lab	3	$91		$16	$6	$22
TOTAL Private Insurance	**60**	**$7,054**	**$4,573**	**$1,635**	**$1,074**	**$2,709**
Medicare Patient						
1662 Anesthesia	7	$1,384		$201	$64	$265
1665 Same day surgery	28	$4,546		$1,065	$866	$1,931
1710 Central supply	5	$255		$126	$33	$159
1715 Pharmacy	16	$469		$127	$28	$155
1722 Lab	5	$135		$26	$11	$37
TOTAL Medicare Payment	**61**	**$6,789**	**$1,767**	**$1,545**	**$1,002**	**$2,547**

a comparison of costs and reimbursement for a same-day surgery laparoscopic cholecystectomy. The first example is a 42-year-old woman with private insurance, and the second is a 70-year-old man with Medicare.

From the previous example, the manager has an understanding that the private insurance carriers truly offset the cost of caring for the Medicare patient, although this margin is narrowing as less is received from private payers. The manager, knowledgeable of payer mix, can determine the financial feasibility of the service that is provided by the same-day surgery facility.

Other Factors Contributing to Reimbursement

Reimbursement is a complex issue. The information provided earlier in the chapter is from a broad perspective and can be generalized to healthcare agencies. Medicare participants are the largest users of healthcare services. In this section, additional information is provided that contributes to Medicare reimbursement. The nurse manager can retrieve this information, in addition to the annual market basket updated fees for Medicare reimbursement, from the CMS website (www.cms.gov).

Operating payments are additional payments to the base DRG reimbursement and vary from large urban (population over 1 million) to other urban and rural hospitals. The reimbursement rate for hospitals has been tied to their quality performance. For example, hospitals that reported successful quality measures for 2008 received 3% increase in reimbursement. Those hospitals that did not report successful quality measures received only a 1% increase in reimbursement. These amounts are adjusted for the area market basket update.

Revenue Budget

Nursing Service Does Generate Revenue

In the healthcare organization—whether hospital, long-term care, home care, or ambulatory settings—nursing services provide organizational revenue. If you are a nurse manager on an inpatient unit, you may hear a finance employee say your unit does not generate revenue. Technically, on an inpatient unit you probably do not have a revenue account—unless you have oncology services, operating room, or a service that can be directly billed. Instead, nursing services on inpatient units are most often included in the room rate charge, and the finance department keeps the records of revenues. However, nursing care does generate and contribute to the revenue generation for the DRG payment in hospitals and for the minimum data set (MDS) reimbursement in long-term care. In this example, revenue becomes muddy because so many disciplines are involved in the patient's care. Remember that patients always come to inpatient units because they need nursing care. Nursing services have traditionally been directly billed in home care as a separate line item. Two states, Maine and Maryland, have recognized nursing's contributions and have specified that hospitals take nursing service out of the room rate charge and list it as a separate item on the patient's bill. More efforts are being made to get nursing taken out of the room rate in hospitals, but to date this has not occurred. This could mean that more inpatient units will be considered profit centers and have a revenue budget.

As noted previously, it is important in the value-based environment that nursing staff give care meeting the reimbursement mandates for protocols, for preventing never events, and for coordinating care so that patients are not readmitted within 30 days. ***Nurse managers have a key role in making sure revenue is not lost in these instances.***

There may be other services or items that can be directly billed, such as operating room procedures, ambulatory services, home care services, drugs, supplies, educational programs, physical or respiratory therapy, consultation services, or wellness programs. In these programs, nurse managers usually have a revenue budget, often called a profit center. In this case, the cost center's services are directly billed to patients. In these settings, the revenue budget is used to make sure that the organization/department/clinic remains viable.

Currently, revenues are reported only occasionally on inpatient cost center budgets. If this occurs, the nurse manager must seek information to learn what these figures represent: Are they billed dollars or are these dollars actually received? Are contractual allowances or discounts included in the revenue figures? Is the figure so unreliable that the nurse manager should just ignore it, or does it provide useful data?

When the nurse manager gets a revenue report for billable supplies or services, most often provided by the finance department, the nurse manager should check the accuracy of the figures and then compare costs and revenue. **Exhibit 15–16** is an example of a detailed nursing unit operations report that includes revenues for inpatient and outpatient sources. Revenue in this type of financial report does not equal true

Exhibit 15–16   Monthly Nursing Departmental Revenue Report by Payer

| | | | 5 North   Nov-0_ | | |
	Actual*	Budget	Variance	Variance %	Favorable/ Unfavorable
INPATIENT REVENUE					
Medicare	167,519	282,683	−115,164	−40.7	U
Medicaid	22,050	34,802	−12,752	−36.6	U
Managed care	29,578	44,515	−14,937	−33.6	U
Commercial	15,004	9,237	5,767	62.4	F
Self-pay	27,293	5,294	21,999	415.5	F
Other	2,406	3,368	−962	−28.6	U
Total	**263,850**	**379,899**	**−116,049**	**−30.5**	**U**
per unit	**782.94**	**796.43**	**−14**	**−1.7**	**U**
OUTPATIENT REVENUE					
Medicare	16,254	9,624	6,630	68.9	F
Medicaid	5,044	3,994	1,050	26.3	F
Managed care	3,388	6,913	−3,525	−51.0	U
Commercial	627	1,031	−404	−39.2	U
Self-pay	1,533	587	946	161.2	F
Other	627	165	462	280.0	F
Total	**27,473**	**22,314**	**5,159**	**23.1**	**F**
per unit	**639**	**970**	**−331**	**−34.1**	**U**
REVENUE TOTAL	**291,323**	**402,213**	**−110,890**	**−27.6**	**U**
per unit	**767**	**804**	**−38**	**−4.7**	**U**

* The *Actual* column represents gross revenue times the ratio of costs to charges from the Medicare/Medicaid report.

reimbursement but is a CCR that is used in the *Medicare Cost Report*. The manager can also note from this report the distribution of payers for the department.

How is this information interpreted? The first column provides the payer source identified in the CCR. Following the reimbursement are the budgeted dollars expected to be collected. The next column is the variance between actual CCR and what was budgeted, or Actual – Budgeted = Variance. Percent variance follows next. This is the percent deviation between the actual column and the budgeted column. The last column shows whether the variance is favorable (F) or unfavorable (U). As you can tell from this report, the revenue total for both in- and outpatient is below the budgeted amount at an unfavorable 4.7%.

The nurse manager must seek information to explain the variation from budget. For this unit, two areas were identified as reasons for the budget variation. First, the census was lower than expected by the budgeted amount, and second, there was decreased reimbursement from contractual agreements that went into effect in the previous month of October. Although nursing management cannot directly affect contractual agreements, nursing does have a strong influence on the census through providing high-quality, safe care the patient and family value as well as by building a trusting relationship with physicians, patients, colleagues, and others in the organization. When everyone acts as an effective team, magic happens.

However, this variance is only a piece of the information the nurse manager has to consider. The manager must also compare the same period last year as well as the year-to-date financials to have the total picture of the unit financial performance. **Exhibit 15–17** provides the fiscal year-to-date financial information for 5 North. This nursing unit is generating 5.2% less than budgeted revenue for the fiscal year to date.

The challenge now is for the nurse manager to be knowledgeable not only of employee and supply expense but also the unit's primary admission and diagnoses, length of stay, complication rates, and reimbursement per DRG. The manager should review the DRG historical admission and discharge history of the unit. Then, the nurse manager can evaluate the unit patient population and identify trends or changes in patient base that may require an expansion of nursing knowledge and skills. In addition, the manager should ask for the following information: length of stay by discharge diagnosis, list of secondary diagnosis, and complications. An analysis of this information will guide the manager to identify areas for improving care to decrease complications (which are costly and are not reimbursed), improve efficiency, decrease supply and manpower costs, and thereby improve the financial performance of the nursing unit.

Exhibit 15–17   Year-to-Date (YTD) Nursing Department Revenue Report by Payer

| | | 5 North | FYTD | Nov-0_ | |
	Actual*	Budget	Variance	Variance %	Favorable/ Unfavorable
INPATIENT REVENUE					
Medicare	1,120,051	1,358,542	−238,491	−17.6	U
Medicaid	205,504	167,253	37,801	22.6	F
Managed care	141,956	213,932	−71,976	−33.6	U
Commercial	67,857	44,392	23,465	52.9	F
Self-pay	50,315	25,440	24,875	97.8	F
Other	12,824	16,187	−3,363	−20.8	U
Total	**1,598,507**	**1,825,746**	**−227,689**	**−12.5**	**U**
per unit	**798.63**	**796.23**	**2.40**	**0.3**	**F**
OUTPATIENT REVENUE					
Medicare	88,162	47,653	40,509	85.0	F
Medicaid	18,805	19,776	−971	−4.9	U
Managed care	32,321	34,229	−1,908	−5.6	U
Commercial	3,615	5,106	−1,491	−29.2	U
Self-pay	5,451	2,907	2,544	87.5	F
Other	4,117	817	3,300	403.9	F
Total	**152,471**	**110,488**	**41,983**	**38.0**	**F**
per unit	**520.38**	**977.77**	**−457.39**	**−46.8**	**U**
REVENUE TOTAL	**1,750,978**	**1,936,234**	**−185,706**	**−9.6**	**U**
per unit	**763.09**	**804.75**	**−41.66**	**−5.2**	**U**

* The *Actual* column represents gross revenue times the ratio of costs to charges from the Medicare/Medicaid report.

Another area that affects the financial performance of a nursing unit is the contractual agreements made between the hospital financial management team, a managed care organization, and a preferred price for supplies based on utilization. *Contractual agreements* are negotiations between the healthcare agency and the health insurer or provider of services and supplies. Contracts may range from the amount paid by the insurer for a specific diagnosis to the amount of supply charges based on utilization. The nurse manager does not have control over contract negotiations but plays a significant role in providing information regarding changes in patient care that influence negotiated reimbursement or prices. In addition, the nurse manager must be aware of the dates of contract renewals to recognize shortfalls during the budget planning process.

Currently, two other factors affect payments. First, as the general population is aging, a higher percentage will be on Medicare. But more significantly, because ACA has indicated that everyone will have insurance, there will be a much higher number of patients on Medicaid. The current depression also places more people at the poverty level, thus adding to Medicaid numbers.

Exhibit 15–17 demonstrates an example of how changes in patient payers and contractual agreements affect the nursing units' budget. In this example, Medicare admissions decreased, private insurance decreased contractual reimbursement, and there was an increase in self-pay patients, which often contributes to indigent care services as well as nonpayment issues. The key factor that cannot be seen in the example is that the private insurance contract negotiations occurred after the budget had been set and a lower reimbursement was negotiated by management as a means to increase patient volume by this carrier. The manager needs to continually evaluate admissions by payer to identify whether the negotiated contract actually increased admissions for the nursing unit.

Predicting Financial Success

The case mix index has been used by hospital administrators to predict financial success since prospective payment was instituted. The nurse manager can use this tool to predict financial success at the nursing unit level. DRGs are divided into 25 major diagnostic categories (MDCs) that include the following information: DRG number, narrative description, relative weight, geometric length of stay, arithmetic length of stay, and outlier threshold. The relative weight is an assigned number that is an indicator of the amount of resources needed to care for the patient with that particular disease process and includes all costs related to the hospitalization (Adams, 1996). The nurse manager should understand that the higher the weight, the more resources needed to care for the patient. The amount of resources needed to treat a particular disease process is the relative weight. A disease requiring many resources, such as total joint replacement, carries a higher weight than atypical chest pain.

From this information, as well as knowledge of supply costs and personnel expense, the nurse manager can be proactive in departmental financial management. Further, the nurse manager can alert the nurse executive and finance department about important reimbursement issues (i.e., lost revenues, higher expenses than revenues). In addition, the nurse manager must realize the hospital's DRG payment rate is also contingent on geographic location, wage index, and patient mix.

The nurse manager should obtain the top 10 DRGs for the nursing unit from the coding department (usually located in Medical Records). By knowing this information, the manager can influence reimbursement on the unit by assisting staff and physicians to document thoroughly for accurate coding.

The manager may choose to select one DRG that is costing more than the reimbursement, establish a multidisciplinary team to evaluate processes of care that may affect patient outcomes and increase cost, and strategize to determine less costly ways to deliver the care safely and efficiently. The utilization review/case manager should play an important role in this function of coding.

Nursing Management Decisions Affect Financial Outcomes

The nurse manager must be cognizant of unit expenses, including personnel and supplies. These are two key areas that nursing can affect to ensure a positive bottom line. The flow of patients into and out of a service area determines the staffing and supplies needed. Nursing must have financial savvy and be creative to manage within this environment.

As previously noted nurse manager involvement is very important in meeting specified protocols, preventing never events, and preventing hospital readmissions within 30 days. These actions can result in revenue not being lost.

In long-term care, reimbursement for Medicaid patients is actually determined by the nurse and depends on how well the nurse has completed the MDS.

Usually, to accomplish a detailed evaluation of cost versus reimbursement, the nurse manager can facilitate an interdisciplinary management team to determine and compare actual costs of the services provided with the reimbursement amount received for those services. The organization and participation on such a team can help all disciplines within the organization to become cognizant of the importance of rectifying systems problems that can contribute significantly to higher costs if left unidentified and unresolved.

Summary

Cost and reimbursement issues are difficult to understand because of the complexity. This is because there are many different ways that costs are calculated and because it is important to know which payer is paying what amount. Hopefully, this chapter has assisted the manager to have an improved understanding of fiscal management for the nursing unit or department and deems him- or herself as the chief executive officer and chief financial officer of his or her area, now recognizing the power of the position in determining successful patient outcomes and a positive bottom line. Note that this chapter is concerned only with assisting the nurse manager in the financial aspects, not with other quality and ethical factors involved.

Note

1. Market basket is an economic term used to indicate a measure of inflation.

Useful Websites

Agency for Healthcare Research and Quality: www.ahrq.gov
Centers for Medicare and Medicaid Services: www.cms.hhs.gov
Henry J. Kaiser Family Foundation: www.kff.org
Select Quality Care Library (SQC Library): www.selectqualitycare.com
Social Security Online: www.socialsecurity.gov
Urban Institute: www.urban.org
U.S. Department of Health and Human Services: www.dhhs.gov

Discussion Questions

1. This chapter discusses the need for an interdisciplinary team approach. Why is this important? Which specific areas/departments should be involved?
2. What is a cost-to-charge ratio? Why should a nurse manager understand this ratio, and how would he or she use it?
3. What challenge does a unit that provides care for special needs patients have in costing out its service?
4. Why do freestanding skilled nursing facilities function more profitably than skilled nursing facilities in acute care organizations?
5. What source is available for the nurse manager to identify reimbursement for Medicare and Medicaid patients?
6. Finance departments regard nursing units as not being revenue generators. Why do you believe they are inaccurate in their assessment?
7. If you were part of the contract agreement negotiations with insurers, what specific contributions would you be able to provide for appropriate reimbursement for services?
8. This chapter hopes to improve your understanding of fiscal management. In your opinion, which factor covered in this chapter would you consider most critical?
9. In the new value-based reimbursement environment, what other measures can a nurse manager take to enhance reimbursement and prevent revenue loss?
10. What are the top ten DRGs in your hospital? Has the administrative team determined if each is cost effective? Is this accurate? If not, how would you determine whether they are cost effective?

Glossary of Terms

Balanced Scorecard and Activity-Based Costing (ABC)—this ratio is more closely aligned with the true costs of caring for the patient. Activity-based costing methodology also resembles performance improvement methods because processes and outcomes are evaluated. The complexity of procedures and tests involved, the intensity of nursing care, the duration of an activity, and the intricacies of operative and postoperative care identify the true costs. In this method, all areas and processes of patient interaction are identified and costs are allocated to the activity center. The balanced scorecard adds the quality dimension to cost and reimbursement data. For instance, cost drivers outside the system, such as patient satisfaction, can be measured and reflected in the overall scorecard.

Capitation—mechanism used by insurers to contain costs by establishing a set payment amount for a population served by a defined healthcare service. Rates are negotiated between the provider and the insurer under a contractual agreement for a year. Reimbursement rates may be for all services offered or for one specific service area, called a "carve out," such as laboratory.

Charges—determined by the allocation of costs to the revenue-producing centers and then projecting an amount needed to recover all the costs.

Costing a Service—all the actual costs expended to provide a specified service, as determined by the interdisciplinary team. This costing exercise should take place for all major services provided within the healthcare organization.

Costs—determined by the organization's financial accounting system, which takes into account actual costs of supplies, manpower, facility, and administration for services provided.

Cost-to-Charge Ratio (CCR)—a ratio determined by dividing the costs by the charges. A ratio under 1.0 (equal costs and charges) is positive and indicates that the organization is making money on the service. A ratio over 1.0 indicates the organization is experiencing a loss—the costs are more than the charges (expected reimbursement). The report is required for all Medicare-certified hospitals, skilled nursing facilities, home health agencies, and renal facilities. The nurse manager should be aware that CCR could lead to misrepresentation of cost when evaluating the profitability of a service.

Operating Payments—additional payments to the base DRG reimbursement that vary from large urban (population over 1 million) to other urban and rural hospitals. In 2009, the reimbursement rate for hospitals was tied to their quality performance (Centers for Medicare and Medicaid Services, 2008). These amounts are adjusted for the area market basket update.

Payment—amount the healthcare agency receives for the services provided. All payers pay differing amounts for the same service depending on the type of payer and the contractual agreement between the agency and the insurer.

Per Diem Approach—a ratio where the indirect costs are divided by the number of patient days to determine per diem costs, and then the indirect costs are allocated equally to all nursing units, which means that the departmental operations report for the obstetric unit and the cardiovascular intensive care unit will have the same dollar amount for indirect expenses even though the obstetric unit had fewer patient days regardless of the actual number of patient days. This method considers all patients the same regardless of intensity of care.

Projection of Reimbursement—calculated by a payment-to-cost ratio that indicates the percentage of costs that are covered by reimbursement.

Volume-Based Measures—a ratio where the indirect costs are assigned according to the volume (which may be visits, admissions, nursing hours per patient day) or machine hours (in radiology and the laboratory).

Volume-Based Environment (first curve)—in the past, reimbursement has been determined by the volume of insured patients. Industrial Age organizational design was used.

Value-Based Environment (second curve)—presently, reimbursement is changing to include organizational performance mandates. When protocols are not met, and when never events occur, insurers are not paying providers for the event or for the hospital stay. Reimbursement is value based.

References

Adams, T. (1996). Case mix index: Nursing's new management tool. *Nursing Management, 27*(9), 31–32.

Carpenter, D. (2003). Soaring spending: No sign of a slowdown. *H & HN: Hospitals and Healthcare Networks, 77*, 16–17.

Centers for Medicare and Medicaid Services. (2008). Proposed fiscal year 2009 payment policy changes for inpatient stays in general acute care hospitals. Retrieved from http://www.cms.hhs.gov/apps/media/press/factsheet.asp?Counter53045

Clancy, T., Kitchen, S., Churchill, P., Covington, D., Hundley, J., & Maxwell, J. (1998). DRG reimbursement: Geriatric hip fractures in the community hospital. *Southern Medical Journal, 91*(5), 457–461.

Cleverley, W. (1987). Product costing for health care firms. *Health Care Management Review, 12*(4), 39–48.

Cleverley, W. (1997). *Financial environment of health care organizations: Essentials of health care finance* (4th ed., Rev.). Gaithersburg, MD: Aspen.

Coughlin, T., & Liska, D. (1997). *The Medicaid disproportionate share hospital payment program: Background and issues* (Series A, No. A-14). Washington, DC: Urban Institute.

Division of Health Care Finance and Policy. (1998). Home health: An emerging challenge in health care. *Healthpoint, 3*, 1–4.

Dunham-Taylor, J., & Pinczuk, J. (2006). *Health care financial management for nurse managers: Applications from hospitals, long-term care, home care, and ambulatory care.* Sudbury, MA: Jones and Bartlett.

Durham, J. (2000). Healthcare's evolution in the technological universe. *Health Management Technology, 21*(4), 91–92.

Easier than ABC: Will activity based costing make a comeback? (2003). *The Economist, 369*, 56.

Ezzati-Rice, T., Kashihara, D., & Machlin, S. (2004). *Health care expenses in the United States, 2000.* (AHRQ Pub. No. 04-0022). Silver Spring, MD: U.S. Department of Health and Human Services.

Finkler, S. (1994). Cost allocation: The distinction between costs and charges. In *Issues in cost accounting for health care organizations* (pp. 81–93). Gaithersburg, MD: Aspen.

Finkler, S., Jones, C., & Kovner, C. (2013). *Financial management for nurse managers and executives.* St Louis, MO: Elsevier.

Health Research and Educational Trust. (2013, April). *Metrics for the second curve of health care.* Washington, DC: American Hospital Association.

Hoffman, F. (1984). Prospective reimbursement. In *Financial management for nurse managers* (pp. 193–203). Norwalk, CT: Appleton-Century-Crofts.

Kane, N., & Siegrist, R. (2002). Understanding rising hospital costs: Key components of cost and the impact of poor quality. Retrieved from http://heartland.org/sites/all/modules/custom/heartland_migration/files/pdfs/14629.pdf

Lane, S., Longstreth, E., & Nixon, V. (2001). *A community leader's guide to hospital finance.* Boston, MA: Access Project.

Lester, J., Bosch, J., Kaufman, J., Halpern, E., & Gazelle, G. (2001). Inpatient costs of routine endovascular repair of abdominal aortic aneurysm. *Academic Radiology, 8*(7), 639–646.

Magnus, S., & Smith, D. (2000). Better Medicare cost report data needed to help hospitals benchmark costs and performance. *Health Care Management Review, 25*(4), 65–77.

Maiga, A., & Jacobs, F. (2003). Balanced scorecard, activity-based costing and company performance: An empirical analysis. *Journal of Managerial Issues, 15*(4), 283–301.

Medicare SNF-PPS Indices [Data file]. Washington, DC: Centers for Medicare and Medicaid Services. Retrieved from http://www.cms.gov/.

Medpac. (2003). *Report to Congress: Medicare payment policy*. Washington, DC: Author.

Nursing Leadership Academy. (2003). *Fundamentals of nursing finance: A foundation for financial leadership (10889)*. Washington, DC: Advisory Board Company.

Popp, A., Scrime, T., Cohen, B., Feustel, P., Petronis, K., Habinak, S., ... Vosburgh, M. (2002). Factors affecting profitability for craniotomy. *Neurosurgery Focus, 12*(4), 1–5.

Ross, T. (2004). Analyzing health care operations using ABC. *Journal of Health Care Finance, 30*(3), 1–20.

Sobun, C. (1999). What does the future hold for Medicare and your reimbursement. *Health Care Biller, 8*(9), 1–4.

Udpa, S. (2001). Activity cost analysis: A tool to cost medical services and improve quality. *Managed Care Quarterly, 9*(3), 34–41.

U.S. Department of Health and Human Services. (1998). *Medicare program: Prospective payment system for hospital outpatient services: Proposed rules* (42 CFR Part 409, et al.). Washington, DC: Health Care Financing Administration Office of Inspector General.

U.S. Department of Health and Human Services, Centers for Medicare and Medicaid Services. (2007). *2007 CMS statistics.* (CMS Pub. No. 03480). Retrieved from http://www.cms.gov/.

U.S. General Accounting Office. (2002). *Skilled nursing facilities: Medicare payments exceed costs for most but not all facilities* (GAO-03-183). Washington, DC: Author.

van der Walde, T., & Choi, K. (2002). *Health care industry market update: Acute care hospitals* (Vol. II). Washington, DC: Centers for Medicare and Medicaid Services.

van der Walde, L., & Choi, K. (2003a). *Health care industry market update: Acute care hospitals*. Washington, DC: Centers for Medicare and Medicaid Services.

van der Walde, L., & Choi, K. (2003b). *Health care industry market update: Nursing facilities*. Washington, DC: Centers for Medicare and Medicaid Services.

van der Walde, L., & Lindstrom, L. (2003). *Health care market update: Home health*. Washington, DC: Centers for Medicare and Medicaid Services.

Weech-Maldonado, R., Neff, G., & Mor, V. (2003). The relationship between quality of care and financial performance in nursing homes. *Journal of Health Care Finance, 29*(3), 48–60.

Young, D. (2007). The folly of using RCCs and RVUs for intermediate product costing. *Healthcare Financial Management: Journal of the Healthcare Financial Management Association, 61*(4), 100–106, 108.

Financial Strategies

Financial strategies, and especially cost-cutting methods, are widely used today. Strategies need to be aligned with a larger issue, strategic management, which is discussed in Chapter 16. Systematic, objective strategic planning, along with the implementation of the plan, drives successful healthcare organizations. The key to successful planning is to make the process a part of the daily operations of the organization. Strategic management is a continuous process of revisiting the system and restoring balance.

Chapter 16 also describes the strategic management process that includes situation analysis, strategic formation, strategic deployment, and strategic management—which encompasses measurement, evaluation, and performance improvement. Directional strategies, mission, vision, values, goals, and objectives provide needed processes for the organization to define and to implement to achieve the desired outcomes. These provide an overall map for staff but will need to be tweaked constantly as changes occur.

Strategic management includes performance measurement. We advocate that the best way to conduct performance measurement is to use balanced scorecards because no metric should ever stand alone. Metrics captured within the organization's balanced scorecard are tied directly to the strategic plan. A primary utility of the balanced scorecard is the tie between strategic management and performance management. Measurement of key financial, quality, market, and operational indicators provides management with an understanding of performance in relation to established strategic goals and graphically displays a snapshot of the institution's overall health. Chapter 16 outlines some common tools and techniques that are useful, such as cost-benefit analysis, break-even analysis, and forecasting models.

Chapter 17 covers a number of financial strategies. In the new value-based reimbursement environment, accompanied by the addition of technology, very different approaches are required in healthcare settings. Using the American Hospital Association's 10 "must-do" strategies, this chapter explores possible ways nurse managers can achieve better financial success in this new environment. It is important to make financial information transparent to all in the organization so that all can contribute to both cost savings and to the best use of the available monies. Chapter 17 also examines the budgeting process and makes suggestions on how to both decentralize and streamline the process: Presently, in some organizations budgeting can waste 30% of administrators' time. In addition, it is important for a nurse administrator to know how to write a business plan, or proposal, that includes the financial information along with what is needed.

In Chapter 18 we turn to another budget strategy: case management. According to the American Nurses Credentialing Center, case management is a dynamic and systematic collaborative approach to providing and coordinating healthcare services in a defined population. It is a process to identify and facilitate options and services for meeting individuals' health needs while decreasing fragmentation and duplication of care, enhancing quality, and achieving cost-effective clinical outcomes. With the increased aged population that has many chronic disease conditions, case management becomes a key force to better manage their care needs. In addition, the last year of life is very expensive (both to the patient and to insurers). Chapter 18 examines some new models and presents trends that integrate and coordinate care, accompanied by increased use of information technologies. In the continuum of care, it is important to provide care in the home as much as possible and to use the least expensive option for care. Better strategies are needed to achieve these goals.

CHAPTER 16

Strategic Management: Facing the Future with Confidence

Sandy K. Diffenderfer, PhD, MSN, RN, CPHQ

The future ain't what it used to be.

—*Yogi Berra*

Effective visioning and decision making are primary tasks of leaders. Teamwork and collaboration are necessary for organizational leaders to make informed decisions and to maintain a viable organization. Seemingly justified by time constraints and the mistaken assessment that issues are minor, nurse managers often make decisions without essential information. By chance, the nurse manager may be successful in the short run, but in the long run the use of intuition—without the benefit of systematic input from stakeholders, pertinent data, and careful planning—most often results in calamity.

The delivery of health care devoid of a systematic process for planning forces managers to "fly by the seat of their pants" through reliance on perceptions and experience. The task of strategic planning and management is to generate accurate information for decision making. Forecasting the future with precision, however, is problematic because contemporary healthcare systems are complex, chaotic, and ever changing. Thus, obtaining accurate information can be a challenge in the healthcare environment where the answers and even the questions seemingly change on a daily basis. Strategic planning and management shifts decision making from intuitive information gathering to systematic and objective investigation and action.

In the midst of contemporary healthcare chaos, as the volume and pace of change continue to accelerate, managers may declare that they have no choice but to spend time and resources "putting out fires." It is surprising that well-adjusted individuals are overwhelmed by change after years of colliding with it. Notwithstanding, Gelatt (1993) observed that change itself had changed. The author described the chaos found in healthcare organizations as *white water change* because change in healthcare had become rapid, complex, turbulent, and unpredictable. Years after Gelatt's (1993) description of change, contemporary healthcare leaders bear witness to unparalleled change in the healthcare environment.

Patnaik (2012) defined *strategic planning* as "visualizing the future and making adequate provisions to deal with the same to meet organizational objectives" (p. 27). The dynamic and complex nature of healthcare mandates that leaders and managers not forsake planning if the organization is to meet key objectives and be positioned for long-term success. The strategic plan must provide an adaptable framework to make ongoing, timely, and dynamic changes to keep pace with the ever-changing healthcare environment. The plan must be designed to be continuous, thus *adaptable* because leaders cannot wait until the next planning cycle to decide how to respond to an unanticipated challenge (Greene, 2009). The plan exists to provide direction "not to prophesize by rigidly fixing unalterable boundaries" (Patnaik, 2012, p. 27) for future actions.

In addition to planning, strategic management is needed. *Strategic management* requires monitoring of key organizational metrics, assessment, evaluation, and continuous improvement to sustain the gains. Successful healthcare leaders use strategic management processes to remain informed about the organization, the market, and the competitive arena. The goal of strategic management is early recognition of environmental changes or the need for internal changes to be proactive rather than reactive. Thus, strategic management is fundamental to organizational success in the ever-changing healthcare environment because the processes provide leaders with direction and momentum for change (Ginter, Swayne, & Duncan, 2013).

Mintzberg and Markides (2000) noted that *strategy* is the art of crafting a unique position in the market. Primary strategy does not need to change often; however, when there is a need to rethink the organization's position, the change should emerge from the ideas and actions of the people in the organization. Once again, the focus is on being proactive rather than reactive.

Nurse managers are situated in the organization between the front-line staff and senior leaders; thus, these individuals are in a unique position to recognize the need for a change in strategy. Nurse managers may be the first stakeholders to recognize when strategies that worked in the past are no longer effective.

Successful organizational leaders understand the need to revise the organization's strategic plan based on feedback from internal as well as external stakeholders. Strategy must be the job of every employee because employees are key internal stakeholders. This is important because the employee's livelihood depends on the success of the organization. In the volatile healthcare market a flat, fully decentralized, bottom-up organizational structure promotes problem solving and innovation. Innovative strategies are more likely to be formulated if everyone in the organization, especially those in the nurse manager role, puts their intellect to the task.

Even though everyone in the organization should be encouraged to come up with new strategic ideas, senior leaders are responsible for the final choices. This is fitting because senior leaders are responsible for the organization's vision. This vision must be congruent with the contemporary healthcare arena. Organizational leaders must determine which ideas will be pursued; otherwise, the result is chaos and confusion. Strategic planning and management enable healthcare leaders to meet the future proactively rather than by responding to the internal and external environment in a haphazard manner. Although strategic planning and management do not eliminate all challenges, the process can drive innovation, integrate the system, and align resources to enable the organization to face the future with confidence.

Strategic planning is a continuous process of revisiting the system and restoring balance. Systematic, objective planning is the key to the development and implementation of plans that drive successful healthcare organizations. Organizational leaders must go beyond large binders with numbers, graphs, charts, and jargon. The data gathered and stored in these binders must be used to improve organizational performance. Often these valuable data—that took many hours of time and significant money to assemble—are considered during the initial phase of the strategic planning cycle, and then are shelved until the next round of strategic planning. If everyone in the organization does not view the strategic plan as a useful document, the organization's culture related to the strategic planning process should be explored.

Although many organizations have separate plans for performance improvement (PI), education, finance, operations, recruitment, and retention efforts would be better spent crafting a single document as the outcome of collaborative teamwork among disciplines and workers. The key to successful planning is to make the process a part of the daily operations of the organization rather than a task to be completed during the planning cycle in preparation for the budget.

Healthcare delivery takes place in complex systems sustained by social networks of internal and external stakeholders (Clancy, 2007). Healthcare employees from different departments and facilities must share information and collaborate to ensure the long-term success of the organization. Transparency fosters innovation and synergy because everyone is aligned with the overall strategies of the organization rather than "playing in their own sandbox." Lack of transparency results in duplication of efforts, increased costs, poor working relationships, and employees working at cross purposes. The resulting chaos and confusion give an appearance of disorganization to external customers.

Because of the complex nature of health care, "silo mentality" is common. Silo mentality is defined as "a mind-set present in some companies when certain departments or sectors do not wish to share information with others in the same company" (Business Dictionary.com, 2010, para. 1). Silo mentality is effective for storing grain because grain silos stand alone; yet even these structures are disappearing from the landscape. Lencioni (2006) described silos as one of the most frustrating aspects of working in an organization. The author stated that these barriers within an organization caused people who are supposed to be on the same team to work against each other and are generally not purposeful but rather the result of leaders failing to provide employees with a compelling purpose for working together. This highlights the importance of the leadership role in creating a common purpose through the organization's mission, vision, goals, objectives, and metrics, all of which are embodied in strategic management.

Healthcare organizational leaders must focus on patient satisfaction as well as patient retention and loyalty. Leaders must know the status of the organization's market share as well as any potential new markets. There may be services that need to be "repackaged" to attract new or evolving markets. These aspects are key factors in competitiveness, profitability, and success of the organization. Choices made by organizational leaders 3 to 5 years ago may no longer be valid and must be continuously questioned. In the past, being decisive was an essential talent often thought to be reserved for those in administrative positions. The healthcare environment of today has replaced the skill of making up one's mind with a *new essential skill of the future—learning how to change one's mind* (Gelatt, 1993). Technologies, customer preferences, and competitors are ever changing, and the organization must be flexible. Successful organizational leaders *question past choices* to determine whether change is necessary. The heart of strategic planning is to devise a systematic, well-balanced process that allows the organization to fit in the environment.

Strategic planning must be objective. The necessity for objectivity was cleverly stated by the nineteenth-century American humorist Artemus Ward, who said, "It ain't so much what people don't know that hurts as what they know that ain't so" (Creative Quotations, 2009). Thus, the facilitator of the strategic planning process must be detached and impersonal rather than engaged in biased attempts to prove preconceived ideas.

According to Mintzberg and Markides (2000), strategy is nothing more than answering three simple, yet difficult questions:

1. Whom should the organization target as customers and whom should it not target?
2. What should the organization offer these customers and what should it not offer?
3. What is the most efficient way to do this?

If the healthcare team does not have clear answers to these three questions, the organization will drift aimlessly until it eventually fails. Team members need clear parameters to guide their actions; these three dimensions help provide the autonomy they need to focus on the key tasks at hand. Without clarity of these three dimensions, organizational efforts will be disjointed because no common understanding of the strategies, goals, and objectives of the business exists.

National and state quality programs outline the essential role of strategic planning within organizations. The 2013–14 Baldrige Performance Excellence Program (National Institute of Standards and Technology [NIST], 2013) *Health Care Criteria for Performance Excellence* strategic planning category represents a total of 85 points toward a possible 1,000 total points distributed across seven categories in the Malcolm Baldrige National Quality Award's scoring system. The strategic planning category consists of two items, strategy development and implementation. The Strategy Development item stresses patient-focused excellence, innovation, and work systems (NIST, 2013). These key strategic issues are fundamental to the organization's strategic planning and management processes.

Although the term *customer* was not used often in health care until recent years, twenty-first-century healthcare leaders recognize the primary customer to be *the patient*. Patient-focused and other customer-focused quality efforts lead to customer acquisition, satisfaction, loyalty, referrals, and organizational sustainability that differentiates a healthcare system from its competitors (NIST, 2013). The ultimate test of quality is customer satisfaction, and to emphasize the role of customer engagement, the point value for Customer-Focused Results in the Malcolm Baldrige National Quality Award's scoring system is 85 points (NIST, 2013). Likewise, Workforce-Focused Results carries a point value of 85 points (NIST, 2013). Areas to consider are those important to the patient such as speed, responsiveness, and flexibility.

In light of the economic forces of healthcare reform, the status quo is not sustainable. *Innovative strategies* are needed for organizations to survive ever-shifting market pressures. Healthcare customers expect **value**, which is a delicate balance between cost and quality. Improvement in work systems contributes to short- and longer-term productivity, cost containment, and the overall well-being of the organization. Finally, organizational and personal learning must be embedded in work systems that are aligned with the organization's strategic plan. This alignment clarifies organizational priorities for employees (NIST, 2013).

The Tennessee Center for Performance Excellence (2009) is an example of a state quality program. The criteria outline that customers are the judge of the organization's quality and performance. Because strategic planning focuses on operational performance and quality as judged by the customer, the first notion is customer-driven quality. Customers of health care are both internal and external to the organization. *Internal customers* include patients and families, physicians, visitors, team members, and volunteers. The employment of physicians has changed physicians from external customers (suppliers of the patients served) to both internal (employees) and external (suppliers) customers. This dual role may conflict when organizational priorities are unclear or when organizational and personal goals are incongruent.

The primary *external customers* of health care are quite complex and consist of suppliers (insurance companies, physicians, labor markets, and donors), consumers (the general public and community), and interfacing organizations (medical profession, teaching and/or other hospitals, boards of directors, health insurances, and drug and supply companies). Additional external influences include licensing, governmental, and regulatory agencies, as well as other healthcare facilities (Bennis & Nanus, 1985). Students who complete clinical assignments in healthcare facilities are also external customers along with faculty and administrators.

Determining the measures customers use when they assess and judge the quality of healthcare services is an important process. Healthcare leaders' perception of quality may be vastly different from customers' perceptions. Nurse managers may believe that achieving zero defects is the priority when, in fact, timeliness is what is most important to the customer. It is important to have multiple listening strategies aimed at assessing how the customer perceives quality. Listening to the customer provides baseline knowledge. Once opportunities to improve are identified, leadership, through strategic planning, must assess and drive improvements. The Joint Commission (TJC, 2013) holds leadership accountable for strategic planning and PI.

It is important that healthcare leaders understand why customers choose particular healthcare services. Providing quality care does not guarantee success; customers must perceive added *value*. Healthcare leaders may erroneously perceive that services are superior in design, service, and cost when, in fact, the services are inefficient, outdated, and ordinary. Unless improvements are made, advances in the market will produce customer dissatisfaction rather than satisfaction with services. Customer satisfaction is paramount to the success of the organization, and capturing this information encompasses a major expenditure. This is true whether the data are captured internally or through an outside vendor such as Gallup (2013) or Press Ganey (2013).

Some healthcare professionals question whether patients and families are qualified to assess healthcare quality. The Internet has eliminated the time-honored adage "We know what is best, after all we have years of education" and has ushered in the age of *informed consumers*. No longer is it acceptable to lecture the patient, "Just do as I say" or "The doctor knows best." Many patients seek healthcare services after an extensive Internet search on the diagnosis and/or treatment(s) in question. Patients and families often arrive for care with an array of scientific literature—indeed, sometimes they are better informed than the clinician is.

An organization's commitment to performance excellence should not be measured by cost but rather viewed as an *investment*. Organizational leaders purchase equipment to improve processes and cycle times. Leaders who make a similar investment in team members receive a much higher return. Boev (2012) found preliminary support for the relationship between nurses' and patients' satisfaction in adult critical care. Thus, successful healthcare organizations recognize and reward team members. If team members are expected to meet the needs of customers, their needs must be met first. This is important because patient satisfaction is now associated with hospital reimbursement (Centers for Medicare & Medicaid Services, 2011).

The Tennessee Center for Performance Excellence (2009) criteria also stress work systems and workforce-related results. Both short-term and longer-term goals of the organization must be determined.

A primary concern is cost competitiveness, which is difficult to attain during economic downturns. It is paramount that healthcare leaders remain committed to the facility's mission and values when deciding how to respond to such crises. Operational capabilities such as speed, responsiveness, and flexibility contribute to the organization's competitive fitness. The strategic plan must align work processes with the strategic direction of the organization by embedding improvement and learning in work processes. This alignment ensures that priorities for improvement and learning reinforce the priorities of the organization.

Comprehensive strategic planning establishes the *organization's strategy* (the plan for achieving the desired end result) and *plan of action* (what the organization must do to get there). Of key importance are the deployment of the plan of action to all business units, how strategic management will be operationalized through identification of key results, and how outcomes are measured and sustained.

The Joint Commission (2013) required leaders to engage in short- and long-term planning. This includes data that measure the performance of the processes and outcomes of care, treatment, and services.

The healthcare system is undergoing tremendous change. Thus, leaders must determine whether decades of habit related to the strategic planning and management process are appropriate given the current volatile environment. Zuckerman (2006) noted that organizations in stable markets may be able to survive using traditional planning practice; nevertheless, the unstable healthcare environment demands a *flexible, ongoing planning process*. Leaders must decide whether to forge ahead with traditional strategic planning or change to a more fluid compressed cycle strategic planning process. Regardless of the decision, it is most important that the organization's mission, vision, and values guide leaders' actions.

Strategic Planning in Health Care

Although the business sector has successfully used strategic planning for the past 50 years, strategic planning has been used in health care only since the 1970s, and then only sporadically (Zuckerman, 1998). According to Ginter, Swayne, and Duncan (2002), the concept of strategic planning was broadened to strategic management during the 1980s when business transformed planning and budgeting beyond the traditional 12-month operating year and began to understand the importance of strategy implementation and control. Prior to this time, healthcare organizations had little impetus for strategic management because the organizations were autonomous, free-standing facilities with cost-plus reimbursement schemes (Ginter et al., 2013).

Zuckerman (2006) reported that a study completed by the Society for Healthcare Strategy and Market Development (SHSMD) of the American Hospital Association and Health Strategies & Solutions, Incorporated, revealed that basic strategic planning in health care appeared sound and effective, well accepted, regular, and integrated and provided direction and focus for the healthcare organizations. However, the author reported that healthcare strategic planning had not evolved past basic processes and had failed to progress to more advanced levels compared to those outside of health care.

On the other hand, Ginter and Swayne (2006) countered that the nuances of the healthcare environment made differences in approaches to strategic planning acceptable. These authors heralded that strategic planning should not be made more rigorous, rather, "the simpler the better" (p. 35). There is no one-size-fits-all strategic planning process for healthcare organizations. To this end, MacPhee (2007) stated that executive leaders must select strategies for the organization that are "realistic, valued, manageable, and locally applicable to employees" (p. 405).

Ginter and colleagues (2013) described the approaches to strategic management as *analytical* and *emergent*. According to the authors, analytical or rational approaches to strategic management involve sequential steps and linear thinking that correspond best with traditional strategic management processes. On the other hand, emergent approaches to strategic management rely on intuitive thinking, leadership, and learning, which correspond with contemporary strategic management processes. Ginter and colleagues (2013) declared that both approaches were valid and useful, and that, indeed, both approaches are required. An overview of contemporary and traditional strategic management processes follows.

Contemporary Strategic Management

Complexity theory provides an explanation for the unpredictability that is inherent in strategic planning (Patneik, 2012). Crowell (2011) described complexity science as "nonlinear, dynamic, often uncertain, and very much relationship-based" (p. 3). The author further stated that complexity leadership ascribes that top-down structures do not necessarily lead to effective outcomes or changed behaviors, rather often the reverse. Complexity theory is particularly relevant to healthcare systems because change is the only constant. Thus, traditional strategic management with a goal of forecasting and monitoring future states is inconsistent with the healthcare environment.

Zuckerman (2006) proclaimed that planners and executives who participated in a survey believed that heathcare strategic planning was effective and provided focus and direction for their organizations. The author noted that in a stable market traditional strategic planning methods worked well; however, in volatile, ever-changing markets such as health care a more nimble approach was needed. Further, he identified that healthcare strategic planning was less rigorous and sophisticated than were the planning processes used by organizations outside of health care.

Zuckerman (2006) offered that state-of-the-art strategic planning encompassed some or all of the following qualities:

1. Systematic, ongoing data gathering, leading to use of knowledge management practices
2. Encouragement of innovation and creativity in strategic approaches
3. More bottom-up than top-down strategic planning
4. Evolving, flexible, continuously improving planning processes
5. A shift from static to dynamic strategic planning (p. 8)

Although these characteristics of a state-of-the-art strategic plan are not new, health care has been slow to break the habit of the traditional strategic plan. Turbulent times in health care provide an opportunity to break from the norm and embrace contemporary strategic planning and management processes.

Several contemporary strategic management processes are found in the literature; some are formal processes, some are less so. Recent authors described emerging trends in strategic planning, for example, the use of nonlinear (Crowell, 2011) compressed, flexible cycles for leaders to be able to quickly respond to the ever-changing environments (Dibrell, Down, & Bull, 2007; Greene, 2009; Lazarus, 2011; Patnaik, 2012; Zuckerman, 2006). Dibrell and associates (2007) found that strategic planning in successful firms had a strong external orientation and built-in flexibility; such flexibility helped managers to respond quickly and effectively to competitive forces. These authors described *strategic flex points* (p. 28) that allowed changes in managers' plans. This planned emergent perspective empowered managers to contact leaders when opportunities or threats were developing to adapt or change the formal strategic plan. The emerging pattern found by these authors was that firms that were able to respond quickly and effectively to external threats and opportunities were more likely to be successful.

Likewise, Greene (2009) described recent seismic events in health care such as the economic crisis, increased market pressures, and healthcare reform as catalysts for change in which decades of habit related to the traditional strategic planning process must be discarded. The author touted the need to address strategy *quarterly* for leaders to ensure that the facility's mission, vision, and values are upheld. A heightened focus on the mission, vision, and values is needed because relentless environmental changes especially related to difficult financial choices may result in a disjoint between the organization's core purpose and decisions that are made for the organization to remain viable.

Lazarus (2011) recommended a commitment to strategic planning and execution that enables leaders to respond quickly to the challenges that lie ahead. He stated, "It is not the big company that acquires the small, *it's the fast that acquires the slow*" (p. 89). The changing healthcare landscape cannot be ignored.

Healthcare planners and executives who recognize the need for a more flexible strategic plan place less emphasis on long-term planning because in such a volatile environment control is merely an illusion. Rather than stand-alone strategic plans, the strategic plan is often linked to business operations including the facility's PI plan (Blatstein, 2012; Lazarus. 2011) and finance and budgeting processes (Blatstein, 2012; Zuckerman, 2006). This decreases silo mentality.

Integrated plans facilitate transparent, focused, and collaborative work among leaders, managers, and team members. Linking the strategic management plan to PI efforts also provides needed metrics to determine the overall state of the organization through the use of a balanced scorecard (BSC) and provides a mechanism for needed improvement through processes such as Lean and Six Sigma. Some authors have noted that these processes are at odds with the complex nature of health care (Vardaman, Cornell, & Clancy, 2012).

Ginter and associates (2013) described the use of both analytical and emergent approaches to strategic management as encompassed in three parts: (1) strategic thinking, (2) strategic planning, and (3) strategic momentum management. These authors stated that strategic thinking is the job of all employees because everyone's work must be reinvented to be in tune with the world. Strategic planning encompasses traditional strategic management activities using strategic thinking and is generally the easiest to complete. Finally, strategic momentum is focused on the strategies that are needed to achieve organizational goals. This integrated approach presents an effective strategic management process.

A strategic planning practice used by the University of Virginia (UVA) School of Nursing (SON) (Harmon, Fontaine, Plews-Ogan, & Williams, 2012) offers promise for effective change in the strategic planning process. These authors described the use of *Appreciative Inquiry (AI)* to formulate the school's strategic plan. Cooperrider and Whitney (n.d.) defined AI as follows:

> Appreciative Inquiry is the corevolutionary search for the best in people, their organizations, and the relevant world around them. In its broadest focus, it involves systematic discovery of what gives "life" to a living system when it is most alive, most effective, and most constructively capable in economic, ecological, and human terms. (para. 1)

Further, Cooperrider and Whitney (n.d.) stated that "AI involves, in a central way, the art and practice of asking questions that strengthen a system's capacity to apprehend, anticipate, and heighten positive potential" (para. 1). Thus, AI provides a positive inclusive approach to strategic planning.

The UVA SON held an AI summit, which is used in business but new to nursing, to achieve rapid positive change and to identify the causes for success (Harmon et al., 2012). The goal was to involve the whole system in the school's strategic plan rather than the traditional committee method that was used in the past. Stakeholders were invited to the AI summit in advance. Using AI principles, the group focused on the positives and potentials rather than problems. "Stories of success" (p. 120) were solicited and shared in small groups, and themes were identified. The themes were shared with the entire group, and participants selected the causes of success. These "moments of excellence" (p. 120) were honed to nine positive core strengths of the SON. This inclusive strategic planning method enabled stakeholders to identify what the SON did best and to design the best possible future (Harmon et al., 2012). Innovative approaches such as the use of AI to guide the strategic planning process provide exemplars of a successful contemporary strategic planning process.

Finally, the complex nature of health care decrees that leaders contemplate systems theory related to strategic planning and management work. Lindberg and Clancey (2010) proclaimed that conventional methods of improvement, for example, Lean and Six Sigma, were under siege because these approaches were not effective in social organizations such as hospitals. Consider the prominence of hospital-acquired infections and the efforts expended toward improvement efforts, yet national statistics document that this patient safety event is pervasive (Reed & May, 2011).

Lindberg and Clancey (2010) proposed that *Positive Deviance (PD)*, which holds that within organizations some individuals or groups have different "deviant" practices that produce better "positive" (p. 152) outcomes. Positive Deviance holds that staff at the point of care understand what works, what does not work, and what the barriers are to safe practice (bottom-up management). The job is to discover the positive deviant practice, and then through widespread engagement spread this best practice throughout the organization and system. This is contrasted to the traditional PI efforts that are deployed in many healthcare organizations as part of strategic management processes (see the section titled "Strategic Management" later in this chapter). Positive Deviance is an example of an *emergent strategic management* process that should be considered by leaders in the contemporary healthcare environment for organizations to be competitive in the market.

A final important motivator for hospitals and providers to transition to a contemporary strategic management process was clearly outlined by the American Hospital Association (AHA, 2011) in the seminal work *Hospitals and Care Systems of the Future*. The authors outlined 10 must-do strategies (p. 4) that hospitals must implement in preparation for the future *value-based market* dynamic, termed the "second curve" (p. 3). Although all 10 strategies link to organizational strategic planning and management, only the most important linkages are discussed here.

Strategy 1 calls for alignment of "hospitals, physicians, and other providers across the continuum" (p. 4), and strategy 5 suggests "joining and growing integrated provider networks and core systems" (p. 17). Likewise, strategy 8, "partnering with payers" (p. 20), further focuses on healthcare alignment. These must-do strategies highlight the need for common ground among stakeholders. As healthcare incentives are aligned, a common mission, vision, and values will be formed. This is challenging work because organizational culture is resistant to change. Hospitals and physicians will move from being competitors to interdependence (p. 13). Likewise, strategy 10, "seeking population health improvement through pursuit of the 'triple aim'" (p. 22), focuses on the increased hospital role in disease prevention, health promotion, and public health initiatives (AHA, 2011). The expectation is seamless care both internal and external to the organization; thus, interdisciplinary collaboration and partnerships are needed. In addition, financial incentives will steer health care from episodic, illness-based care to a focus on wellness and healthy lifestyles.

The second and third strategies focus on using evidence-based practices to improve quality and patient safety and efficiency through productivity and financial management (AHA, 2011). Strategy 7 is related: "strengthening finances to facilitate reinvestment and innovation" (p. 19). These strategies provide a stimulus for a *flexible* (to remain current) strategic management process because new evidence is available daily. In the present state, termed the "first curve" (p. 14), improvement and sustainability of core measures are used. In the second curve (p. 14), when value-based purchasing is fully implemented, measurement, analysis, and decreased variation in clinical care are the focus in an effort to improve quality (AHA, 2011). The use of a balanced scorecard approach ensures that one aspect of the business does not suffer diametrically aligned with improvements in another. These strategic planning metrics will become increasingly important as leaders balance the duty to maintain regulatory mandated process and outcome metrics while seeking to understand *value as defined by the patient*. As margins tighten, financial health is needed to pay for work and equipment that is necessary to reach the goals of related strategies (AHA, 2011).

"Developing integrated information systems" (AHA, 2011, p. 4) is the fourth strategy. Leaders must ensure that storage and analysis of data including real-time information across the continuum are effective. The emphasis is on data mining and use of data for improvement in patient care. The costs associated with obtaining and maintaining integrated computer systems are concerning, especially in the current state of healthcare financial instability. Of interest is that the AHA (2011) reported, "The interviews revealed that the organizations who installed IT systems have found that literacy, cultural, and work flow barriers were much more critical than the cost barrier to successful implementation" (p. 16).

All employees must be valued and engaged in the work of the organization. Strategy 6, "educating and engaging employees and physicians to create leaders" (p. 18), focuses on the need for leaders and effective *managers of change*—the only constant in health care. As the healthcare system becomes integrated and the focus shifts to population-based health rather than episodic illness care, leadership skills will be needed to engage all stakeholders.

Strategy 9 addresses organizational planning: "advancing an organization through scenario-based strategic, financial, and operational planning" (AHA, 2011, p. 21). Traditional strategic planning (discussed later), which is future focused, is ineffective in turbulent markets such as the ever-changing current healthcare environment. Thus, leaders must plan for a variety of potential situations (AHA, 2011). Potential scenarios include natural disasters, reimbursement cuts, loss of a large community employer, and so forth. Strong financial and operational considerations are needed because there are many potential new circumstances. "Scenario-based analysis includes a market environmental scan, analysis of internal capabilities, identification of the unknown, development of key scenarios, and plans to implement the necessary strategies" (p. 21). Whereas many of these tactics are used in traditional strategic planning, the emphasis is on flexibility. This is particularly important as collaboratives and partnerships are formed. Again, the emphasis is on a *flexible* strategic plan because the future is unknown. In addition, the need for integrated operational, financial, educational, quality, and strategic plans is clear.

Traditional Strategic Management

The traditional strategic management process traces the following map: (1) situation analysis, (2) strategy formation, (3) strategy deployment, and (4) strategic management, which encompasses measurement, evaluation, and PI. **Exhibit 16–1** outlines the traditional strategic management process. Blatstein (2012) noted that the real value of the process was not the strategic plan, rather the journey that participants take in exploring the future. Such planning reveals future possibilities not previously recognized and helps to shape the future for the organization.

Exhibit 16–1   Traditional Strategic Management Process

Situation Analysis	Strategy Formation	Strategy Deployment	Strategic Management
External environmental analysis: • Opportunities • Threats	Directional strategies: • Mission • Vision • Values • Goals and Objectives	Culture	Goals and Objectives
Internal environmental analysis: • Strengths • Weakness	Adaptive strategies	Structure	Measurement • Balanced Scorecard
• Mission • Vision • Values • Goals	Market entry strategies	Resources	Evaluation standards
	Competitive strategies		Performance Improvement

Situation Analysis

Situation analysis, the initial stage of strategic planning, is the process of determining the current state of the organization. Although historical data are an asset in determining the current state, leaders should resolve to avoid the trap of focusing on the analysis of past performance. Zuckerman (1998) described this phenomenon as "analysis paralysis," a serious problem that can bog down the strategic planning process. Undue emphasis on past performance can result in loss of focus and momentum. Key players may become disinterested, and buy-in may be lost.

Leaders must focus on *results*, not "busy work." There will always be those in the group who insist on more and better data; however, profiling key business drivers for the organization should be captured and analyzed on an ongoing basis, thus negating the need for overanalysis of historical data. Rarely are data needed beyond the past 5 years.

Key issues to consider include which factors are within the control or influence of the organization and how external forces affect the competitive position of the organization. During this step, a literature search is typically completed related to strategic planning approaches (Blatstein, 2012). Understanding and analyzing the current situation are accomplished through three interrelated processes: external environmental analysis, internal environmental analysis, and the development of the organization's mission, vision, values, and goals. These processes are not separate and distinct but rather overlap, interact with, and influence one another.

External Environmental Analysis

The first process, *external environmental analysis*, focuses on determining the current position of the organization within both the general environment and the healthcare environment. This profile is the beginning of a forward-looking process that considers market trends and forecasts (Zuckerman, 1998). To understand the *external environment*, the organization must look outside its boundaries (beyond itself) to identify and analyze issues taking place outside the organization. These issues represent opportunities and threats and assist in identifying "what the organization should do." This analysis is needed because available resources, competencies, and capabilities influence success in the external environment.

DeSilets and Dickerson (2008) suggested the following basic questions, "Do you have an area of expertise worth promoting?" "Are you undercapitalized?" "Is your market growing or shrinking?" (p. 196).

Opportunities and threats influence strategy formation and represent fundamental issues that can directly affect the success or failure of the organization. It is insufficient to simply be aware of these issues; healthcare leaders need to understand the nature of the opportunities and threats before they affect the organization. Organizational leaders must have an effective method for scanning the external environment for pertinent information. Factors to be considered include legislative and political changes, economic modifications, social and demographic shifts, new technology, and competitive market changes (Ginter et al., 2002). Additional external factors that have the potential to affect the business based on the type of healthcare organization are also important to assess.

Review of legislative, political, and regulatory trends is necessary to determine any major environmental influences that may affect the future performance of the organization. Regulatory and legislative changes in both public and private healthcare organizations will continue as these entities struggle to ensure healthcare access, patient safety and privacy, and cost management. Major trends should be profiled for the past 3 to 5 years. Forecasting, using alternative scenarios, should be identified and discussed (Zuckerman, 1998) with a focus on minimizing negative impacts and maximizing potential benefits.

Economic trends and forecasts should be exercised with caution and overanalysis should be avoided. Only the broadest trends and variables that affect the organization should be considered. Nevertheless, shifts in the national economy cannot be ignored because the impact is realized at the local level. Although minor shifts in economic performance are of minimal consequence to the strategic planning process, local trend analysis may identify geographic segments with potential for future penetration (Zuckerman, 1998).

Demographic changes, such as an aging population and increased life span, must be considered because these factors directly affect healthcare organizations. Major population shifts can indicate geographic areas that may be targeted for future market growth. Social trends, such as a more ethnically diverse and better educated population, affect the provision of services as well. Critical shortages of nurses, pharmacists, physical therapists, and other healthcare professionals necessitate a focus on retention and recruitment efforts.

Technology needs continue to escalate. Increasingly, technology allows healthcare settings to be seamlessly connected across providers and levels of care. Confidentiality of healthcare data is a major concern. Healthcare organizations need to leave the chisel and stone technique with cartoon characters such as Fred Flintstone and rather rise to the opportunity to provide seamless patient medical records.

Primary market research is completed by focusing on competitive and market changes external to the organization. This information helps to determine the organization's competitive position in the market. Market research is completed through interviews, focus groups, and surveys. Targets of this research include senior leaders of competitor organizations, community leaders, primary employers, and those knowledgeable of the market situation. The primary task is to generate information, thereby decreasing the uncertainty that comes with the managerial art of decision making. Research means literally to "search again," a process whereby one looks at the data to understand all that needs to be known about a subject (Zikmund, 2003). Although caution must be exercised so that this aspect of the process does not take an undue amount of time and resources and is not overemphasized, leaders must know the market. At times, research reveals information not readily apparent and key to success in the market.

> The secret of business is to know something nobody else knows.
>
> —*Aristotle Onassis*

A parallel matrix is helpful when analyzing the external environment. This matrix allows visualization of competitively relevant threats with external opportunities. **Exhibit 16–2** provides an example parallel matrix.

Internal Environmental Analysis

Recall that available resources, competencies, and capabilities influence success in the external environment. *Internal environmental analysis* involves an extensive review of internal processes, culture, structure, and technology to reveal strengths and weaknesses. Strengths are those things that the organization does well, not only from the viewpoint of the organization's employees but from the customer's viewpoint (DeSilets & Dickerson, 2008). *Weaknesses* represent organizational vulnerabilities and include processes that are not functioning at the desired level and are in need of PI project work. Nevertheless, resources are finite, and thus targeted projects should link to the organization's strategy.

According to the 2013–14 Baldrige *Health Care Criteria for Performance Excellence* (NIST, 2013), *work systems must be agile*, that is, systems must be able to adapt quickly and effectively because the healthcare environment is ever changing. Analysis of internal processes should entail little more than review of PI activities and results, assuming that the organization links the efforts of PI with the organization's strategic plan (Lazarus, 2011). This also assumes that organizational leaders prioritize and fund PI efforts based on criteria that link projects to organizational strategy (Lazarus, 2011). Such linkage is often not the case; recall the discussion earlier in this chapter regarding silo mentality. Nevertheless, if PI efforts and strategic planning and management are not linked, additional time and effort must be spent reviewing the results of key internal processes and outcomes.

Shirey (2011b) noted that the *influence of organizational culture* when executing strategy cannot be underestimated. Thus, cultural norms must be considered early in the strategic planning process. This is important because culture is enduring and difficult to change (Shirey, 2011b). These proclamations are linked to the results of a Wharton School study (Hrebiniak, 2005) that documented that managing change was often the most important factor for successful execution of organizational strategy. Further, Hrebiniak (2005) noted that many leaders in the study held that the ability to change was synonymous with the ability to manage change of the organizational culture. Leaders must consider whether selected strategies that require change have an impact on the culture of the organization. For example, if a strategy is selected by leaders without input from employees in an organization with a history of effective shared

Exhibit 16–2 External Environment Parallel Matrix	
Nurse's Heaven Hospital Strategic Plan 20XX Opportunities and Threats	
Opportunities	**Threats**
No competitors offer wound management services	Increased competition from larger medical center serving the same population
The hospital owns six vacant physician offices; five new physicians are needed	Larger medical center recently constructed five new physician offices that are connected to the facility

governance, the change may not be embraced; thus, execution may be sabotaged and the selected strategy may fail or the change may not be sustained. Finally, Hoffman (2007) reported that the results of a study with an international sample of 75 companies (57.7% response rate) concluded that culture had little relationship to planning. However, the strength of the planning–performance relationship varied by culture. The study provided beginning evidence of a systematic planning–performance relationship among companies from different cultures.

Review of the *structure of the organization* during the internal environmental analysis may reveal strengths or weaknesses. For example, the traditional hierarchical bureaucratic organizational structure continues to be prevalent especially in large healthcare organizations and systems. Bureaucracies were originally developed to promote efficiency and production during the Industrial Age when divisions of labor and a centralized formal structure promoted production (Yoder-Wise, 2010). However, contemporary knowledge workers desire autonomy and the authority to act at all levels of the organization. Thus, flat or participatory management structures and shared governance models demonstrate that leaders trust employees' to act appropriately and that employees embrace accountability. This is important in turbulent environments such as health care where being proactive may facilitate customer satisfaction.

As healthcare systems become internally integrated (radiology, nursing, laboratory, pharmacy, and other ancillary departments), the interface often becomes a logistical nightmare. No one technology system has "one-stop shopping," whereas one system might excel in a key feature but may be deficient in another. Furthermore, the technology competitor probably excels in a different key aspect of an integrated system. Most practitioners no longer complete laborious manual record reviews and "paper and pen" documentation. Nevertheless, the cost of technology is a growing concern, especially considering the economic climate.

In the internal environmental analysis phase, Gelatt (1993) cautioned against *info-mania*. He described info-mania as the idolizing of information. *Info-maniacs* worship facts. There is sure to be at least one member of the leadership team who demands more and more facts even when the team is drowning in information, for example, "Exactly how many admissions did Dr. X have 3 years ago?" "Four years ago?" "Five?" Caution is advised because focusing only on facts leaves little time or energy for innovation. Generating more information than the human mind can process is dysfunctional. Healthcare leaders must understand the competitive relevance of identified issues. Weaknesses require strategies to minimize the vulnerability of the organization, whereas strengths must be optimized to maximize their impact. This information provides a foundation for strategy formulation (Ginter et al., 2002). Plotting strengths and weaknesses on a parallel matrix (**Exhibit 16–3**) provides a visual for evaluating the competitive advantages relative to strengths and the competitive relevance of weaknesses.

The real voyage of discovery consists not in seeking new landscapes, but in having new eyes.

—Marcel Proust

Exhibit 16–3 Internal Environment Parallel Matrix

Nurse's Heaven Hospital Strategic Plan 20XX Strengths and Weaknesses

Strengths	Weaknesses
Convenient ground level parking	Lack of sufficient parking Monday-Friday
Patient-oriented team members	Team member turnover rate exceeds regional average

Zuckerman (1998) explained that *primary market research* serves to gather information regarding the organization's strengths and weaknesses as it relates to its competitors and to involve leadership in the strategic planning process. Leaders should begin by reviewing any recent market research that is available and gathering information through interviews, focus groups, and surveys. Primary target groups for market research include board members, physicians, health professionals, management staff, and other key stakeholders of the organization.

Many organizations use *focus groups* to solicit *stakeholder input* (Krueger, 1988; Morgan, 1993). Focus groups incur significant cost (time and money); thus, priority is given to key customer groups such as patients, families, team members, community members, and physicians. A focus group consists of a small group of individuals (6–10), usually with similar interests, who participate in an unstructured, free-flowing interview with a skilled facilitator. The facilitator begins by introducing the topic with the goal of uncovering core issues related to strategic planning. A recorder documents key statements for management to consider in strategy development. Caution must be used, however, because focus groups may not represent the entire population.

Drenkard (2001) documented the success of the Inova Chief Nurse Executive team in using large group interventions to convene and engage nurses across a large healthcare system in northern Virginia. This method involved the entire system and used a key mass of people affected by the change. This critical mass participated in (1) understanding the need for change, analyzing the current state, and deciding what needed to be changed; (2) generating ideas about how to make the needed changes; and (3) implementing and supporting the change. The Inova Chief Nurse Executive team sponsored six large group events to engage the several hundred nurses in the workforce. These sessions provided time for interaction, development of the strategic plan, and networking for the involved nurses.

Mission, Vision, Values, and Goals

The mission, vision, values, and goals of the organization ultimately affect the strategy that is adopted. A clear understanding by all employees of these foundational underpinnings cannot be overemphasized. MacPhee (2007) stressed that change strategies begin with an analysis of the mission and vision. The mission and vision provide a framework for analysis of personal and organizational values. The author stated that "the vision and mission can also be a springboard for personal values examination and a means to build a stronger organizational culture with shared values and a collective identity" (p. 408). This is especially important considering the rapid pace of change in the healthcare market where organizations are competitors one day and the next day, organizations within a merged system.

According to Ginter and colleagues (2002), the organization's *mission* is the articulation of the external opportunities and threats and the internal strengths and weaknesses. Simply, the mission is the reason the organization exists. Chapman (2003) noted that the organization's mission needs to matter. The mission of the organization must not be just clichéd words framed on the wall. Likewise, healthcare organizations need volcanic vision statements that eliminate old patterns of mediocrity. The *vision* is the view of the future based on the understanding of environmental forces. Chapman (2003) described three elements of effective mission and vision statements: clear and easy to remember, a call for dramatic improvement in the lives of others, and proclamation by leaders who, through example, demonstrate a passionate commitment to making the statements come alive.

The core *values* constitute the fundamental truths that the organization holds dear and reflect the philosophy of the organization. Examples include honesty, integrity, customer service, and commitment to excellence. *Goals* specify the major direction of the organization and provide actionable linkage to the mission. The mission, vision, values, and goals are considered a part of the situation analysis because they are influenced by the results of both external and internal environmental analyses.

Strategy Formation

The first step in the traditional strategic planning process, situation analysis, involves data gathering. *Strategy formation* uses these data for decision making. These decisions are critical to the success of the organization because they become the organization's strategy. Ginter and associates (2013) described four types of strategies: directional, adaptive, market entry, and competitive.

Directional Strategies

Although the mission, vision, values, goals, and objectives are part of the situation analysis, they are also part of strategy formation because they provide the broadest direction for the organization—*directional strategies*. The mission, vision, values, and goals indicate what the organization wants to do. These strategies reflect the critical success factors within the particular service category, in this case, health care. Critical success factors are applicable to all competitors and take into account the external environment. In other words, they define what the organization must accomplish to stay in business. These strategies provide initial direction for the organization and guidance when making key organizational decisions. The reciprocal relationship (adapted from Ginter et al., 2002, p. 177) of directional strategies is shown in **Exhibit 16–4**.

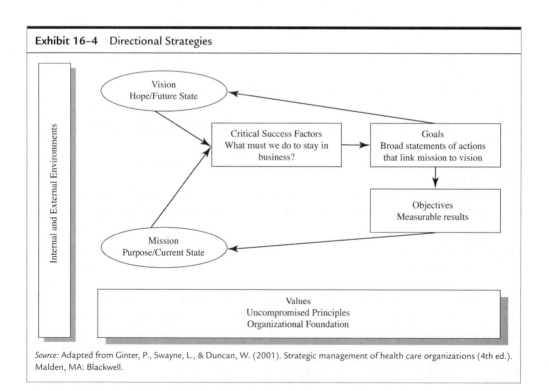

Exhibit 16–4   Directional Strategies

Internal and External Environments

Vision
Hope/Future State

Critical Success Factors
What must we do to stay in business?

Goals
Broad statements of actions that link mission to vision

Objectives
Measurable results

Mission
Purpose/Current State

Values
Uncompromised Principles
Organizational Foundation

Source: Adapted from Ginter, P., Swayne, L., & Duncan, W. (2001). Strategic management of health care organizations (4th ed.). Malden, MA: Blackwell.

Mission

The organization's *mission* should articulate the organization's purpose or reason that it exists. The mission statement describes what makes the organization distinct and reflects the expectations of stakeholders, those who have an interest in the business. In short, the mission defines the organization and describes what it does. The mission statement must be more than an attractive wall hanging. The mission must be communicated and lived by all team members in the organization, especially team members who work directly with customers.

Vision

The organization's *vision* describes the optimal future state of the business. The vision should create a mental picture of what the organization will be when leaders and team members accomplish their mission. It describes the hope for the future—what should the organization be 5 years from now? Time and effort link the mission (what the organization is today) and vision (what it will be in the future). The vision should be stated in clear, simple terms that provide a challenge and leave no doubt as to the importance of the vision. Stakeholders should be able to understand the vision and commit it to memory. The vision should be inspiring and is generally not stated in quantitative terms. Though the vision should stand the test of time, it should be constantly challenged and revised when necessary.

Values

Values represent the basic principles, fundamental beliefs, and tenets of team members and define what they deem important to the organization. Values state uncompromised principles that are timeless and do not change with the ever-changing climate of business operations. Some organizations use the terminology "guiding principles" to refer to values. Values guide beliefs, attitudes, and behaviors and provide the foundation for operating the business. Key business decisions should be measured against the values of the organization so that the organization never loses sight of its purpose.

Goals

Goals are more specific than the mission and vision. Nevertheless, goals are broad statements that provide direction for team members and link the mission to actions necessary to reach the desired future state of the organization—the vision. Blatstein (2012) stated that goals answer the question, "Where do I want to go?" (p. 33). The author described the importance of a "Big Hairy Audacious Goal (BHAG)" (p. 33), a stretch goal for the organization that is difficult to achieve. The BHAG motivates leaders to consider opportunities and obstacles for the future. During the discussions of the BHAG, as leaders reach common ground related to the goal, leaders gain insight about what motivates and inspires others. This work enables leaders to work together better as a team (Blatstein, 2012). Goals that focus on activities unrelated to the organization's critical success factors have the potential of diverting leadership attention and team member energy. The number of goals should be limited for the same reasons. Goals should be stated in easily understood terms so that team members can readily link what they need to do with the mission and vision for the organization, for example, the following:

- Expand Women's Services to encompass all key aspects of the business
- Position Nurse's Heaven Hospital as a strong community hospital with a focus on primary care
- Develop a comprehensive healthcare system including primary care, radiation therapy, skilled nursing facility, home health, and durable medical equipment

Objectives

For the desired outcome of goals to be achieved, *objectives* are designed to make each goal operational. This is an important step because objectives provide a mechanism for quantifiable results or outcomes to measure success. Objectives describe the results to be achieved, when and by whom, and are measurable. Examples of objectives for the preceding goals are as follows:

- The director of Women's Health will direct the completion of renovations of the existing unit by December 31, 20*XX*.
- The chief executive officer will recruit six hospitalists by August 31, 20*XX*.
- The chief nursing officer will recruit/hire 20 team members for the skilled nursing unit by November 30, 20*XX*.

The mission, vision, values, goals, objectives, and the external and internal environmental analyses depict the essence of the organization. These entities provide a basis for strategy formation, and thus it is important that this work be completed with careful thought and analysis.

Adaptive Strategies

Whereas directional strategies provide general guidance, *adaptive strategies* are more specific and describe the process for carrying out the directional strategies. Directional strategies are the ends, whereas adaptive strategies are the means. Adaptive strategies describe how the organization will expand, contract, or maintain its scope of services (Ginter et al., 2002). These are the strategies most visible to those outside the organization.

Expansion Strategies

Expansion strategies include diversification, vertical integration, market development, product development, and penetration (Ginter et al., 2002). *Diversification* occurs at the corporate level when markets outside the organization's core business offer potential for significant growth. Because the organization is venturing outside the core business, diversification is generally considered a risky venture. Diversification is most often seen in health care when there are opportunities in less-regulated markets.

There are two types of diversification (Ginter et al., 2002): related and unrelated. In healthcare organizations, *related diversification (concentric)* includes related products and services such as home health, hospice, or radiation treatment. *Unrelated diversification (conglomerate)* includes businesses in the general environment such as a laundry, restaurant, or office buildings and those within the healthcare industry such as pharmaceuticals, medical supplies, or insurance. Selecting markets and products that complement one another can reduce risk. Nevertheless, unrelated diversification has been found to be generally unsuccessful in generating revenue for healthcare organizations. Ginter and Swayne (2006) warned that unrelated diversification may not be realistic in health care because such organizations have a dominant core business (patient care) that is capital and human intensive, and thus it is difficult for healthcare organizations to be successful outside the core business.

Vertical integration is the second corporate-level expansion of adaptive strategies. The purpose of vertical integration in health care is to enhance the continuity of care while simultaneously managing the channel of demand for healthcare services. Healthcare organizations that use vertical integration grow the business along the channel of distribution of core processes (Ginter et al., 2002). Vertical integration can reduce supply costs and enhance integration. A successful example would be the inclusion of technical education programs for team members in critically short supply such as nursing assistant and technicians. Vertical integration was the fundamental adaptive strategy of the 1990s. This rapid change was realized as hospitals joined networks or systems in an effort to secure resources, increase capabilities, and gain greater bargaining power with purchasers and healthcare plans (Ginter et al., 2002). Nevertheless, Ginter and Swayne (2006) recommended caution when considering vertical integration for the same reasons listed earlier regarding unrelated diversification.

Market development occurs at the division or strategic service unit level and focuses on entering new markets with existing products or services. The purpose of this strategy is to add volume through geographic expansion of the service area or by expansion into new market segments within the present geographic area (Ginter et al., 2002). *Horizontal integration* is a type of market development that grows the business by acquiring or affiliating with competitors. Horizontal growth of healthcare systems in the 1980s and early 1990s created multihospital systems. Many of the expected benefits such as reduction of duplication of services, economics of scale, improved productivity, and operating efficiencies did not materialize, and horizontal integration strategies slowed in the late 1990s (Ginter et al., 2002). In addition, Ginter and Swayne (2006) stated that service area limited market development (expansion) for many services because technologies are often developed by those outside the organization, for example, drug companies and equipment manufacturers.

Product development also occurs at the division or strategic service unit level and involves the introduction of new products or services to existing markets. Whereas related diversification is the introduction of a new product, product development refines, complements, or extends existing products or services such as women's health or cancer treatment. Product development may be used when customer requirements are changing, technology is changing, or when there is a need to create differentiation advantage (Ginter et al., 2002).

Penetration strategies, like market and product development, focus on increasing volumes and market share. Market penetration is an aggressive marketing strategy centered on extending existing services. This strategy is used when the present market is growing and expected revenues are high (Ginter et al., 2002).

Contraction Strategies

When the organization needs to decrease the size or scope of operations at either the corporate or divisional level, four *contraction strategies* are considered. Divestiture and liquidation occur at the corporate level, and harvesting and retrenchment occur at the divisional level (Ginter et al., 2002).

When a service unit is viable yet a decision to leave the market and sell an operating unit is made, *divestiture* occurs. Generally, the divested business unit has value and will continue to be operated by the purchasing organization (Ginter et al., 2002). This strategy has become common over the past decade as healthcare organizations carve out noncore business. Examples of noncore healthcare business that may be divested include pharmacy, laboratory, and radiology. Business units may be divested for several reasons, including industry decline, the need for cash to fund priority operations, or marginal performance. Services too far from the core business may be divested in an effort to focus on business at hand, or management expertise for the particular service may not be available within the leadership group.

Liquidation is the selling of assets of an organization that can no longer operate. In contrast to divestiture, liquidation assumes that the operating unit cannot be sold as a viable operation (Ginter et al., 2002). Some assets, of course, may still have value, such as buildings and equipment. Reasons for liquidation include bankruptcy, the need to dispose of nonproductive assets, the need to reduce assets, or the emergence of expensive new technology that will make the current technology obsolete.

Harvesting occurs when the market has entered long-term decline or there is a need for short-term cash (Ginter et al., 2002). For example, despite a strong market position, revenues are expected to decline industry-wide over the next years. The unit will be allowed to generate as much revenue as possible;

however, no new resources will be invested in the business. This allows for an orderly exit from the market by planned downsizing. Harvesting has occurred with many small rural hospitals that could not maintain or improve their financial positions because of the lack of physician and community support, an aging population, and the migration of the young to urban areas.

Retrenchment occurs when the market has become too diverse, and there is a decline in profitability as a result of increasing costs (Ginter et al., 2002). Although the market is still viewed as viable, costs are too high. Retrenchment involves redefinition of the market if it is too spread out geographically. Costs such as personnel or facility assets that are marginal or nonproductive are reduced.

Recall, however, the role of the organization's mission as related to contraction strategies. Ginter and Swayne (2006) noted that contraction strategies may be limited in healthcare organizations because services may be mandated, needed by the community, or core to the organization's mission.

Maintenance-of-Scope Strategies

When current strategies are appropriate and few changes are needed, the organization may use *maintenance-of-scope strategies* to *maintain* the existing market position. This does not mean that the organization does nothing but rather pursues either enhancement or status quo strategies (Ginter et al., 2002). Carefully crafting the PI process through direct linkage to resources and performance measures will ensure that processes remain in control or that those that do not perform well are evident to leaders and managers.

When the organization is progressing toward its vision yet nevertheless improvements are needed, *enhancement strategy* may be used. This may entail quality improvement efforts directed toward improving organizational processes or reducing costs. This is a time for innovation and redesign of timeworn systems. The focus should be on those identified as most important to key customers such as patients and families.

Status quo is based on the assumption of a mature market when growth has ceased. The goal is to maintain the market share. When using the status quo strategy, organizations may attempt penetration or market/product development (Ginter et al., 2002).

Market Entry Strategies

The three major strategies to enter a market include: purchase, cooperation, and development. *Market entry strategies* are not ends in themselves, but rather adaptive strategies that may be used to bring market strategies to fruition (Ginter et al., 2002).

Purchase Strategies

There are three *purchase market entry strategies*: acquisition, licensing, and venture capital investment. *Purchase strategies* enable a healthcare organization to enter the market quickly. Each strategy places different demands on the organization (Ginter et al., 2002).

When healthcare organizations purchase an existing organization, organizational unit, or a product or service, *acquisition entry strategy* is used. Acquisition takes place at the corporate or divisional level. The acquisition may be integrated into existing operations, or it may operate as a separate unit. Acquisitions often flounder because it is difficult to integrate existing culture and operations. Often, it takes several years post acquisition to combine two organizational cultures. Despite the difficulties of integrating cultures, the synergy realized by the creation of a comprehensive healthcare system has demonstrated that acquisition is an effective purchase strategy.

Licensing avoids the time and market risks of technology or product development (Ginter et al., 2002). When licensure is used as a strategy, proprietary technology is usually not purchased and therefore the organization is dependent on the licensor for support and upgrade. Healthcare organizations frequently use licensing strategies for implementation of clinical documentation systems. This strategy lowers the financial and market risk of technologies outside the core business.

Venture capital investment is a low-risk option whereby healthcare organizations purchase minority investment in a developing enterprise. This provides an opportunity to "try out" and, possibly later, enter into new technology. Examples include life science portals for bioinformatics, home-based healthcare services for elderly adults, and cardiology arrhythmia management companies (Ginter et al., 2002).

Cooperation Strategies

According to Ginter and associates (2002) mergers, alliances, and joint ventures—*cooperation strategies*—were the most popular strategies of the 1990s. Cooperation strategies enable organizations to carry out adaptive strategies.

Although similar to acquisitions, in a *merger* two organizations combine through a mutual agreement to form a single new organization (recall that in an acquisition a healthcare organization purchases an existing organization, organizational unit, or a product or service). Merger strategies are used to accomplish horizontal integration by combining two similar organizations, or vertical integration, by creating an integrated delivery system. Reasons for mergers include improving efficiency and effectiveness (combining resources and exploiting cost-reduction strategies), enhancing access (broader services), enhancing financial position (gaining market share), and overcoming concerns of survival (enduring in an aggressive market). As with acquisitions, the major hurdle in a merger is the integration of two separate organizational cultures. Because a new organization is formed, mergers are often more difficult to navigate than acquisitions are. In a merger, a totally new organizational culture must be developed. If mergers are to be successful, work groups must be formed to reformulate the mission, vision, and core values of the new organization. Merger of two organizational cultures into one takes years to complete (Ginter et al., 2002).

Alliance strategies entail arrangements among existing organizations to achieve a strategic purpose not possible by any single organization. Alliances include federations, consortiums, networks, and systems. Alliances attempt to strengthen competitive position while the organizations maintain their independence. Healthcare organizations often form an alliance to achieve economies of scale in purchasing. Examples include Premier and Voluntary Hospitals of America (Ginter et al., 2002). Although not a merger or acquisition, alliances have many of the same issues with conflicting cultures.

Joint ventures are used when risks are too high or the project is too large or too expensive to be done by a single organization. In a joint venture, two or more organizations combine resources to accomplish a designated task. The most common healthcare joint ventures are

- Contractual agreements
- Subsidiary corporations
- Partnerships
- Not-for-profit title-holding corporations

In a *contractual agreement*, two or more organizations contract to work together toward specific objectives. *Subsidiary corporations* form a new corporation, usually to operate non–healthcare activities. A partnership is a formal or informal arrangement between two or more parties for mutual benefit of the organizations involved. *Not-for-profit title-holding corporations* form tax-exempt title-holding corporations to provide benefits to healthcare organizations engaged in real estate ventures. The dynamic healthcare environment mandates that organizations engage in joint ventures to lower costs (Ginter et al., 2002).

Development Strategies

Organizations may enter new markets through internal resources. There are two types of *development entry strategies*: internal development and internal ventures.

> **Internal development:** Organizations use internal development for products or services closely related to existing products or services. The organization maintains a high level of control through the use of existing resources, competencies, and capabilities. Although internal development presents an image of a growing organization, there is a time lag to break even, and obtaining significant market share against strong competitors is difficult (Ginter et al., 2002).

> **Internal ventures:** In contrast to internal development, internal ventures are most appropriate for products or services that are unrelated to the current products or services. Nevertheless, congruence of internal ventures with the organization's mission, vision, and values must be considered. Internal ventures set up separate, relatively independent entities within the organization. An example of an internal venture is a hospital that develops home health care through an internal venture (Ginter et al., 2002). Success of this strategy is mixed because the organization's internal climate is often unsuitable for the venture.

In the final stage of strategic formation, a *gap analysis* examines the difference in the current state and the desired state, or vision for the future. Gap analysis is the process of examining how large a leap must be taken to meet the vision and what must be done to make the leap. If organizational leaders set their vision too narrow, they will find their current state meets the vision but lacks incentive to aspire for higher and greater things. Their task is accomplished, and the planning process ends. With this in mind, leaders must communicate the vision in a somewhat revolutionary manner. The vision should inspire team members to perform their best because there is no room for mediocrity in healthcare vision. The desired outcome of the gap analysis is a strategic plan that has a reasonable probability of success. To accomplish this, priorities must be established and resources allocated to narrow the gap between the current state and the desired state. This process establishes the groundwork for the strategies necessary to ensure the desired outcome (Drenkard, 2001).

Planning encompasses stewardship of the organization and its resources. Care must be taken to articulate the core assumptions about the nature of the market, the competitions, and the organization; otherwise, a gap will exist between the aspirations of the organization and the way the organization actually behaves. When what we do day to day is in contrast to what we say we do and hope to be, a paradox exists that leads to team member frustration. For example, does the organization value creativity or discipline? Is the focus on short-term or long-term goals? Quality or the bottom line? Although conflicts occur in every organization, successful organizations meet the challenge and reconcile aspirations and actions as part of the strategic planning process (Solovy, 2002). Decisions regarding resources must be made with the core value—what the patient needs or values and what is best/safest for the patient—as the focal point of the organization. The financial bottom line is a secondary priority to safe care. When the financial bottom line is the priority, money is wasted.

An additional gap can also exist between management's view of the organization and the team members' view. Team members are closer to the core business (patient care), and thus their input must be sought as part of the planning process. A planned process whereby each business unit can share information and seek guidance and clarification facilitates buy-in and avoids duplication of efforts. The alternative, top-down, directive approach may result in a high-quality strategic plan, but team members who have input into planning more readily accept the expected outcomes and so become more vested in work processes. Thus, the process includes a system of notification for team members as to the status of their suggestions and how they were evaluated, or if their ideas were not used, feedback is given to team members as to the rationale.

It is imperative that healthcare leaders understand and focus on their core business. Focusing on the core business provides a clear strategic vision—the big picture—in contrast to scattered plans that steal time and energy with little to show except charts and graphs. Successful organizations focus their strategy on their core rather than on the industry's competitive factors. One method of assessing the health of the organization's strategic planning process is to consider the time spent focusing on the competition. If more time is spent analyzing competitors than focusing on the core business, the process is off task. The primary priorities are the processes and outcomes that the organization must do well to remain in business and those things that the organization does particularly well. Healthcare dollars are scarce. Across-the-board investing often signals that competitors are setting the organization's agenda. Conversely, when an organization's strategy is formed reactively as it tries to keep up with competitors, it loses its uniqueness (Kim & Mauborgne, 2002).

Strategy Deployment

Failure to implement the strategic plan is the most common flaw in the planning process (Zuckerman, 1998). Martin (2010) warned that "a mediocre strategy well executed is better than a great strategy poorly executed" (p. 66). Thus, carefully crafted strategies are useless if sufficient time is not spent developing the plan for *strategy deployment* (Shirey, 2011b). Zuckerman (1998) emphasized that team members may be overwhelmed with managing the day-to-day crises, leaving little time to implement strategic objectives. In addition, if the objectives are not specific, team members may lack the direction needed to meet the established goals. Communication of the strategic plan must be coordinated throughout the entire organization both vertically and horizontally. To provide direction at the work level, goals and objectives must be established for each business unit and ought to link to the overall plan for the organization. This linkage provides guidance and consistency in decision making and enables managers and team members to understand the present and plan for the future. All team members must be able to articulate how "what they do" fits into the overall plan for the organization.

For each goal and objective, *at least one person should be assigned as the primary individual responsible for planning, implementing, and monitoring progress.* This is often a member of senior leadership. Specific target dates are assigned to provide a timeline for expected progress. If realization of goals involves intradepartmental work processes, PI teams may be assigned. Senior leadership should establish specific dates to review progress toward each goal. Accountability is accomplished (and rewarded, or otherwise) through linkage between the goals and objectives of the strategic plan and individual team member evaluation criteria. **Exhibit 16–5** provides an excerpt from a strategic planning matrix.

Exhibit 16–5   Sample of Strategic Planning Matrix

Nurse's Heaven Hospital			Strategic Plan 20XX		
Goal	Objective	Actions	Measure/ Benchmark	Target Date	Responsible Party
Expand Women's Services to encompass all key aspects of the business	Complete renovations of the existing unit by 12/31/XX	1. Monitor progress daily 2. Facilitate weekly construction progress meeting 3. Facilitate monthly medical staff meetings 4. Facilitate biweekly team member meetings	1. Phase I complete by 08/31/XX 2. Phase II complete by 10/31/XX 3. Complete Phase III by 12/31/XX Benchmark: There Medical Center, Anywhere, USA	12/31/20XX	Director of Women's Health

Culture

The *culture* of the organization includes the shared assumptions, values, and behavioral norms of the group. These assumptions and values remain constant over time, even when membership of the organization changes, and are the basis for an informal consciousness (Ginter et al., 2002). This is significant in the current climate of mergers, acquisitions, and buy-outs. The shared values of team members may not reflect the values of the organization. When this occurs, the customary way of doing things (behavioral norms) may sabotage the strategic plan. To ensure congruency, shared assumptions (mission—who we are) must support the organizational vision and goals (what we want to accomplish). If the plan is in conflict with the culture, deployment will be a challenge. Unfortunately, if the culture is in significant conflict with the strategic plan and a strong subculture exists, change will be difficult because team members may prefer to "do things the way we have always done them."

Ginter and Swayne (2006) warn that healthcare organizations have a unique culture related to power. These authors noted that healthcare organizations and hospitals, in particular, have a history of hierarchical power that hampers planning and participation from those closest to the patient. To be cognizant of the assumptions, values, and behavioral norms of team members, successful leaders are involved in the day-to-day operations of the organization. Healthcare leaders must schedule regular visits to each business unit. In addition, regular visits to all stakeholders are imperative. It is not acceptable to attempt to lead from the office or through computer technology. Email, voice mail, video conferencing, and other technologies do not take the place of face-to-face contact, nor do they reflect a complete picture of the culture of the organization. Insights gleaned from involvement with stakeholders and the day-to-day operations of the organization provide vital insight during the situation analysis. Leaders must assess whether the directional strategies are still appropriate and reflect the culture of the organization. *Considering the organizational culture is perhaps the most crucial aspect in the deployment of the strategic plan.*

It is important to consider strategies that assist in developing a culture that is adaptive to change. Involving stakeholders in the strategic planning process cultivates an environment of trust and respect. Buy-in from those involved in the processes and outcomes of care is worth the extra time necessary to glean these insights. This input is especially pertinent during the shaping of directional strategies—mission, vision, values, and goals. Cultural assessment during the situation analysis may determine that additional implementation strategies are necessary to maintain or change the organizational culture. As previously mentioned, the roles of nurse leaders position them to be acutely aware of the "pulse" of the organization. Nurse leaders and managers must feel comfortable expressing views different from those in senior leadership. An atmosphere of trust encourages risk taking and is necessary for innovation to occur. If trust is absent, personal safety and security become the priority, and the status quo will be maintained despite an elaborate strategic plan. In addition, time and money may be wasted on endeavors that do not reflect current customer needs.

Maintaining a climate of trust and respect, one that encourages risk taking and innovation, is hard work. Leaders must "walk the talk." Saying one thing while doing another (or, even more critical, rewarding another) creates confusion. The directional strategies, mission, vision, values, and goals must be communicated often, both verbally and in writing. Prominent posting in both common areas and each business unit is essential. Additional successful strategies include having the mission appear on all meeting agendas and minutes, on stationery, and on laminated cards for team members. The key strategy for maintenance of an organizational culture that is adaptive to change is to live it as reflected in the daily business of the organization.

Structure

Ginter and associates (2002) described three basic organizational structures: functional structure, divisional structure, and matrix structure. Similar to organizational culture, structure must not impede the overall strategy.

Functional organizational structures organize activities around mission-critical functions or processes. This is the most prevalent organizational structure for organizations with a relatively narrow focus such as healthcare organizations. Departments are organized according to their function, such as clinical services, finance, marketing, or information systems. Organizations that are structured around mission-critical functions may consider clinical services as the center of the functional structure with other sections of the organization organized around clinical processes such as registration, radiology, laboratory, and so forth (Ginter et al., 2002).

Health care is highly specialized, and expertise within the specialty is highly valued. Functional structures can foster efficiency; however, this type of structure can also result in silo mentality. Functional structure slows decision making, makes coordination of work difficult, and inhibits communication as each department looks after its own interest without the realization of how its processes affect others.

Divisional structures are common in healthcare organizations that have grown through diversification, vertical integration, or market or product development (Ginter et al., 2002). Divisional organizations attempt to break down larger, diverse organizations into more manageable and focused sections. This division is especially important when structures of the organization are in different geographic locales, and thus have a different environment and unique customers. Divisional structures have difficulty in maintaining a consistent image and purpose. Divisional structures may additionally require multiple layers of management and duplication of services, thus increasing costs. Organizations that choose divisional structures must carefully coordinate strategic business unit activities.

Matrix structures organize activities around problems to be solved rather than functions, products, or geography (Ginter et al., 2002). The nurse manager may have a dual reporting structure, to the vice president of Women's Health (product) as well as to the vice president of Nursing Services (functional). Thus, the nurse manager is responsible to the vice president of Nursing for nursing care and to the vice president of Women's Health when working on the women's health product line. In some matrix structures, the reporting relationships follow a project or program, and the relationship ends when the project is complete. Matrix structures foster creativity and innovation; nevertheless, they are difficult to manage because priorities can become confused. Thus, matrix structures require expert coordination and communication.

Resources

Deploying the selected strategies uses four key resources: financial, human, information systems, and technology (Ginter et al., 2002). Analysis of *financial resources* was a key factor in the internal environmental analysis. In addition, finance provided key input for strategy formation. Once strategies have been decided, finance is the vehicle to implement them. Leaders should require that major purchase requests be submitted with documented links to the strategic plan. Major projects require capital investment, which generally must be approved by the governing body.

Human resources must be considered before deployment of the strategic plan. There are several questions to consider: Will additional training be required? Are additional team members needed? Will there be a need for team members with different skills and experiences? This is a critical time to complete an organizational learning needs assessment with all team members. This provides a bridge between the strategic plan, education plan, and PI plan. Multiple plans should be consolidated into one master strategic plan. This is less confusing for team members and assists with unified communication of the organization's plan for improvement.

Although *information resources* are crucial to develop the internal and external environmental analysis, they are equally important in the deployment of the strategic plan. As previously mentioned, clinicians can no longer be expected to complete laborious paper documentation. Likewise, leaders must be able to extract data entered into clinical documentation systems with relative ease, thereby negating the need for manual data extraction. A shared drive on the organization's computer system assists in ease of review of the strategic plan. Key business drivers selected as part of the organization's balanced scorecard should also be available on a shared computer system (balanced scorecards are discussed in more detail later in this chapter). Large binders containing the organization's plans, placed on the highest shelf and never used, are dinosaurs.

The strategies selected drive the needed technologies. *Strategic technology* is concerned with the type of organization, the sophistication of the equipment, and management of the technology used *within* the organization (Ginter et al., 2002). Healthcare organizations are high-technology organizations. Equipment becomes obsolete as quickly as it is installed. This is an area of increasing concern for healthcare leaders because it represents major expenditures for the organization.

Strategic Management

Goals and Objectives

Exhibit 16–5 demonstrates a sample strategic planning matrix. Senior leaders ensure that team members remain focused by assigning specific dates/times for review of the status of each goal and objective. Someone once said, "People respect what you inspect." An additional pertinent adage is, "You are what you measure." Although these statements are poor examples of transformational leadership, the adages unfortunately hold true. Assessment of efforts toward meeting established goals and objectives not only keeps leaders aware of the status of planning efforts, but it also provides team members the opportunity to "show off" their hard work. This personal time and attention by senior leaders demonstrate that the strategic plan is more than a "dusty binder on the shelf" but is rather a working document that ebbs and flows with the organization.

Follow-up reviews can be assigned by target date or minimally twice per year. Typically, quarterly reports are assigned to assess whether the work is proceeding as planned or whether adjustments need to be made based on current reality. Assigning quarterly due dates for status reports on alternate months assists in time and agenda management for senior leaders as well as busy team members. Responsible parties should be forwarded a reminder of the date, time, and place of the meeting as well as the report expectations (i.e., verbal, written, visuals). Presenters should be instructed on the amount of time allotted for their presentation. To assist team members to prepare for the meeting, it is helpful if a general format is established. Beware, however, because being too prescriptive can stifle creativity. **Exhibit 16–6** demonstrates a quarterly report matrix for follow-up of progress toward established goals and objectives.

Exhibit 16–6 Sample Goals and Objectives Quarterly Report Matrix

| | Nurse's Heaven Hospital Strategic Plan 20XX Goals and Objectives Report Matrix | | | | | | | | | | | |
Goal	Jan	Feb	Mar	Apr	May	Jun	Jul	Aug	Sept	Oct	Nov	Dec
A	X			X			X			X		
B		X			X			X			X	
C			X			X			X			X

Measurement: Balanced Scorecard

Kaplan and Norton (1996) of the Harvard Business School developed scorecards (also known as dashboards, instrument panels, and data display devices) in 1991. The utility of the *balanced scorecard (BSC)* remains unchanged—the provision of a strategic management and performance management tool. Measurement of key financial, quality, market, and operational indicators provides management with an understanding of performance in relation to established strategic goals and graphically displays a snapshot of the institution's overall health (Health Care Advisory Board, 1999).

Selection of critical metrics is key because the Health Care Advisory Board (2002) noted in its study of hospital downturns that inadequate performance measurement was the cause of 10% of financial flashpoints—unexpected, dramatic declines in total margin and cash flow. As organizations grow increasingly complex, it is critical that leaders have easy access to accurate data that provide a view of overall organizational performance rather than being inundated with mountains of disparate reports from the various business lines and departments.

Successful BSC implementations have been documented using the process shown in **Exhibit 16–7** (Health Care Advisory Board, 1999).

Theurer (as cited in Health Care Advisory Board, 1999) recognized that the following pitfalls should be avoided when creating indicators for a BSC: (l) lack of context (measures should tie to strategic goals and drive organizational strategy and resource allocation), and (2) lack of benchmark data (seeing how the organization ranks against a peer group).

Leadership must empower employees and provide sufficient resources to develop unit-level performance measures. Without sufficient resources, the staff will simply recycle existing measures. Bureaucratic uniformity squelches the individualized nature of each unit and should be avoided so that each unit can be measured based on its unique attributes. Indicators must be used as tools for continuous improvement, not as tools to punish poor performance. Leadership should provide positive reinforcement when improvements are made. The Health Care Advisory Board (1999) noted that dashboards should be *limited to* 15 to 30 standards of measurement. Drill-down data should be reserved for situations when a more comprehensive assessment is warranted.

Performance Improvement

Performance improvement is a systematic, organization-wide approach to improving the processes and outcomes of the healthcare system. Performance improvement shifts the focus from individual performance to the performance of the organization's systems and processes. Although individual performance must be maintained, only those team members who are unwilling or unable to change (a very small percentage of the workforce) are penalized. There are four basic tenets of PI: *customer focus, continuous improvement of processes, team member involvement,* and *use of data and team knowledge to improve decision making*. To be successful, PI effects must be embraced by senior leaders and must involve all departments and team members in clinical as well as nonclinical areas. Performance improvement efforts are a part of the strategic planning process, not a separate function orchestrated to comply with regulatory standards.

Exhibit 16–7 Balanced Scorecard Implementation/25- to 26-Month Process

	J	F	M	A	M	J	J	A	S	O	N	D	J	F	M	A	M	J	J	A	S	O	N	D	J	F
Commitment from senior leadership; senior leadership education before initiation prevents ambiguity	X	X	X	X	X	X	X	X	X	X	X	X	X	X	X	X	X	X	X	X	X	X	X	X	X	X
Strategic planning retreat (critical); involving the entire organization	X	X																								
Select strategic planning committee; identify objectives for each perspective in the balanced scorecard			X	X																						
Strategic planning committee communicates with staff					X	X																				
Revise scorecard based on staff input							X																			
Revised scorecard deployed to staff								X	X																	
Each unit/department and employee develops scorecard that supports facility scorecard								X	X																	
Strategic planning committee reviews departmental and individual scorecards; suggests revisions										X	X															
One-year mark; senior leaders formulate 3- to 5-year plan based on finalized scorecard												X														
Departmental and organizational progress reviewed quarterly; identify opportunities to improve													X	X	X	X	X	X	X	X	X	X	X	X		
Evaluation committee assesses staff performance based on the individual balanced scorecards. Based on the results: retention, promotion, salary increases, and rewards																									X	X
Strategic planning committee revises the balanced scorecard and 3- to 5-year plan based on results of the metrics																									X	X
Cycle continues in the following years																										

Collecting Data: Quantitative Methods

The process for measurement, assessment, and PI is designed to assist the organization to use resources effectively in the provision of quality patient care. Performance improvement activities focus on interrelated factors, governance, managerial support, and clinical processes, which affect patient outcomes and the financial viability of the facility. Data collection in the form of clinical measurement, assessment, and improvement activities should focus on the flow of patient care and assess how well the processes in which individuals participate are performed, coordinated, integrated, and improved. When a problem or opportunity to improve care is identified, action is taken, and the effectiveness of the action is assessed. Results of PI activities are used primarily to improve patient care processes. When the results of PI activities are relevant to the performance of an individual, the results are used as a component in the evaluation of the individual's capabilities.

Priority for data collection is given to those aspects of care evaluating the following areas:

1. **High risk:** Patients who are at risk of serious consequences or are deprived of substantial benefit if the care is not provided correctly (including providing care that is not indicated or failing to provide care that is indicated)
2. **High volume:** Aspect of care occurs frequently or affects large numbers of patients
3. **Problem prone:** Aspect of care has tended in the past to produce problems for staff or patients
4. **High cost:** Aspect of care is resource intensive
5. **Top money loser:** Care provided has been documented to lose money for the facility
6. **Regulatory requirement:** Outcome data required by regulatory agencies
7. **Key indicators of quality:** Include core processes and those identified by customers

Measures are used to capture PI data. A *measure* is a variable relating to the structure, process, or outcome of care. Measures are selected based on the organization's key business drivers (what must be done well to remain in the business), for example, identifiers of key quality characteristics and customer satisfaction, strategic management goals and objectives, assessment of performance relevant to functions, the design and assessment of new processes, measurement of the level of performance, and stability of important existing processes. An *operational definition* of each measure must be well defined for ease and reliability of data collection. *Measures of process* are often standards of care or practice. Measures of process include objective criteria based on authoritative sources and supported by the best available clinical and PI literature. Quality control measures are also documented as required by regulatory agencies.

To be useful, data must be transcribed to information through data display, interpretation, and analysis. Tools for analyzing data over time include line graphs, run charts, or control charts. These tools allow the nurse manager to look for trends or patterns in the data.

Line Graphs

Line graphs aid in assessment of trends or changes in performance. These simple graphs indicate whether a process is working and may reveal areas in need of improvement. The data are plotted as the events occur over time. The horizontal axis (x) is used to plot time, for example, days of the week, months of the year, and so forth. The vertical axis (y) is used to plot the observed level of performance. Once the data points are plotted on the graph, lines are drawn connecting point to point enabling visualization of trends. Line graphs are used when data collection is still in the early stages before sufficient data are available to complete a control chart (usually 24–30 data points). Nevertheless, at least 10 to 12 data points are needed to have a meaningful graph. If it is discovered that a problem occurs at identified times, an in-depth analysis as to the cause and resolution may be undertaken.

The line graph in **Exhibit 16–8** demonstrates data collected for an identified compliance issue for the months of October 20*XX* through February 20*XX*. Five data points connected by a line provide visualization of the compliance rate that ranges from 24% to 43%. At this early stage of data collection, visualization for a beginning analysis is possible; however, additional data points are required before construction of more sophisticated graphs (run charts and control charts).

Run charts are used when the nurse manager requires a more sensitive analysis of data over time than is available with a line chart. Although run charts are more sophisticated than line charts are, they do not have the benefit of assessment of statistical process control. Typically, run charts are used until sufficient data points are available for assessment of statistical process control (SPC). In addition to the data point connections, an arithmetic mean is calculated and plotted on the graph.

There is natural variation in everything. An objective of statistical process control is to analyze this variability and to assign causes. A key question is whether the variation is normal or abnormal. This is done by establishing the limits of chance variation. Variation beyond these limits is the result of designated causes. Common cause (normal) variation is derived from random, expected differences in the process, whereas special cause (abnormal) variation is outside what is expected and is derived from identifiable reason(s)/change(s) in the process.

An example of common cause variation related to charting omissions is that related to layout of forms and time constraints of healthcare workers. Special cause variation is variation caused by computer downtime (unless, of course, the computer is down as much as it is up) when workers must use paper charting.

Deciding when to follow up on common cause variation depends on the nature of the data. If variation results from common cause, the result of work inherent in complex processes, and the results are satisfactory, then monitoring rather than additional study may be all that is needed. This may be true of charting. Although 100% compliance would be ideal, it is probably not achievable.

Leaders must decide how much variation (deviation from the mean) in the process is acceptable. This is usually done based on the nature of the process and outcomes deemed key to the organization. Most often

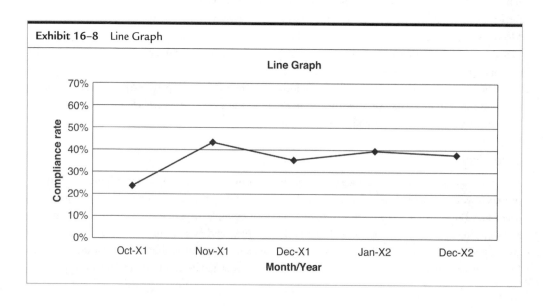

Exhibit 16–8   Line Graph

healthcare leaders strive to decrease variation in processes where there is potential for adverse patient care. If significant variation in the process is unsatisfactory, such as medication errors, patient falls, or nosocomial infections, the process needs to be studied (for example, using a rapid-cycle PI team).

Responding to special cause variation as if it were common cause can create false alarms and/or increase costs (time is money). The quest for reasons for special cause may lead to blaming individuals for poor results. These investigations often waste resources, create resentment, and may increase variation, for example, targeting one department with low satisfaction scores for 1 month with the expectation of "improving or else." If the identifiable cause is apparent, there may be no need to work on the process. Unfortunately, facilities often react to special cause variation because of pressure from regulatory agencies. The best way to deal with special cause variation is to design quality into the process—prevent adverse events rather than study them.

The run chart in **Exhibit 16–9** provides a visual cue of an error rate plotted for 12 months from April 20*XX* through March 20*XX*. The mean is documented as 0.42. Two data points are worthy of analysis, May and June 20*XX*. What is the root of these two data points, both on the upper side of the mean with successive increase—special cause or common cause? Although this run chart provides more information than a line chart does, a control chart is constructed to assess for statistical process control. *Statistical process control* is a method for monitoring the control or extent of variation in a process or outcome. The goal is to reduce variation, thus increasing the desired result.

Control charts are specialized run charts that also allow visualization of data over time. Control charts are used when the nurse manager wishes to discover how much variability in a process is caused by random variation (process design) and how much is caused by special cause variation (unique actions/events) to determine whether a process is in statistical process control. Control charts are borrowed from manufacturing where predictable results are required. In health care, as in manufacturing, there should not be a high degree of variation in the product. In health care, the primary product is patient care. Because these are typically called control charts in manufacturing, we use this term here as well.

A mean (arithmetic average) is established for each data set/chart. Healthcare organizations typically calculate the upper and lower control limits at three standard deviations above and below the mean.

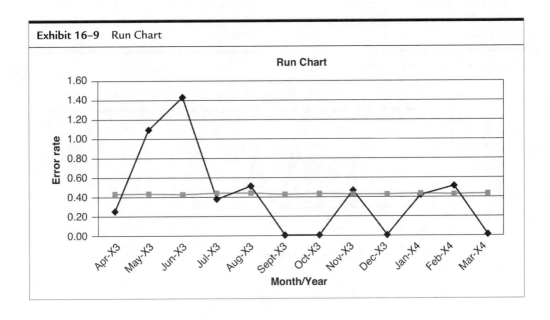

Exhibit 16–9   Run Chart

Data points outside of the established control limits are to the result of a special cause. These data points represent deviations from the way the process normally operates (Goal/QPC, 2008). A fluctuation in the data within the established control limits results from variation in the process resulting from common causes within the system (design, choice).

Criteria for interpreting control charts are as follows:

1. **Outside of the control limits:** A data point that falls outside the control limits on the chart, either above the upper control limit or below the lower control limit.
2. **Shift:** Eight or more consecutive points either all above or all below the mean. Values on the mean are skipped and the nurse continues to count. Values on the mean do not make or break a trend.
3. **Trend:** Six points all going up or all going down. If the value of two or more successive points is the same, the point is ignored when counting; like values do not make or break a trend.
4. **Two out of three:** Two out of three consecutive points in the outer third of the chart (greater than two standard deviations). The two out of three consecutive points could be on the same side or on either side of the mean.

The control chart in **Exhibit 16–10** demonstrates a medication error rate for August 20*XX* through March 20*XX*. The mean is 0.90 with an upper control limit (three standard deviations above the mean) of 2.69 and a lower control limit of 0.00 (a negative error rate is not possible). All data points are within the control limits. No shifts (eight or more consecutive points all above or below the mean) or trends (six points all going up or all going down) are identified. The two-out-of-three criterion (two out of three consecutive points in the outer third of the chart) is not demonstrated. Nurse managers needing more in-depth information regarding control charts are referred to Lighter and Fair (2004) *Quality Management in Health Care: Principles and Methods* specifically related to the determination of the types of data and corresponding appropriate control charts.

Matrix

A *matrix* is used to show combinations of data. Examples include unit statistics such as admissions, nursing hours per patient day, percentage of occupancy, medication error rate, and overall rate of patient satisfaction for an obstetrical unit over a period of months. In **Exhibit 16–11**, the months are documented

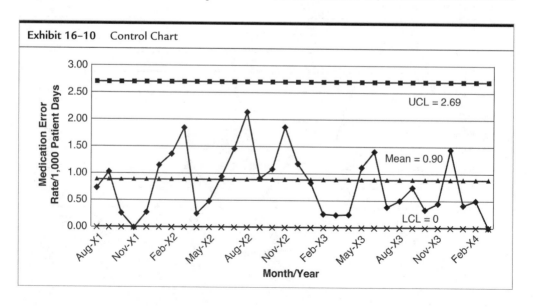

Exhibit 16–10   Control Chart

Exhibit 16–11	Matrix Chart											
OB Unit	Jan	Feb	Mar	Apr	May	Jun	Jul	Aug	Sep	Oct	Nov	Dec
Admissions	650	653	640	600	590	575	555	602	643	670	675	700
Nursing Hours/ Patient Day	5.9	6.0	6.1	6.3	6.6	6.8	7.0	6.7	5.8	5.9	5.7	5.5
Percent Occupancy	.75	.76	.74	.68	.67	.65	.63	.68	.74	.78	.79	.81
Medication Error Rate	1.5	1.0	.75	.54	.45	.16	.05	.50	1.45	1.3	1.7	.10
Overall Patient Satisfaction	.85	.88	.89	.90	.96	.97	.98	.95	.86	.81	.80	.78

in the matrix heading with the measures listed down the left side. This chart provides the data, but it is not as easy to spot anomalies or trends using this method.

The data in Exhibit 16–11 could be used to assess relationships between data sets, for example, overall patient satisfaction and nursing hours per patient day. Does patient satisfaction decrease as nursing hours per patient day decrease? Yes, in this example. Do medication errors increase when nursing hours per patient day decrease? Yes, in this example. Each data set is compared with a different data set for identification of applicable relationships. Relationships are sometimes difficult to discern using a matrix for comparison. A multiple-line graph demonstrates a better visual of relationships between data sets.

Multiple-Line Graph

Relationships of the data captured in a matrix may be better visualized in a *multiple-line graph*. What do the data show happens with the rate of overall patient satisfaction when nursing hours per patient day decrease? Does patient satisfaction increase as nursing hours per patient day increase? Are data relationships more readily apparent during certain months of the year? Spreadsheet software can be used to convert matrix data to a multiple-line graph easily. Caution should be exercised to not display too many indicators on the same graph, thus making it difficult to interpret. Color coding the lines to correlate with data elements assists in analysis of data relationships.

The multiple-line graph in **Exhibit 16–12** allows for easy visualization of the relationship between a decrease in nursing hours per patient day and subsequent increase in medication error (September and October). Each applicable data set from the matrix may be plotted on a multiple-line graph to discern relationships.

Cost-Benefit Analysis

Comparison of the benefits and costs of a proposed endeavor is completed through cost-benefit analysis. *Cost-benefit analysis* is a budgeting technique once used primarily by the government. However, it is becoming increasingly popular as organizational leaders realize the impact their business has on society and the community they serve. Cost-benefit analysis is also an analytical technique that compares the social costs and benefits of a proposed program against the costs of the venture under consideration. If the benefits outweigh the costs, a positive cost-benefit is expected, and it makes sense to spend the money; otherwise, it does not. Criteria for evaluation in a cost-benefit analysis include project goals, benefits and costs, discounting cost and benefit flows at an appropriate rate, and completing a decision analysis (Finkler, 2001).

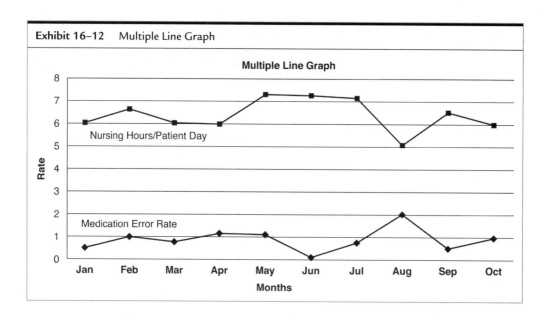

Exhibit 16–12   Multiple Line Graph

The first step in cost-benefit analysis is to determine the goals of the project—what does the organization hope the project will accomplish? What would the community gain if the project comes to fruition? Identifying goals and objectives clarifies the expected benefit for those served. Examples include less travel time for patients in need of cancer treatment or local education resources for high-risk mothers.

Once project goals and objectives have been determined, project benefits must be determined. All losses and gains expected to be experienced by society are included, expressed in dollar terms. Losses incurred to some sections of society are subtracted from the gains that accrue to others. The benefits include only those things that are a direct or indirect result of the project. Alternative strategies are considered so as to choose the option with the greatest net benefit or ratio of benefit to cost (Finkler, 2001). Leaders would not include benefits that are a reality whether or not the project is realized. For example, although cancer treatment may be available at a tertiary medical center 100 miles away, the dollar costs related to the benefit of not having to travel such a long distance are included in the analysis but not the benefits of cancer treatment because they are already available.

Costs must be estimated as part of the cost-benefit analysis. All costs must be considered including opportunity costs because when a decision is made to do something, other alternatives are sacrificed. For example, an increase in inventory requires extra cash. The cash used will not be available for use somewhere else in the organization (another opportunity). This is a critical consideration in cost-benefit analysis (Finkler, 2001). In the cancer treatment example, the facility may have to forgo a transplant program to finance the cancer treatment program. This opportunity cost should be estimated. These calculations include the time value of money.

Project costs and benefits often occur over a period of years. Money has different value over time. If a project has a $2 million start-up cost that will be paid back through revenue over a 5-year period, the $2 million is worth more today than over the next 5 years. This comparison of benefits and costs over time is referred to as discounting cash flow. *Discounting cash flow* uses an interest rate (discount rate) to convert all cost and benefits to their value at the present time (Finkler, 2001). The methodology for the discounting method is beyond the scope of this chapter. Nurse managers requiring in-depth information related to long-term financing are referred to in Finkler (2001).

To complete the decision analysis, estimated costs and benefits are compared with each other in the form of a ratio—benefits divided by costs. If the resulting metric is greater than 1, the benefits exceed the costs and the project is desirable. The greater the benefit-to-cost ratio, the more advantageous the project (Finkler, 2001).

Break-Even Analysis

Healthcare leaders must seek out projects or ventures to improve financial stability or to subsidize loss leaders, services that lose money but provide a community need. *Break-even analysis (BEA)* determines the minimum volume of services that a program must provide to be financially self-sufficient. This tool is useful for determining profitability of a new venture. Break-even analysis is used in situations in which there is a specific price associated with the service (Finkler, 2001). A break-even analysis is an essential part of a business *pro forma*.

This seems like a simple endeavor—if the reimbursement per unit of service is greater than the cost, the new endeavor would be expected to make a profit. On the other hand, if the expected reimbursement is less than the cost, the new endeavor will lose money. However, cost per unit depends on volume. When volume is low, the cost per unit will be higher. As volumes increase, the venture may become profitable. Thus, it is imperative that the organization understand at what point *revenues (money expected to be received) will be equal to expenses (cost to provide the service)*. This is the break-even point.

To grasp the steps in calculating the break-even-point equation, key terminology must be understood:

- *Total revenue* is the average price multiplied by the number of units.
- *Total expenses* include fixed and variable costs.
- *Fixed costs (FC)* are costs that do not change as volume changes within the relevant range (range of activity that would be reasonably expected to occur in the budget period).
- *Variable costs (VC)* vary in direct proportion to volume. When calculating expenses, variable cost is expressed in variable cost per unit.

Finkler (2001, p. 107) described the following calculation to find that break-even point. In this example, 1,000 cesarean deliveries at a total cost of $2,500 per cesarean delivery generate $2,500,000 in total revenue. The break-even point (at cost of $2,500 per case) is 450 cesarean deliveries—the point at which total revenue equals total expenses. **Exhibit 16–13** provides a visual example of the break-even point for cesarean deliveries.

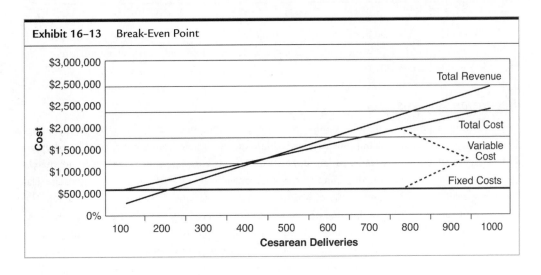

Exhibit 16–13   Break-Even Point

Recall that the break-even point occurs when the total revenues equal the total expenses, thus the break-even point is calculated as follows:

> *Total revenue = P (price) × Q (volume)*
> *Total expenses = V (Variable costs [VC] × Volume [Q]) + Fixed costs (FC)*

> *P × Q = (VC × Q) + FC*
> *$1,125,000 × 450 cases = $625,000 ÷ 450 (recall that variable cost is per case)*
> *× 450 cases + $500,000*
> *($1,125,000 = 450 cases at $2,500/case)*
> *($625,000, the variable cost = $1,125,000 total cost − $500,000 fixed cost)*

The next step is to subtract (VC × Q) from both sides of the equation:

> *(P × Q) − (VC × Q) = FC*
> *$1,125,000 × 450 cases − ($625,000 ÷ 450 × 450 cases) = $500,000*

Next, factor out the Q from the left side of the equation:

> *Q × (P − VC) = FC*
> *450 cases × ($1,125,000 − $625,000 ÷ 450 cases) = $500,000*

The resulting formula is as follows:

> *Q = FC ÷ P − VC*
> *Q is the quantity needed to break even.*
> *450 cases = $500,000 ÷ $1,125,000 − $625,000 ÷ 450 cases*
> *Q = 450 cases*

To summarize, BEA is used to determine the volume at which a service neither makes or loses money. Volume is vital to profitability because healthcare prices are often fixed, whereas average cost is not fixed (Finkler, Jones, & Kovner, 2013).

Regression Analysis

Understanding regression analysis is imperative for successful budgeting and strategic planning. Nurse managers must understand how to effectively predict a variable (for example, cost) based on an independent variable (for example, patient days). Without this knowledge, nurse managers are merely guessing as to whether their nursing unit can remain financially viable. *Regression analysis* is a statistical technique available in computer software used to forecast the relationship between two variables. The independent variable is typically plotted on the x-axis of a scatter graph and the dependent variable is plotted on the y-axis. The computer software requires the user to enter the data for the x and y values. After entering these data, little more than a command to compute the regression is required. It is important that nurse managers not be intimidated by this technique but rather become familiar with its use in the planning process. Guessing is not suitable for professionals charged with meeting the needs of suffering society.

Regression measures the linear association between a dependent (criterion) and an independent variable (predictor). Regression assumes that the dependent variable is predictively linked to the independent variable. Regression analysis is particularly valuable for forecasting because it attempts to predict the values of a continuous, interval-scaled, dependent variable from the independent variable. For example, the number of full-time equivalent (FTE) team members (the dependent variable) might be predicted on the basis of patient days (the independent variable). Forecasting in this manner is crucial to anticipate staffing needs as volumes fluctuate. Nurse managers may seek input from the finance department related to regression analysis.

Collecting Data: Qualitative Methods

Brainstorming

A *brainstorming* session is used to understand an issue, understand the impact the issue may have on the organization, or generate ideas for strategic alternatives. Brainstorming enhances communication, generates new ideas and alternatives, sparks creativity, and stimulates innovation. Members of the group present ideas with brief explanations; however, dialogue and evaluation of the ideas are not undertaken at this juncture (Goal/QPC, 2008). The ideas are usually recorded on flip charts. Team members are encouraged to verbalize ideas no matter how impossible they may seem at first.

There are two methods for brainstorming: structured (each team member gives ideas in turn) and unstructured (team members give ideas as they come to mind) (Goal/QPC, 2008). Structured and unstructured brainstorming can be done silently or aloud. Brainstorming supports breakthrough thinking and organizational change. This is important because creative thinking is needed for change because imaginative ideas are not always available when most needed (Shirey, 2011a). Group dynamics, however, can be problematic. To obtain the best thinking from the group, a facilitator specially trained in group techniques is recommended for brainstorming sessions.

Focus Groups

Similar to brainstorming, *focus groups* are convened to reach conclusions regarding environmental issues. Focus groups were discussed earlier in this chapter as a mechanism for generating information during the internal environmental analysis. Experts in the areas related to the identified issue provide leadership and the opportunity to discuss important issues. In addition, focus groups provide a venue to gain new insight and fresh alternatives (Ginter et al., 2002). This insight empowers and equips the experts with ideas for alternative actions if necessary.

Nominal Group Technique

Another problem-identification and problem-solving method for groups is called *nominal group technique (NGT)*. In nominal group technique, team members independently generate a written list of ideas regarding the issue. After members have been given sufficient time to generate their list, each member takes turns reporting one idea at a time to the entire group. New ideas generated are recorded on a flip chart for consideration. Members are encouraged to build on the ideas of fellow team members. When all ideas have been exhausted, the team discusses the ideas, and then team members privately vote by ranking the ideas in order of preference. After the ideas are ranked, the group discusses the vote, and voting continues until consensus is reached. The advantage of nominal group technique is that everyone has equal status and power, ensuring representation of the group. In addition, nominal group technique eliminates the biases of those in a leadership position (Ginter et al., 2002).

Nominal group technique allows a team to quickly come to consensus regarding the importance of issues, problems, or solutions by individual rankings into a team's final priorities (Goal/QPC, 2008). Because all team members participate equally, commitment is built into the team's choice. It is especially useful for reserved team members because it places them on equal footing with more dominant team members.

Delphi Technique

The *Delphi technique* uses a structured group decision-making technique based on repeated use of rating scales to obtain opinions about a decision. Computer software is available that summarizes the results, making the process easier and faster. Members of the group first explore the issue individually and then design a questionnaire for a larger group. The results are tabulated and given back to the group for discussion. The process continues with progressively focused questionnaires. The process is repeated until members of the group reach consensus regarding the issues and a decision is reached.

Alternately, the process may begin in a more free-flowing style with team members initially identifying important issues. This individual brainstorming technique is particularly valuable when team members are unable to meet in a group setting. Key themes are then put into a questionnaire for ranking by team members. After team members rank issues, the questionnaire is sent out again to all members for further input. This process continues as many times as necessary to reach consensus on key issues.

The Delphi technique is particularly valuable for obtaining input from team members during the strategic planning process when face-to-face conversation is not possible but input is valued. An advantage of the Delphi technique is the protection of anonymity, making the technique particularly useful for issues where there is significant disagreement. The technique is particularly useful for groups that have historically failed to communicate effectively. The Delphi procedures offer a systematic method that ensures team member opinions are considered (Gordon, 2002).

Scenario Development: Tree Diagrams

To implement an identified strategy, tasks must be mapped for implementation during *scenario development*. *Tree diagrams* are used to break broad goals, graphically, into increasing levels of detailed actions so that a stated goal can be accomplished (Goal/QPC, 2008). This tool encourages team members to expand their thinking while simultaneously linking the team's overall goals. Tree diagrams assist team members to move theory to reality.

The first task is to choose the goal statement. Alternately, the team may have been assigned a goal on which to work. If the team selects the goal, care must be taken to create, via consensus, a clear, action-oriented statement. Team members must have intimate knowledge of the goal topic.

Next, major tree headings, or subgoals, are selected. These subgoals may be established first through brainstorming and then by using the nominal group technique. These subgoals are the major means of achieving the goal statement. The first level of detail must remain broad so that it does not jump to the lowest level of task. After working from the goal statement and first-level detail, the team proceeds through the three levels of detail. Some subgoals are simple, whereas others require more breakdown. At each level the facilitator queries the group as to whether or not something obvious has been forgotten. An additional important question for the team is whether these actions result in accomplishment of the given goal or subgoal. *Sticky notes* may be used to create the levels of detail because they can easily be moved around. Lines are drawn when the tree is finished. The tree can be oriented from left to right or top to bottom.

The tree diagram is an effective communication tool. This technique allows for input from direct caregivers. The team's final task is to revise, add, or delete goals or subgoals as deemed appropriate (Goal/QPC, 2008). **Exhibit 16–14** is an example of a tree diagram for a healthcare organization.

Gantt Charts

Project management is critical as new ventures or programs are pursued. Complex projects require that successive activities be completed in a timely fashion. Several commercial computer software programs are available; however, a simple Gantt chart can be constructed with materials at hand.

A *Gantt chart* displays activities or goals in a matrix format. The time frame is displayed on the horizontal axis, and the activities to be completed for the project are documented on the vertical axis. If dates are especially important (i.e., when one phase of the project must be completed on a specific date for the next phase to begin), project leaders may designate specific dates on the chart. **Exhibit 16–15** shows a sample Gantt chart for a PI team. Gantt charts are also useful as a planning tool for new managers. It is easy for time to get away, and before a new manager may realize it, evaluations are past due or reports are due the next day without adequate time to prepare. Managers may also use a Gantt chart to pace themselves so that they do not get overwhelmed—everything cannot be done in a week's time. Planning activities throughout the year decreases stress and the need to fight fires on a daily basis. Gantt charts are especially helpful for nurse leaders who are visual learners because one can see what and when items need to be completed.

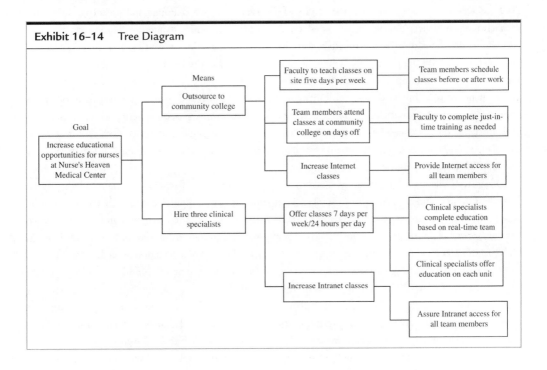

Exhibit 16–14   Tree Diagram

Exhibit 16–15   Sample Gantt Chart for a Performance Improvement Team

Activities	Jan	Feb	Mar	Apr	May	Jun	Jul	Aug	Sept	Oct	Nov	Dec
Select process	X											
Charter team	X											
Collect baseline data	7											
Analyze baseline data		15										
Select improvement		28										
Plan the improvement			5									
Do the improvement			10									
Check the results			31									
Act to maintain the gain				X	X	X	X	X	X	X	X	X

Evidence-Based Practice

Recent empirical research related to the efficacy of the strategic planning process is unclear (Falshaw, Glaister, & Tatoglu, 2006; Kaissi, Begun, & Hamilton, 2008; Wilson & Eilertsen, 2010; Zuckerman, 2006). Zuckerman (2006) reported the results of a survey in which planners and executives identified their current strategic planning efforts as effective; nevertheless, when compared to strategic planning efforts outside of health care, the practices were less rigorous and did not employ best practices. Kaissi and coworkers (2008) reported a study in which the sample was limited to hospitals in the state of Texas. Hospitals within the sample reported that 87% had a strategic plan, and most reported that physicians and their board were involved. Responsibility for the plan was assigned to the chief executive officer in approximately one-half of the organizations. Three strategic planning processes were positively associated with financial performance: having a strategic plan, having the chief executive officer responsible for the plan, and involvement of the board. Further longitudinal studies were recommended to evaluate relationships between planning and performance.

Of concern related to empirical evidence to support the efficacy of strategic planning is a study by Falshaw, Glaister, and Tatoglu (2006) of 113 companies in the United Kingdom that examined the relationship between strategic planning and financial performance. The researchers found no relationship between formal planning processes and company performance. Limitations of the study included concerns with measurement validity and time lag of efforts. A longitudinal study was recommended.

It is imperative that hospital leaders use evidence to guide leadership practices and not just to maintain practice because of tradition. Although the study is dated, Tapinos, Dyson, and Meadows (2005) examined the relationship between strategic planning processes and the success of strategy development through a survey of strategic planning systems. These researchers found that performance measurement was one of the four primary factors in strategic planning processes. Such metrics were used more often in large organizations and those who operated in rapidly changing environments (for example, health care). The results of the study supported the transition from traditional strategic planning processes to more contemporary processes. Tapinos, Dyson, and Meadows (2005) stated that organizational complexity related to size and rate of market change created variation in the impact of performance measurement in strategic planning because complexity increased the need for information. Performance measurement had significant influence related to achievement of organizational goals and the effectiveness and efficiency of the strategic planning process. Finally, to a large extent, approaches for measuring organizational performance lacked effective feedback loops to strategic planning. These researchers recommended additional research related to the link between performance measurement and strategic planning.

Of heightened interest considering the turbulence in healthcare financing are the results of a survey completed by Wilson and Eilertsen (2010) regarding whether strategic planning assisted organizations during the recent economic crisis. These authors noted that organizations that embraced strategic planning were better situated to pursue opportunities for growth in times of crisis. Likewise, small organizations were better able to pursue growth than were large organizations for which defensive actions were more common during crisis. Participants in the survey recommended that organizational leaders (1) strengthen strategic thinking through scenario planning and listening and analysis of market and client trends, (2) decrease the time lag for review of the strategic plan, (3) make a stronger connection between the organization's strategic plan and resource allocation, (4) increase leadership engagement, and (5) develop strategic action through improved change and performance management and through improved communications. Finally, the authors suggested a more serious commitment to strategic planning and use of the planning principles for decision making during crises. It is important for leaders to take advantage of opportunities rather than focus on defensive actions (Wilson & Eilertsen, 2010). This report strengthens the case for more effective strategic planning in health care especially because financial constraints continue to dominate the landscape.

Shoemaker and Fischer (2011) reported a successful nursing evidence-based strategic planning process that encompassed the journey to Magnet Recognition. The framework was based on a BSC and the Magnet domains. Blatstein (2012), a strategic planning facilitator, consultant, and teacher, reported on a research methodology that used a strategic planning approach that focused on four areas. These foci were "development of a core purpose, values, Big Hairy Audacious Goal (BHAG), and envisioned future" (p. 31). The author declared that good strategic planning entailed the answer to the following questions, "1) who am I?; 2) where do I want to go?; and 3) how am I going to get there?" (p. 32). This strategic planning process focused on the intellectual journey, learning, and empowerment of participants as well as integrated organizational plans and metrics. These reports provide evidence of effective strategic planning processes.

Role of the Nurse Manager

Nurse managers are situated in a unique position to recognize the need for change in the organization. Sandwiched between the front-line staff and senior leaders, nurse managers may be the first to recognize the need for changes in strategy. Nurse managers stimulate their team members by cultivating a positive culture of performance excellence and a corresponding reward system. The challenge is to define the parameters within which team members can experiment and be innovative. Nurse managers uphold the organization's value system and maintain systems that focus on the core business of patient care. Managers ensure that strategies are in tune with the current needs of customers and are balanced so that one strategy does not suffer at the expense of another. They must be sensitive to important changes and continuously inquire of all their customers as to whether their needs are being met. Of key importance is that nurse managers maintain the system by ensuring issues get picked up quickly and senior leaders are made aware before issues escalate into a crisis. Effective nurse managers do not just herald problems but offer solutions as well. Nurse managers bind the organization together within the *internal environment* so that team members are galvanized into action. Managing a nursing unit is not an easy task and is certainly not for the faint of heart.

Gelatt (1993) defined the skills needed to continually adapt, innovate, and change. "This 'flexpert' is open-minded, comfortable with uncertainty, delighted with change, and capable of unfreezing and refreezing beliefs, knowledge, and attitudes" (pp. 11–12). *Flexperts* understand that the inability to shift paradigms not only restricts flexibility but causes the individual to become out-of-date, inaccurate, and in need of revision. Culture, communities, experiences, and healthcare organizations change constantly and make old paradigms dysfunctional.

As nurse managers look toward the future, strategic planning fosters a sense of positive uncertainty that assists team members in the acceptance of change, ambiguity, uncertainty, and inconsistency. As Chapman (2003) stated in *Radical Loving Care*, "Our Vision statements need to be engraved in our hearts, not just on plaques" (p. 110). Committed leadership begins with those who make up the majority of caregivers in health care: nurses.

Discussion Questions

1. Because visioning and effective decision making are primary tasks of leaders, discuss mechanisms that nurse managers can use to ensure that they make the best decisions.
2. Describe positive and negative aspects of abandoning traditional healthcare strategic planning processes and adopting a contemporary approach.
3. Discuss the process of external and internal environmental analyses, and then speculate scenarios that may result if these steps in strategic planning are omitted or are not done well.
4. Reflect on the mission, vision, values, and goals of a healthcare organization and provide examples of how individual employees, departments, and work units support all four of these as a foundation for directional strategies.
5. Describe how leaders can positively affect organizational and unit culture in the current healthcare environment, and then consider how the culture affects relationships, learning, change, and innovation.
6. Consider a healthcare organization and discuss measures that might be selected for a balanced scorecard. Explain the rationale for selection of each measure and describe how leaders could ensure a balance of measures. Next, discuss how leaders can remain informed regarding the current status of the organization considering at a minimum volume, financial, quality, and satisfaction measures.
7. Using the measures selected in discussion question 6, explain tools and techniques that could be used to display and analyze the data.
8. Qualitative tools and techniques are often dismissed in healthcare organizations. Select one qualitative method and discuss how the technique could be used to drive improvements.
9. Describe how nurse leaders and managers could contribute to evidence-based practice related to healthcare strategic planning.
10. Think about the role of the nurse manager, and discuss the importance of the role to employees and the overall organization.

Glossary of Terms

Acquisition Entry Strategy— when healthcare organizations purchase an existing organization, organizational unit, or a product or service.

Adaptive Strategies—how the organization will expand, contract, or maintain their scope of services (the means). They include expansion strategies, contraction strategies, and maintenance-of-scope strategies.

Alliance Strategies—arrangements among existing organizations to achieve a strategic purpose not possible by any single organization.

Appreciative Inquiry (AI)—the art and practice of asking questions that strengthen a system's capacity to apprehend, anticipate, and heighten positive potential.

Balanced Scorecard (BSC)—measurement of key financial, quality, market, and operational indicators that provides management with an understanding of performance in relation to established strategic goals and graphically displays a snapshot of the institution's overall health.

Brainstorming—a thinking process used to understand an issue, the impact the issue may have on the organization, or generate ideas for strategic alternatives.

Break-Even Analysis (BEA)—determination of the minimum volume of services that a program or service must provide to be financially self-sufficient.

Contraction Strategies—strategies that decrease the size or scope of operations.

Cooperation Strategies—where the organization enters into mergers, alliances, and joint ventures.

Cost-Benefit Analysis—comparison of the benefits and costs of a proposed endeavor.

Culture—the shared assumptions, values, and behavioral norms of the group or organization.

Delphi Technique—a structured group decision-making technique based on repeated use of rating scales to obtain opinions about a decision.

Directional Strategies—initial direction for the organization and guidance when making key organizational decisions. They include mission, vision, values, goals, and objectives (the end).

Diversification—at the corporate level when markets outside the organization's core business offer potential for significant growth. Related diversification (concentric) includes related products and services. Unrelated diversification (conglomerate) includes businesses in the general environment.

Divestiture—when one leaves a market and sells an operating unit.

Divisional Structures—attempt to break down larger, diverse organizations into more manageable and focused sections.

Emergent Strategic Management—relies on intuitive thinking, leadership, and learning, which correspond with contemporary strategic management processes.

Enhancement Strategies—when the organization is progressing toward its vision yet nevertheless improvements are needed.

Expansion Strategies—strategies to expand services.

External Customers—in health care these consist of suppliers (insurance companies, physicians not employed by the organization, labor markets, and donors), consumers (the general public and research community), and interfacing organizations (medical profession, teaching hospitals, boards of directors, health insurances, and drug and supply companies). Additional external influences include licensing, governmental, and regulatory agencies, in addition to other healthcare facilities.

External Environment—the issues outside an organization's boundaries that represent opportunities and threats and that after analysis assist in identifying what the organization should do.

Focus Groups—groups convened to reach conclusions regarding environmental issues.

Functional Organizational Structures—structures that organize activities around mission-critical functions or processes.

Gantt Charts—graphics that display activities or goals in a matrix format.

Goals—statements that specify the major direction of the organization and provide actionable linkage to the mission.

Harvesting—when the market has entered long-term decline or there is a need for short-term cash.

Horizontal Integration—when the business grows by acquiring or affiliating with competitors, such as multihospital systems.

Internal Customers—in health care these include patients and families, physicians (when employed by the organization), visitors, team members, and volunteers.

Internal Development—a development strategy for products or services closely related to existing products or services.

Internal Environment—internal processes, culture, structure, and technology that, when reviewed and analyzed, reveal strengths and weaknesses.

Internal Ventures—when products or services that are unrelated to current products or services are started within the organization.

Joint Ventures—when two or more organizations combine resources to accomplish a designated task; a strategy used when risks are too high or the project is too large or too expensive to be done by a single organization.

Licensing Strategy—a strategy of paying for use of proprietary technology that is not purchased; therefore, the organization is dependent on the licensor for support and upgrade.

Line Graphs/Multiple-Line Graphs—charts that aid in assessment of trends or changes in performance (quantitative).

Liquidation—selling of organizational assets.

Maintenance-of-Scope Strategies—when current strategies are appropriate and few changes are needed, the organization may elect to maintain the existing strategies.

Market Development—entering new markets with existing products or services.

Market Entry Strategies—adaptive strategies used to bring market strategies to fruition. The three major strategies to enter a market are purchase, cooperation, and development (internal development and internal ventures).

Matrix—a type of chart used to show combinations of data.

Matrix Structures—structures that organize activities around problems to be solved rather than functions, products, or geography.

Merger—when two organizations combine through a mutual agreement to form a single new organization.

Mission—the articulation of the external opportunities and threats and the internal strengths and weaknesses of an organization.

Nominal Group Technique (NGT)—when team members independently generate a written list of ideas regarding an issue. After members have been given sufficient time to generate their list, each member takes turns reporting one idea at a time to the entire group.

Objectives—descriptions of the results to be achieved, when and by whom, that are measurable.

Penetration Strategies—strategies that focus on increasing volumes and market share.

Performance Improvement (PI)—a systematic, organization-wide approach to improving the processes and outcomes of the healthcare system.

Product Development—the introduction of new products or services to existing markets.

Purchase Strategies—when healthcare organizations purchase an existing organization, organizational unit, or a product or service.

Regression Analysis—a statistical technique available in computer software used to forecast the relationship between two variables. Multiple regression allows for the simultaneous investigation of two or more independent variables on a single interval-scaled or ratio-scaled dependent variable.

Retrenchment—when the market has become too diverse and there is a decline in profitability as a result of increasing costs.

Scenario Development—a technique used to implement an identified strategy where tree diagrams are used to break broad goals graphically into increasing levels of detailed actions so that a stated goal can be accomplished.

Situation Analysis—the initial stage of strategic planning; the process of determining the current state of the organization. This is accomplished through three interrelated processes: external environmental analysis, internal environmental analysis, and the development of the organization's mission, vision, values, and goals.

Status Quo—the assumption of a mature market when growth has ceased. The goal is to maintain the market share.

Strategic Management—a process that fulfills the need for knowledge of the organization, the market, and the competitive situations healthcare leaders face and provides for ongoing, dynamic changes in the strategic plan as needed.

Strategic Planning—to devise a systematic, well-balanced process that allows the organization to fit in the environment. It stresses patient-focused quality and operational PI. It is a continuous process of revisiting the system and restoring balance.

Strategy Deployment—implementing the strategic objectives. This includes culture, structure, and resources.

Strategy Formation—gathering data and using these data for decision making. There are four types of strategies: directional, adaptive, market entry, and competitive.

Values—the fundamental truths that the organization holds dear and that reflect the philosophy of the organization.

Venture Capital Investment—a low-risk option where organizations purchase minority investment in a developing enterprise.

Vertical Integration—grows the business along the channel of distribution of core process such as an acute facility adding home care or long-term care.

Vision—the view of the future based on the understanding of the environmental forces.

References

American Hospital Association, 2011 Committee on Performance Improvement. (2011, September). *Hospitals and care systems of the future*. Chicago, IL: Author.

Bennis, W., & Nanus, B. (1985). *Leaders: The strategies for taking charge*. New York, NY: Harper & Row.

Blatstein, I. M. (2012). Strategic planning: Predicting or shaping the future? *Organizational Development Journal, 30*(2), 31–38.

Boev, C. (2012). The relationship between nurses' perception of work environment and patient satisfaction in adult critical care. *Journal of Nursing Scholarship, 44*(4), 368–375.

BrainyQuote. (2013). *Aristotle Onassis.* Retrieved from http://www.brainyquote.com/quotes/authors/a/aristotle_onassis.html

BusinessDictionary.com. (2010). *Silo mentality.* Retrieved from http://www.businessdictionary.com/definition/silo-mentality.html

Centers for Medicare & Medicaid Services. (2011, November). *Hospital value-based purchasing program.* Retrieved from http://www.cms.gov/Outreach-and-Education/Medicare-Learning-Network-MLN/MLNProducts/downloads/Hospital_VBPurchasing_Fact_Sheet_ICN907664.pdf

Chapman, E. (2003). *Radical loving care.* Nashville, TN: Vaughn.

Clancy, T. R. (2007). What we can learn from complex systems science. *Journal of Nursing Administration, 37*(10), 436–439.

Cooperrider, D. L., & Whitney, D. (n. d.). *What is Appreciative Inquiry?* Retrieved from http://appreciativeinquiry.case.edu/intro/whatisai.cfm

Creative Quotations. (2009). *Artemus Ward.* Retrieved from http://www.creativequotations.com/one/1839.htm

Crowell, D. M. (2011). *Complexity leadership: Nursing's role in health care delivery.* Philadelphia, PA: F. A. Davis.

DeSilets, L., & Dickerson, P. (2008). SWOT is useful in your tool kit. *Journal of Continuing Education in Nursing, 39*(5), 196–197.

Dibrell, C., Down, J., & Bull, L. (2007). Dynamic strategic planning: Achieving strategic flexibility through formalization. *Journal of Business and Management, 13*(1), 21–35.

Drenkard, K. (2001). Creating a future worth experiencing: Nursing strategic planning in an integrated healthcare delivery system. *Journal of Nursing Administration, 31*(7–8), 364–375.

Falshaw, J. R., Glaister, K. W., & Tatoglu, E. (2006). Evidence on formal strategic planning and company performance. *Management Decision, 44*(1), 9–30.

Finkler, S. (2001). *Financial management for public, health, and not-for-profit organizations.* Upper Saddle River, NJ: Prentice Hall.

Finkler, S. A., Jones, C. B., & Kovner, C. T. (2013). *Financial management for nurse managers and executives* (4th ed.). St. Louis, MO: Elsevier Saunders.

Gallup. (2013). *Gallup.* Retrieved from http://www.gallup.com/home.aspx

Gelatt, H. B. (1993, September–October). Future sense: Creating the future. *Futurist, 27*(5), 9–13.

Ginter, P., Swayne, L., & Duncan, W. (2002). *Strategic management of health care organizations* (4th ed.). Malden, MA: Blackwell.

Ginter, P. M., & Swayne, L. E. (2006). Moving toward strategic planning unique to healthcare. *Frontiers of Health Services Management, 23*(2), 33–37.

Ginter, P. M., Swayne, L. E., & Duncan, W. J. (2013). *The strategic management of health care organizations* (7th ed.). San Francisco, CA: Jossey-Bass.

Goal/QPC. (2008). *The memory jogger II healthcare edition: A pocket guide of tools for continuous improvement* . Salem, NH: Author.

Gordon, J. (2002). *Organizational behavior: A diagnostic approach* (7th ed.). Upper Saddle Ridge, NJ: Prentice Hall.

Greene, J. (2009, November). The new pace of strategic planning. *H&HN: Hospitals & Health Networks, 83*(11), 31–32, 34.

Harmon, R. B., Fontaine, D., Plews-Ogan, M., & Williams, A. (2012, March–April). Achieving transformational change: Using Appreciative Inquiry for strategic planning in a school of nursing. *Journal of Professional Nursing, 28*(2), 119–124.

Health Care Advisory Board. (1999). *Balanced scorecards.* Retrieved from http://www.advisory.com

Health Care Advisory Board. (2002). *Avoiding financial flashpoints: Foreseeing and preventing decline in hospital and health system fortunes.* Retrieved from http://www.advisory.com

Health Care Advisory Board. (2006). *Effective use of dashboards to analyze hospital success.* Retrieved from http://www.advisory.com

Hoffman, R. C. (2007). The strategic planning process and performance relationship: Does culture matter? *Journal of Business Strategies, 24*(1), 27–48.

Hrebiniak, L. G. (2005). *Making strategy work: Leading effective execution and change.* Upper Saddle River, NJ: Wharton School.

The Joint Commission. (2013). *Comprehensive accreditation manual for hospitals.* Oakbrook Terrace, IL: Joint Commission Resources.

Kaissi, A., Begun, J. W., & Hamilton, J. A. (2008, May/June). Strategic planning processes and hospital financial performance. *Journal of Healthcare Management, 53*(3), 197–209.

Kaplan, R., & Norton, D. P. (1996). *Translating strategy into action: The balanced scorecard.* Boston, MA: Harvard Business School.

Kim, W., & Mauborgne, R. (2002). Charting your company's future. *Harvard Business Review, 80*(6), 76–83.

Krueger, R. (1988). *Focus groups: A practical guide for applied research.* Newbury Park, CA: Sage.

Lazarus, I. R. (2011, March/April). What will it take? Exploiting trends in strategic planning to prepare for reform. *Journal of Healthcare Management, 56*(2), 89–93.

Lencioni, P. (2006). *Silos, politics, and turf wars: A leadership fable.* San Francisco, CA: Jossey-Bass.

Lighter, D., & Fair, D. (2004). *Quality management in health care: Principles and methods* (2nd ed.). Sudbury, MA: Jones and Bartlett.

Lindberg, C., & Clancey, T. R. (2010, April). Positive Deviance: An elegant solution to a complex problem. *Journal of Nursing Administration, 40*(4), 150–153.

MacPhee, M. (2007). Strategies and tools for managing change. *Journal of Nursing Administration, 37*(9), 405–413.

Martin, R. L. (2010). The execution trap. *Harvard Business Review, 88*(10), 64–71.

Mintzberg, H., & Markides, C. (2000). Commentary on the Henry Mintzberg interview. *Academy of Management Executive,* 39–42.

Morgan, D. (1993). *Successful focus groups: Advancing the state of the art.* Newbury Park, CA: Sage.

National Institute of Standards and Technology. (2013). *2013–2014 health care criteria for performance excellence.* Gaithersburg, MD: Author.

Patnaik, R. (2012). Strategic planning through complexity: Overcoming impediments to forecast and schedule. *IUP Journal of Business Strategy, IX*(1), 27–36.

Press Ganey Associates. (2013). *Press Ganey.* Retrieved from http://www.pressganey.com/index.aspx

Quotations Page. (2013a). *Marcel Proust.* Retrieved from http://www.quotationspage.com/search.php3?Search=&start search=Search&Author=proust&C=mgm&C=motivate&C=classic&C=coles&C=poorc&C=lindsly

Quotations Page. (2013b). *Yogi Berra.* Retrieved from http://www.quotationspage.com/search.php3?Search=&startsear ch=Search&Author=Yogi+Berra&C=mgm&C=motivate&C=classic&C=coles&C=poorc&C=lindsly

Reed, K., & May, R. (2011, March). *HealthGrades patient safety in American hospitals study.* HealthGrades. Retrieved from https://www.cpmhealthgrades.com/CPM/assets/File/HealthGradesPatientSafetyInAmericanHospitalsStudy2011.pdf

Shirey, M. R. (2011a). Addressing strategy execution challenges to lead sustainable change. *Journal of Nursing Administration, 42*(1), 1–4.

Shirey, M. R. (2011b). Brainstorming for breakthrough thinking. *Journal of Nursing Administration, 41*(12), 497–500.

Shoemaker, L. K., & Fischer, B. (2011). Creating a nursing strategic planning framework based on evidence. *Nursing Clinics of North America, 46,* 11–25.

Solovy, A. (2002). The paradox of planning. *Healthcare & Healthcare Network, 76*(9), 32.

Tapinos, E., Dyson, R. G., & Meadows, M. (2005). The impact of performance measurement in strategic planning. *International Journal of Productivity and Performance Management, 54*(5/6), 370–384.

Tennessee Center for Performance Excellence. (2009). Criteria for performance excellence. Retrieved from http://tncpe.org/what_we_do/criteria.php

Vardaman, J. M., Cornell, P. T., & Clancy, T. R. (2012). Complexity and change in nurse workflows. *Journal of Nursing Administration, 42*(2), 78–82.

Wilson, J. W., & Eilertsen, S. (2010). How did strategic planning help during the economic crisis? *Strategy & Leadership, 38*(2), 5–14.

Yoder-Wise, P. S. (Ed.). (2010). *Leading and managing in nursing* (5th ed.). St. Louis, MO: Elsevier Health Sciences.

Zikmund, W. (2003). *Business research methods* (7th ed.). Mason, OH: South-Western.

Zuckerman, A. M. (1998). *Healthcare strategic planning: Approaches for the 21st century.* Chicago, IL: Health Administration.

Zuckerman, A. M. (2006). Advancing the state of the art in healthcare strategic planning. *Frontiers of Health Services Management, 23*(2), 3–15.

Financial Strategies

Janne Dunham-Taylor, PhD, RN

OBJECTIVES

- Identify financial strategies for survival in the value-based environment.
- Appropriately identify and deal with financial issues and processes that impede effectiveness.

Nurse administrators need to be equal partners in the financial and budgeting process and develop financial and budget strategies—*attaching numbers and monetary amounts to strategies*. Identifying strategies is part of the administrative *and* leader roles, always supporting the basic value of giving patients what they desire with available dollars. Financial strategies are interconnected with all other strategies and decisions in the organization. Obviously, the best strategies are developed when all stakeholders are involved in the process. Although some strategies must be identified by the executive group (including a nurse executive) or other departments, nursing can identify and carry out many strategies that not only help the organization, but also better serve the patient. Everyone in the organization must continually identify financial strategies, and then implement, evaluate, and make improvements to them as successes and failures occur.

We are moving into the second-curve, value-based environment from the old volume-based reimbursement environment (first curve) that was only concerned with the number of insured patients being treated. Now this focus is no longer enough because *reimbursement can be lost if certain quality measures are not met. In addition, a percentage of reimbursement for the next year is lost if a facility's performance ratings decline.* The following environmental factors are driving this change:

- Demand-altering demographic changes
- Employer, government, and consumer pressure to curb the unsustainable increase in healthcare spending
- Shift in financial incentives away from fee-for-service reimbursement in favor of value-based payments that reward positive outcomes and efficiency
- Rise in provider accountability for the cost and quality of health care
- Consistent demand to reduce care fragmentation by redesigning care delivery
- Increased transparency of financial, quality, and community benefit data
- Projected shortages of nurses, primary care physicians, and other healthcare providers in regard to population demand
- Persistent introduction of high-cost medical technology and pharmaceutical advances
- Difficulty in raising capital to meet the strategic needs for new facilities, medical technology, and information systems
- Uncertainty about federal and state healthcare reform legislation and regulation
- Overall decline in reimbursement
- Recognition and challenge to variations in care provision and, as a result, cost (American Hospital Association [AHA], 2011, p. 8)
- Viability of the US economy

As these events occur, health systems can ignore them and keep on doing things the same way, or they can prepare for the second curve (which is already occurring) to ensure success in the new environment. The present belief is that hospitals "will evolve to become part of 'care systems' or 'integrated networks,' encompassing everything from home-based chronic care management to inpatient acute treatment" (AHA, 2011, p. 10).

Thus, to survive in this new second-curve environment, we need to make major changes in the way we do business. "The second curve is concerned with value: the cost and quantity of care necessary to produce desired health outcomes within a particular population" (AHA, 2011, p. 8). According to the American Hospital Association (AHA) Committee on Performance Improvement and the Health Research and Educational Trust (HRET), it is imperative we modify "core models for business and service delivery" (p. 3). This is exciting because they recommend valuing nurse leaders (as well as physicians) at the point of care.

The American Hospital Association (AHA, 2011, 2013) identified 10 "must-do" strategies to be successful in the second-curve environment. The 10 must-do strategies for success in the new value-based environment are:

1. Aligning hospitals, physicians, and other providers across the continuum of care
2. Utilizing evidenced-based practices to improve quality and patient safety
3. Improving efficiency through productivity and financial management
4. Developing integrated information systems
5. Joining and growing integrated provider networks and care systems
6. Educating and engaging employees and physicians to create leaders
7. Strengthening finances to facilitate reinvestment and innovation
8. Partnering with payers
9. Advancing an organization through scenario-based strategic, financial, and operational planning
10. Seeking population health improvement through pursuit of the triple aim (p. 11) (The Institute for Healthcare Improvement [2007] identified the triple aim "to encourage hospitals to simultaneously focus on population health, increased quality, and reduction in health care cost per capita" [p. 22].)

These 10 strategies provide clues to all healthcare administrators, as well as nurses, on how to ensure success in this present unstable environment. This entire text has been designed to help nurse administrators better achieve the second curve. The goal is for the outcomes of financial strategies to achieve cost savings or reorganize available monies in a more effective way. But they also may cost additional dollars. Technology is a good example of this. Financial strategies need to be carefully crafted to achieve financial success in the second-curve environment.

Our best resources for needed strategies are the patients and the leaders at the point of care. In this new environment, administrators serve patients and leaders at the point of care. This is a new perspective that many administrators have not presently adopted. It will take a lot of work from the board down to change for success to be achieved.

There is an infinite number of possible strategies. This chapter discusses some, but please add to this list. Certain strategies work more effectively in one setting but not as well in another because all facilities have particular quirks or differences.

Complexity Issues

> Growth in organizational complexity is more than a perception; it is a reality with sound theoretical underpinnings. The ramifications of growing complexity are immense. Beyond a certain level, organizational complexity can decrease both the quality and financial performance of a health system. (Clancy, 2010, p. 248)

Clancy suggests some strategies that we can keep in mind as we deal with this. Black swans, one example of complexity, are unexpected events. The first strategy is to "be prepared for the unexpected" (Clancy, 2010, p. 248). This is why it is important to have "highly reliable systems, standardized protocols, and checklists" and make sure these are tightly controlled to prevent errors.

The second strategy is to "limit combinatorial complexity." Healthcare organizations are already too complex. Then, when something happens, we add to the complexity by using quick fixes, which only worsen the situation and make it more complex. It is so important to use systems thinking and involve all stakeholders in solutions that decrease complexity. The idea is to *simplify*. Each of our actions and those of staff leaders need to decrease complexity as much as possible. For instance, organizational processes should be simplified. Otherwise, as complexity increases, it becomes exponential, creating even more serious problems (errors, reimbursement loss, etc.)—and lower bottom lines.

The third strategy is to "use creative destruction—the systematic evaluation and elimination of nonessential activities" (Clancy, 2010, p. 249). This is why hospitals are getting into the Lean movement. The problem here is that we cannot just do this in a meeting with a group of administrators present. Staff actually doing the work need to be involved. Patients need to be involved. Physicians and other departments need to be involved. These are all important stakeholders in strategy development. Otherwise, the Lean movement just creates more complexity because someone does not realize that what he or she is changing has other harmful side effects that were not considered in the process. The same thing happens when quick decisions are made to deal with budget crises instead of carefully planning ahead for these events.

The fourth strategy is "don't give up" (Clancy, 2010, p. 249). For instance, the exponential growth of technology can be overwhelming. The good news is that technology helps us do our work better. The bad news is that it makes things more complex. It may be best not to purchase a new technology that has just been developed, but to wait until it has been used a bit and some of the initial glitches have been resolved. The idea is not to give up on expensive technology but to let it progress a bit before purchasing and to make a careful decision to determine the expense, time, and effort needed to implement the technology.

Providing What the Patient Values

The most important strategy is to be sure that ***everyone listens to the patient, making the patient the leader in choosing what will happen***. Often patients need our expertise before they can make decisions about their care, so regular dialogue with front-line staff and physicians is critical.

Because the first and fifth must-do strategies are concerned with the continuum of care, let's think about this from the nursing perspective. Presently, a first-curve volume issue is the cost strategy where ***the patient is moved to the least expensive setting***. For instance, we move a surgical patient quickly from the recovery room, to the intensive care unit, to stepdown or general care unit, to skilled nursing unit, to home with home care. This saves money, but continuity is lost and errors happen because the patient has different people caring for him or her in each setting. Patients hate this as do the front-line caregivers. We need to *reexamine this practice*. Surely there is a better solution. Some organizations are experimenting with units where a patient stays in the same place with the same front-line staff throughout an episode of care in a hospital. That is a start. However, the overall continuum of care is still not achieved as the patient is moved to rehab, long-term care, or the home—each time experiencing different caregivers. Often caregivers in one setting do not think about, and prepare the patient for, continuing care in the next setting or in the home. How can we better achieve this?

In the second curve, *achieving the continuum of care with as little duplication as possible* has great value to the patient, saves costs and staff time, increases quality, and achieves better patient outcomes. Healthcare providers need to become more aware of the entire continuum (not get stuck in the silo that only includes the present location) and perceive how their patients might be affected by the home environment. Insurers are attempting to force the issue by not covering readmission within 30 days of discharge.

There is another continuum issue. Because so many healthcare dollars are spent on elderly adults with chronic conditions, providers need to figure out better ways to treat people at home, or in the least expensive environment, and to *teach patients and families how to deal more effectively with chronic conditions that will prevent the need for more expensive care*. Also, we know that currently 25% of Medicare dollars is spent on services for 5% of beneficiaries in their last year of life.

As providers, we need to find out what the patient values (eliminating many unnecessary procedures patients do not want) and figure out better ways to provide treatment in the home rather than in more expensive settings. Note that this will also help patients financially. A "Mount Sinai School of Medicine study found that out-of-pocket expenses for Medicare recipients during the five years before their death averaged about $39,000 for individuals, $51,000 for couples, and up to $66,000 for people with long-term illnesses like Alzheimer's" (Wang, 2012).

Ensuring Quality and Safety

Another must-do strategy is concerned with *using evidenced-based practices to improve quality and patient safety*. Finding needed evidence and using it to identify best clinical, administrative, and educational practices is a continual process. As we find new knowledge, we need to change our behaviors accordingly. The information is worthless unless we use it. This means we need to be constantly looking for evidence pertaining to all areas of our practice (clinical, administrative, and educational). *All staff, including administrators, need to be proficient in finding and using pertinent information to improve work outcomes.*

The next step is to *incorporate the information that is useful into our work*. "Translation science is the process of incorporating research findings into practice" (Russell-Babin, 2009, pp. 29–30). This second step is critical (Cadmus et al., 2008). Yet studies show:

> Nurses do not consistently implement evidence-based best practices [EBP]. . . . Although nurses believe in evidence-based care, barriers remain prevalent, including resistance from colleagues, nurse leaders, and managers. Differences existed in responses of nurses from Magnet versus non-Magnet institutions as well as nurses with master's versus nonmaster's degrees. Nurse leaders and educators must provide learning opportunities regarding EBP and facilitate supportive cultures to achieve the Institute of Medicine's 2020 goal that 90% of clinical decisions be evidence-based. (Melnyk, Fineout-Overholt, Gallagher-Ford, & Kaplan, 2012, p. 410)

Within organizations, one of our responsibilities as nurse administrators is to achieve both steps ourselves as well as to encourage staff to do the same. "Anecdotal reports from nurses support that engaging in EBP renews the professional spirit of the nurse" (Melnyk et al., 2012, p. 410). Research supports that EBP reduces morbidities, mortality, and medical errors. Gale and Shaffer (2009) found the following:

> Top reasons to adopt EBP [evidence based practice] were having personal interest in the practice change, avoiding risk of negative consequences to the patient, and personally valuing the evidence. Top barriers to EBP were insufficient time, lack of staff, and not having the right equipment and supplies. (p. 91)

Other barriers were "a lack of EBP knowledge and skills, a perception that EBP is time [consuming], a belief that EBP is burdensome, and organizational cultures that [do not] support evidence-based care" (Melnyk et al., 2012, p. 411).

In Melnyk and associates' (2012) study, respondents indicated the following enhancements would promote EBP:

- An online resource center where best evidence-based practices are housed and experts are available for consultation
- Tools that can help implement EBP with patients (some embed this in the electronic medical record)
- Online education and skills-building modules in EBP

- An online distance continuing education EBP fellowship program with expert EBP mentors
- Access to an EBP mentor
- Regular web seminars conducted by experts in EBP (p. 412)

Leadership interventions are a critical factor with nurses using evidence (Gifford et al., 2012). Wells, Free, and Adams (2007) describes an internship program to teach staff nurses EBP.

Besides needing to pay attention to the evidence, serious quality and safety issues plague the healthcare environment. Consider the following:

> Every time you walk into a hospital or clinic in the United States, you take your life in your hands. Whatever your condition, you will probably be cared for by people who are overworked and hobbled by wasteful systems. With 15 million incidents of medical harm in the U.S. every year, such as drug errors, wrong-site surgeries and infection, there is a good chance you will be hurt in this interaction. Medical professionals like us are horrified every time we cause harm, but even the best intentions do not change facts.
>
> Governments can tweak payment systems and probably get some temporary fiscal relief. But until we focus reform efforts on where most of the money goes, which is healthcare delivery, we will remain stuck in a revolving door of near disaster and narrow escapes. To get to the point where all people have access to high-quality healthcare, affordably, we must focus our attention on how the healthcare delivery system determines cost and quality. Then we need to change that delivery model entirely.
>
> In fact, hospitals, physicians, and nurses—all of healthcare—must change. First, we must emphasize the science of medicine over the art. This means turning to evidence-based medicine, which is already underway in some sectors. But we are also talking about evidence-based delivery, work that has barely begun. (Toussaint & Gerard with Adams, 2010, pp. 1–2)

Systems problems that cause quality and safety issues must be fixed and are best resolved by involving *all* the stakeholders in identifying incremental changes (including the costs of these changes) to improve a situation. The idea is to decrease complexity, to find *a simpler way*. Stakeholders try each small incremental change, celebrating the successes. Or, as glitches or other unintended events happen (often this is a sign that complexity has been increased—something was not identified in the strategy), they go back to the drawing board and try another solution.

One of the best examples of an interdisciplinary group discussing giving the patient only what is valued is presented in *On the Mend: Revolutionizing Healthcare to Save Lives and Transform the Industry* (Toussaint & Gerard with Adams, 2010). Here an interdisciplinary group (including physicians and patients) examined *processes* and changed the way they were providing care.

The idea is that everything we do in health care is a series of processes. These processes include time wasters that do not improve giving patients what they value (and that increase complexity). Some procedures completed are not what patients actually wanted done. And there are so many errors occurring. Bureaucracies only create additional complexity where more errors will occur, and this is what has happened in health care. We desperately need to simplify processes and question every step. Is each step necessary? Are there other simpler ways we could accomplish the work, yet still achieve what the patient values? Little by little we can fix the system.

In *On the Mend*, the authors describe outcomes they have achieved. Note that they did not achieve this all at once.

> [By examining and changing processes], we have made life better for our patients. In 2002 for instance, mortality rate for coronary bypass surgery at ThedaCare was nearly 4%—about 12 deaths per year. After several improvement projects in cardiac surgery over seven years, in which we typically removed 40% of wasted time and effort with each pass, cardiac mortality was reduced to near zero. Also, a

patient's average time spent in hospital fell from 6.3 days to 4.9 and the cost of a coronary bypass declined 22%. Teamwork like this has saved us more than $27 million and ThedaCare has passed those savings along, becoming the overall lowest-price healthcare provider in Wisconsin. (Toussaint & Gerard with Adams, 2010, p. 3)

Another quality and safety issue is *missed care*, first identified by Kalisch (2009). Missed care is when we skip doing basic nursing care and patients get infections, bedsores, and other problems. This occurs when RNs and aides do not value their work enough to ensure that this care is completed, and when staff nurses are not working carefully with aides or do not have the time because staffing is inadequate. Aides take pride in their work, too, and should be valued and involved in fixing the problem. Otherwise, it really hurts our patients and affects the bottom line.

Another problem is *duplication*. For example, we may have five or six people all taking histories from and performing physicals on the same patient. In addition, we do not use the history and physical—as well as other information—already completed by the facility that just transferred the patient to us. Or transfer information is lacking.

Interruptions are another issue in need of new strategies. Interruptions are common in health care and detract from critical thinking, causing errors. We need to implement strategies that decrease interruptions such as instructing the medication nurse to wear a certain vest that signifies he or she is not to be interrupted or employing technology to better deal with communicating about patient issues.

Along with interruptions, *finding caregivers* is a big time waster. For instance, sometimes a nurse calls or pages a physician who is unavailable. Then, the physician calls the nurse and finds it hard to track down the nurse. Systems like Vocera or computerized documentation systems that link the practice setting with the physician's office can facilitate this interprofessional communication and save caregivers time.

Quality and safety are enhanced by having *adequate numbers of staff* to do the work. If this is not so, it is an important issue to deal with. Cite the evidence: Adequate staffing makes a difference in patient outcomes and reimbursement.

Evidence shows that hiring a higher number of registered nurses (RNs) is actually *less expensive* than hiring a higher number of nursing assistants or licensed practical nurses. (We tend to think the opposite because RN salaries are higher than the salaries of nursing assistants and LPNs, but the evidence shows this is not so.) For those with a bottom-line mentality, this may be hard to fathom. You will hear, "But nursing assistant salaries are less than an RN salary. How can this be true?" Expenses are lower when there is a higher RN ratio and there is enough support staff present to facilitate the RN function. This is true across the healthcare continuum.

Another factor with quality and safety is making sure that the *staff is there when needed* and not there when there is less to do. For instance, perhaps certain staff members are very busy at peak times but do not have enough to do at other times. Yet we continue to schedule them in the same way. It is better to schedule someone to come in only for the peak times.

To counteract this issue, Martha Jefferson Hospital in Charlottesville, Virginia, implemented a program that provided a nurse refresher program to inactive nurses and then hired them as admission-discharge-teaching nurses to help with these functions throughout the facility. This was a win–win situation because the patients got better care, hospital stays were shortened, and staff morale improved (Blankenship & Winslow, 2003). Other hospitals schedule older nurses on shorter shifts to achieve a similar goal.

In nursing, we need to examine whether *12-hour shifts* should be used. Many errors are caused because nurses are not alert, are sleep deprived, and so forth when they work 12-hour shifts. On the other hand, nurses like these longer shifts because they get more days off—or more days to work prn at another facility—which only makes them more error prone.

Another strategy is to either provide a wellness program or obtain employee discounts at local facilities that **enhance employee health and well-being.** This can also be achieved by supporting leaders at the point of care using specific strategies identified elsewhere in this discussion.

Workarounds are another issue that can indicate certain processes or technology routines are cumbersome. Staff figure out ways to work around the issues. Some workarounds are positive where staff are trying to help patients get the care they need in cumbersome environments. Other workarounds are negative, for instance, avoiding safety guidelines when staffing is inadequate. Strategies—both in identification of issues and in ways to better deal with these issues—are needed.

These are fixable issues but must become important from the top down in an organization. Many of these are more appropriately fixed using a shared governance structure. Everyone needs to walk the talk and support the basic value(s) in every strategy or action that is taken.

This may also involve *environmental changes*; for example, when elderly adults have to walk long distances to lab or X-ray, having or building or remodeling services to be close by parking areas can be ideal. Sometimes services need to be updated and the available space changed. A current change for nurses involves ways to get more materials/supplies/technology at the bedside to save walking time of nursing staff.

Improving Efficiency Through Productivity and Financial Management

The fourth AHA must-do strategy concerns efficiency in productivity and financial management, which are interwoven with the seventh strategy, strengthening finances to facilitate reinvestment and innovation. Although part of accomplishing these strategies is the role of the finance department, nurses can contribute to both efforts.

One financial issue has been identified as RNs being pulled away from patients for more than 50% of their time to perform work not related to patients, *non-value-added time.* This costs millions of dollars per unit each year. It is a prime example of processes gone awry. Nurses want to spend more time with patients; patients value time with their nurses. So, why do nurses have to waste time on the non-value-added activities? This is where practice councils can be very helpful. If operating correctly, they can identify and make changes at the bedside that are immediate, that provide what patients value, that provide higher-quality care and safety, and that meet reimbursement mandates.

Such issues have prompted some hospitals to form a new department, the *Value Analysis Department.* "Its mission is twofold: to ensure that a facility's processes are of superior quality and that these processes are financially appropriate" (Russell, 2013, p. 53). Whether this requires a new department or not (does this create more complexity?), all in the organization need to examine and work out better ways to accomplish the work that support nurses being at the bedside more often.

In financial management, we need to move out of the old linear, ineffective, outmoded, authoritarian model where finance and nursing personnel do not discuss issues together and where finance personnel give nurse managers the same budget amounts with a bit more added for inflation or a percentage taken out for budget cuts. The nurse managers should question everything. To meet second-curve reimbursement demands, this is *not* an acceptable way of dealing with financial issues.

It is better to identify a fixed annual budget, but with the caveat that it will continue to be tweaked as changes occur so that the organization can best meet environmental challenges. In the second curve, it is important for *financial information to be transparent and shared with all staff.* In this environment, *all staff need to be cost conscious.* It is important to take into account which departments are already more cost conscious so that they are *not penalized* when budget cuts are necessary. Having all equally share across-the-board cuts—that often happen in more authoritarian, linear systems—is not the best way to meet budget challenges in the second curve.

Budget cuts happen regularly in health care as reimbursement amounts continue to decline. For instance, government reimbursement for Medicaid and Medicare services gives back only cents on the dollar. This means that the reimbursed amount is less than half (and even less with Medicaid) of that expended by the healthcare facility. Other insurance plans follow suit, taking similar measures, asking for larger discounts each year.

Budget cuts also result from not meeting performance measures and making poor business decisions, such as giving too great a discount to insurance carriers, losing contracts with insurance companies, rescuing physician offices running at a deficit, providing poor leadership, or operating consistently at a loss yet never taking any measures to improve the situation. As healthcare organizations have increased in complexity there are more costs, but the outcomes do not reflect the expenditures. Strategies identified need to decrease complexity, not add to it.

An important budget strategy needs to include a ***plan for how to handle different financial scenarios***, such as being at 100% occupancy when only budgeted for 80%, being 20% under the anticipated occupancy rate, or having to decrease costs by 5% or 10%. We know that these situations occur, so involving all stakeholders in developing a plan to handle these situations *before* they occur is wise management. This is a much more thoughtful way of making decisions and results in better outcomes—a second-curve strategy. When nothing is done until everyone is in the middle of the crisis, poor outcomes result.

In the budget process, *nursing needs to be a majority player* with other departments. When all stakeholders are involved in the process, staff can identify ways to save money that administrators never thought about, and this results in more effective plans.

As we work with budgets, our worldview—our silos (**Exhibit 17–1**)—influences our choices and, perhaps unintentionally, inhibits the potential reality. Let's examine some examples.

One silo is that *resources are scarce*. This is not surprising because, as discussed elsewhere, *accounting and financial theories are based on scarcity*:

> Accounting and finance are applied areas of microeconomics. The theory of economics forms the foundations upon which all financial management is ultimately built. The essence of economics is that society has *a limited amount of resources*, with competing demands for them. The economic system attempts to allocate those resources in an optimal fashion. (Finkler & Kovner, 2007, p. 3)

Compare this way of thinking with the quantum view, where the world is composed of energy fields. In the quantum view, we need to be careful about our thoughts because they create our reality. Wouldn't it be better to choose *abundance* rather than *scarcity*? Perhaps our present cost-cutting dilemmas have been caused by too many people thinking there are limited resources! We probably would make different decisions if we thought resources were abundant. In this book, we choose abundance. *Many financial people will have difficulty with this concept because their education and their work environment have always emphasized scarcity.*

Another silo is *doing things the way we have always done them*. Because the environment is always changing, this is actually the kiss of death. We cannot avoid change.

A third silo is *bottom-line thinking*. We advocate the importance of providing what the patient values first to stay viable. The bottom line is always second if we want to survive as an organization. If this is the mentality in an organization, *this will need to be changed to achieve adequate reimbursement*.

In the quantum view, we are all interconnected. Thus, we cannot *separate financial decisions from other organizational decisions*. Any action we take affects everyone else. This means that everyone in the organization needs to be aware of and involved in working with budgets/finances, as well as using and discovering financial strategies.

Each of these issues is a basis for discussion and, if resolved, will achieve better outcomes for everyone, including the bottom line.

The importance of interdisciplinary groups composed of staff, administrators, physicians, and patients working together to identify and implement financial strategies cannot be overemphasized because each of us possesses only a partial answer. **Exhibit 17–2** identifies some possible strategies. The more we can work as a team and as equal players, the more effective our strategies will be. This is why it is so important for all administrators and staff to do regular rounds, support nurse leaders and physicians at the point of care, and only provide what the patient values because they provide a more accurate picture of what is actually happening in the trenches.

Exhibit 17–1   World View Financial Beliefs

Traditional Beliefs
- Resources are scarce.
- Do things the way we have always done them.
- Use bottom-line thinking.
- Financial decisions are separate from the rest of the organization.

Quantum View
- Resources are abundant.
- Change will always happen. We cannot escape it.
- The bottom line comes second, behind what the patient values.
- Financial decisions need to be made within the context of the total organization.

Exhibit 17–2   Possible Budget Strategies

- Providing care the patient values
- Fixing organizational processes that decrease complexity, i.e., Non-value added time, missed care, workarounds, duplication, interruptions, finding caregivers, having adequate staffing consistently
- Educating each staff member on importance of pay for performance issues
- Educating each staff member on new reimbursement requirements
- Providing more budget transparency
- Fixing the budget process
- Providing more effective bottom-up leadership
- Having everyone do regular rounds as top priority
- Supporting nurse managers
- Having adequate staffing
- Encouraging staff to be leaders
- Having shared governance councils
- Increasing interdisciplinary collaboration
- Improving case management by involving all staff
- Improving communication everywhere
- Using best evidence—clinical, leadership, and organizational
- Appropriately using technology
- Fixing environmental issues
- Creating a cost-conscious environment
- Getting everyone involved in spotting changes/new trends
- Employing advanced practices nurses
- Eliminating disruptive/abusive behaviors
- Identifying issues causing moral distress for clinicians and deal with them

What Not to Do

Let's turn to some things to avoid because they increase complexity unnecessarily. First, many of the slash-and-burn strategies presently used are *not* advocated here. People who advocate *slash-and-burn cost cutting* would do well to heed some research published in the *Harvard Business Review*: **"Companies with few or no layoffs performed significantly better than those with large numbers of layoffs"** (Rigby, 2002). In addition, research shows that **companies with similar growth rates that did not downsize consistently outperformed those that did downsize**. In addition, costs are associated with layoffs:

- Severance packages
- Temporary declines in productivity or quality
- Rehiring and retraining costs

Thoughtless approaches are implemented without considering future consequences. This research shows that *greater cost savings are realized by dealing with the more knotty organizational and leadership problems* and that downsizing and layoffs can actually be more expensive in the long run.

Another strategy we do *not* advocate is to resort to *quick-fix solutions* such as suddenly reorganizing or reengineering/restructuring when in a budget crunch or when faced with personnel problems, problem departments, or systems issues. Two common ways to restructure and reorganize are inpatient bed consolidation by reaggregation of the patient population with increased outpatient or freestanding facility solutions, and downsizing and cutting present staff positions.

Making quick-fix decisions that restructure the organization most often result in increased complexity, layoffs, people in new jobs not understanding their additional responsibilities, missed care, errors, decreased patient satisfaction, and survivor issues with those left. They have drastic effects on both the remaining workforce and on efficiency in general. Most often, the result is inefficiency, realized in elevated costs and other expensive short-term and long-term effects—not to mention patient harm.

A short-term effect of redesign is that the *survivors* need to be oriented to assume the duties of displaced personnel. This means that a less effective, less efficient staff are not only dealing with the acquisition of new duties—and the resultant creation of more patient safety issues—but are also experiencing *survivor sickness*. Burke (2002) describes survival sickness as having the following characteristics: "low morale, decreased commitment, and increased cynicism, mistrust, and anger. Affected caregivers may question the effectiveness of their facility's functioning, describe their work environment as deteriorated, and believe that this deterioration threatens patient's well-being" (p. 41). Not to mention they make more errors, miss care, and exhibit other characteristics of low-quality care. These are the short-term effects, but it does not stop there.

How well the organization supports staff during times of restructuring directly affects retention of the remaining staff. A long-term effect, along with additional costs, may be a subsequent increase in staff turnover rates resulting from restructuring. Sometimes it is easier to be the person who is displaced than to be one of the remaining staff on a unit or in a department. Based on these facts, it is very important for the nurse administrator and other healthcare organization officials to provide support for the survivors.

Actually providing survivor support is a tall order. It is best if administrators continually communicate with staff about the changes that will take place as well as why the changes are necessary. *Once staff trust is lost, it is very difficult to regain.* In addition, staff morale suffers when layoffs or restructuring occurs, and teamwork probably is affected within and between departments. Burke (2002) advocates taking the following steps to improve staff involvement that deal more effectively with survivor issues:

- Create focus groups or hold employee meetings to discuss the restructuring, particularly what went right and solutions for what went wrong. (Note here that it would have been better to do focus groups and employee meetings as part of the planning process for redesign in the first place.)

- Develop education programs to help employees adjust.
- Identify employee concerns through surveys (or have everyone start doing rounds!).
- Formulate new communication strategies for better transparency.
- Reevaluate jobs to better reflect new responsibilities.

Both reorganization and reengineering were meant to happen in a carefully crafted way, following dialogue and careful planning by all stakeholders involved. Instead, they have actually been used to provide quick fixes that then create further problems. Meanwhile, the original issues were not resolved, complexity is increased, and the situation actually worsens. Is it any wonder that in this frenzy there are additional costs incurred that were not considered?

> It is both obvious and worthy of emphasis that if we are going to improve cost and service performance in [healthcare organizations], we must begin by looking at how we use our employees—how many there are, what kinds, what we ask them to do, how we organize them, and how in reality they spend their time and the institution's resources. . . . For [healthcare organizations], the value added is the sum of all personnel-related expenses. . . . Not all costs are created equal. . . . What is needed is a framework that recognizes the differences between costs and the different strategies to which each might or might not be susceptible. As a result, operations strategists devised a conceptual model for thinking about costs: the cost performance hierarchy. (Lathrop, 1993, pp. 24–27)

The performance hierarchy asks three questions.

1. What is done? Evaluation includes: census and admission rates; variability of external demand; intensity of care required/severity of illness; quality of care objectives; service offerings; and location.
2. How is it done? Here one would examine organizational structure, management processes, operating policies and systems, capacity management, physical size and layout, equipment deployment, and skill mix.
3. How well is it done? Evaluation includes quality measurements, productivity levels, work pace, and skill level. (Lathrop, 1993, p. 28)

The Budget Process: Is It Flawed or Effective?

Another strategy is the budget process itself. In our interconnected world, the best budget process involves *everyone* in the organization—including patients, families, and physicians. The budget is *transparent* and shared with staff. The budget process is *participative* but extends beyond just participation. The process is most effective when all involved are *equal partners* and use dialogue (both sharing information and listening to others). This approach is much more effective than an authoritarian, or top-down, method of communication. Therefore, everyone from the housekeeper or nursing assistant through the physician and the board chair is involved in the decision-making process (this includes the strategic plan)—with the patients and their families being the pivotal, or most important, part of this process. Physicians have to be included because physician practice patterns can have a direct effect on increasing or decreasing the budget. Nurses need to be involved in this all along the way.

We recommend being *honest* about budgets. The problem with dishonesty is that lies beget more lies, and once you have been found out, your believability is ***gone***. Trust, once lost, is extremely difficult to regain or, realistically, is probably never regained! Integrity is essential.

Honesty can become a problem in an organization if everyone is playing games. If you, a manager, have been honest and have been diligent about holding down costs yet no one else has been held accountable, when there are budget cuts you may be expected to cut the same percentage as those who have not been accountable. Your unit then becomes *penalized* for being more effective! Thus, it is very important to stress with your supervisors and the finance department right from the start that you are holding down costs and request that they take this into account if there is a budget cut. In certain organizations it is important to get this agreement in writing.

Historically, a *flawed budget process* has been used. This process started in the 1920s when large companies used the process "as a tool for managing costs and cash flows" (Hope & Fraser, 2003, p. 113). Then, in the 1960s:

> Companies used accounting results not just to keep score but also to dictate the actions of people at all levels of the company. By the early 1970s, a new generation of leaders schooled in the finer arts of financial planning had begun to rely on financial targets and incentives—in lieu of such benchmarks as productivity and marketing effectiveness—to drive performance improvement. (p. 113)

This caused serious problems in the 1980s and 1990s when companies started paying more attention to sales targets than to satisfying customers. Suddenly, money was running the game rather than supporting it.[1] Unfortunately, some healthcare organizations continue to use this flawed process today.

Hope and Fraser (2003) report that budgeting can take up to *30% of management's time*! This time commitment becomes even more overwhelming when mergers and reorganization occur. This is expensive time that does not really accomplish much in the way of outcomes. In fact, many harmful games can result. Consider the following from Jensen (2001) in the *Harvard Business Review*:

> CORPORATE BUDGETING IS A JOKE, and everyone knows it. It consumes a huge amount of executives' time, forcing them into endless rounds of dull meetings and tense negotiations. It encourages managers to lie and cheat, lowballing targets and inflating results, and it penalizes them for telling the truth. It turns business decisions into elaborate exercises in gaming. It sets colleague against colleague, creating distrust and ill will. And it distorts incentives, motivating people to act in ways that run counter to the best interests of their companies.
>
> The sad thing is, these shenanigans have become so common that they're almost invisible. The budgeting process is so deeply embedded in corporate life that the attendant lies and games are simply accepted as business as usual, no matter how destructive they are. . . .
>
> As soon as you start motivating unit and department heads to falsify forecasts and otherwise hide or manipulate critical information, you undermine the salutary effects of budgeting. Indeed, the whole effort backfires. You end up with uncoordinated, chaotic interactions as people make decisions on the basis of distorted information they receive from other units and from headquarters. Moreover, since managers are well aware that everyone is attempting to game the system for personal reasons, you create an organization rife with cynicism, suspicion, and mistrust. When the manipulation of budget targets becomes routine, moreover, it can undermine the integrity of an entire organization. (pp. 96–97)

Another similar perspective is presented by Hope and Fraser (2003):

> Budgeting, as most corporations practice it, should be abolished. . . . Companies . . . cling tenaciously to budgeting—a process that disempowers the front line, discourages information sharing, and slows the response to market developments until it's too late. . . . In practice, they marshal the power of computer systems to uncover mind-numbing levels of detail and, using the budget as a benchmark, demand to know why a sales team has rung up higher-than-normal telephone charges, for instance, or why it has underspent the quarter's entertainment allowance. And where is "all the authority of the chairman" when the team finds it can't meet the budget's sales targets? Fearing the consequences, the team will lean on customers to order goods they have every intention of returning. And if by some chance the team thinks it will exceed its targets, it will press customers to accept delivery in the next fiscal period, delaying valuable cash flows.

> In extreme cases, use of the budget to force performance improvements may lead to a breakdown in corporate ethics. [They then discuss several failed companies where, for example, employees had to be 2% under budget, with nothing else being acceptable.] Other failed companies had tight budgetary control processes that funneled information only to those with a "need to know."
>
> A number of companies have recognized the full extent of the damage done by budgeting. They have rejected the reliance on obsolete data and the protracted, self-interested wrangling over what the data indicate about the future. And they have rejected the foregone conclusions embedded in traditional budgets—conclusions that render pointless the interpretation and circulation of current market information. (pp. 108–109)

Bart's (1988) research on gamesmanship found several *budget games that managers played*: understating volume estimates, not declaring/understating price increases, not declaring/understating cost reduction programs, and overstating expenses for advertising, consumer promotions, trade-related issues, and market research. These budget manipulations resulted in "'cushion,' 'slush fund,' 'hedge,' 'flexibility,' 'cookie jar,' 'hip/back pocket,' 'pad,' 'kitty,' 'secret reserve,' 'war chest,' and 'contingency' funds" (p. 286). This occurs because usually senior management does not have the time to find the cushions or because others were not as familiar with the product and did not realize the true costs.

Another game that is played with budgets is the *spend it or lose it* mentality that goes on at the end of the budget year. In this game, a manager knows that any money left in the budget will be lost at the end of the fiscal year, so the manager decides to find things to spend the money on just before the fiscal year closes.

Bart's (1988) research also examined *companies where games were not played*. Here "there was a good deal of trust between senior management and product managers" (p. 290). Honesty was valued. In fact, trust and honesty were so important one manager said,

> The moment I betray my . . . manager, I've had it in this company. My bosses will be angry with me for being unfair. And [people reporting directly to me] will never take my word at face value again. They'll start to play games with me and I'll have to try and catch them . . . and that sure can waste a lot of time! (p. 291)

Today, hopefully, we are using more participative, customer-oriented processes. This results in flatter structures and rapid responses to market changes and stays closer to the customer—emphasizing public relations, empowering workers to make appropriate decisions as they do their work, and sharing information, including information about budget expenses and revenues. All this enhances our systems so that employees have all the tools present to do their work more effectively. Yet, if we still use the cumbersome, flawed, historic budget process, we do not achieve any of these objectives.

That is why we advocate different, newer processes that include dialogue, honesty, and transparency.

Some companies have done away with the budget and the budget process. They *replace the traditional budget with rolling forecasts*:

> Alternative goals and measures—some financial, such as cost-to-income ratios, and some nonfinancial, such as time to market—move to the foreground. And business units and personnel, now responsible for producing results, are no longer expected to meet predetermined, internally selected financial targets. Rather, every part of the company is judged on how well its performance compares with its peers' and against world-class benchmarks.
>
> In companies using these standards of performance, business units become smaller, more numerous, and more entrepreneurial. Strategy becomes a grass-roots endeavor. The aggregate result of many small teams exploiting local opportunities is a much more adaptive organization.
>
> But that's not to say these companies abandon their high expectations. They don't naively assume that everyone who is given more autonomy will improve his or her performance. In fact, they

require employees to do something much tougher than meet a fixed target. They ask them to chase a will-o'-the-wisp, to measure themselves against how well comparable groups inside and outside the company will turn out to have done in the same period, given the economic conditions prevailing at the time. Because employees won't know whether they've succeeded or by how much until the period is over, they must use every ounce of their energy and ingenuity to ensure that their performance is better than that of their peers. Business units ... can measure their progress against comparable units within the company through the use of a few key financial measures. In order to measure themselves against external peers, they can use operational benchmarks based in industrywide best practices. . . .

Abandoning budget targets . . . frees a business to give a wide variety of emerging information its due. . . . This shifts the emphasis from meeting short-term promises to improving our competitive position year after year. The result is much more accurate interpretation of our results. (Hope & Fraser, 2003, pp. 109–110)

Hope and Fraser (2003) report that the focus has shifted from detailed budget plans to trend analyses and 3-month rolling forecasts for five to eight quarters. Managers, along with the finance department, are expected to constantly revise the forecasts. Instead of the cumbersome, detailed traditional budget approach, these forecasts include only "key variables, such as orders, sales, costs, and capital expenditures, which means they can be compiled relatively easily and quickly, sometimes by a single person in a single day" (p. 112). This way, the budget information is constantly updated and takes the latest economic trends and customer usage patterns into account. Information is open to all in the organization. Playing budget games becomes difficult, and everyone receives more accurate, updated information for appropriate strategic planning.

Here's how rolling forecasts usually work. Let's say that in the middle of March 2003, a company creates a five-quarter forecast that covers the period from the beginning of April 2003 through the end of June 2004. From the moment it is completed, new data start coming in. Once three months' worth is in hand, the process begins again. A new five-quarter forecast updates the projections for the period covered by the previous forecast and creates a brand-new projection for the quarter farthest in the future, July-September 2004.

Volvo relies on several types of rolling forecasts. Every month, it orders up a "flash" forecast that looks three months ahead, informing managers about current demand and helping them determine whether, for example, price promotions should be introduced or curtailed. Every quarter, a 12-month forecast updates the managers' working assumptions about customer behavior and economic trends. And every year, two additional forecasts—one looking four years ahead, one looking ten years ahead—help managers assess the company's market positioning and determine schedules for phasing out old models and phasing in new ones. (Hope & Fraser, 2003, p. 112)

Companies using this approach have discovered that they can *save up to 95% of the time they originally spent going through the historical budget process.* For those of us used to traditional budgets, this can be a difficult change to picture. Instead of anticipating the budget for the next year, longer term goals, often rolling forecasts that project for the next couple of years, are identified. Then, the manager reviews the forecasts every quarter. The quarterly review helps managers to continually assess the action plan and to change it as new developments occur. Elements measured include both hard and soft performance data such as profits, cash flows, cost ratios, customer satisfaction, and quality. The organizations became *radically decentralized and needed a much smaller corporate structure* to support the front-line managers. Hope and Fraser (2003) describe companies that use this method:

In an empowered organization, people are free to make mistakes and equally free to fix them. Managers have wide discretion in making decisions; as a result, they can obtain resources more quickly than in traditional companies and without having to document need quite so elaborately, partly because they are accountable for the profitability of their units and can therefore be expected to shed any excess in the event that demand falls. . . . And employees, because they don't require much supervision, don't need the extensive central services that most organizations provide. Eliminating those services has a dramatic effect on a company's cost structure. . . .

Without budget expectations to worry about, staff members can do something with the nonconforming customer and market information they collect—other than hide it. The reporting of unusual patterns and trends as they unfold helps the business avoid shortages or overages and formulate changes in direction. Instead of being imposed from above, strategy seeps up from below. (pp. 110–111)

Creating a Cost-Conscious Environment

Materials and supply costs, rising daily in health care, need to be examined. These costs are second only to the cost of staffing. One way to decrease supply costs is by exercising more reasonable use of supplies by nursing staff. Nurse managers responsible for creating and maintaining their unit's fiscal budgets can provide substantial decreases in costs by controlling supply expenditures. An overall decrease in the organization's fiscal budget may be realized as each individual unit's supply budget is trimmed for efficiency. Staff need to understand the importance of charging patients appropriately for supplies. Missed charges mean less money. Budget transparency is the key here. Trimming and charging are happening using a process involving staff who directly use the supplies. In fact, in a positive environment where staff are empowered, they will think of better ways to save costs than supervisors or finance can achieve.

As we become more conscious of supply costs as managers, it is important to *involve staff* in this issue.

> We must also communicate to patients, nurses, and physicians that [healthcare organizations] no longer can afford to give things away. Someone always ends up paying. Nurses are trained to help people, to be generous and giving. For example, a nurse may give a patient a bunch of sterile pads rather than instructing him to go to the local pharmacy. Even those who mean well can put a [healthcare organization] out of business. (Lefever, 1999, p. 30)

Inefficiencies mount up. For unit-based cost savings to occur, staff should be involved in the formulation of the department's fiscal budget and know the overall organization's financial targets. They see monthly reports showing whether they are meeting the budget goals. Staff then have a better sense of how they are contributing to either cost inefficiencies or to cost containment without compromising quality. After all, practice behaviors can affect the cost of delivering patient care.

To maximize efficiency of supply usage by staff it is important to take an *educational approach* to the issue. Krugman and colleagues (2002) reported a successful multidisciplinary financial education research project taken by a western tertiary teaching hospital. In this project, nurses, resident physicians, pharmacists, and nursing students integrated fiscal knowledge into practice. This study measured baseline financial knowledge regarding charges, reimbursement, and regulatory issues before implementing several initiatives. The team then developed a variety of initiatives to target knowledge deficits. A logo was created and used as a symbol for identifying financial articles published quarterly in the hospital newsletter. Subcommittees addressed the institution's financial problems. Efforts began with various educational activities, such as videos and the purchase of a financial software program for nursing leadership.

The post survey showed that the subjects' financial knowledge improved. Targeted educational interventions proved successful. Financial outcomes included an increase in captured patient charges, improved documentation of services rendered, and decreased materials loss and wastage. This study was indicative of the positive effects that can be realized from awareness campaigns and educational activities involving staff and physicians (Krugman et al., 2002, p. 277).

An additional finding was that often nurses had negative attitudes toward cost-effectiveness, associating it with a *bottom-line orientation* that resulted in staffing reductions, pay cuts, longer work hours, and diminished resources. Do you see all the damage a bottom-line orientation actually does? Because of these negative attitudes, nurses may not be as cost effective in their nursing practice.

Invisible costs for unused supplies from packs and trays, obsolete and slow-moving inventory, pilferage, giveaways, and uncontrolled usage indicate waste and are a prime target for nurse managers who wish to correct supply budget variances. First, nurse managers must determine how and where the major waste is occurring. They can do this by reviewing the unit's present inventory of supplies and determining whether there are opportunities for efficiency in areas where practice creates costly waste. For example, when physicians who no longer have patients in the department request supplies from that department, this is considered waste. Correcting this waste may be as simple as revising or providing guidelines to standardize supply usage. Decreasing types of stock that are not used frequently not only decreases the number of dollars required for the department's supply budget but also provides more space for pertinent supplies.

As the financial resources available for purchase of supplies, linen, and equipment have dwindled as a result of low reimbursements, there has been more *hoarding* of supplies and equipment. Although hoarding provides staff with immediate access to the resources they need for patient care, staff do not realize that they add to their supply and equipment problems overall. *Overstocking and hoarding cost money.* Tying up financial resources for purchase of more and more supplies because of stockpiling can actually build to a point where the whole facility is not efficient in the management of materials. For example, hoarding of IV pumps (or linen, monitors, or wheelchairs) only creates the need to purchase more IV pumps for the facility—a big, unnecessary expense. This "lost" inventory would be less costly if left in circulation throughout the healthcare organization.

In actuality, *hoarding is a symptom of a larger systems problem.* Instead of hiding and storing more inventory for the unit, it is much more cost efficient to bring together a group of stakeholders from appropriate departments to work out a better solution. The solution needs to have *the right numbers at the right times in the right place.*

This systems strategy is also a useful way to examine supply and equipment fluctuations as patient volume changes. For instance, if the patient census, or acuity, has decreased, the nurse manager, as well as other appropriate departmental managers, could check to see whether the inventory usage has also decreased. A *periodic survey and inventory* of all nursing units in a facility can help with these issues.

In addition, nurse administrators can periodically review overall monthly budget costs for linen, supplies, and equipment. Sudden variances in this budget could indicate hoarding, creating the need for purchases to counteract the decreases in certain areas. (Hoarding, if it persists a long time, may not appear as an increase in the budget but must still be dealt with to achieve cost-effectiveness.) Close interaction with departments, such as the laundry, central supply, and materials management, could shed light on areas of concern. These are process issues. Complexity is involved and the processes need to be simplified.

Educating staff about supply costs so that they can adjust inventories to meet patient demands is extremely important. The staff should realize that they have a direct responsibility to achieve efficiency and, if something is not working, to express their concerns to the appropriate managers so that problems can be fixed. Everyone, including the nurse manager, needs to be involved in achieving better efficiencies.

One common purchasing approach is to have supplies delivered only as they are needed: the *just-in-time* philosophy. The idea behind this is to save money by not stockpiling and to avoid having too much already present at the facility. In health care, a service industry, where we are not making the same widgets every day, it can be difficult to anticipate which patients with which medical or surgical problems will need supplies each day. It is difficult to anticipate emergencies. So, it is best to be moderate with this approach.

Another purchasing strategy is to join a *purchasing collaborative* such as VHA or Premier. Organizations that join get materials and supplies at lower costs because purchases are made by the entire group. Still, local services are needed, such as laundry, but when an organization can purchase as part of a larger system, costs can be decreased.

Being part of a larger system has advantages. This is one reason why so many stand-alone hospitals have joined with *larger hospital systems*. Then, even in local purchases, they can get better discounts. Another reason is that, when dealing with Medicare and other insurance companies, the negotiation of contracts, as well as submitting claims, is complicated and time consuming. Being part of a larger group more effectively deals with all this.

Standardization of supply usage can also provide cost savings. For example, the standardization of items placed in sterile trays and packs for labor and delivery procedures on obstetrical units, in emergency rooms, or in surgery departments may be warranted. Meeting with the physicians up front to elicit their input on the design of the new trays is a must. The changes need to satisfy their needs as well as provide efficiency. Otherwise, more waste could occur.

Sales representatives from supply vendors who are providing the most efficient contracts for their supplies may be especially helpful in the design of these new packs and trays. Attending healthcare supply trade fairs may also provide the nurse administrator with excellent information concerning the newest and most efficient items available to be placed in the packs. Price wars from vendors may be advantageous in acquiring the most items of quality for the least amount of money. In other words, cost comparison is a must (still keeping quality in mind).

Because the cost of medical supplies and equipment is one of the major budget items associated with health care, it is imperative for nurse administrators to be knowledgeable in the latest trends affecting the purchasing of these supplies. Having knowledge and being able to *talk the talk* with purchasing managers are essential skills for nurse managers to have an influence on the buying practices of their units and the institution as a whole. This is also why it is an advantage to send nurse managers and staff to seminars and trade shows.

Developing Integrated Information Systems

Where is the wisdom we have lost in knowledge?
Where is the knowledge we have lost in information?

—Thomas Stearns Eliot

We cannot ignore that we are in the Information Age. Complexity is growing at an exponential rate as can be seen with technologies: "computer processing power and storage capacity, the number of healthcare providers using various types of medical technology in hospitals, healthcare information on the intranet, and the decline in medical devices size" (Clancy, 2010, p. 247).

> In his book, *The Nature of Technology*, Arthur defines technology from 3 perspectives: 1) as a means to fulfill a human purpose, 2) an assemblage of practices and components, and 3) a collection of devices and engineering practices available to a culture. Three definitions are needed because each points to technology in a different sense or category from the others.
>
> Note that practices, as opposed to just physical devices, are considered a form of technology because they also are a means to fulfill a human purpose.
>
> Therefore, processes and methods can be considered a form of technology if we include the devices that execute them.

> In today's healthcare environment processes, methods and technology are all linked. Changes in technology impact the process, and changes in the process impact the technology. (Clancy, 2010, pp. 247–248)

This is certainly an example of complexity. As new technology becomes available it increases organizational complexity. This benefits organizations but at the same time creates additional challenges and expenses.

Remember the saying, *high tech, high touch*? The touch part in health care continues to be important, even as we add more technology. Remember the old research on the failure-to-thrive babies? The problem was that they were not being lovingly touched. So, we must always *balance* the information/technology with wisdom/knowledge and with the touch aspect of health care.

Another issue in the Information Age is that there is so much information available it is not humanly possible to ever know it all. And we must not become a slave to it. As expressed in the quote at the beginning of this section, we still need wisdom, and we still need our knowledge, judgment, and experience as we do our work. The issue is that we need the wisdom and knowledge *along with* the information. The information provides us with a useful *tool*—additional evidence—to add to, or correct, our present knowledge and wisdom. As we are involved in each administrative, educational, or patient situation there are still individual differences that we must account for before we determine what to do (Matney, Brewster, Sward, Cloyes, & Staggers, 2011). We still need to make decisions based on all these factors.

Technology creates more complexity in additional ways. Now there is usually an IT or Information Technology department (or personnel) in healthcare organizations. As more organizations added technology, issues resulted when end users did not understand or resisted technology use or the technology was not adapted to the organization in a usable way. IT programmers did not understand healthcare nuances and healthcare providers did not understand the intricacies of the technology.

This resulted in a new nursing role—an *informatics nurse specialist (INS)* who has healthcare experience and who also understands the technology (Huryk, 2011; McLane & Turley, 2011). Informatics nurse specialists are assets to the organization. They are involved with technology decisions and purchases, implementation, and updates and changes needed in the technology and they act as a liaison between IT and the nursing staff.

The American Nurses Association (ANA) provides the *Scope and Standards of Nursing Informatics Practice* (ANA, 2007). ANA defines nursing informatics as follows:

> Nursing informatics is a specialty that integrates nursing science, computer science, and information science to manage and communicate data, information, and knowledge in nursing practice. Nursing informatics facilitates the integration of data, information, and knowledge to support patients, nurses, and other providers in their decision-making in all roles and settings. This support is accomplished through the use of information structures, information processes, and information technology.
>
> The goal of nursing informatics is to improve the health of populations, communities, families, and individuals by optimizing information management and communication. This includes the use of technology in the direct provision of care, in establishing effective administrative systems, in managing and delivering educational experiences, in supporting life-long learning, and in supporting nursing research. (p. vii)

There are now master's degree programs available in nursing informatics, and in 2005 the American Nurses Credentialing Center (ANCC) established a certification process for a Certified Professional in Health Information and Management Systems.

In 2007, the Alliance for Nursing Informatics (ANI) was formed (see www.allianceni.org/). This is a collaborative effort with academia, practice, industry, and nursing specialties to provide a unified voice for nursing informatics. It is cosponsored by the American Medical Informatics Association (AMIA) and the Healthcare Information and Management Systems Society (HIMSS) (Murphy, 2010).

Health information technology (HIT) can be a *huge expenditure*, and the decision to purchase it should be made carefully. For instance, electronic medical record (EMR) systems—also called EHRs (electronic health records)—can cost millions of dollars. Many healthcare organizations, especially small or rural facilities, are not purchasing these systems because of the high cost. Interestingly, in the 2011 HIMSS survey, 600 nurse informaticists prioritized three issues as being most important in not implementing HIT: (1) lack of integration/interoperability (this was the top barrier), (2) lack of financial resources (this had been the top barrier in the past), and (3) lack of administrative support (Sensmeier, 2011). Other downsides are increased security and privacy risks (Gallagher, 2013). AHA (2011) reported that "organizations who installed IT systems have found that literacy, cultural, and work flow barriers were much more critical than the cost barrier to successful implementation" (p. 16).

For those who have purchased an EMR system, most think that the upfront cost of purchasing and implementing computerized charting is offset by the cost efficiency it provides. Streamlined documentation is vital in the overall medical records process to provide accuracy and ease of access to required records, to provide safety checks, to document the time and cost of nursing care, and to meet regulatory guidelines and justify insurance payments. Consider coding, for instance. In a paper system, a lot of time is spent searching through mounds of paper to obtain coding information. Computerized charting decreases the turnaround in reimbursement for hospital stays by providing a fast, efficient retrieval of the pertinent coding information.   .

> [HIT] promotes (1) accurate and complete information about a patient's health for patient-centered care based on patient characteristics and preferences; (2) better coordination of the care; (3) evaluation of outcomes; (4) a way to securely exchange information with patients, providers, and caregivers; and (5) information to enable early diagnosis, minimize duplication, reduce errors, and provide safer care. (Wilson & Newhouse, 2012, p. 395)

It provides clinical decision support and reduces reliance on memory by pushing reminders and alerts to providers (Clancy & Anteau, 2008, p. 159).

Waneka and Spetz (2010), in a review of the HIT literature, found the following:

- HIT improves the quality of nursing documentation.
- HIT reduces medication administration errors.
- Nurses are generally satisfied with HIT and have positive attitudes about it.
- Nurse involvement in all stages of HIT design and implementation, and effective leadership throughout these processes, can improve HIT. (p. 509)

Another advantage for the EMR system purchase is the growing competition. For example, health maintenance organizations now cover some 67 million Americans. Kaiser Permanente, the nation's largest health maintenance organization, spent $1 billion for information technology that will achieve better care as well as document that the care was given (Schonfeld, 1998, p. 111). Then, it marketed this to employers to show that their care would be safer because of this technology. This was prompted when employers, such as General Motors and Xerox, started ranking health plans by cost and quality to give their employees the best possible health care. To give a health maintenance organization the edge in the saturated market, low-cost care was not enough. Higher standards and quality of care must also accompany the lower cost.

The fourth AHA must-do strategy is to develop integrated information systems. Presently, most information systems do not interface with other systems. For instance, the human resources department has information about nurses in its database system that the nursing department has in its scheduling technology. The information has to be put into each system separately because the two systems do not interface with one another (they are not integrated). This duplicates work (a time waster), and, as something is changed in one system, it might not be changed in the other system, so errors occur.

Because the EMR system is so expensive, and because only about 12% of hospitals had by then purchased an EMR system, in 2009 the American Recovery and Reinvestment Act (ARRA) created the Medicare and Medicaid Electronic Health Records Incentive Programs that provided billions of dollars in incentive payments to eligible professionals and hospitals that adopted EMRs. To be eligible for funds, providers had to comply with *meaningful use* (MU) criteria (Smith & Bolton, 2013). MU

> is an umbrella term for rules and regulations that hospitals and providers must meet to qualify. . . . MU criteria included using a certified HER for functions that both improve and demonstrate the quality of care, such as e-prescribing, electronic gathering and exchange of health information; and submission of quality measures to CMS. (Wilson & Newhouse, 2012, p. 396)

In stage II of the meaningful use legislation, providers are to electronically make personal health information available to more than half of their patients. In addition, providers will "ensure that more than 10% of their patients view, download, or transmit their health information to a 3rd party. They will also have to demonstrate that they provide more than 10% of their patients with EHR-generated educational resources" (Wilson, Murphy, & Newhouse, 2012, pp. 493–494). If this goal is not met, funding will be taken back from a facility. So far, though adoption of EMRs and MU "accelerated between 2010 and 2011, meeting the stage I criteria still remains a challenge for most organizations" (p. 495).

Gomez (2010) and Vondrak (2012) gave recommendations to consider when upgrading or installing an EMR system (not included here). Stakeholders should consider the following before purchasing technology:

- All stakeholders need to be involved in evaluating the technology.
- How useful is it? Is it easy to use?
- What are the costs (purchase, installation, maintenance, other equipment needed, implementation costs, technology updates, and internal personnel and maintenance costs including implementation)? Is it worth the money expended?
- Does it interface with other technology?
- Does it have or require a backup system? A maintenance system? Is downtime needed for this?
- Can it be updated easily?
- Is there system support from the company it was purchased from? Is house support needed?
- Have work environment issues been considered? (Where will it be located, is a cart or table needed, do users sit or stand while using?)
- How secure is it (so it does not violate privacy/confidentiality requirements)? Is it safe?
- Can the people using it actually get a chance to try it and evaluate it?
- How do others who have already purchased the system evaluate it?
- What are the pros and cons about the purchase of this technology?
- Figure a cost benefit analysis of this purchase before making the purchase decision.

Another popular HIT has been the *computerized physician order entry* (CPOE) technology where physicians enter orders into a computer system. This is an improvement over trying to read their writing. Reasons to use these have been: "to improve patient safety and quality of care, decrease costs, and reduce the risk of medical errors" (Cowan, 2013, p. 27). However some unintended consequences have occurred: (1) communication decreased between physicians and nurses, and (2) staff figured out workarounds and did not use the program as it was intended. Another issue is that "excessive reminders, alerts, and warning messages have been associated with alert fatigue wherein the care professional disregards the message" (p. 29). The next development is electronic interdisciplinary care plans (Jones, Jamerson, & Pike, 2012). All this has increased complexity.

There are a number of issues with technology. For example, sometimes the technology purchased is not complete, such as a partial EMR system that is used for charting but not for MD orders. So, staff have to go back and forth with paper versus electronic entries and use both systems for documentation. This can easily duplicate work, take more time, and cause errors.

Sometimes there is not adequate testing before implementation and huge issues result that cannot be immediately fixed. This creates staff frustration that gets passed on to patients. Staff figure out workarounds (ways to get around the limitations) that may create more errors and safety issues.

Technology implementation has spawned another nursing role, that of *superuser bedside nurses*. These are nurses who, during implementation of technology such as the EMR system, are present around the clock for go-live events to help end users more effectively use the new technology. Sometimes when confronted with new technology, end users can discover workaround activities that avoid the system and create unsafe practices. Observation and support on the part of the superusers are strategies to achieve safer practices (Rosenberg & Rodik, 2012).

Many of the large EMR systems need downtime for backup and upgrading activities, for fixing misfunctions, and for when there is no electricity. This can create other problems for staff. For instance, we now have a new generation of nurses who do not know how to use a paper chart. Yet often a paper chart is what is used during technology downtime. Thus, now we need mock downtime so that the organization can more effectively deal with these situations.

Communication technology has gained importance for use in healthcare organizations. A popular device is Vocera, which enables a hands-free way for staff to communicate on a unit. The downside is that it is an interruption and, when improperly used, can violate Health Insurance Portability and Accountability Act (HIPAA) confidentiality (Dunphy, MacNairn, Finlay, Wallace, & Lemaire, 2011).

Technology has enabled telehealth capabilities so that people in their homes or in rural communities can directly interact with health providers. This is more convenient for patients and achieves cost savings. One of the most exciting new uses of telehealth is in the form of telemergency services, including triage services, which bring the benefits of fast and efficient emergency care to underserved rural areas. Electronic or telephone links can connect patients at distant sites with physicians and nurse practitioners for care. Telehealth has become an enormous source for giving care to patients.

Fox and Duggan report that 81% of U.S. adults use the internet and 59% say they have looked online for health information in the past year. 35% of U.S. adults say they have gone online specifically to try to figure out what medical condition they or someone else might have (2013).

Phone consultations can save as much as $50 to $240 per member and also save the customers time. Nurses with physician backup can provide services.

Educating and Engaging Employees and Physicians to Create Leaders

The sixth AHA must-do strategy is about creating *leaders at the point of care*. This includes physicians and nurses as well as other employees. In the second curve, the most important place in the healthcare environment is the point of care. We have often gotten the word *leader* confused with *administrator*. Anyone can become a *leader* when two or more people get together. An *administrator* possesses the position in the organizational chart that determines who has overall responsibility for certain areas.

Here, in the second-curve environment, **leaders at the point of care are the most important people in the organization**. Administrators *support* these leaders to give the care. This is not to say that administrators should not be leaders as well, but their role is administrative, supporting leaders at the point of care. This is an enormous change for healthcare administrators who have not been educated to behave in this manner.

Many first-curve administrators (as well as most of the U.S. population) view the CEO as the most important person in the organization. So, having leaders at the point of care is a major shift in many people's perspectives.

Just saying this is the case is not enough: Actions speak louder than words. Administrators need to live this perspective and show in all their actions that those at the point of care are the most important. This is why everyone (including administrators) needs to do regular rounds. That is where the action is. To accomplish this, administrators may need to evaluate the necessity of many of the meetings they schedule. Some are excellent and promote team functioning; others do not. ***Rounds need to replace many meetings because the people in the meetings are often not in touch with what is happening at the bedside***.

Effective leadership is very important wherever it occurs, at any level in the organization. Effective leadership includes the ability to value empowerment of others. Unless one has achieved Stage 4 in Hagberg's power scale, empowerment will not occur.

Nurse managers need to encourage and empower all staff to be leaders at the point of care, and they must support these leaders. For some nurse managers, this is a new way of thinking. Their support is pivotal to the success of this second-curve strategy. They can support a positive culture and environment because this results in the best outcomes, including reimbursement.

Many times nurse managers are not given *adequate orientation and mentoring* or have too many duties to perform realistically. When this is the case generally everyone loses.

Another issue is that sometimes there are *too many full-time equivalents (FTEs)* reporting to a nurse manager. We recommend that 35–50 FTEs is ideal. And the nurse manager role needs to be supported by charge nurses on every shift, as well as an assistant nurse manager or comanager who provides more consistent coverage on a unit. Patient, nurse, and physician satisfaction result from effective leadership on the part of managers. The nurse manager—along with all the staff—need to be *valued and supported by higher levels of administration*. (Upper levels of management may need to change to achieve this goal.) Positive management results in positive outcomes—and positive bottom lines.

Other actions that support leaders at the point of care include valuing the staff nurse who needs to be in equal partnership with the physician, promoting clinical autonomy, increasing messy communication, encouraging collaboration between all disciplines at the point of care, encouraging innovation, and promoting interdisciplinary shared governance. In addition, it is helpful to give staff ways to more effectively resolve conflicts that will invariably occur. Systems thinking is preferred, with all in the organization understanding how interconnected everything is. There needs to be ongoing dialogue among everyone throughout the organization with the players having *equal* importance in the dialogue. All the players—this includes nursing and finance—have key information that, when shared, results in better decisions. The best decisions are always based on what patients value. Ultimately, better finances are realized.

In the second curve where nurses at the point of care are given more autonomy, some hospitals give RNs the responsibility to *ensure appropriate admissions*. One system used at the Mayo Clinic's Luther Midelfort Health System in Eau Claire, Wisconsin, follows:

> At least three times a day staff nurses or clerks on each unit fill out a simple form via the hospital's Intranet indicating the Unit's current patient volume and staffing situation. The computer assigns a numerical value to "anecdotal data," entered by the unit staffer and generates a "traffic light" color—red, orange, yellow, or green—signaling the unit's capacity. The unit's assigned color is posted on the Intranet's

"status board" and is immediately available to nursing supervisors. Nurses have the ability to override the assigned color if they disagree with the computer's assessment. Each unit designates its own nurse or nurses to evaluate the computer-generated assessment; very often the charge nurse or another direct-care nurse with a leadership role is given the assignment. The nurses' "capping trust"—the authority the system grants them to restrict unit admissions—cannot be overridden by doctors or administrators. . . . [This] has not only improved throughput . . . but also contributed to increased job satisfaction among nurses and a percent drop in the hospital's RN vacancy rate. (Connolly, 2002)

Disruptive/abusive behaviors are another issue that needs attention in organizations. Everyone (including physicians) needs to give respect to others in words and actions. Differences of opinion are grist for the mill for needed changes. But disruptive or abusive behaviors should not be tolerated, with appropriate action being taken with offenders. In positive environments, positive outcomes are achieved.

When caregivers experience *moral distress* administrators need to deal with the issue. When everyone is doing rounds, it will become evident that caregivers feel moral distress around certain issues. It helps to have an ethics committee, medical staff support, and a practice council that can examine these issues. If the distress is a result of an issue such as inadequate staffing, administration must take action to resolve the problem.

In the Institute of Medicine (IOM) and Robert Wood Johnson Foundation (RWJF) report *Future of Nursing: Leading Change, Advancing Health,* published in 2010, the second and third recommendations support the AHA must-do strategies. The second recommendation is: "Nurses should achieve higher levels of education and training through an improved education system that promotes seamless academic progression." As RNs assume leadership positions at the point of care, additional education such as achieving the BSN, MSN, DNP, and PhD degrees enhances the abilities of both nurse administrators and RNs to achieve the AHA strategies.

The third IOM/RWJF recommendation is: "Nurses should be full partners with physicians and other healthcare professionals in redesigning healthcare in the United States." This goal is important to best achieve the 10 must-do AHA strategies. In the first curve, physicians and top-level administrators often considered themselves in a one-up position with nurses. In the second curve, the best results are achieved when equal partnership is valued by all groups.

Partnering with Payers

The eighth AHA must-do strategy, partnering with payers, is an important activity for the executive group and the finance department. Accountable care organizations can achieve this goal, but some healthcare organizations will choose not to be involved in this arrangement. Nursing indirectly influences reimbursement, however, because the performance standards include patient outcomes and achieving pay-for-performance goals.

Scenario-Based Strategic, Financial, and Operational Planning

The ninth AHA must-do strategy is involved with scenario-based strategic planning. In the first curve, this was an activity that the executive group accomplished with board approval. Often, it was not even shared with staff. In the second curve, it is most effective when all in the organization are involved in contributing to strategic planning, understanding it, and tweaking it as needed at the point of care, even though the executive group has overall responsibility for setting the course. Because change is always happening, a strategic plan is not carved in stone but is created with the idea that it will change as the environment changes.

Scenarios are an important addition in the second curve. When those at the point of care try out various scenarios as situations occur with patients, they find that some scenarios are very successful and some are not. Keeping the successful strategies, sharing them across the organization, and implementing them at different points of care provide administration with data on what is most likely to succeed in a strategic plan. Of course, regular rounds are also a must so that executives keep in touch with patient issues.

Achieving Population Health Improvement Through Pursuit of the Triple Aim

The 10th AHA must-do strategy proscribes that health providers at all levels pursue the triple aim. The triple aim, as defined by the Institute for Healthcare Improvement in 2007, is "to encourage hospitals to simultaneously focus on population health, increased quality, and reduction in health care cost per capita" (p. 22). This includes doing more health promotion and disease prevention activities with patients, as well as being more involved in public health of the community. All of the preceding strategies can help healthcare providers achieve the 10th strategy.

It is interesting that serving populations has recently come into focus as Doctorate in Nursing Practice (DNP) programs discuss population health and assign capstone activities to achieve better patient and organizational outcomes. Most often these activities increase quality and also save money.

Writing a Business Plan

Because budget strategies can result in making changes, especially if they alter the way money is spent, nurse managers must be able to effectively express needed changes in an organized, professional fashion that emphasizes not only what needs to happen but the costs involved. Hence this section on writing a business plan or a proposal.

Business plans and proposals can be used to request a needed piece of equipment, explain a different way of implementing patient care, or design a new service. A business plan example is found in the Appendix. The plan or proposal can be given to a supervisor, the nurse executive or director of nursing, or, after consultation with the nurse executive, the finance department personnel, the executive team, or even the board.

The business plan or proposal should present *actual data and costs* as well as provide a thoughtful rationale for the solutions. It should be readable and concise—executive team members prefer one-page executive summaries. The first step is to prepare a thoughtful business plan or proposal for the nurse executive, as discussed here.

Generally, a business plan reflects changes in the way services are delivered and involves a shift in the way money is spent. Alternately, the plan or proposal may request that the budget reflect different monetary amounts within certain categories based on changes in the patient population. The plan might also be more extensive and ask for several different, or more updated, pieces of equipment to provide a service—such as new cardiac monitors—or request new technology such as an electronic medical record system for the entire facility or system. Because nurses are involved with patients, the plan may even suggest providing a new, innovative service that the nursing staff and the nurse manager have identified that is not presently provided.

A business plan or proposal has more credence if it is typed neatly using word processing software and can be illustrated effectively with Power Point or other graphic computer programs. The plan needs to be carefully thought out so that it leads the reader through understanding a problem, provides the reader with the proposed solution to deal with the problem, and presents the reasons why this proposed solution is the best way to solve the problem. At times, it may be best to present several solutions that may cost different amounts of money, giving the pros and cons of each one.

Think of to whom the plan will be presented. What is their perspective on the situation to which your proposal refers? What information will they need to know? What background information might be helpful to include in the plan? Be clear about what is requested and what the impact or effect will be on the whole organization. Be organized in the delivery and present a reasonable solution to the problem. Plans should include the following:

- **Title:** Be sure to include the name of the person who wrote the proposal. Sometimes it is helpful to give additional background information to the reader.
- **Definition:** Define the proposed item, change, service, or program.
- **Rationale:** Why is it needed? Why is this the best item, or way, to do the service? Discuss advantages—how this proposal saves costs or increases safety—and disadvantages. Here you may need to outline other alternatives you have considered.
- **Implementation plan:** Specify what needs to happen. Provide timelines and costs.
- **Costs/benefits:** Show the actual costs and, if appropriate, how this will change existing costs. Often, this can be presented more clearly using a spreadsheet, table, pie chart, or bar graph.
- **Evaluation plan:** How will you evaluate the effectiveness of this proposed item or service?

Note

1. For more on this subject, see the book coauthored by Tom Johnson, *Relevance Lost: The Rise and Fall of Management Accounting*.

Discussion Questions

1. For each of the 10 must-do strategies, describe an action or change you can make in your department to better prepare for the second curve.
2. Describe the effectiveness of the budget process where you work. What is very positive about it? What needs to be improved? What could be done to improve it?
3. Name 10 financial strategies that would improve the finances at your work.
4. Select one strategy from question 1, and describe how you would introduce the action or change you propose in the workplace. Then, map out what would need to happen for it to be implemented.
5. How does complexity influence budget strategies and their implementation? Give examples.
6. Write a business plan for a change or piece of equipment or new process needed at your work.

References

American Hospital Association, 2011 Committee on Performance Improvement. (2011, September). *Hospitals and care systems of the future*. Chicago, IL: Author.

American Nurses Association. (2007). *Scope and standards of nursing informatics practice*. Silver Spring, MD: Nursebooks.org.

Bart, C. (1988). Budgeting gamesmanship. *Academy of Management Executive, 11*(4), 285–294.

Blankenship, J., & Winslow, S. (2003). Admission-discharge-teaching nurses: Bridging the gap in today's workforce. *Journal of Nursing Administration, 33*(1), 11–13.

Burke, R. (2002). The ripple effect. *Nursing Management, 33*(2), 41–42.

Cadmus, E., Kilgallen, M., Wynen, E., Holly, C., Chamberlain, B., Gallagher-Ford, L., & Steingall, P. (2008). Nurses' skill level and access to evidence-based practice. *Journal of Nursing Administration, 38*(11), 494–503.

Clancy, T. (2010). Technology and complexity: Trouble brewing? *Journal of Nursing Administration, 40*(6), 237–249.

Clancy, T., & Anteau, C. (2008). Coordination: New ways of harnessing complexity. *Journal of Nursing Administration, 38*(4), 158–161.

Connolly, A. (2002, May). Luther Midelfort: Granting RNs authority to restrict admissions streamlines patient flow. *Boston Business Journal.*

Cowan, L. (2013). Literature review and risk mitigation strategy for unintended consequences of computerized physician order entry. *Nursing Economic$, 31*(1), 27–31.

Dunphy, H., MacNairn, I., Finlay, J., Wallace, J., & Lemaire, J. (2011). Hands-free communication technology: A benefit for nursing? *Journal of Nursing Administration, 41*(9), 365–368.

Finkler, S., & Kovner, C. (2007). *Financial management for nurse managers and executives* (4th ed.). St. Louis, MO: Elsevier.

Fox, S. & Duggan, M. (2013). *Health Online 2013.* Washington, DC: Pew Internet and American Life Project. Retrieved http://www.pewinternet.org/Reports/2013/Health-online.aspx

Gale, B., & Schaffer, M. (2009). Organizational readiness for evidence-based practice. *Journal of Nursing Administration, 39*(2), 91–97.

Gallagher, L. (2013). Security risk! Accessing and sharing data. *Nursing Management, 31*(3), 22–27.

Gifford, W., Davies, B., Graham, I., Tourangeau, A., Woodend, A., & Lefebre, N. (2012). Developing leadership capacity for guideline use: A pilot cluster randomized control trial. *World Views on Evidence-Based Nursing.* Sigma Theta Tau International.

Gomez, R. (2010). Automation: HER upgrade considerations. *Nursing Management, 28*(12), 35–37.

Health Research & Educational Trust. (2013, April). *Metrics for the second curve of health care.* American Hospital Association. Retrieved from http://www.hpoe.org/future-metrics-1to4

Hope, J., & Fraser, R. (2003). Who needs budgets? *Harvard Business Review, 81*(2), 108–115.

Huryk, L. (2011). Interview with an informaticist. *Nursing Management, 29*(11), 44–48.

Institute of Medicine. (2011) *The future of nursing: Leading change, advancing health.* Washington, DC: National Academies Press.

Jensen, M. (2001). Corporate budgeting is broken—let's fix it. *Harvard Business Review, 70*(10), 94–101.

Jones, K., Jamerson, C., & Pike, S. (2012). The journey to electronic interdisciplinary care plans. *Nursing Management, 30*(12), 9–12.

Kalisch, B. (2009). Nursing and nurse assistant perceptions of missed nursing care: What does it tell us about teamwork? *Journal of Nursing Administration, 39*(11), 485–493.

Krugman, M., MacLauchlan, M., Riippi, L., & Grubbs, J. (2002). A multidisciplinary financial education research project. *Nursing Economic$, 20*(6), 273–278.

Lathrop, J. (1993). *Restructuring health care: The patient-focused paradigm.* San Francisco, CA: Jossey-Bass.

Lefever, G. (1999). Invisible costs, visible savings. *Nursing Management, 30*(8), 29–32.

Matney, S., Brewster, P., Sward, K., Cloyes, K., & Staggers, N. (2011). Philosophical approaches to the nursing informatics data-information-knowledge-wisdom framework. *Advances in Nursing Science, 34*(1), 6–18.

McLane, S., & Turley, J. (2011). Informaticians: How they may benefit your healthcare organization. *Journal of Nursing Administration, 41*(1), 29–35.

Melnyk, B., Fineout-Overholt, E., Gallagher-Ford, L., & Kaplan, L. (2012). The state of evidence-based practice in US nurses: Critical implications for nurse leaders and educators. *Journal of Nursing Administration, 42*(9), 410–417.

Murphy, J., (2010). Nursing informatics: The intersection of nursing, computer, and information services. *Nursing Economic$, 28*(3), 204–207.

Rigby, D. (2002, April). Look before you lay off. Downsizing in a downturn can do more harm than good. *Harvard Business Review,* 20–21.

Rosenberg, S., & Rodik, J. (2012). Bedside nurses go-live: And informatics. *Nursing Management, 30*(6), 44–46.

Rosenfeld, B. (2000). A remote possibility. *Cost & Quality, 6*(4), 38–39.

Russell, J. (2013). Nurses as value analysis facilitators. *Nursing Management, 31*(2), 53–55.

Russell-Babin, K. (2009). Seeing through the clouds in evidence-based practice. *Nursing Management, 39*(11), 26–33.

Schonfeld, E. (1998). Can computers cure health care? *Fortune, 137*(6), 111–116.

Sensmeier, J. (2011). Transformation through it. *Nursing Management, 29*(7), 35–39.

Smith, J., & Bolton, L. (2013). What is meaningful use and what are the implications for the future of health care? *Nurse Leader, 18*(2) 20–21.

Toussaint, J., & Gerard, R., with Adams, E. (2010). *On the mend: Revolutionizing healthcare to save lives and transform the industry.* Cambridge, MA: Lean Enterprise Institute.

Vondrak, K. (2012). Healthcare reform, health IT, and EHRs: The nurse executive's role. *Nursing Management, 30*(12), 46–51.

Waneka, R., & Spetz, J. (2010). Hospital information technology systems' impact on nurses and nursing care. *Journal of Nursing Administration, 40*(12), 509–514.

Wang, P. ((2012, December 12). Cutting the high cost of end-of-life care. CNNMoney. Retrieved from http://money .cnn.com/2012/12/11/pf/end-of-life-care-duplicate-2.moneymag/index.html

Wells, N., Free, M., & Adams, R. (2007). Nursing research internship: Enhancing evidence-based practice among staff nurses. *Journal of Nursing Administration, 37*(3), 135–141.

Wilson, M., Murphy, L., & Newhouse, R. (2012). Patients' access to their health information: A meaningful-use mandate. *Journal of Nursing Administration, 42*(11), 493–496.

Wilson, M., & Newhouse, R. (2012). Meaningful use: Intersections with evidence-based practice and outcomes. *Journal of Nursing Administration, 42*(9), 395–398.

Wellmont Health System Bristol Regional Medical Center

Proposal for Neuro/Surgical Step-Down Units

Prepared by Velvet Vanover, MSN, RN, CCRN
Clinical Manager, Wellmont Health System

December 10, 2003
Wellmont Health System
Bristol Regional Medical Center

Proposal for Neuro/Surgical Step Down Units

History: The three intensive care units (30 beds total) are remaining full at all times. Intensive care patients often have to wait either in the emergency department or on a medical/surgical unit for a patient to be transferred out before they can be admitted to the Intensive Care Unit. This causes delays in patient treatment, increases nursing demands on the medical/surgical unit, and increases length of stay.

Proposal: Formation of two - 4 bed Neuro/Surgical Step-Down Units to be located on the existing nursing units of 2 East and 2 West. Creation of these step down units would allow patients to be moved out of the intensive care units.

2 East

The four existing, camera monitored, beds would be upgraded to become a full Neurological/Surgical Step Down Unit. The primary patient would be the complex neurological/surgical patient that no longer meets the criteria of a critical care unit, but requires more intensive observation, intervention, and treatment than can be offered by a medical/surgical floor.

2 West

The four existing beds currently utilized as step down beds would be upgraded to become a full Surgical Step-Down Unit. The primary patient would be the complex surgical patient that no longer meets the criteria of a critical care unit, but requires more intensive observation, intervention, and treatment than can be offered by a medical/surgical floor.

The development of two step-down units would increase both the efficiency and quality of care presently offered to patients at the hospital. Other advantages include: decreased length of stays in the SICU, smoother transitions to Medical/Surgical areas, supported "fast tracking" for discharge home, and increased patient/family satisfaction. In addition, there would be increased physician satisfaction by providing additional options and alternatives for the most appropriate patient care.

The purpose of each of the Step-down units would be to provide specialized care for neurological/surgical patients who require close clinical and technical observation with rapid interventions. Patients may require continuous monitoring of one or more of the following: Cardiac, NIBP, pulse oximeter, A-line, and/or CVP line.

The Step-down units will be staffed on a nurse (RN) patient ratio of 1:4.

In addition, Patient Care Technicians will be assigned to assist in patient care.

They will be responsible for assisting with the collection of vital signs to include temperature, pulse rate, respiratory rate, and blood pressure. The RN will be responsible for monitoring vital signs more frequently than every 4 hours.

Patients

Three patient types would benefit from these step-down units.

1. Patients that are currently admitted to an intensive care unit but do not fully meet the requirements of an ICU. These patients require closer observation than a medical/surgical unit can offer.
2. Patients admitted for elective surgical procedures that require multiple care units. These patients would benefit by avoiding the surgical intensive care unit. They could be admitted and return post-operatively to the same room. This would result in increased patient satisfaction, increased communication, and ultimately may decrease the length of stay.
3. Patients that have had appropriate lengths of stay in the surgical intensive care and no longer require the same level of care. At the same time this patient still requires more care and observation than is offered on a medical/surgical unit.

Physicians

Physicians have voiced many concerns regarding the current patient flow. Among those concerns are: the costly delays in transfers from the surgical intensive care unit; the skill levels of nurses on the medical/surgical floors; and the nurse/patient ratios. Specific specialties concerns are:

1. Neurosurgeons feel additional education is needed for nursing staff to include close observation and assessment for rapid patient changes. In addition, they would like to have access for cardiac and pressure monitoring of the neurosurgical patient.
2. Surgeons site concerns over delays in transfers out of the intensive care units; consistency in the nurse/patient ratio; lack of cardiac monitoring in the current step-down area; and inability of staff to do basic critical drips and arterial lines.

Staff

Both nurse managers on 2 East and 2 West feel that a staffing nurse/patient ratio of 1 to 4 would be possible without increasing the current FTEs on those units. There would need to be assurance of an assigned nurse for those beds without overflowing into the other medical/surgical beds. Additional needs for staff would include:

1. Education in both cardiac and arterial line monitoring.
2. Education in critical thinking.
3. Education in assessment and observation of the neurological and surgical patient.

Benefits of Developing Step-Down Units

Improved Patient Outcomes

- Increased continuity of care through same caregivers and decreased transfers.
- Increased patient satisfaction and compliancy through consistent patient teaching.
- Increased observation and assessment for quick interventions.
- Increased family participation consistent with Planetree.

Improved Operating Efficiency

- Increased and appropriate use of intensive care units by eliminating admission or allowing earlier discharge from those units to step-down units.
- Financial savings by having step-down beds to move patients to when order for transfer is written.
- Increased telemetry monitoring capabilities.
- Increased rate difference on 2 East and 2 West for monitored beds.
- Increased use of present staff at higher level of care.

Improved Physician Relationships

- Fulfillment of request by physicians for step-down areas with guaranteed staffing patterns.
- Increased physician satisfaction by providing competent, quality patient care.
- Increased relations with neurosurgeons by meeting patient acuity needs.
- Increased loyalty for patient admissions to Wellmont-Bristol Regional Medical Center.

Enhanced Market Shares

Development of two, 4-bed step-down units would increase patient flow and allow increased market shares in the neurological patient and intensive care patient. Additional step-down beds would free up intensive care beds that are often in short supply. This would eliminate the need for possible diversion to another facility. An increase in the number of neurological surgical patients would occur because of the additional beds available as well as increased care levels.

Financials

Initial Investment

4 Monitors	$55,712.10	
Rewiring	$1,000.00	
Education	+ $17,145.60	(16 hrs educ × $17.86 avg hourly salary ×
Subtotal	$73,857.70	60 nurses = $17,145.60)

Step Down Charge	$607.50	
Average Room Rate	− $370.00	
	$237.50 increase per room per day	

8 beds at	$4,860.00 per day	(Step Down Rate)
8 beds at	− $2,960.00 per day	(Private Rm. Rate)
	$1,900.00 per day	

$1,900.00 × 365 = $69,350.00 increased revenue per year

Salary Comparison

SICU salary cost per pt. day (2:1 ratio)	$857.28 per day*
SDU salary cost per pt. day (4:1 ratio)	$428.64 per day
Salary Savings	$428.64 per day
8 patient beds per day	$857.28 per day Salary Savings

*Fixed cost of Manager, Clinical Educator, and Unit Coordinator approximately same for all units. Ergo, does not influence salary cost.

Reimbursement Issues

Case Mix of Patient Population:	65% Medicare/Medicaid/TennCare
	35% Managed Care*

*Self pay/Worker's Comp and other payers included in Managed Care %.

A. Medicare/Medicaid/TennCare

Pays at flat rate per stay. Savings to be achieved by providing the service at a lower cost to WBRMC would be seen in saved salary dollars.

$857.28/day Salary Savings × 365 days × 65% Payer Mix = $203,389.68 year savings.

B. Managed Care

Pays at per diem rate or % of charges rate. Per diem rate change would result in loss of charges to organization. Changing from ICU rate to step down rate equals $528.00 loss per day.

$528.00 loss per day × 8 beds × 365 days per year × 35% payer mix = $539,616.00 loss per year *

*This would only be if all 8 patients would have been in ICU.

Impact: $539,616.00 Loss
                              − $203,389.68 Savings
                                $336,226.32 Loss per year to Organization

Total Financial Impact   Initial Investment $73,857.77
                              + Loss Revenue $336,226.32
                                $410,084.09 Loss

1st Year Increased Revenues $69,350.00
Salary Saving Per Year   + $312,907.20
                                $382,257.20

1st Year =   Loss of $27,826.89
After 1st year =   Revenue of $23,319.12 per year

TITLE: ADMISSION AND DISCHARGE CRITERIA NEURO/SURGICAL STEP-DOWN
              UNIT
PURPOSE: To facilitate the increased care of the complex neuro/surgical patient requiring continu-
              ous observation, assessment, and intervention but not requiring intensive critical care.
OBJECTIVES: To deliver safe, effective, quality care to acutely ill neurological and/or surgical patients.
              To participate in collaborative interdisciplinary healthcare teams.
              To maintain a competent, highly trained nursing staff to provide acute care utilizing the
              nursing process.
GUIDELINES:

Medical Staff Management:

The attending physician will retain authority and responsibility for the admission, transfer, and discharge
of the patient except where special problems are designated to the care of consultants.

Nursing Management:

The nurse manager of the 2 East and 2 West units will have (24 hr) responsibility for each of their 4 bed
step-down units.

Admission Criteria:

Admission to the surgical step-down unit will be based on the following criteria:

a. The acuity status of the patient based upon the patient classification system.
b. Technology required for monitoring the patient.
c. The needs of the patients requiring the following:
    1. Ongoing observation and assessment.
    2. Monitoring of NIBP, Cardiac Rhythms, Temp, Arterial lines, and/or CVPs.
    3. Frequent monitoring of vital signs.
    4. Administration and monitoring of intravenous drips**:
    Dobutamine
    Low-dose Dopamine

Lidocaine
NTG
Nipride
Neosynephrine
Cardizem
Labetolol

**Levophed, Epinephrine, and High-dose Dopamine should only by used in the ICUs.

CHAPTER 18

An Overview of Case Management

Susan L. Rasmussen, PhD, RN, and Patricia A. Hayes, PhD, RN

OBJECTIVES

- Describe reasons for the need to redesign healthcare delivery.
- Trace the development of models of case management and healthcare delivery and characteristics making them desirable.
- Describe programs developed to reduce acute care expenses and, at the same time, deliver quality care.
- List implications of the Patient Protection and Affordable Care Act on healthcare delivery in acute and long-term care.

Introduction

Case management, a healthcare delivery strategy, has experienced increasing attention since it was implemented with managed care in the 1980s and 1990s to rein in healthcare costs. Diagnosis-related groups, utilization review, case management, and discharge planning were developed to ensure that hospitalized patients were treated effectively and efficiently and discharged from this most expensive healthcare setting. Effort was initiated to identify and assist high-risk, high-cost Medicare and Medicaid enrollees, and persons with complex conditions, for transition from hospital to home to provide care in a less expensive setting and avoid unnecessary medical costs.

Although the rate of healthcare spending has been reduced, the cost of healthcare reached $2.6 trillion in 2010 (Henry J. Kaiser Family Foundation, 2012, p. 14). With 17.9% of the gross domestic product funding the healthcare industry (Carper & Machlen, 2013), questions about the quality of health care remain. While leading the world in research and cancer treatment, the United States has fewer physicians and hospital beds and higher prevalence of chronic diseases (Organisation for Economic Co-operation and Development, 2013) at a time when its baby boom population is retiring.

Because half of the $2.6 trillion in healthcare costs was spent on 5% of the population, focus on identifying this smaller but more expensive group seems warranted and identification is not difficult. In 2010, mean healthcare expenses for persons 65 years of age and older were $10,274 with Medicare paying 25.7% of total healthcare expenses, and mean expenses for persons younger than 65 years of age were $3,866 (Carper & Machlen, 2013). Because more than 60% of people 65 years of age and older have multiple chronic conditions (Smith et al., 2008), this population is likely to benefit from case management for chronic conditions and potential complications requiring future hospitalization.

Health care for uninsured children and adults as well as disabled and aged persons in the United States is funded by Medicaid, a joint program of federal and state governments. The total outlay for Medicaid in 2010 was $404.1 billion, of which the federal government paid $272.8 billion and states contributed $131.3 billion (Office of the Actuary, 2012). Medicaid health services cost per person was estimated at $6,775 in 2010 (Office of the Actuary, 2012, p. iii). Estimated per capita spending for children ($2,717) and adults ($4,314) was much lower than that for aged ($15,495) and disabled ($16,963) beneficiaries (Office of the Actuary, 2012, p. 13). Total cost for disabled persons receiving Medicaid was $160.7 billion, while cost for aged Medicaid recipients was $73.7 billion. Although aged and disabled persons compose only 27% of Medicaid enrollees, they received nearly 67% of funds (Office of the Actuary, 2012, p. 14). Long-term care costs to Medicaid (i.e., nursing home services, home health care, intermediate care facility services, and home and community-based services) reached $118 billion in 2010. The remaining 34% of Medicaid funds for children and adults will be the source of funds for the uninsured to be covered with implementation of the Patient Protection and Affordable Care Act of 2010 (PPACA) with some additional funding. In addition to Medicaid, many of the disabled and aged groups receive Medicare, making them "dual-eligible."

It is clear the current system of funding is not tenable in the economic climate that exists and a more equitable arrangement for long-term and chronic care is needed. To "bend the curve" of rising costs long term, savings in addition to reduced spending will be needed. Changes to compensation include bundling of hospital readmissions with the first admission and all care for chronic conditions, accountable care organizations that accept capitation, pay for performance linking measures of patient care quality to payment, and coordinated care (Cutler, 2010, pp. 1133–1134). Change from an acute care model to one focused on chronic care management, health maintenance, and preventive interventions could provide the older age group more appropriate care and increased quality of life and reduce long-term costs.

These issues have brought about a major reimbursement change—from a volume-based reimbursement system to a value-based reimbursement environment (American Hospital Association [AHA], 2011; Health Research and Educational Trust, 2013). Of the 10 "must-do" strategies identified by the AHA to survive in the value-based environment, the first strategy is: "Aligning hospitals, physicians, and other providers across the continuum of care" (p. 4).

Within the continuum of care, case management is not necessary for every hospitalized patient. Although many persons enter the hospital for procedures and surgeries and these admissions and physician charges account for 31% of expenditures (Carper & Machlen, 2013), most of these patients benefit from protocols designed to manage acute care and are discharged with instructions and appointments, and they recover without incident. However, case management is critical for certain patients, especially those with many chronic illnesses. According to the American Nurses Credentialing Center (ANCC, 1998):

> Case management is a dynamic and systematic collaborative approach to providing and coordinating healthcare services to a defined population. It is a participative process to identify and facilitate options and services for meeting individuals' health needs, while decreasing fragmentation and duplication of care and enhancing quality, cost-effective clinical outcomes. (p. 3)

The majority of certified and noncertified case managers have nursing backgrounds, with a small percentage of case managers having social work backgrounds (Tahan & Campagna, 2010, p. 188). This fact is understandable because nursing care in the home and concern for the health care of acutely and chronically ill populations have been demonstrated through nurse advocacy from battlefields to tenements (Buhler-Wilkerson, 2001). Building on a rich history in public health nursing and social work, case management has evolved since the turn of the century from community service coordination to approaches that coordinate and deliver healthcare services across the care continuum. With the passage of the Patient Protection and Affordable Care Act of 2010 (PPACA) (see www.gpo.gov/fdsys/pkg/BILLS-111hr3590enr/pdf/BILLS-111hr3590enr.pdf), case managers have the opportunity for even greater responsibility for care coordination of acute and subacute care, home care, and long-term care. This evolution has coincided with the development of new models of healthcare delivery and standards for case management practice. The models are diverse, growing in number, and changing as healthcare systems continue to transform.

Within this context of evolving models, the terms *case management*, *care management*, and *care coordination* have been used interchangeably and clarification is necessary because of the provisions of PPACA. The definitions of *case management* often lack consensus. However, two major definitions have emerged, one specific to the discipline of nursing and the other more interdisciplinary in focus. *The ANCC definition cited earlier is grounded in the nursing process and focuses on collaboration and client populations as important elements for nursing case management.*

The interdisciplinary definition developed by the Case Management Society of America describes case management as a "*collaborative process of assessment, planning, facilitation, care coordination, evaluation, and advocacy for options and services to meet an individual's and family's comprehensive health needs through communication and available resources to promote quality, cost-effective outcomes*" (Case Management Society of America, n.d.). The major difference between the two definitions is *ANCC's focus on the health needs of populations* and *CMSA's focus on the health needs of individuals and/or families.*

Other definitions include *care management* defined by Mechanic (2004) as programs that use various types of knowledge and information to improve medical practice and aid patients' self-management of illness to improve health status as well as reduce hospitalization and other unnecessary costly medical care (McDonald et al., 2007, p. 43). The definition of *care coordination* broadens the focus somewhat by including numerous skilled and knowledgeable participants who are dependent on each other to carry out tasks that aid in patient care and who rely on sharing of information to manage and integrate activities to deliver appropriate healthcare services (McDonald et al., 2007, p. 39). Case management, however, identifies a person whose responsibility is "to oversee and coordinate care delivery [targeted to] high-risk patients [with a] diverse combination of health, functional, and social problems"(McDonald et al., 2007, p. 43).

Common *goals for case management models* include the following:

- Quality of care demonstrated by therapeutic and beneficial patient outcomes
- Length of stay focused on cost control through rapid movement of inpatients through the system
- Resource utilization achieved through protocols or case management plans derived from research and evaluation of patient outcomes
- Prevention and disease management
- Continuity of care achieved through the integration of services across the illness episode by a familiar case manager (Flarey, 1996; Taylor, 1999; Zander, 2009)

How organizations operationalize these goals depends on the case management model they select to guide their particular case management delivery system. In the current climate of controlling healthcare expenditures while delivering quality care for a population with increasing numbers of chronically ill and uninsured or underinsured individuals, models of healthcare delivery have been introduced that have influenced the PPACA and the continuum of care.

Models of Case Management in Nursing and Healthcare Delivery: Past and Present

In the last two decades, many models of case management have appeared in the literature. A number of models have come and gone, primarily because they lacked sound theoretical underpinnings or failed to generate research findings that supported the core concepts within the models. The progression of nursing case management knowledge is described and synthesis of key case management models is provided in textbooks such as those by Cohen and Cesta (2005) and Flarey and Blancett (1996).

It should be noted that *utilization review (UR)* programs were instituted by insurance companies in the period of the 1970s and 1980s to retrospectively analyze patient medical records to determine whether days of acute care hospitalization could be "carved out" if they lacked medical necessity. This caused friction between UR nurses, physicians, and hospitals (Powell & Tahan, 2010; Shockney, 2010). By the late 1980s, reviews were done concurrently by utilization management (UM) nurses hired by the hospital in an effort to manage care across the healthcare continuum and use resources more effectively. This was used to insure reimbursement and to educate the patient and family (Powell & Tahan, 2010; Shockney, 2010). Independent utilization management nurses were hired later to evaluate the reasons for discharge delays and problems associated with transfer to other levels of care (Shockney, 2010). By the early 1990s, case management was introduced. Nurses were hired to handle specific populations of patients with complex needs requiring chronic care and to ensure that cost-effective, quality care was delivered safely and at an appropriate level (Shockney, 2010). The link between reimbursement and case management should not be forgotten when analyzing the models developed.

Nursing Case Management Models

Case management models have been categorized into *within-the-walls (hospital-based)* and *beyond-the-walls (community-based)* classifications. Fitting into these classifications are two models introduced in the 1980s that have been studied extensively, adopted, and/or adapted by healthcare organizations across the country: the New England Medical Center Hospitals, a within-the-walls model, and the Carondelet St. Mary's Hospital (often referred to as the Arizona model), a beyond-the-walls model. Both models have a strong theoretical basis, and research data have shown the models to be effective in controlling institutional costs by achieving decreased hospital lengths of stay and decreased readmissions while maintaining quality patient care (Ethridge, 1997; Ethridge & Lamb, 1989; Zander, 1988a).

The New England Medical Center Hospitals model, developed by Zander in 1985 (Zander, 1988b, 1988c) was the first initiation of within-the-walls case management. According to Zander, the model structures care of clients experiencing acute illness episodes. The focus of this conceptual model is on outcomes; it is a synthesis of primary nursing care and nursing process and introduced critical pathways and case management plans as essential guides in structuring the episode of care. Unit-based primary care was selected as a core concept because it was known to facilitate nursing accountability, continuity, and satisfaction for patients. Case management adopted the nursing process as a problem-solving strategy using a critical pathway for a specific condition/surgery as a method for structuring, coordinating, and assessing patient progress or variance. Critical pathways have proven to be one of the most innovative concepts of the model and have been widely adapted (Renholm, Leino-Kilpi, & Suominen, 2002), becoming a symbol of case management. Zander (1988b) defines a critical pathway as follows:

> A tool that helps practitioners manage an episode of care for a patient population or condition by providing a timeline of the expected course of care with expected patient outcomes. The critical pathway is designed to improve quality of patient care and promote efficient utilization of resources. (p. 28)

In this model, the case management plan is conceptualized as a comprehensive document. The document is designed to function as a tool that integrates the nursing process and the critical pathway and to deal with variance analysis (deviations from the pathway). In addition, the document is used to record the relationship of caregiver interventions with patient outcomes along a timeline. This plan enables primary nurse case managers to coordinate a patient's entire episode of care across hospital units and to identify those patients who are not progressing toward discharge as anticipated. Although these protocols provide direction, nurse case managers must recognize that the individual needs of some patients will necessitate variance. Early identification of such individuals will be critical in the world of capitated acute care and readmission penalties.

In the New England Medical Center case management model, a primary nurse formulates a case management plan and becomes the patient's primary caregiver. If the patient transfers to another hospital unit, a new primary nurse is assigned to deliver direct care and the initial primary nurse continues to administer the patient's case management plan. Care coordination is facilitated through team meetings, case consultation, and interdisciplinary communication, focused by critical pathways. Because the model is grounded in primary nursing and nursing process, it has been applied easily to a variety of within-the-walls settings.

Zander (1996) describes the episode of illness as finite and the continuum of care as infinite. This infinite continuum linking within-the-walls and beyond-the-walls models will, in the future, focus on wellness/prevention services that promote higher levels of care (Zander, 1996) requiring more nurse case managers skilled in developing and using critical pathways across the continuum of health care and in applying them to direct care for populations of clients (Zander, 2002).

In 1985, Carondelet St. Mary's Hospital developed the first beyond-the-walls case management model (Ethridge, 1987). Changing reimbursement patterns, resulting from Medicare cost-containment measures and the growing number of clients enrolled in managed care, resulted in patients being discharged while still in the early stages of recovery, and the need to provide care after discharge emerged. Nurse administrators at St. Mary's created the professional nurse case management model to offer case-managed nursing services to chronically ill and high-risk clients across hospital and community settings, moving care beyond the acute episode of illness into the continuum of care. The goals of the model are to offer case-managed services that improve and promote a person's health or peaceful death and assist individuals to learn new ways of managing their illness situations.

The nurse case manager–client relationship is the concept in the model most integral to achieving quality and cost outcomes. Outcomes include "improved self-care skills, fewer hospitalizations, and enhanced quality of life" (Lamb & Stemple, 1994, p. 12). These outcomes will be seen in other models as well. Evidence from the studies suggests that the emphasis placed on building caring therapeutic nurse–client relationships that motivates clients to engage in self-care strategies and thereby improves functional performance.

St. Mary's used these outcome data to negotiate managed care contracts and, as a result, launched the first nursing health maintenance organization (HMO). Contracts were negotiated using a capitated reimbursement system that extended community case management services to approximately 22,000 HMO members who were experiencing chronic illnesses, disease complications, and recurring institutionalizations. Preliminary findings showed that nursing case management reduced hospitalizations and home health visits to below the national average, increased knowledge of health-promoting behaviors over time, and motivated more than 50% of the HMO enrollees to attend annual health screening programs that contributed to decreased health risks (Ethridge, 1997).

In this integrated delivery model, one professional nurse case manager may work for several months (or years) with a chronically ill HMO member, coordinating care for him or her in the hospital, in the long-term care facility, in the home, or in wellness centers located within retirement complexes. Professional nurse case managers procure needed resources, provide screening, counsel, make referrals to physicians, and engage in wellness education. This broader approach to nursing practice acknowledges the interconnectedness of life and illness situations and recognizes the individual without losing sight of the evolving whole. This integration of care carries over to the models of care influencing care even today.

Both models are prototypes for within- and beyond-the-walls case management models and demonstrate case management's effectiveness in lowering use and cost of services. These innovative professional practice models restructured case management and the case manager role, proved successful in affecting continuity of care and health maintenance, ensured accountable resource use, achieved cost-containment goals, and effectively bridged transitions among hospital-based units and integrated healthcare networks.

In the aftermath of the prospective payment system, both of these models stopped being replicated and case management focused on utilization review and discharge planning in the hospital and ceased to exist as a continuum into the community (Daniels, 2011; Zander, 2008). Hospitals downsized their workforce and programs to reduce costs leading to the end of many primary care nurse units.

Disease Management and the Chronic Care Model

This introduction of managed care has influenced health care since the late 1990s. Because of the increased emphasis on care coordination in healthcare delivery models, a review of their development and components may provide background for current direction in health care and provisions of the PPACA. *Disease management (DM)* is primarily a medical model of care of persons with a specific disease and was coupled with the *Chronic Care Model (CCM)* (Wagner, Austin, & Von Korff, 1996) to meet demands for cost constraints and performance monitoring of chronic conditions (Wagner, Davis, Schaefer, & Von Korff, 1999). Because of DM's close alignment with the medical model, adoption was more easily accomplished in practice settings and specialty clinics. Todd and Nash (1997) cite factors in which DM succeeded: understanding a disease's usual course, targeting persons with a specific chronic disease likely to benefit from intervention, focusing on prevention and/or disease resolution, increasing compliance through patient education, providing continuity of care across healthcare settings, establishing integrated data management systems, and aligning incentives.

Efforts to provide disease-specific programs of care coordination have been based on the *patient navigator role* introduced at Harlem Hospital to facilitate access to care and diagnosis and treatment for women with abnormal breast cancer screening (Pedersen & Hack, 2010) with other programs identified for other cancers (Redwood, Provost, Perdue, Havercamp, & Espey, 2012) and tobacco cessation (Lubetkin, Lu, Krebs, Yeung, & Ostroff, 2010). Nurses, social workers, and peer counselors who have a previous diagnosis of cancer are trained and act as patient care navigators (Pedersen & Hack, 2010) through complex healthcare systems.

Patient navigator programs will be reimbursed under section 3510 of the PPACA and could be important to accessing chronic care in rural communities (Bolin, Gamm, Vest, Edwardson, & Miller, 2011). The Patient Navigator program was added to the Public Health Service Act and the requirement of minimum core proficiencies for patient navigators was added to the PPACA (Moy & Chabner, 2011). Limits to this program are related to the authorization of a sum to be determined by Congress but that does not guarantee appropriate funding with the current financial climate (Moy & Chabner, 2011).

However, DM continued to use the existing system of acute care delivery, and Wagner and his associates (1996) recognized that the management of chronic illness resulted in fragmentation of care even in integrated acute illness management systems. Adaptation to new healthcare demands and the introduction of the CCM included *addition of evidence-based practice guidelines, multidisciplinary team approaches, patient education, outcome measures, and feedback to stakeholders including patients, providers, and health plans* (Center on an Aging Society, 2004). A survey of 72 programs using DM found that self-management support was not included, and, because of specialist care of the selected diseases, there were limited links to primary care (Wagner et al., 1999).

The CCM was designed within a managed care organization (MCO) with Wagner and colleagues (1996) employing systems theory to redesign primary care practice, employ self-management as a goal of patient education, provide expert support to ensure delivery of effective interventions, and use information technology to provide reminders and analyze outcomes. Population-based approaches to managing various chronic conditions (i.e., asthma, diabetes, and congestive heart failure) were developed and tested (Bodenheimer, Wagner, & Grumbach, 2002a, 2002b). A critical element of the CCM is the coordination of care using information systems that signal need for preventive care or diagnostic tests, provide flow sheets of results, and report on benchmark attainment (Bodenheimer et al., 2002a). Self-management of chronic conditions by patients was recognized as important to the prevention of complications and hospital admissions as well as reducing costs to the HMO and the patient. Referral to community resources and group appointments are followed as patient progress toward self-management is tracked. The CCM has been studied in a number of primary care settings (Wagner, 2010; Wagner et al., 2001) and for a variety of chronic illnesses (Stellefson, Dipnarine, & Stopka, 2013; Suter, Hennessey, Florez, & Newton Suter, 2011). The Joint Commission's Disease-Specific Care Certification is based on the CCM elements, and the National Committee for Quality Assurance granted the CCM its Quality Award (Suter et al., 2008).

Medical Home and Patient-Centered Medical Home Models

Imitation or adaptation of a model often provides evidence of its utility. While the CCM was implemented in MCOs primarily for chronically ill adults, pediatricians had developed the "medical home" model for chronically ill children with elements similar to CCM. The American Academy of Pediatrics (AAP) defined the medical home model as providing preventive care, ambulatory and inpatient care for acute illnesses, care over an extended period to provide continuity, and care by subspecialty consultants in addition to advocacy efforts with schools and community agencies and a central record and database containing a child's medical information accessible wherever needed (American Academy of Pediatrics [AAP], 1992).

Later the American Academy of Family Physicians and American College of Physicians joined the AAP and the medical home effort, calling the model the Patient-Centered Medical Home (PCMH), and described a physician-led team of professionals who provide a "whole person" approach to ongoing, comprehensive care situated in primary care. Wagner and associates (2005) questioned the PCMH focus on physician communication versus patient self-management with chronic illness and noted that the various definitions of patient-centered medical home are more focused on changing the physician mind-set than the need for a change in practice design.

The medical home model attracted the attention of Medicare, and demonstration projects were performed incorporating many CCM components (Hennessey, Suter, & Harrison, 2010). Kuraitis (2007) noted similarities in the DM and medical home because of the presence of coordination of care. Princell, a master's prepared nurse, describes the role of care coordinator in a patient-centered medical home as focused on the needs of chronically ill patients, their health risks, barriers to care, and self-management planning (Henderson, Princell, & Martin, 2012, p. 56). Stephens (2012) describes the added value nurse practitioners' skill sets can bring to management of chronic illness in PCMH and CCM practice. Further, description of the relation of the medical home model to DM uses American College of Physician terminology very similar to the CCM with patient registries, population-based protocols, practice guidelines, teaching of disease self-management skills, and feedback to physicians about their performance (Kuraitis, 2007), possibly indicating the adoption of components.

To address new needs, new roles were designed. The *practice facilitator* addresses quality improvement and helps the primary care practice become a PCMH while the *care manager* is involved with direct patient care through patient education for self-management and coordinates care with other providers, settings, and services (Taylor, Machta, Meyers, Genevro, & Peikes, 2013, p. 80). In summary, coordination of chronic illness care requires specialized clinical and organizational skills that include careful monitoring of the multidisciplinary team's activities, knowledge of disease management, and patient self-management education that advanced practice can provide coupled with excellent information technology and systems organization as well as compatibility with all the stakeholders.

Home Hospital

Because overcrowding of emergency departments, inadequate numbers of hospital beds, and iatrogenic complications of hospitalization are occurring, programs that deliver acute care to the chronically ill older adult at home have been studied at Johns Hopkins University. The *Home Hospital (HH)* program established criteria for selection of persons presenting at the emergency department (ED) who might be candidates for acute care at home (Leff et al., 1999). Community-dwelling persons 65 years of age and older with community-acquired pneumonia (CAP), chronic heart failure (CHF), chronic obstructive airways disease (COAD), or cellulitis were selected for the study. Persons consenting for HH care were examined by the HH *physician* in the ED and then transferred from the ED to home with the *nurse coordinator*. The nurse coordinator spent an extended period of time directly supervising care for at least 24 hours and arranging temporary nursing visits, placement of Lifeline equipment, diagnostic tests, medications, and other equipment and oversight of care (Leff et al., 1999). The HH physician would visit the patient each day and was available 24 hours a day. Charges were 53% less than those of similar persons admitted to the hospital, and HH patients were significantly more satisfied with healthcare provider interactions and overall impression of care (Leff et al., 1999).

In a later multisite study using three Medicare-managed healthcare systems (i.e., an independent practice association, a for-profit multispecialty physician group, and a not-for-profit Medicare-managed care plan) and a Veterans Administration medical center, costs were compared for all patients (Frick et al., 2009). Costs were found to be lower when Hospital-at-Home was available for patients with CHF and COAD but not for patients with CAP or cellulitis with the thought that cost was related to the nursing cost in the home (Frick et al., 2009, p. 53). No nursing costs were provided for the hospital charges. A study performed in an integrated healthcare system found patient costs of Hospital-at-Home to be 19% lower than hospital costs for inpatients, but the authors noted that bundling reimbursement and billing methods were aimed at providing care at home (Cryer, Shannon, Van Amsterdam, & Leff, 2011).

Sinha, Bessman, Flomenbaum, and Leff (2011) conducted a systematic review of the literature to determine a best practice model of ED case management for older adults living independently in the community who frequently visit the ED. Their review of 34 articles identified eight core competencies needed in an effective emergency practice model including geriatric case management during and beyond the ED visit: an evidence-based practice model, nursing clinical delivery involvement or leadership, high-risk screening, focused geriatric assessment, initiation of care and disposition planning in the ED, interprofessional and capacity-building work practices, post-ED follow-up with patients, and establishment of evaluation and monitoring processes.

A multisite study of the *Guided Care Model* in eight primary care practices built on these competencies and demonstrated fewer hospital readmissions and home healthcare episodes (Leff & Novak, 2011). Using many of the elements of the CCM, the Guided Care Model has marketed materials for practices, patients, and a certificate for nurses (Leff & Novak, 2011) to aid in the implementation process in primary care.

Alternatives to Nursing Home

The transition from hospital often means a move to a nursing facility for older adults. While the nursing home is less expensive than the hospital, it is not cheap. Programs have been studied to provide older adults services in their homes that will allow them to stay there as long as they are safe. *Aging in Place*, a program developed by the School of Nursing of the University of Missouri (Marek, Stetzer, Adams, Popejoy, & Rantz, 2012), and the *Program of All-Inclusive Care for the Elderly (PACE)*, a program for dual-eligible persons or persons who may pay for the program services but are certified by their state as requiring nursing home care, have both demonstrated that the provision of Medicare home health, Medicaid home and community services, and intensive care coordination have been less costly than the nursing home (Marek et al., 2012; Wieland, Kinosian, Stallard, & Boland, 2013). Because remaining in their home is a desire of most elderly adults, these programs will most likely see expansion.

Nursing Homes

Nursing homes are also developing into community health centers where persons come for rehabilitation after joint replacement, memory care, and not solely custodial care. High acuity, complexity, and instability of many patients discharged from the hospital to the nursing home may result in readmission penalties that are part of PPACA. These patients' needs signal the need for careful transition planning. Problems that must be addressed include the massive amount of paperwork that accompanies patients that nursing home staff must decipher as the patient waits. More than 10% of all medication errors have occurred in transition to the nursing home (Goins, 2012, p. 51), and because many of the transfers are occurring late in the day or late on Friday, the opportunity for missing medications and lack of equipment may cause gaps in care leading to mistrust by the patient.

Transfers from the nursing home to the hospital are not without problems of accurate documentation and provision of a person-centered report to the hospital staff. Goins (2012) sees nurse practitioners hired by the nursing home as key to reducing hospital readmission because they are familiar with the patients but are not reimbursable by Medicare and Medicaid if hired by the nursing home. *Quality improvement programs* such as Interventions to Reduce Acute Care Transfers (INTERACT) provide staff with information that aids in early identification of status changes and reduces acute admissions that may result in complications as well as costs (Goins, 2012).

Today, rising healthcare costs and older adults living longer with multiple chronic diseases have resulted in new emerging models of case management. Many of the new models embrace ideas of the old. For example, Daniels (2011) developed a case management model that targeted acute care populations in hospital settings. In this model, the professional case management organizations including the Case Management Society of America (CMSA), the Commission for Case Management Certification (CCMC), and the American Case Management Association provide the frameworks through which the case managers will provide patient care. Many of the roles and functions of the case manager in this model were adopted from the New England Medical Center case management processes of advocating care for individuals across the hospital continuum.

Practicing Case Management: Role and Functions of a Case Manager

A common response when one speaks of case management and the case manager role as new strategies for healthcare delivery is that nurses have been case managing clients for years. However, this response fails to recognize the unique body of knowledge and skills that underpins the functional role of case management. *Case managers see the big picture of client care*. That is, they must fully integrate the total spectrum of acute to chronic phases of care within clients' lived experience rather than simply possessing knowledge and skills limited to direct care delivery in one setting.

Practicing from this perspective requires nurses to have expert knowledge and skills in the following *case management domains*:

1. Providing direct care
2. Procuring community resources
3. Coordinating care across hospital units and healthcare delivery networks
4. Evaluating healthcare services for cost-effectiveness
5. Building positive nurse–client long-term relationships

In the *first domain*, *providing direct care*, the case manager's knowledge and skills include assessment and planning. Because knowledge development in clinical nursing is grounded in holistic assessment and care planning, nurses are well prepared to assess the interrelationships among medical, psychological, social, and behavioral components of clients' illness situations. These assessment findings are used to plan, intervene, and reassess how the components affect the client.

Although assessment and planning are already core functions of nursing, from a case management perspective assessment is an ongoing, continual process that seeks to understand patients' illness situation within the context of their total healthcare experiences. This expanded view of assessment provides consistency between planning and delivering care because care of case-managed clients often occurs at multiple points of service.

Thus, nurses practicing as case managers must shift their thinking and knowing from a focus on delivering and managing episodes of illness events within one service setting to providing and managing care within a *broader service context, one that includes the community*. This change of focus does not come easily and role ambiguity may lead to ethical dilemmas, role conflict, and job dissatisfaction (Gray, White, & Brooks-Buck, 2013; Smith, 2011). Skills required in disease management and case management necessitate more advanced training that incur time and expense by the nurses and the institution (Tomcavage, Littlewood, & Sciandra, 2012) and may need academic programs' curricular consideration. Stephens (2012) notes the value of using advanced practice nurses in care coordination. Thinking and knowing from a community perspective require a nurse case manager to develop new levels of community consciousness and a new level of community connection to provide direct care more effectively.

Community awareness and connection also enable a case manager to *procure and manage resources*, the *second domain*. Knowing what resources are available in the community for case management clients as well as building relationships with referral agencies that provide these resources are essential functions of a case manager (Berg-Weger & Tebb, 1998; Mick & Ackerman, 2002). Knowledge of community agencies and resources is important in filling gaps in care left by family support systems and insurance. Resource identification and service planning may involve skills in linking clients to needed services such as transportation to medical appointments, assistive devices, home health care, meal delivery, skilled nursing services, personal emergency response systems, and restorative therapies (Schraeder, 2001). Wise allocation of resources, a goal of case management, requires a case manager to make sound clinical judgments about client needs and use of resources.

Coordinating care and services across healthcare units and healthcare delivery networks, the *third domain*, is a key role of the case manager. Here the case manager must design tools that define case management responsibilities and interventions. A case manager often uses tools such as screening tools, critical pathways, case management plans, and protocols to support clinical reasoning, goal and outcome development, and to coordinate care across provider settings. Coordinating care entails tracking a client's progress, monitoring for early signs of problems, gathering and analyzing data, and communicating the results to healthcare organizations, providers, and consumers (Lagoe, 1998).

Recognizing the skills of case managers in assessment, Meek (2012) encourages case managers to be proactively involved in the transformation process as hospitals and private practice systems become accountable care organizations (ACOs) and work to develop predictive models that reduce risk associated with readmission and negative outcomes. Specialized knowledge enables nurse case managers to assist analytic teams in developing various predictive statistical models. Because case manager knowledge of *perceived* "feeling and functioning" and self-care is based on factors that population health management sees as more important in predicting readmission than disease-related factors, nurse case managers can identify characteristics of at-risk patients who may need a longer stay or modification of the critical path (Meek, 2012, p. 18).

Instead of focusing attention on the acute episode of hospitalization and facilitating discharge, case managers will need to view their case load as an entire population's health, take responsibility for care across multiple healthcare settings, and be prepared as advanced practice nurse case managers to help move health systems to the ACO model (Meek, 2012), *as well as meet the AHA value-based reimbursement priorities*. Professional case managers have demonstrated skills in continual assessment, administration of case management tools, interpretation of data, and communication and have been stewards of healthcare resources and dollars that add to client satisfaction by reducing the frustration that comes from negotiating care at multiple service sites (Berg-Weger & Tebb, 1998; Kegel, 1996; Lagoe, 1998; Lamb & Stemple, 1994; Salazar, 2000). Clearly, nurse case managers and their social work colleagues (Fink-Samnick, 2011) are in a unique position to make a difference in this time of rapid change.

Successful performance depends on excellent communication with other disciplines, especially physicians. Efforts to *improve communication and collaboration between physicians and case managers* were the focus of a summit convened in 2003 by the CMSA. Physicians and case managers from across the country attended. Barriers and solutions to effective communication were identified and used to establish a framework for successful collaboration between the two groups. Despite the discussions and consensus, issues remain in communication between physicians and case managers (Smith, 2011).

In a case study whole systems analysis of nurses who cared for persons with long-term conditions in the United Kingdom, researchers suggest that the Chronic Care Model is evident in policies adopted in the United Kingdom and nursing practice has been constrained by roles and services based on power differential and care based on diagnostic categories rather than integrated needs of patients (Procter, Wilson, Brooks, & Kendall, 2012). Successful self-management by patients was accomplished by *community matrons* (similar to community health nurses in the United States), but the authors suggested that the success was associated with individual nurse determination and might not be sustainable because nurse autonomy depended on having a champion in the local medical leadership (Procter et al., 2012). This concern about the inability of the nurse to function to the extent of scope of practice because of medical practitioners is echoed by Sinha and associates (Sinha et al., 2011).

The most important function of the nurse case manager is to *coordinate a multidisciplinary plan that moves clients across the continuum of care*, whether between hospital units or into other service settings (Novak, 1998). Lack of coordination within and among healthcare settings contributes to increased hospital readmission rates and costs of care (Burns, Lamb, & Wholey, 1996). To overcome ineffective coordination requires strong skills to negotiate with payers and providers to ensure smooth transitions and to sustain continuity of care for clients.

Transitional care refers to "actions that are designed to ensure the coordination and continuity of healthcare as patients transfer between locations and different levels of care" (Bennett, Probst, Vyavaharkar, & Glover, 2012). The transition from hospital to home can result in fragmented care, miscommunication, medication errors, and inadequate follow-up. One in five Medicare recipients discharged from the hospital is readmitted in 30 days. Half do not see a doctor for follow-up before being readmitted (Jencks, Williams, & Coleman, 2009). Coordination has not happened. Hand-offs or handovers of patients' information and care between healthcare providers and agencies rely on a shared view of the patient that may not exist because of the time and condition the patient presents and the services required of the care provider (Balka, Tolar, Coates, & Whitehouse, 2010, p. 211). Because data required may be needed in several output configurations by various contacts—insurance companies, Medicare, physician, home health agency, hospital, pharmacy—data formats that include demographic information should be introduced that reduce the need for the patient repetition of information (Balka et al., 2010), a source of non-valued-added time.

Eichler (2013) suggests that because the Medicare population has many comorbidities, there is a need for careful assessment and accurate coding to ensure reimbursement because a readmission may be the result of another condition or disease progression. After discovering that a screening tool for persons at risk of readmission did not identify a high percentage of readmitted patients, Eichler (2013) recommends short pilots of screening tools to identify at-risk patients should be performed before adoption and she questions the adequacy of the callback strategy if the screening tool is not accurate.

In an analysis of 21 randomized controlled clinical trials of interventions for chronically ill adults transitioning from acute care to other settings, 9 studies reported positive effects on one measure of readmission

(Naylor, Aiken, Kurtzman, Olds, & Hirschman, 2011). The authors note outcomes (i.e., quality of life, functional status, and survival) and cost-effectiveness of the 9 studies with reduced readmissions were cited, although many did not include the intervention's cost in the analysis or using dual-eligible, cognitively impaired, or medically underserved populations (Naylor et al., 2011). Six of the 9 studies effective in reducing readmission had an in-person home visit, and studies that reduced readmissions through 6 to 12 months after discharge had a focus on self-management (Naylor et al., 2011). Two studies reported significant reduction in readmission with interventions involving discharge management and follow-up for patients having common medical and surgical conditions and persons with congestive heart failure, while the third intervention had a significant decrease in readmission used telehealth (Naylor et al., 2011). Despite attention to the components of the transitional care provisions of the PPACA, none of the studies matched all the components. Use of health information technology and coordination of community resources were not evaluated in most studies (Naylor et al., 2011).

The *fourth* knowledge *domain* is *managing financial matters*. There are two aspects to this role: the first is to understand the payer systems, and the second is to develop and apply methods for evaluating quality service and cost-effective care. *Understanding common payer systems*, such as HMOs, preferred provider organizations, point-of-service plans, and Medicare and Medicaid, is essential. By being aware of the advantages and disadvantages of the numerous reimbursement methods within payer delivery systems, the case manager can bridge the gap between provider and payer and effectively coordinate care and secure services for clients. With the development of payer–provider partnerships in accountable care organizations (ACOs), shared goals to improve quality as well as decrease expenses could see inpatient and insurance company case managers having less adversarial and more collaborative patient care discussions (Claffey, Agostini, Collet, Reisman, & Krakauer, 2012).

Case managers working with specific populations learn the criteria for eligibility, benefits, and the specific process for accessing services from payer sources commonly used in these populations. Maneuvering through the provider and payer system requires the case manager to assess the client's existing healthcare coverage and determine whether it is adequate or whether other sources of funding for services are available. Knowing how the process works helps when communicating with individuals in charge of referral authorization and prevents unnecessary or excessive charges. With the prospect of bundled charges and fee-for-performance, some capitation negotiations may be required that include development costs.

The second aspect of this knowledge domain is concerned with the case manager's responsibility *to build his or her knowledge about the financial performance of the case management program(s) and to build support for case management services*. To accomplish these functions, a case manager needs to design outcomes and use cost analysis methods to evaluate the cost-effectiveness of case management services. A case manager must understand financial and budgeting methods and be able to apply outcome measures that result in a valid, reliable, and thorough assessment (Kleinpell-Nowell, 1999; Terra, 2007). In her article, Kleinpell-Nowell (1999) compiles a helpful list of commonly used outcome measures and sources of research-based outcome instruments appropriate for evaluating case management effectiveness.

A cost-analysis evaluation considers factors such as external performance referents, including benchmarking, or comparing the assessment results with those of another organization(s), to add validity to evaluation findings (Ketchen, Palmer, & Gamm, 2001). In the view of Ketchen and colleagues (2001), it is only when compared with a point of reference that cost-benefit analysis findings have meaning. This method may also reveal additional insights about the strategy used, or additional strategies to use, to facilitate cost containment. Using performance referents external to the organization can affect the future viability of a particular healthcare delivery strategy such as case management. For example, integrated hospital delivery systems that case manage high-risk patient populations with chronic conditions could compare their cost-benefit analysis performance with licensed external disease management organizations specializing in case managing similar populations of patients. Efficiency and quality will be judged according to benchmarks established by payers such as Medicare and Medicaid, and care coordinators will be compared.

Another method of assessing performance considers both financial and operational measures. The balanced scorecard provides management with financial measures that can inform on results of previous actions taken, whereas operational measures (i.e., customer satisfaction, internal processes, and the organization's innovation and improvement activities) provide some information about the future financial performance (Kaplan & Norton, 1992). As hospital networks and ACOs plan for the future with PPACA, care coordination will play a major role in financial and operational measures. Case managers must be prepared not only to show cost-effectiveness but provide data that will demonstrate focus on benchmarks and customer and employee satisfaction. Although it will be important to show reduced costs, improved outcomes and more expansive goals will indicate potential (Meliones, 2000). The ability to assist development of predictive models as well as collect measures of customer involvement using validated instruments such as the Patient Assessment of Chronic Illness Care (PACIC) (Glasgow et al., 2005) will be valuable to the institution's demonstration of care coordination.

It is challenging to have the knowledge and skills necessary to practice in a cost-effective manner and to have expertise in choosing appropriate outcome performance measures and tools that assess the future financial performance of case management. When successfully managed, the role of case manager can be sustained and case management remains a vehicle for the delivery of quality cost-effective care in a managed care financing system.

The focus of the *final* knowledge *domain* of case management is *building meaningful nurse–client relationships*. Although nurse theorists' works have long touted the importance of building meaningful nurse–client relationships, a current research refocus examines client relationships in the nursing case management process. The result has been that nurse case managers have become more concerned, or need to be more concerned, with the importance and benefits of forming relationships with clients. For example, McWilliam, Stewart, Brown, Desai, and Coderre (1996) explored the experiences of individuals living with chronic illness. The researchers discovered that clients wished to be involved in mutual knowing (mutual relationships) between client and nurse and believed that being known enhanced their personal knowledge and in turn their ability to follow through with self-care. The authors concluded that more attention needed to be placed on continuity of the caregiver rather than on the continuity of the care plan.

Lamb and Stemple (1994) discovered that clients who believed they were in partnerships felt empowered to assume an active role in their health care, thus resulting in renewed efforts to become involved in health maintenance and promotion strategies. These authors grounded their research in Newman's theory of expanding consciousness, which describes a nurse as one who "enters into a partnership with the client with the mutual goal of participating in an authentic relationship, trusting that in the process of its evolving, both will grow and become healthier in the sense of higher levels of consciousness" (Newman, 1986, p. 68).

Patient-centeredness is one of the goals of high-quality care (AHA, 2011; HRET, 2013; Institute of Medicine, 2001), and all of the models of care include the importance of interactions in which the patient is viewed as a "whole person," not a collection of disease processes or risk factors, and should be involved in self-care and decision making (Wagner et al., 2012, p. 249). The PCMH model has received increased interest because of the personal physician and the continuity of that connection extending to multiple healthcare providers on the patient's team (Henderson et al., 2012).

Practicing case management from this perspective enables clients to become partners with case managers and meets one of the goals of case management—to optimize the client's self-care ability (Taylor, 1999).

Creating an atmosphere that builds respectful relationships requires a case manager to develop and use the skills of active listening and being present; these skills enable clients to become their own "insider-experts in self-care" (Lamb & Stemple, 1994, p. 12).

Self-management for a patient includes "developing knowledge of condition(s) and treatment; medication management and adherence; self-monitoring of disease symptoms; management of the effects of disease on physical, emotional, and social role function; reducing health risks; preventative maintenance; and working collaboratively with health care providers" (Battersby et al., 2010, pp. 561–562). This requires more than 15 minutes before discharge. Principles identified that are associated with case managers improving self-management include assessment of clinical severity, functional status, and barriers to self-management; collaborative problem solving; self-management support (SMS) by various providers; use of a variety of SMS formats (i.e., individual, group, telephone, self-instruction); ongoing follow-up and reminders; use of goal-directed and guideline-based programs; links to community-based self-management programs that are evidence-based; and use of multifaceted interventions rather than ones with a single component (Battersby et al., 2010).

On the whole, the five knowledge domains of the case manager role outlined here describe the new knowledge and skills needed to perform the role of case manager, contrasted with the basic practice of nurses. As nursing case management has evolved, there have been increased opportunities for nurses to move from basic nursing practice into this expanded role, which provides more autonomy and possibly more job enrichment (Goode, 1995; Reimanis, Cohen, & Redman, 2001).

Case Management Certification

The *case management certification* process ensures a common baseline of knowledge and gives the professional and public assurance of a certain degree of competence and higher quality of case management services. The need for advanced training and expertise is viewed as important in the transformation of healthcare systems to ACOs (Tomcavage et al., 2012) and may be valuable to networks in reducing the issues of role function of care coordination (Smith, 2011). The demand for board-certified case managers has increased, with 36% of employers requiring board certification as compared to 26% of employers in 2004 (Sminkey, 2012). There are numerous licensure, certification, and certificate programs available for case managers working in various fields of health care. Listing each is beyond the scope of this chapter; rather, three key certifications are described.

The *Commission for Case Manager Certification (CCMC)* is an independent credentialing agency that sponsors and oversees one of the major case management certifications. The CCMC, nationally accredited by the National Commission for Certifying Agencies, is the only national accreditation body for private certification organizations in all disciplines. Since the CCMC began certifying case managers in 1993, more than 24,000 case managers have earned the Certified Case Manager (CCM) credential. This credential is designed as an adjunct to other professional credentials in health and human resources.

The CCM examination is research based and covers competencies and job functions in six major domains of knowledge as listed previously. With the expectation that case managers function as care coordinators, competency measures within the certification examination are collected to "identify essential activities, knowledge, skills, and abilities deemed important and common practice by case managers" (Tahan & Campagna, 2010, p. 246). Case management practices, healthcare management and delivery, principles of practice, psychosocial aspects, healthcare reimbursement, and rehabilitation were identified as important content in the knowledge domain, whereas case management process and services, resource utilization and management, psychosocial and economic support, rehabilitation, outcomes, and ethical and legal practices were important activity components (Tahan & Campagna, 2010). The CCMC study guide is available through the CMSA (www.ccmcertification.org/node/428).

The *American Nurses Credentialing Center (ANCC)*, the credentialing arm of the American Nurses Association, offers a second method of certification (ANCC, 2013). In 1997, the center began certifying nurse case managers, providing them with the RN-BC credential. Candidates for the exam must have a current, active registered nurse license. An applicant for the certification examination must have 2 years of full-time registered nurse experience, a minimum of 2,000 hours of clinical practice in case management in the past 3 years, and 30 hours of continuing education in nursing case management over the past 3 years. The framework for Nursing Case Management used by ANCC consists of the following five components: assessment, planning, implementation, evaluation, and interaction. The ANCC has published a review book and resource (Leonard & Miller, 2012) to assist with preparation for the national examination (see www.nursesbooks.org/Main-Menu/Certification/ANCC-Resources/NursingCaseMgmt-4thEdition.aspx).

Both the CCMC and ANCC require ongoing continuing education for recertification, which is required every 5 years. Professional development and clinical practice hours must be documented for recertification.

Certification for case management administrators (CMAC) is sponsored by the Center for Case Management and can be obtained from the Credentialing Advisory Board (see http://cfcm.com/resources/certification.asp). Eligibility for the certification exam occurs by meeting one of three broad requirements: a baccalaureate or higher degree with experience as a case manager, a certification in a core specialty, and/or being a faculty member in an academic setting teaching graduate-level courses or content in case management. The exam covers content about high-risk populations, assessment, strategy development, leadership, strategic planning, human resource management, and outcome management.

Trends and Issues Influencing Case Management

There are three trends or issues influencing case management: the economic downturn, the value-based reimbursement environment and the Patient Protection and Affordable Care Act. The value-based reimbursement environment has changed reimbursements to reflect more quality/continuum issues (as discussed previously with the ACO example). This will only increase in the future.

The Patient Protection and Affordable Care Act is the issue that will have a great impact on health care in general and case management specifically. The law is complex as is the current healthcare system and further modification will be needed as time passes. Already there is concern that changes will not control costs of insurance, with the average cost of a family health insurance premium equaling 50% of household income by 2021 and exceeding income by 2033 (Young & DeVoe, 2012). Elimination of inefficient programs will need to occur rapidly and rapid turnaround time is anticipated for demonstration projects. Implementation of programs that have demonstrated increased quality, reduced costs, and promoted population health will need to be disseminated quickly as well.

Due for full implementation in 2014, aspects of the PPACA have already rolled out: coverage for young people until 26 years old on parents' insurance; states are expanding the number covered on Medicaid; access to insurance for uninsured persons, including children, with preexisting conditions is available; lifetime limits on insurance coverage are eliminated; and free preventive health for seniors has begun (see www.healthcare.gov/law/timeline/full.html).

The opening of the healthcare exchanges will make it possible for many uninsured persons to choose coverage, but states' reluctance to manage the exchanges could place an added cost burden on the federal government. Because there is an anticipated increase in persons needing coverage and these persons are likely to have existing healthcare issues, there will be a need for primary care providers and infrastructure to implement electronic health record (EHR) systems and data collection to demonstrate quality care using evidence-based interventions. Not to be forgotten, rural and small medical practices question their ability to afford the Patient-Centered Medical Home model (Baxter & Nash, 2012; Bolin et al., 2011).

Accountable Care Organizations

Several sections of the PPACA directly affect case management because they address redesign of healthcare delivery systems. Development of accountable care organizations (ACOs) under the PPACA requires collaboration of payers and providers to transform the current fee-for-service payment system to pay-for-performance with services under Medicare (Claffey et al., 2012; Hart, 2012). Programs are under way with examples of private and public funding with virtual ACOs including providers and hospitals, integrated ACOs that include insurance and delivery roles (i.e., Geisinger Health System and Kaiser Permanente), and Medicare ACO that allow care outside the ACO (Hart, 2012). The Medicare Shared Savings Program was revised to include sharing of Medicare savings with the ACOs earlier, reducing the number of quality measures that ACOs must meet, informing the ACOs of the Medicare beneficiaries likely to be in the ACOs, and allowing community health centers and rural health clinics to lead ACOs (Hart, 2012, p. 24).

Claffey and associates (2012) describe one effort of a private insurer and an independent physician association to combine care management and data analysis capabilities of the payer with the clinical practice of a multispecialty provider organization with Medicare beneficiaries. The payer provided a stipend to cover medical director and care coordinators' design time, fee-for-service reimbursement plus enhanced per-member per-month payment for reaching quality and efficiency metrics at the end of the calendar year, the stratified population database, an embedded care manager to work with practice care coordinators (who were nurse practitioners or physician assistants), and an on-site resource specialists from the local Agency on Aging (Claffey et al., 2012).

DuBard, Cockerham, and Jackson (2012) report on the collaboration of a "state-wide, community-based, physician-led program to establish access to primary care medical homes for vulnerable populations and equipping those medical homes with the multidisciplinary support needed to assure comprehensive, coordinated, high-quality care" (p. 34). Medicaid enrollees with multiple chronic conditions, low literacy, polypharmacy, low socioeconomic status, and multiple physicians accounted for a quarter of the Medicaid recipients but used 80% of Medicaid funds. Services included using face-to-face encounters with care managers; ensuring an outpatient appointment quickly after discharge including transportation; reviewing medication management with network clinical pharmacy; providing patient and caregiver education about conditions using a variety of methods; producing an individualized self-management notebook (includes personal health record, educational resources, and tracking system for disease self-management); data support and information exchange with hospitals serving Medicaid patients; developing cross-agency partnerships; and innovating and leveraging local partnerships (DuBard et al., 2012, pp. 35–37). Success of the program has led to an increased per-member per-month management fee that allows embedding of care management and pharmacy support services in those hospitals and practices seeing large volumes of Medicaid enrollees with complex conditions. Over 12 months, the recipients of transitional care enrolled in the medical home were less likely to be readmitted than were nonenrollees (DuBard et al., 2012, p. 38).

Cost and Prevention of Readmissions

Identification of at-risk and high-risk persons for increased care needs or readmission to the hospital will fall to case managers. Again, available screening tools may require pilots to determine whether the tool has specificity for the population (Eichler, 2013). Development of tools will be needed for various populations and regions. Older adults with the greater incidence of multiple chronic illnesses are more likely to come to the ED (Sinha et al., 2011). Efforts to place case managers at entry points to hospitals (i.e., EDs) have been useful in reducing ED costs and improving follow-up in primary care community care programs, but not in reducing hospital admissions (Kumar & Klein, 2012, p. 9). One study of uninsured persons using an ED at least six times in a year implemented a drop-in group medical appointment, direct phone access to the nurse case manager, small group life skill and support sessions, and individual sessions after the group medical visit (Crane, Collins, Hall, Rochester, & Patch, 2012). After a year, ED and inpatient mean charges per person went from $1,167 the 12 months prior to enrollment to $230 since enrollment and some participants had part-time employment and stable housing (Crane et al., 2012). Annualized direct costs of the program including physician time was $66,000 (Crane et al., 2012, p. 188).

The dynamic nature of health care has set the stage for the many new trends and issues now emerging in case management. After a decade of movement into fully integrated delivery systems, healthcare organizations have created interdependent interactive structures designed to coordinate care across the continuum, with the goal of containing cost and maintaining or increasing quality. By default, if not by design, case management has emerged as the primary strategy to coordinate services, to provide care, and to communicate across these multiorganizational systems. This trend provides an unprecedented opportunity for nurses to showcase their leadership and their accomplishments in using nursing case management as a model to both promote quality and achieve cost reductions in health care.

The implementation of an evaluative study of coordinated care programs, sponsored by the Centers for Medicare and Medicaid Services, was implemented by the Mathematica Policy Research organization. This study has the potential to generate measurable data that confirm nursing case management's successful impact on cost and quality. Fifteen integrated healthcare delivery systems from across the country were selected in January 2004 to participate. Two-thirds of these systems use case managers to coordinate care. They design and initiate interventions with physicians and a mix of other healthcare professionals for chronically ill Medicare-recipient clients. The participating institutions have designed some very innovative programs that require new, advanced skills for practice. For instance, many programs use telemedicine, in-home monitoring devices, and the Internet for counseling and interactive communication with clients. The electronic links allow important client data to be sent to the case manager for evaluation and action, or to be shared with the primary physician for redesign of medical care. Further, tracking client data may help to transition clients more efficiently across organizations' multiple service settings. The organizations and case managers participating in this study hope that coordinating services across the continuum and using new technologies will produce outcomes that reflect a decrease in fragmented care, an increase in client knowledge and self-care, improved client satisfaction, and, of course, a reduction in Medicare expenditures for chronically ill individuals. (The final reports for the demonstration project can be accessed at http://mathematica-mpr.com/publications/SearchList2.aspx?jumpsrch=yes&txtSearch=evaluation%20of%20coordinated.)

The Centers for Medicare and Medicaid Services demonstration projects have been funded for 4 years and evaluated every 2 years. This pattern is expected to change in an effort to find effective programs and implement them and save taxpayer funds. Funding of studies for 1 year is anticipated with short turn-around for results to be reported so that decisions about implementation can be made.

As presented earlier, the Chronic Care Model research findings have included various federal programs. Self-management support, community resources, and delivery system design are areas in which nursing case management can play a role. Advanced practice nurses will be important as providers of preventive care/self-care management education. It is imperative that nurse case managers advocate the use of case management models that move beyond functions of medical necessity to models with nursing functions that reflect the values of health embedded within the discipline of nursing's theories. Only in this way can we hope to shape healthcare policy. Thus, we advocate that case management models emphasize the values of nursing and are guided by nursing theories.

Technology and the Internet

The inclusion of monitoring devices, electronic links, and the Internet as sources of information reflects a trend throughout healthcare systems, both public and private. From a case management perspective, Internet connectivity has the power to link case managers to clients' insurance plans, pharmacies, and physician offices; to electronic health records to track previous medical and nursing information about clients from the multiple service sites within the integrated system (Robinson, 2001); and to evidence-based guidelines for interventions in chronic illness.

The advent of the Internet has also propelled consumers toward greater use of technology (Adams, 2000). 81% of U.S. adults use the internet and 59% say they have looked online for health information in the past year. 35% of U.S. adults say they have gone online specifically to try to figure out what medical condition they or someone else might have. These figures suggest that consumers seek information beyond that provided by health caregivers, leading to the need to correct or clarify understanding.

Nurse case managers could develop and share a collection of reliable Internet sites with their client populations to answer questions about their healthcare situations or to connect them with others who are experiencing similar illness situations. Adams (2000) believes that case managers could deliver care as an integrated package of personal services, combined with education and knowledge tailored to the patient, via the Internet. Discussions of the many revolutionary new ways e-health, telehealth, and other technologies can be used to improve healthcare delivery in general and case management in particular can be found in a number of publications (Frick et al., 2009; Lillibridge & Hanna, 2009; Marineau, 2007; Reed, 2005).

The phenomenal growth of case management information systems and Internet technology has fostered a new culture of health care, one that empowers healthcare providers and consumers to track clinical decisions, access and compare information (Mastrian, 2007; Meadows, 2001). It will eventually move all healthcare professionals to embrace these tools to gain greater access to information, obtain better clinical outcomes (Carver, 2001; McGonigle, Mastrian, & Pavelekovsky, 2007), and meet the expectations of their clients. The Medicare and Medicaid Electronic Health Record (EHR) Incentive Program was designed to encourage implementation of electronic health record (EHR) as a means of linking goals to information, tracking indicators of performance, and providing access to patient medical information across different platforms (Gordon & Geiger, 1999) to reduce fragmentation of healthcare delivery. Although practices were encouraged to adopt EHR, incentives were insufficient for many rural and small practices to consider purchase.

Trends toward fully integrated health systems delivering coordinated care using multiple information technologies as mechanisms to both facilitate and measure the effectiveness of this care do produce serious issues, however.

Patient Health Information

With the widespread use of Internet technology in healthcare organizations, protecting data confidentiality has become a major issue. This public consumer concern prompted legislators to enact the Health

Insurance Portability and Accountability Act (HIPAA) of 1996, an effort designed to achieve better electronic security of personal health information (Waldo, 2000). HIPAA legislation provides standards and regulations for information transmitted or exchanged electronically and how it affects any organization, provider, or payer that handles individually identifiable health information. Under these HIPAA rules, the case manager may need to obtain written authorization from the individual before requesting or transmitting information from providers or payers and most definitely needs to identify which transactions do or do not meet the HIPAA guidelines. Whether this will create barriers to the continuum model of case management, such as delaying the coordination of care and resource access, and delaying or preventing electronic information exchange, is still unclear.

Encryption, although important for protected health information in EHR systems, may interfere with the use and compatibility of telemedicine and telehealth as remote health care is expanded and more products are introduced. Implications related to professional credentialing are expected with teleprograms and interventions occurring across state lines via Internet—legislation is already attempting to reduce barriers to interstate physician practice (Fink-Samnick, 2012). Fink-Samnick cautions that unintended consequences of EHR include more work for clinicians, demands for system changes, conflict between electronic and paper-based systems, negative user emotions, new kinds of errors, and downloading of EHRs to unprotected personal mobile devices (Fink-Samnick, 2012, p. 38).

Transitions in Health Care

The trend toward providing coordinated care across the continuum and over the life span of clients is congruent with the client's expectations and satisfaction with health care (Dunn, Sohl-Kreiger, & Marx, 2001; Lamb & Stemple, 1994) and better ensures reimbursement in the new value-based environment. Transitions in care delivery present critical moments for case managers in how case managers and healthcare organizations aid client transitions from one site to another. This has become an issue for both providers and clients. The Institute of Medicine (2001) report identified gaps in safety and care as patients transfer to different levels of care. Stanton (2008) consulted 10 experts in the field of case management to determine future trends. The experts identified transitions of care as an area of major concern and as an area in which case management can have the greatest impact.

The medical home model and, more recently, the Patient-Centered Medical Home model have identified mechanisms for coordination of care with physician-led multidisciplinary teams incorporating many of the elements suggested by Wagner and associates (2012). Coordination may take place in the primary care setting by a patient health coach who is responsible for much of the health teaching and patient scheduling. How this model will interface with community resources and hospitals is unclear. If PCMHs form ACOs with payers and hospital networks, there is the possibility of greater coordination of transitions to and from hospitals.

The literature suggests that clients prefer one provider across all settings and that this approach is the best method for clinical integration and coordination of all aspects of care (AHA, 2011; HRET, 2013; Lamb & Stemple, 1994; McWilliam et al., 1996). Patients who see the same provider have demonstrated prescribed medication compliance, improved identification of medical problems, fewer hospital admissions, and lower overall costs (Wagner et al., 2012, p. 245). At this time, however, case managers and organizations rarely follow this approach; rather, it is more common to link hospital-based case managers with community-based case managers. Within this type of system, case managers need to be adept at sharing information about the client's past and current illness situations to ensure both continuity and satisfaction with care as the client transitions from the illness episode to the continuum of care. The shared information or handoff needs to include the client's preferences and successful strategies for promoting a relationship that fosters client goal attainment and produces client satisfaction outcomes.

Case Manager Preparation

Preparation of nurses to practice case management using both continuum delivery models and effective technology is an ongoing concern. It is generally agreed among nurse researchers and educators that there is a need for formal educational preparation of the nurse case manager, including preventive healthcare perspectives (Hallberg, 2004) and appropriate computer skills for the role. Presently, inadequacies in the academic approach continue (Cicatiello, 2000; Hallberg, 2004; Halstead, 2000; Sowell & Young, 1997). Agreement ends and disagreement begins, however, when these nurse scholars discuss curricula content and debate which educational level, undergraduate or graduate, is required to prepare case managers for entry into practice.

Because more than 30% of the current certified case managers do not possess a baccalaureate degree (Tahan & Campagna, 2010), concern about preparation for the task of care coordination and negotiating role, function, responsibilities, and reimbursement for care may become an issue (Sminkey, 2012). Aging of the current workforce and the desire for increased numbers of certified case managers cause concern about having sufficient qualified case managers to handle the changing focus from episodic care to longer term health management (Sminkey, 2012).

Nursing has the knowledge and skills, but willingness to establish curricular change and changing standards of preparation may be needed. The reality is that all nurses need content and clinical practice experiences in case management and need to acquire skills in accessing information and managing databases via the Internet (Halstead, 2000; Stanton, 2008). Often, both staff nurses and advanced practice nurses are expected to become members of interdisciplinary case management teams and to make client care decisions based on case management concepts and electronic client data. To assist in forming predictive models, case managers will require statistical and financial background currently not included in undergraduate and most graduate programs.

Sowell and Young (1997) believe that to meet the changing job expectations the baccalaureate graduate should have the expertise to be an effective case management team member, with knowledge of both data-based clinical paths and the quality/financial issues that influence care coordination. The advanced practice nurse graduate, on the other hand, must obtain the expertise needed to perform the case manager role for a caseload of clients within a specialized target population. This view of case management education reflects the current trend in schools of nursing (Haw, 1996).

According to Haw's (1996) national survey of case management education in universities, 95% of nursing schools are beginning to prepare the undergraduate in basic case management concepts and processes including community resource referral, health team collaboration, client progress monitoring, and technology health services (Halstead, 2000). Haw's survey (1996) also indicates that the emphasis in graduate case management education is on role performance behaviors, and therefore the graduate curriculum incorporates many more clinical practicum experiences than are offered in undergraduate education. Findings and conclusions by Haw suggest that nurse educators view the case manager role as an advanced practice role even though employers usually list the undergraduate degree as a requirement for hire. In the end, whether case management education is included at the undergraduate level or graduate level, there is an overall trend toward more formal case management preparation in nursing academia (Haw, 1996; Stanton, Swanson, Sherrod, & Packa, 2005). The need for care coordination in primary care and the need to manage care of increased numbers of newly insured individuals may require the combination of roles from the *nurse practitioner*.

Workforce readiness was recently addressed by the executive director of the CCMC, Patrice Sminkey. Her concerns center around the need to prepare case managers to practice in new models and learn new roles, requiring academic curricula grounded in the latest trends in case management. She recommends that faculty use the findings from the CCMC role and function study (Tahan & Campagna, 2010) to develop the curricula (Sminkey, 2012). When 16 million new clients gain access to primary health care in 2014 through the Patient Protection and Affordable Care Act, it is predicted that new models for primary care services within a coordinated health system will be needed. Case management practice models and case managers will need additional knowledge and skills to meet this challenge.

Health System Redesign

Finally, the emerging value-based reimbursement era of coordinating care across continuums creates issues for both integrated health system providers and case managers alike. It has been established that case managers need skills in accessing and managing patient care data across many different settings. Accurate tracking of patient visits, patient outcomes, and costs is necessary to plan for the delivery of services and the allocation of resources across the continuum. As case managers acquire these skills, there is mounting pressure for integrated healthcare delivery systems to provide these data. However, case management information systems that accurately track these data are costly (Mastrian, 2007; Noone & McKillip, 1996), and purchasing these new technologies requires sufficient profit margins. Unfortunately, *integrated healthcare systems* that are coordinating much of their services in community rather than acute care settings are discovering that capitated reimbursement practices by commercial and federal payers have reduced their profit margins (Lamb & Zazworsky, 2000). Unless financial incentives are aligned with service coordination initiatives, the trend toward coordinating care across the continuum by case managers cannot be sustained.

Planned collaboration of a provider organization and a health plan led to the transformation from a fee-for-service payment system to an accountable care organization (ACO) as developed in the Medicare Shared Savings Program and Pioneer Accountable Care Organization model (Claffey et al., 2012). A financial agreement that included current fee-for-service reimbursement plus an increased per-member per-month payment for achieving quality and efficiency benchmarks at the end of each calendar year was negotiated.

Three areas provided the focus of the two agencies: dedicated case management resources, data reporting, and quality measurement. A payer's case manager was embedded in the provider organization and implemented health risk assessment and predictive modeling along with the care coordinator clinical judgment to assess patient needs.

Selection of metrics caused the provider to institute use of diabetes and ischemic vascular disease measure bundles that would improve population health management and provide the payer with historical data on which to establish risk profiles. Attainment of benchmarks resulted in payment of negotiated incentive money to the practice (Claffey et al., 2012). Similar incentives with PPACA funds are planned for meaningful use of EHRs and meeting the quality outcomes and core measures.

Ongoing research initiatives by the federal government are encouraging. The studies suggest that coordinating care across the continuum for Medicare patients does successfully reduce healthcare costs; thus, future capitated reimbursement structures may increasingly cover these services and be sufficient to support the cost of developing and maintaining data systems. The current economic situation may change this occurrence.

Anticipating the Future of Case Management

The rapid and ongoing transformation of healthcare systems in response to the value-based reimbursement changes and PPACA has made anticipating the future of case management as unpredictable as the ever-changing patterns of a kaleidoscope. However, this change also creates an environment where nursing case management can flourish. As healthcare systems pursue their goals of bundling costs, practice redesign, and chronic care management, case management can become a dominant strategy selected by these systems to meet their goals. (For example, hospitals could use case management more effectively to prevent 30 day re-admissions.) It is easy to imagine that in the future accountable care organizations' care coordinators will oversee large populations' benchmarks, and case managers will provide for safe, seamless transitions with the help of community-based case managers, fostering client trust and confidence in both the healthcare system and the case management approach.

Further twisting of the kaleidoscope offers a view of a future in which all clients are insured, their health is managed, and the role of the care coordinator or patient coach includes an emphasis on risk assessment and preventive care provided to Medicare beneficiaries accompanied by implementation of delivery of care after discharge that reduces recidivism. The overall trend of managed care toward expanded benefits that include complementary alternative medicine, prevention, and long-term care in the home supports this vision.

Consumers today are beginning to demand that health care address their health as well as prepare them for self-management of their conditions. These expanded benefits for consumers support and subsidize the future development of wellness models of case management.

Health managers will be expected to provide care in a variety of settings and at various levels of care; the goal will be to manage population health risks in community primary care rather than in acute care settings. In the near future, case managers will be challenged to provide ways to offset the depersonalization and threat to nurse–client relationships caused by the greater use of technology for assessment and lack of communication with clients.

In the end, the shape that case management takes will depend on the diligence of both integrated delivery systems and case managers to search for new possibilities; and to reflect, question, and create images of care that capture the client's perspective. This reflection and partnership between the system and case manager will create a new kaleidoscope of colors and patterns, encompassing health management models that illuminate a bright future for both care providers and clients.

Discussion Questions

1. What components of the PPACA do you feel benefit your institution most?
2. How could certification in case management benefit high-risk, high-cost patients in your hospital, network, or practice?
3. What is case management participation in a fully integrated healthcare delivery system? How do you participate in this process?
4. What measures should be instituted to secure patient protected health information (PHI) and EHRs? What precautions should be taken in use of the Internet in healthcare settings, and what policies should be developed regarding use of personal electronic devices such as smartphones with patient information?
5. What role will PPACA legislation play in case management in the future?
6. What factors should be included in a predictive model for readmission?
7. How will the value-based reimbursement environment influence case management in the future?

Glossary of Terms

Aging in Place—a program developed by the School of Nursing of the University of Missouri to transition patients from hospital to home.

Care Coordination—numerous skilled and knowledgeable participants who are dependent on each other to carry out tasks that aid in patient care and who rely on sharing information to manage and integrate activities to deliver appropriate healthcare services.

Care Management—programs that use various types of knowledge and information to improve medical practice and aid patients' self-management of illness to improve health status as well as reduce hospitalization and other unnecessary costly medical care.

Care Manager—the healthcare provider involved with direct patient care through patient education for self-management and who coordinates care with other providers, settings, and services.

Case Management—a term that has two major definitions. The ANCC definition is grounded in the nursing process and focuses on collaboration and client populations as important elements for nursing case management. The Case Management Society of America is an interdisciplinary definition: a "collaborative process of assessment, planning, facilitation, care coordination, evaluation, and advocacy for options and services to meet an individual's and family's comprehensive health needs through communication and available resources to promote quality, cost-effective outcomes."

Case Management Domains:

1. **Providing direct care**
2. **Procuring community resources**
3. **Coordinating care across hospital units and healthcare delivery networks**
4. **Evaluating healthcare services for cost-effectiveness**
5. **Building positive nurse–client long-term relationships**

Case Management Models—models of case management that have been categorized into within-the-walls (hospital-based) and beyond-the-walls (community-based) classifications.

Case Management Certification—certification that can be obtained from the Commission for Case Manager Certification (CCMC) or the American Nurses Credentialing Center (ANCC).

Chronic Care Model—redesigned primary care practice by adding the following components to the DM model: evidence-based practice guidelines, multidisciplinary team approaches, patient education, outcome measures, and feedback to stakeholders such as patients, providers, and health plans. The goal for patients is self-management by providing expert support to ensure delivery of effective interventions and use of information technology to provide reminders and analyze outcomes. Population-based approaches to managing various chronic conditions (i.e., asthma, diabetes, and congestive heart failure) were developed and tested. A critical element of the CCM is the coordination of care using information systems that signal the need for preventive care or diagnostic tests, provide flow sheets of results, and report on benchmark attainment.

Disease Management (DM)—primarily a medical model of care of persons with a specific disease.

Guided Care Model—a best practice model of emergency department case management for older adults living independently in the community who frequently visit the ED. This model identified eight core competencies for effective geriatric case management during and beyond the ED visit: an evidence-based practice model, nursing clinical delivery involvement or leadership, high-risk screening, focused geriatric assessment, initiation of care and disposition planning in the ED, interprofessional and capacity-building work practices, post-ED follow-up with patients, and establishment of evaluation and monitoring processes.

Home Hospital (HH)—a program that established criteria for selection of persons presenting at the emergency department who might be candidates for acute care at home. These patients were examined by the HH physician in the ED and then transferred from the ED to home with the nurse coordinator. The nurse coordinator spends an extended period of time directly supervising care for at least 24 hours and arranging temporary nursing visits, placement of Lifeline equipment, diagnostic tests, medications, and other equipment and oversight of care. The HH physician visits the patient each day and is available 24 hours a day.

Patient Navigator Role—introduced at Harlem Hospital to facilitate access to care and diagnosis and treatment of patients. Nurses, social workers, and peer counselors who have a previous diagnosis of cancer are trained and act as patient care navigators through complex healthcare systems. Patient navigator programs will be reimbursed under section 3510 of the PPACA and could be important to accessing chronic care in rural communities.

Practice Facilitator—a person who addresses quality improvement and helps the primary care practice become a PCMH.

Program of All-Inclusive Care for the Elderly (PACE)—a program for dual-eligible persons or persons who may pay for the program services but who are certified by their state as requiring nursing home care to transition patients from hospitals to home.

Transitional Care—actions that are designed to ensure the coordination and continuity of health care as patients transfer between locations and different levels of care.

Utilization Review (UR)—procedures instituted by insurance companies in the 1970s and 1980s to retrospectively analyze patient medical records to determine whether days of acute care hospitalization could be "carved out" if they lacked medical necessity.

Value-Based Environment (Second Curve)—presently, reimbursement is changing to include organizational performance mandates. When protocols are not met, and when never events occur, insurers are not paying providers for the event or for the hospital stay. Reimbursement is value based.

Volume-Based Environment (First Curve)—in the past, reimbursement has been determined by the volume of insured patients. Industrial Age organizational design was used.

References

Adams, J. (2000). Applying e-health to case management. *Lippincott's Case Management, 5*(4), 168–171.

American Academy of Pediatrics. (1992). The medical home. *Pediatrics, 90*(5), 774.

American Hospital Association, 2011 Committee on Performance Improvement. (2011, September). *Hospitals and care systems of the future.* Chicago, IL: Author.

American Nurses Credentialing Center. (1998). *Nursing case management catalogue.* Washington, DC: Author.

American Nurses Credentialing Center. (2013). Nursing case management. Retrieved from http://www .nursecredentialing.org/Certification/NurseSpecialties/CaseManagement.html

Balka, E., Tolar, M., Coates, S., & Whitehouse, S. (2010). Socio-technical challenges in implementing safe patient handovers. In C. Nohr & J. Aarts (Eds.), *Information technology in health care: Socio-technical approaches 2010* (pp. 206–212). Fairfax, VA: IOS Press.

Battersby, M., Von Korff, M., Schaefer, J., Davis, C., Ludman, E., Greene, S. M., . . . Wagner, E. H. (2010). Twelve evidence-based principles for implementing self-management support in primary care. *Joint Commission Journal on Quality and Patient Safety, 36*(12), 561–570.

Baxter, L., & Nash, D. B. (2012). Implementing the Patient-Centered Medical Home model for chronic disease care in small medical practices: Practice group characteristics and physician understanding. *American Journal of Medical Quality.* doi:10.1177/1062860612454451

Bennett, K. J., Probst, J. C., Vyaharkar, M., & Glover, S. (2012). Missing the handoff: Post-hospitalization follow-up care among rural Medicare beneficiaries with diabetes. *Rural and Remote Health, 12*(2097).

Berg-Weger, M., & Tebb, S. (1998). Caregiver well-being: A strengths-based case management approach. *Journal of Case Management, 7*(2), 67–73.

Bodenheimer, T., Wagner, E. H., & Grumbach, K. (2002a). Improving primary care for patients with chronic illness. *Journal of the American Medical Association, 288*(14), 1775–1779.

Bodenheimer, T., Wagner, E. H., & Grumbach, K. (2002b). Improving primary care for patients with chronic illness: The Chronic Care Model, part 2. *Journal of the American Medical Association, 288*(15), 1909–1914.

Bolin, J. N., Gamm, L., Vest, J. R., Edwardson, N., & Miller, T. R. (2011). Patient-centered medical homes: Will health care reform provide new options for rural communities and providers? *Family & Community Health, 34*(2), 93–101.

Buhler-Wilkerson, K. (2001). *No place like home: A history of nursing and home care in the United States.* Baltimore, MD: Johns Hopkins University Press.

Burns, L., Lamb, G., & Wholey, D. (1996). Impact of integrated community nursing services on hospital utilization and costs in a Medicare risk plan. *Inquiry, 33*, 30–41.

Carper, K., & Machlen, S. R. (2013). Statistical brief #396: National health care expenses in the U.S. civilian non-institutionalized population, 2010. Retrieved from http://meps.ahrq.gov/mepsweb/data_files/publications/st396/stat396.shtml

Carver, T. (2001). Continuum-based care coordination via the Web. *Care Management, 17*(2), 14–20.

Case Management Society of America. (n.d.). What is a case manager? Retrieved from http://www.cmsa.org/Home/CMSA/WhatisaCaseManager/tabid/224/Default.aspx

Case Management Society of America. (2010). *Standards of practice for case management* (Rev. ed.). Little Rock, AR: Author.

Center on Aging Society. (2004, January). *Disease Management Programs: Improving health while reducing costs?* (Issue Brief No. 4). Washington, DC: Georgetown University. http://ihcrp.georgetown.edu/agingsociety/pubhtml/management/management.html http://ihcrp.georgetown.edu/agingsociety/pdfs/management.pdf

Cicatiello, J. (2000). A perspective of health care in the past—insights and challenges for a health care system in the new millennium. *Nursing Administration Quarterly, 25*(1), 18–29.

Claffey, T. F., Agostini, J. V., Collet, E. N., Reisman, L., & Krakauer, R. (2012). Payer–provider collaboration in accountable care reduced use and improved quality in Medicare Advantage plan. *Health Affairs, 31*(9), 2074–2083.

Cohen, E., & Cesta, T. (2005). *Nursing case management* (4th ed.). St. Louis, MO: Elsevier Mosby.

Crane, S., Collins, L., Hall, J., Rochester, D., & Patch, S. (2012). Reducing utilization of uninsured frequent users of the emergency department: Combining case management and drop-in group medical appointments. *Journal of the American Board of Family Medicine, 25*(2), 184–191.

Cryer, L., Shannon, S. B., Van Amsterdam, M., & Leff, B. (2011). Costs for "Hospital at Home" patients were 19% lower with equal or better outcomes compared to similar inpatients. *Health Affairs, 31*(6), 1237–1243.

Cutler, D. (2010). Analysis and commentary. How health care reform must bend the cost curve. *Health Affairs, 29*(6), 1131–1135.

Daniels, S. (2011). Introducing HCM v 3.0: A standard model for hospital case management. *Professional Case Management, 16*(3), 109–125.

DuBard, C. A., Cockerham, J., & Jackson, C. (2012). Collaborative accountability for care transitions: The Community Care of North Carolina transitions program. *North Carolina Medical Journal, 73*(1), 34–40.

Dunn, S., Sohl-Kreiger, R., & Marx, S. (2001). Geriatric case management in an integrated care system. *Journal of Nursing Administration, 31*(2), 60–62.

Eichler, D. (2013). Patient screening and callbacks to prevent readmissions: A process improvement project. *Professional Case Management, 18*(1), 25–31.

Ethridge, P. (1987). Nurse accountability program improves satisfaction, turnover. *Health Progress, 68*, 44–49.

Ethridge, P. (1997). The Carondelet experience. *Nursing Management, 28*(3), 26–28.

Ethridge, P., & Lamb, G. (1989). Professional nursing case management improves quality, access and costs. *Nursing Management, 20*(3), 30–35.

Fink-Samnick, E. (2011). Understanding care corrdination: Emerging opportunities for social workers. *New Social Worker, 18*(3), 18–20.

Fink-Samnick, E. (2012). Are we there yet? Professional licensure strives to sync with practice reality. *Professional Case Management, 18*(1), 37–40.

Flarey, D. (1996). Case management: Delivering care in the age of managed care. In D. Flarey & S. Blancett (Eds.), *Handbook of nursing case management*. Gaithersburg, MD: Aspen.

Flarey, D., & Blancett, S. (Eds.). (1996). *Handbook of nursing case management*. Gaithersburg, MD: Aspen.

Fox, S. (2006). *Online health search, 2006*. Washington, DC: Pew Internet and American Life Project. Retrieved from http://www.pewinternet.org/Reports/2006/Online-Health-Search-2006.aspx

Fox, S. & Duggan, M. (2013). Health Online 2013. Washington, DC: Pew Internet and American Life Project. Retrieved http://www.pewinternet.org/Reports/2013/Health-online.aspx

Frick, K. D., Burton, L. C., Clark, R., Mader, S. I., Naughton, W. B., Burl, J. B., . . . Leff, B. (2009). Substitutive Hospital at Home for older persons: Effects on costs. *American Journal of Managed Care, 15*(1), 49–56.

Glasgow, R. E., Wagner, E. H., Schaefer, J., Mahoney, L. D., Reid, R. J., & Greene, S. M. (2005). Development and validation of the Patient Assessment of Chronic Illness Care (PACIC). *Medical Care, 43*(5), 436–444.

Goins, T. W., Jr. (2012). Transitions to and from nursing facilities. *North Carolina Medical Journal, 73*(1), 51–54.

Goode, C. (1995). Impact of a CareMap and case management on patient satisfaction and staff satisfaction, collaboration, and autonomy. *Nursing Economic$, 13*(6), 337–348.

Gordon, D., & Geiger, G. (1999). Strategic management of an electronic patient record project using the balanced scorecard. *Journal of Healthcare Information Management, 13*(3), 113–123.

Gray, F. C., White, A., & Brooks-Buck, J. (2013). Exploring role confusion in nurse case management. *Professional Case Management, 18*(2), 66–76. doi:10.1097/NCM.0b013e31827a4832

Hallberg, I. (2004). Preventive home care of frail older people: A review of recent case management studies. *Journal of Clinical Nursing, 13*(6b), 112–120.

Halstead, J. (2000). Implementing web-based instruction in a school of nursing: Implications for faculty and students. *Journal of Professional Nursing, 16*(5), 273–281.

Hart, M. A. (2012). Accountable care organizations: The future of care delivery? *American Journal of Nursing, 112*(2), 23–26.

Haw, M. (1996). Case management education in universities: A national survey. *Journal of Care Management, 2*(6), 10–23.

Health Research and Educational Trust. (2013, April). *Metrics for the second curve of health care.* Retrieved from http://www.hpoe.org/future-metrics-1to4

Henderson, S., Princell, C. O., & Martin, S. D. (2012). The Patient-Centered Medical Home. *American Journal of Nursing, 112*(12), 54–59.

Hennessey, B., Suter, P., & Harrison, G. (2010). The home-based chronic care model: A platform for partnership for the provision of a patient-centered medical home. *Caring, 29*(2), 18–24.

Henry J. Kaiser Family Foundation. (2012). Health care costs: A primer—key information on health care costs and their impact. Retrieved from http://www.kff.org/insurance/upload/7670–03.pdf

Institute of Medicine, Committee on Quality of Health Care in America. (2001). *Crossing the quality chasm: A new health system for the 21st century.* Washington, DC: National Academy Press.

Jencks, S. F., Williams, M. V., & Coleman, E. A. (2009). Rehospitalizations among patients in the Medicare fee-for-service program. *New England Journal of Medicine, 360*(14), 1418–1428.

Kaplan, R. S., & Norton, D. P. (1992, January/February). The balanced scorecard—measures that drive performance. *Harvard Business Review, 70*(1), 71–79.

Kegel, L. (1996). Case management, critical pathways, and myocardial infarction. *Critical Care Nurse, 16*(2), 97–114.

Ketchen, D., Palmer, T., & Gamm, L. (2001). The role of performance referents in health services organizations. *Health Care Management Review, 26*(4), 19–26.

Kleinpell-Nowell, R. (1999). Measuring advanced practice nursing outcomes. *AACN Clinical Issues, 10*(3), 356–368.

Kumar, G. S., & Klein, R. (2012). Effectiveness of case management strategies in reducing emergency department visits in frequent user patient populations: A systematic review. *Journal of Emergency Medicine, 44*(3), 717–29. doi: 10.1016/j.jemermed.2012.08.035.

Kuraitis, V. (2007). Disease management and the medical home model. Competing or complementary? *Disease Management and Health Outcomes, 15*(3), 135–140.

Lagoe, R. (1998). Basic statistics for clinical pathway evaluation. *Nursing Economic$, 16*(3), 125–131.

Lamb, G., & Stemple, J. (1994). Nurse case management from the client's view: Growing as insider-expert. *Nursing Outlook, 42*(1), 7–14.

Lamb, G., & Zazworsky, D. (2000). The Carondelet case management program. In E. Cohen & T. Cesta (Eds.), *Nursing case management* (3rd ed.). St. Louis, MO: Mosby.

Leff, B., Burton, L., Guido, S., Greenough, W. B., Steinwachs, D., & Burton, J. R. (1999). Home hospital program: A pilot study. *Journal of the American Geriatrics Society, 47*, 697–702.

Leff, B., & Novak, T. (2011). It takes a team: Affordable Care Act policy makers mine the potential of the Guided Care Model. *Generations, 35*(1), 60–63.

Leonard, M., & Miller, E. (2012). *Nursing case management review and resource manual.* Silver Spring, MD: American Nurses Credentialing Center.

Lillibridge, J., & Hanna, B. (2009). Using telehealth to deliver nursing case management services to HIV/AIDS clients. *Online Journal of Issues in Nursing, 14*(1), 9–16.

Lubetkin, E. I., Lu, W., Krebs, P., Yeung, H., & Ostroff, J. S. (2010). Exploring primary care providers' interest in using patient navigators to assist in the delivery of tobacco cessation treatment to low income, ethnic/racial minority patients. *Journal of Community Health, 35*(6), 618–624.

Marek, K. D., Stetzer, F., Adams, S. J., Popejoy, L. L., & Rantz, M. (2012). Aging in Place versus nursing home care: Comparison costs to Medicare and Medicaid. *Research in Gerontological Nursing, 5*(2), 123–129.

Marineau, M. (2007). Telehealth advanced practice nursing: The lived experiences of individuals with acute infections transitioning in the home. *Nursing Forum, 42*(4), 196–208.

Mastrian, K. (2007). Tips, tools and techniques. *Professional Case Management, 12*(3), 181–183.

McDonald, K. M., Sundaram, V., Bravata, D. M., Lewis, R., Lin, N., Kraft, S. A., . . . Owens, D. K. (2007). *Closing the quality gap: A critical analysis of quality improvement strategies* (Vol. 7, Care Coordination). Rockville, MD: Agency for Healthcare Research and Quality.

McGonigle, D., Mastrian, K., & Pavelekovsky, K. (2007). Information systems and case management practice series, part II: case management information systems goals, benefits, and system selection or development. *Professional Case Management, 12*(4), 239–241.

McWilliam, C., Stewart, M., Brown, J., Desai, K., & Coderre, P. (1996). Creating health with chronic illness. *Advances in Nursing Science, 18*(3), 1–15.

Meadows, G. (2001). The Internet promise: A new look at e-health opportunities. *Nursing Economic$, 19*(6), 294–295.

Mechanic, R. (2004, May). Will care management improve the value of US healthcare. In *11th Background Paper for the Annual Princeton Conference. Available at*: http://healthstat.net/publications/documents/CareManagement2004_002.pdf http://healthforum.brandeis.edu/research/pdfs/CareManagementPrincetonConference.pdf

Meek, J. A. (2012). Affordable Care Act: Predictive modeling challenges and opportunities for case management. *Professional Case Management, 17*(1), 15–23.

Meliones, J. (2000, November–December). Saving money, saving lives. *Harvard Business Review*, 57–67.

Mick, D., & Ackerman, M. (2002). New perspectives on advanced practice nursing case management for aging patients. *Critical Care Nursing Clinics of North America, 14*, 281–291.

Moy, B., & Chabner, B. A. (2011). Patient navigator programs, cancer disparities, and the Patient Protection and Affordable Care Act. *The Oncologist, 16*, 926–929.

Naylor, M. D., Aiken, L. H., Kurtzman, E. T., Olds, D. M., & Hirschman, K. B. (2011). The importance of transitional care in achieving health reform. *Health Affairs, 30*(4), 746–754.

Newman, M. (1986). *Health as expanding consciousness*. St. Louis, MO: Mosby.

Noone, C., & McKillip, C. (1996). Data management through information systems. In D. Flarey & S. Blancett (Eds.), *Handbook of nursing case management*. Gaithersburg, MD: Aspen.

Novak, D. (1998). Nurse case managers' opinions of their role. *Nursing Case Management, 3*(6), 231–237.

Oermann, M., Lesley, M., & Kuefler, S. (2002). Using the Internet to teach consumers about quality care. *Journal of Quality Improvement, 28*(2), 83–89.

Office of the Actuary, C. f. M. a. M. (2012). *2011 actuarial report on the financial outlook for Medicaid*. Retrieved from http://www.cms.gov/Research-Statistics-Data-and-Systems/Research/ActuarialStudies/downloads/MedicaidReport2011.pdf

Organisation for Economic Co-operation and Development. (2013). Statistics. Retrieved from http://www.oecd.org/statistics

Pedersen, A., & Hack, T. F. (2010). Pilots of oncology health care: A concept analysis of the patient navigator role. *Oncology Nursing Forum, 37*(1), 55–60.

Powell, S. K., & Tahan, H. A. (2010). *Case management: A practical guide for education and practice* (3rd ed.). Philadelphia, PA: Wolters Kluwer/Lippincott Williams & Wilkins.

Procter, S., Wilson, P. M., Brooks, F., & Kendall, S. (2012). Success and failure in integrated models of nursing for long term conditions: Multiple case studies of whole systems. *International Journal of Nursing Studies*. doi:10.1016/j.ijnurstu.2012.10.007

Redwood, D., Provost, E., Perdue, D., Havercamp, D., & Espey, D. (2012). The last frontier: Innovative efforts to reduce colorectal cancer disparities among the remote Alaska Native population. *Gastrointestinal Endoscopy, 75*(3), 474–480.

Reed, K. (2005). Telemedicine: Benefits to advanced practice nursing and the communities they serve. *Journal of the American Academy of Nurse Practitioners, 17*(5), 176–180.

Reimanis, C., Cohen, E., & Redman, R. (2001). Nurse case manager role attributes: Fifteen years of evidence-based literature. *Lippincott's Case Management, 6*(6), 230–242.

Renholm, M., Leino-Kilpi, H., & Suominen, T. (2002). Critical pathways. *Journal of Nursing Administration, 32*(4), 196–201.

Robinson, J. (2001). The end of managed care. *Journal of the American Medical Association, 285*(20), 2622–2632.

Salazar, M. (2000). Maximizing the effectiveness of case management service delivery. *Case Manager, 11*(3), 58–63.

Schore, J., Peikes, D., Peterson, G., Gerolamo, A., & Brown, R. (2011). *Fourth report to Congress on the evaluation of the Medicare Coordinated Demonstration Project*. Princeton, NJ: Mathematica Policy Research.

Schraeder, C. (2001). Discharge planning. *Hospital Case Management, 9*(10), 155–156.

Shockney, L. D. (2010). Evolution of patient navigation. *Clinical Journal of Onology Nursing, 14*(4), 405–407.

Sinha, S., Bessman, E. S., Flomenbaum, N., & Leff, B. (2011). A systematic review and qualitative analysis to inform the development of a new emergency department–based geriatric case managment model. *Annals of Emergency Medicine, 57*(6), 672–682.

Sminkey, P. (2012). The next half of the battle: Workforce readiness for board certified case managers. *Professional Case Management, 17*(3), 132–133.

Smith, A. C. (2011). Role ambiguity and role conflict in nurse case managers: An integrative review. *Professional Case Management, 16*(4), 182–196; quiz 197–198. doi:10.1097/NCM.0b013e318218845b

Smith, A. W., Reeve, B. B., Bellizi, K. M., Hearlen, L. C., Klabunde, C. N., Ansellem, M., . . . Hayes, R. D. (2008). Cancer, comorbidities, and health-related quality of life of older adults. . *Health Care Financing Review, 29*(4), 41–56.

Sowell, R., & Young, S. (1997). Case management in the nursing curriculum. *Nursing Case Management, 2*(4), 173–176.

Stanton, M. (2008). The "wins" of change: Evaluating the impact of predicted changes on case management practice. *Professional Case Management, 13*(3), 161–168.

Stanton, M., Swanson, M., Sherrod, R., & Packa, D. (2005). Case management evolution: From basic to advanced practice role. *Lippincott's Case Management, 10*(6), 274–284.

Stellefson, M., Dipnarine, K., & Stopka, C. (2013). The Chronic Care Model and diabetes management in US primarycare settings: A systematic review. *Prevention of Chronic Disease, 10*, E26. doi:10.5888/pcd10.120180

Stephens, L. (2012). Family nurse practitioners: "Value add" in outpatient chronic disease management. *Primary Care, 39*(4), 595–603. doi:10.1016/j.pop.2012.08.008

Suter, P., Hennessey, B., Florez, D., & Newton Suter, W. (2011). Review series: Examples of Chronic Care Model: The home-based Chronic Care Model: Redesigning home health for high quality care delivery. *Chronic Respiratory Disease, 8*(1), 43–52. doi:10.1177/1479972310396031

Suter, P., Hennessey, B., Harrison, G., Fagan, M., Norman, B., & Suter, W. N. (2008). Home-based chronic care. An expanded integrative model for home health professionals. *Home Healthc Nurse, 26*(4), 222–229. doi:10.1097/01.nhh.0000316700.76891.95

Tahan, H. A., & Campagna, V. (2010). Case management roles and functions across various settings and professional disciplines. *Professional Case Management, 15*(4), 245–277.

Taylor, E. F., Machta, R. M., Meyers, D. S., Genevro, J., & Peikes, D. N. (2013). Enhancing the primary care team to provide redesigned care: The roles of practice facilitators. *Annals of Family Medicine, 11*(1), 80–83.

Taylor, P. (1999). Comprehensive nursing case management: An advanced practice model. *Nursing Case Management, 4*(1), 2–10.

Terra, S. (2007). An evidence-based approach to case management model selection for an acute care facility. *Professional Case Management, 12*(3), 147–157.

Todd, W. E., & Nash, D. (1997). *Disease management—a systems approach to improving patient outcomes.* Chicago, IL: American Hospital Publishing.

Tomcavage, J., Littlewood, D., & Sciandra, J. (2012). Advancing the role of nursing in the Medical Home Model. *Nursing Administration Quarterly, 36*(3), 194–202.

Wagner, E. H. (2010). Academia, chronic care, and the future of primary care. *Journal of General Internal Medicine, 25*(Suppl. 4), S636–638. doi:10.1007/s11606-010-1442-6

Wagner, E. H., Austin, B. T., & Von Korff, M. (1996). Organizing care for patients with chronic illness. *Milbank Quarterly, 74*(4), 511–544.

Wagner, E. H., Bennett, S. M., Austin, B. T., Greene, S. M., Schaefer, J. K., & Vonkorff, M. (2005). Finding common ground: Patient-centeredness and evidence-based chronic illness care. *Journal of Alternative and Complementary Medicine, 11*(Suppl. 1), S7–15. doi:10.1089/acm.2005.11.s-7

Wagner, E. H., Coleman, K., Reid, R. J., Phillips, K., Abrams, M. K., & Sugarman, J. R. (2012). The changes involved in Patient-Centered Medical Home transformation. *Primary Care, 39*(2), 241–259. doi:10.1016/j.pop.2012.03.002

Wagner, E. H., Davis, C., Schaefer, J., Von Korff, M., & Austin, B. (1999). A survey of leading chronic disease management programs: Are they consistent with the literature? *Managed Care Quarterly, 7*(3), 56–66.

Wagner, E. H., Grothaus, L. C., Sandhu, N., Galvin, M. S., McGregor, M., Artz, K., & Coleman, E. A. (2001). Chronic care clinics for diabetes in primary care: A system-wide randomized trial. *Diabetes Care, 24*(4), 695–700.

Waldo, B. (2000). HIPAA: The next frontier. *Information Systems and Technology, 18*(1), 49–50.

Wieland, D., Kinosian, B., Stallard, E., & Boland, R. (2013). Does Medicaid pay more to a Program of All-Inclusive Care for the Elderly (PACE) than for fee-for-service long-term care? Journal of Gerontology Series A Biological Scence Medical Science, 68(1), 47–55. doi:10.1093/gerona/gls137

Young, R. A., & DeVoe, J. E. (2012). Who will have health insurance in the future? An updated projection. Annals of Family Medicine, 10(2), 156–162.

Zander, K. (1988a). Nursing group practice: The Cadillac in continuity. *Definition, 3*(2), 1–2.

Zander, K. (1988b). Managed care within acute care settings: Design and implementation via nursing case management. *Health Care Supervisor, 6*(2), 24–43.

Zander, K. (1988c). Nursing care management: Strategic management of cost and quality outcomes. *Journal of Nursing Administration, 18*(5), 23–30.

Zander, K. (1996). The early years: The evolution of nursing case management. In D. Flarey & S. Blancett (Eds.), *Handbook of nursing case management*. Gaithersburg, MD: Aspen.

Zander, K. (2002). Nursing case management in the 21st century: Intervening where margin meets mission. *Nursing Administration Quarterly, 24*(5), 58–68.

Zander, K. (2008). *Hospital case management models*. Marblehead, MA: HCPro.

Zander, K. (2009). The six core functions of case management. *Center for Case Management, 24*(1), 1–3.

Finance and Accounting Issues

Although a nurse manager may never need to learn accounting and finance basics, we have included some beginning information about them in this book. We hope this helps the nurse manager to have a greater appreciation for the finance side of the organization. It is helpful for nurse managers to be able to read financial statements for healthcare organizations, explained in Chapter 19, as well as to learn more about certain financial ratios commonly used in healthcare organizations, as described in Chapter 20. For a more detailed background in these topics, nurse managers can enrol in accounting or finance courses.

Accounting for
Healthcare Entities

Paul Bayes, DBA Accounting, MS Economics, BS Accounting

OBJECTIVES

- Provides the reporting of the finance side of the organization.
- Helps the nurse manager to read a detailed financial statement to include Balance Sheet, Income Statement and Cash Flow Operating Activities.

Introduction

Accounting has been called the language of business because accounting information provides direction for action. Healthcare organizations can be classified as either for-profit or not-for-profit, but much of the information is the same and requires similar decision making. Each organization has assets and liabilities. The difference occurs in the area defined as either stockholder's equity (for-profit) or unrestricted, temporarily restricted, and permanently restricted funds (not-for-profit).

The financial synopsis of management's actions is contained in the financial statements (see this chapter's appendix for examples of a profit-oriented and not-for-profit entities). Excerpts from these statements are used as examples throughout this chapter. Years ago, it was uncommon for healthcare entities to have financial problems. However, changing economic conditions and revenue-limiting measures by third-party providers (insurance companies/government) require healthcare entities to take a more proactive look at the financial condition of their business. The failure to do so may result in what has happened to many "dot-coms" as well as established companies in recent years.

Financial statements are required every year, and publicly traded healthcare entities must also issue quarterly financial statements. These financial statements consist of the statement of financial position (balance sheet), the *income statement* (also called statement of *financial activities*—income and expenses or statement of earnings), and statement of cash flows. In recent years, more attention has focused on the statement of cash flows because cash is the lifeblood of a business. To be an informed decision maker, you must understand how to use financial statements, but you do not necessarily have to know how to prepare these financial statements. Thus, the focus of this chapter is on the understanding and use of financial information.

Accounting Framework

One of the basic frameworks of for-profit accounting is the accounting equation: Assets = Liabilities + Equity. *Assets* are those items that provide future cash flow or have future economic benefit. If you were to prepare a personal financial statement for a bank loan, you would list those items that have value (assets) and can be sold in case of default on the loan. For business organizations, assets are used to generate revenue for the firm. *Liabilities* are claims on the assets of an organization. The claims are those of creditors who have provided resources such as buildings and equipment but have not been fully paid. In the example of a personal loan, liabilities include credit card, car, or home mortgage balances. The difference between the assets and liabilities of an organization is the equity, or in the personal loan application example, *net worth*. Examples of these items follow. All amounts are in millions except for earnings per share.

In not-for-profit organizations, the result of subtracting liabilities from assets is called *net assets* or *fund balances*. Not-for-profit entities return the excess amount to the sponsoring organization if they cease to continue stated purposes. The accounting framework for a not-for-profit organization would be Assets = Liabilities + Net assets or fund balances. Examples of these differences are illustrated as follows.

Statement of Financial Position (Balance Sheet)

Assets

The *balance sheet*—consisting of the assets, liabilities, and equity—is a snapshot of the healthcare entity and is dated for a 1-day period of time. The assets, liabilities, and equity or fund balances reflect only the amounts as of a certain date. Traditional examples use December 31 as the ending day, but firms have other ending time periods. The asset portion of Hospital Anywhere USA, which is dated as of December 31, appears in **Exhibit 19–1**. Complete financial statements are found in the appendix.

Assets may be classified as current versus long term or, more specifically, current assets, property and equipment (*tangible assets*), investments, and *intangible assets* such as patents. *Current assets* are those items that will be used to generate revenue in either 1 year or the operating period, whichever is longer (most often this is 1 year).

Generally, the first item listed on the statement of financial position is cash, although many times it is combined with temporary investments, which are considered *cash equivalents*. Temporary investments are cash equivalents because they can be sold quickly with little or no loss in value. This is the reserve needed to meet the operational needs of the organization such as salaries and to meet other obligations as they arise.

An important source of future cash is generically identified as *accounts (patients) receivable*. These may be represented by amounts owed by either patients to which the organization has provided services or by claims filed with third-party providers such as insurance companies. These provide future cash flows, and therefore it is imperative these insurance claims are filed quickly and accurately. Reducing the collection period provides cash more quickly for operations. This amount is often reported as a "net" number, reflecting amounts that will not be collected or reductions from third-party providers.

Exhibit 19–1   Asset Section of Balance Sheet

(Dollars in millions)		
Assets	2004	2003
Current assets		
Cash and cash equivalents	$314	$190
Accounts receivable, less allowance for doubtful accounts of $1,583 and $1,567	2,211	1,873
Inventories	396	383
Income taxes receivable	197	178
Other	1,335	973
Total current assets	**4,453**	**3,597**
Property and equipment at cost		
Land	793	813
Buildings	6,021	6,108
Equipment	7,045	6,721
Construction in progress	431	442
Total property and equipment	**14,290**	**14,084**
Accumulated depreciation	(5,810)	(5,594)
	8,480	8,490
Investments of insurance subsidiary	1,371	1,457
Investments in and advances to affiliates	779	654
Intangible assets, net of accumulated amortization of $785 and $644	2,155	2,319
Other	330	368
Total assets	**$17,568**	**$16,885**

Other current assets of the organization consist of *inventory* items such as drugs in the pharmacy, surgical supplies, items maintained at nursing stations, and drinks and/or food in the cafeteria. The alternative inventory cost measures are not discussed in this text. The income taxes receivable account is the equivalent of receiving a tax refund but waiting for the check.

Property and Equipment

The largest item on a for-profit healthcare entity's balance sheet is probably *buildings* and *equipment*. This may also be defined as *tangible assets*. *Land* on which a healthcare facility is located is one item included in this section. Land is not written off, unless there is something that impairs value such as pollution of the land site. Other tangible assets, such as buildings and equipment, have skyrocketing costs because of the complexity of equipment and more rigorous building codes and regulations. Buildings are the physical facilities in which patient services are provided. Equipment may be items such as x-ray and computed tomography (CT) machines or less complex items such as patient beds. The increased costs require either the availability of large amounts of funds for purchases (cash) or credit-granting sources. *Construction in progress* is an account indicating buildings that have not been completed but are being built. The account indicates progress toward completion. *Depreciation* is an accounting charge wherein the balance of the equipment and buildings is systematically written off over a period of time. *Accumulated depreciation*, which is the sum of the annual depreciation charges, is then subtracted from the plant and equipment balance, providing a net figure. This number does not relate to current market value but rather is book value only, which is the original cost minus accumulated depreciation.

Investments

Investments are classified as long term in nature in that they are held for income purposes. These may be a result of using excess cash to either invest in items such as other organizations, joint ventures, purchase stocks, or bonds of other organizations or donations received from external parties. As in the case of Hospital Anywhere USA, they are investments in other organizations (affiliates of Hospital Anywhere USA) or loans made to affiliate organizations.

Intangible Assets

Intangible assets generally are those items that have no physical presence but do have value in the form of legal rights to use or sell an asset. One example is patents that have been developed by employees of the organization. Use of a patent may provide a strategic advantage over competing facilities or may reduce your firm's costs below that of competitors. One item that is harder to define as an intangible asset is *goodwill*. Goodwill occurs when an entity purchases another organization and there is an excess amount paid for the net assets of the purchased entity that exceeds market value. This excess amount is goodwill.

Most intangible assets are also systematically written off over a period of time like that of depreciation but the process is called *amortization*. Goodwill must be evaluated each year, and a determination must be made for impairment of value. If value declines, goodwill must be reduced ("written down") by this amount.

Liabilities

To begin our discussion of liabilities, please refer to **Exhibit 19–2**.

Exhibit 19–2 Liabilities Section of Balance Sheet		
(Dollars in millions, except for per share amount)		
Liabilities	**2004**	**2003**
Current liabilities		
Accounts payable	693	657
Accrued salaries	352	403
Other accrued expenses	1,135	897
Government settlement accrual	840	
Long-term debt due within 1 year	1,121	1,160
Total current liabilities	**4,141**	**3,117**
Long-term debt	5,631	5,284
Professional liability risks, deferred taxes and other liabilities	2,050	2,104
Minority interests in equity of consolidated entities	572	763
Forward purchase contracts and put options	769	
Total liabilities	**13,163**	**11,268**

Current Liabilities

Accounts payables are claims on assets. These are short term in nature and are generally expected to be paid in 30 to 120 days based on the type of claim but can be unpaid up to 1 year. The purchase of operating supplies such as surgical staples and food items are examples.

Accrued liabilities (i.e., salaries) are those that have been incurred in the course of business but have not yet been paid. For example, if employees are paid on the fifth of the month for effort in the previous month, then it is an accrued expense. Employers owe employees for services provided but have not yet made payment. Accounting recognizes expenses when incurred, not necessarily when paid. Other accrued expenses could include interest incurred on debt but not paid or taxes owed to government entities.

Most organizations finance equipment or a building that requires a large outlay of resources over a long period of time, with some financing arrangements lasting up to 40 years. Each year as that portion of the debt becomes due in the current year, it is considered a current liability.

Long-Term Liabilities (Debt)

Long-term debt examples include such items as mortgages and bonds issued to borrow money. This debt is not paid in the current year or operating period. Other items identified as long-term debt could include professional liability risks such as unsettled lawsuits resulting from malpractice claims and employee work-related injuries. *Deferred taxes* are the differences between income reported in financial statements and that paid to the U.S. Treasury.

Stockholder's Equity

For-profit corporate firms raise funds by issuing either *preferred or common stock*. **Exhibit 19–3** provides an example. These stocks represent ownership shares in an organization. Both stocks generally have a par value and sell for more than this base amount (capital in excess of par value). The *par value* is arbitrarily established as a low amount and is used for accounting records.

Exhibit 19-3   Stockholder's Equity Section of Balance Sheet

	(Dollars in millions)	
Stockholder's equity:		
Common stock $.01 par; authorized 1,600,000,000 voting shares 50,000,000 nonvoting shares; outstanding 521,991,700 voting shares and 21,000,000 shares and 21,000,000 nonvoting shares—2004 and 543,272,900 voting shares and 21,000,000 nonvoting shares—2003	5	6
Capital in excess of par value		951
Other	9	8
Accumulated other comprehensive income	52	53
Retained earnings	4,339	4,599
Total stockholder's equity	4,405	5,617
Total liabilities and stockholder's equity	**$17,568**	**$16,885**

Preferred stock is not used as extensively as common stock but is one possible source of funds. The stock gets its name from the preference over common stock in either payments of dividends or distribution of liquidation proceeds in case of the firm ceasing business. Three additional financial items are found in the stockholder's equity section of Hospital Anywhere USA.

The final item found on the statement of financial position is *retained earnings*. The name is misleading because there is no actual money in this account. Retained earnings is an account used by the accounting function to balance the books at the end of the year. The amount carried to retained earnings is the difference between all revenue sources, expenses and costs, and dividends paid. The equivalent section of the stockholder's equity of a not-for-profit is called a fund balance.

Income Statement

The *income statement* is a financial statement that captures information about revenue sources, expenses, and costs of doing business during a period of time. For example, a yearly income statement would be labeled for the year ended. Hospital Anywhere USA shows years ended December 31, 2004, 2003, and 2002 (**Exhibit 19–4**).

Most revenue sources come from providing patient services. The problem with these sources is that the amount billed is not the amount received. For example, using the prospective payment system established in the early 1990s, many of the major insurance companies pay only between 50% and 60% of the amount billed. For Medicare and state health plans, such as Medicaid, this amount is even lower—it could be as low as 25%. This has led to major changes in the accounting of healthcare providers, such as more accuracy in billing. If a claim is filed with a third-party provider, payment must be received as soon as possible. Many healthcare providers found that claims collection was taking as many as 90 days. This means services were provided, resulting in expenditures, but the healthcare provider has only a piece of paper representing a claim. Many providers have improved their claims collection through improved accuracy of coding and by using electronic filing. The sooner the payment is received, the sooner the healthcare entity can use the funds to pay its own claims for services provided by creditors and purchase new equipment or replacement equipment for improved diagnosis.

Exhibit 19–4	Income Statement		
(Dollars in millions)			
	2004	2003	2002
Revenues	**$16,670**	**$16,657**	**$18,681**
Salaries and benefits	6,639	6,694	7,766
Supplies	2,640	2,645	2,901
Other operating expenses	3,085	3,251	3,816
Provision for doubtful accounts	1,255	1,269	1,442
Depreciation and amortization	1,033	1,094	1,247
Interest expense	559	471	561
Equity in earnings of affiliates	(126)	(90)	(112)
Settlement with federal government	840	0	0
Gains on sales of facilities	(34)	(297)	(744)
Impairment of long-lived assets	117	220	542
Restructuring of operations and investigation related costs	62	116	111
Total expenses	**16,070**	**15,373**	**17,530**

Additional revenue may take the form of providing services for other healthcare facilities or through the investment of funds. One example of additional services is that of a healthcare facility, such as Healthy Hospital, doing laundry service for other hospitals. One section of Hospital Anywhere USA asset section illustrated the category called investments. Revenues from invested funds in the form of interest or dividends can also supplement basic operations.

Reductions in payments by third-party providers, including government entities, have forced many healthcare facilities to establish an active foundation so that additional funds are directed to the foundation. These additional sources of funds can be used to either cover shortfalls in revenues or can be invested to provide interest or other forms of additional revenue.

Costs and Expenses

Deductions from the revenue sources take the form of either costs or expenses. *Costs and expenses*, in the income statement, are those items used up or incurred in the generation of revenues. For Hospital Anywhere USA, the largest of these expenses is generally salaries and benefits paid to employees.

The second largest category of expenses is *supplies and services*, as shown in **Exhibit 19–4**. Each patient for whom services are rendered requires some use of supplies (i.e., forms for patient information, swabs for testing, testing supplies, or food and beverages provided through food services).

The third largest item is the *provision for doubtful accounts* (bad debt expense/provision for bad debts), which is the adjustment for patient services that are expected not to be collected. Bad debt expense is the charge for not being able to collect patient accounts. Charges filed with third-party payers are reduced according to payment schedules established by these firms. This reduces the amount of revenue from the gross (full) amount billed to the net amount. The amount over that paid by the third-party payers is expected to be collected from the patient to whom services were provided. This refers to deductibles and copayments, which are amounts the patient pays over the reasonable and customary charges. However, with Medicare and Medicaid patients, it is illegal to go back and bill the patients for whatever Medicare and Medicaid doesn't pay. In some cases, the patient will not be able to make payments. These must be taken as further charges in the form of bad debts.

Depreciation is a deduction allowed by the Internal Revenue Service. This is a paper and pencil amount (accounting) and is not an actual use of cash sources. Once a building or piece of equipment is acquired, it may be "written off" over a designated period of time. The cost of the equipment is allocated to a specific time period and is used to reduce the net revenue and thus reduce taxes. For example, if a piece of diagnostic equipment having a 10-year life span is purchased for 5 million dollars, using one of the many methods allowed for the calculation of depreciation (straight-line), the depreciation amount per year would be $500,000 ($5,000,000 ÷ 10 years = $500,000 depreciation per year). As stated previously, this reduces income and will lead to fewer taxes being paid.

Depending on the size of the healthcare facility, additional costs may be incurred.

Cash Flow

As stated previously, cash is the lifeblood of a business. The *cash flow statement* shows one part of the financial stability of a firm. If all transactions were cash based, then this statement would be easy to prepare and interpret. For-profit entities are required by generally accepted accounting principles (GAAP) to report on an accrual basis. This means that revenue must be reported when earned, not necessarily when payment is received, and expenses are recognized when incurred, not paid. This requires several estimates during the reporting period. For example, if a service has been provided and a healthcare entity has a reasonable expectation of collection and can identify the amount to be collected, then it must be reported as revenue. Cash for the service may not be received until the next period.

If employees are paid every Friday and the reporting period ends on Thursday, then salaries must be accrued. For simplicity let us assume those salaries are $100,000 per week and no one works on the weekends. Each week the healthcare entity makes cash payments of $100,000 until the final week of the year. Since the reporting period ends on Thursday, the firm owes the employees $80,000 (4 days of pay) for services rendered. This amount must be recorded as an expense in the current period but does not require cash expenditure until the next reporting period.

The *bad debt expense* must likewise be estimated at the end of the year. The total amount of bad debts will not be known until all efforts to collect an account have been exhausted. This requires recognition of the bad debt expense for the reporting period (quarterly or yearly). The estimate is based on past experience in collection of accounts receivable, necessitated by adjustments for economic conditions. If 2% of the accounts receivable have been identified as bad in previous years and there was a major plant closing in the current reporting period, it could be expected that the amount collected would decrease and the bad debt expense would increase.

Preparation of the cash flow statement requires a thorough knowledge of the financial statements. Taking the cash balance at the beginning of the period and subtracting the ending cash balance provides the change in cash. The cash flow statement provides information explaining why cash changed. Financial statement items causing changes in cash are identified as operating, financing, and investing activities.

Operating Activities

Operating activities focus on the current portion of financial statements. They are the most important part of the cash flow analysis. Operating activities focus on the cash inflows and outflows from events that occur in the current operating period (**Exhibit 19–5**). Financing and investing activities can provide funds but are limited to the extent of the time to which they can provide cash flow. There are upper limits on

Exhibit 19–5 Cash Flow Operating Activities Section			
	(Dollars in millions)		
Cash flows from continuing activities	**2004**	**2003**	**2002**
Net income	$219	$657	$379
Adjustments to reconcile net income to net cash provided by continuing operating activities			
Provision for doubtful accounts	1,255	1,269	1,442
Depreciation and amortization	1,033	1,094	1,247
Income taxes	(219)	(66)	351
Settlement with federal government	840	0	0
Gains on sales of facilities	(34)	(297)	(744)
Impairment of long-lived assets	117	220	542
Loss from discontinued operating assets	0	0	153
Increase (decrease) in cash from operating assets and liabilities			
Accounts receivable	(1,678)	(1,463)	(1,229)
Inventories and other assets	90	(119)	(39)
Accounts payable and accrued expenses	(147)	(110)	(177)
Other	71	38	(9)
Net case provided by continuing operating activities	**$1,547**	**$1,223**	**$1,916**

the amount of debt that can be issued (borrowed) on stock that can be sold. Likewise, there is a limited amount of investments that can be sold to provide cash inflow. There is also a limit on the number of long-term assets that can be sold, and much like personal debt, there is a limit to the amount of money that can be borrowed.

Cash flow can be calculated in two ways, but the one preferred by most entities starts with the net income or loss from the income statement. All current assets and liabilities from the balance sheet must be analyzed to determine the impact on cash flow. If accounts receivable increases, how is cash impacted? Cash would decrease. If the amount of current assets represented by accounts receivable increases, you now have more paper and less cash coming in. From the perspective of the income statement, when services were provided you recorded the item as income. Net income is therefore higher than the cash generated from revenue, leading to the adjustment in net income on the cash flow statement. The same is true for all other current assets. There is an inverse relationship between the change in current assets and the impact on cash flow. If current assets increase, they will be deducted from net income. Or, vice versa, if current assets decrease, they will be added back to net income.

Current liabilities have the opposite effect. If any current liability increases, this adds to the cash balance. What is the impact on cash if current liabilities increase? The firm has acquired either goods or services without having a cash outflow. The cash balance is improved by acquisition of assets without having a cash outflow. All current liabilities have a direct relationship with the impact on cash flow. Increases are added to net income, and decreases are subtracted from net income. The result of adding or deducting changes in current assets and liabilities to net income provides cash flow from operating activities.

Financing Activities

The second portion of the cash flow statement is the *financing activities*, which focuses on long-term liabilities (those having a due date of longer than 1 year) or equity in the form of common or preferred stock (**Exhibit 19–6**). If long-term liabilities increase during the year, it provides cash inflow. The firm is borrowing money to use in the business. If long-term liabilities decrease, then this implies that the liabilities are being paid off, leading to a decrease in cash. Stock operates in the same manner. If either the common or preferred stock accounts increase, then the implication is that stock is used to finance firm activities. If they decrease, then stock is being repurchased and cash is leaving the firm. Likewise the payment of dividends on stock decreases cash outflow.

Investing Activities

The last part of the cash flow statement concerns the *investing activities* of an organization, as shown in **Exhibit 19–7**. This focuses mainly on the long-term assets of a business. If these assets are sold, cash inflows occur. On the other hand, if long-term assets are acquired, then cash is presumed to decrease.

Exhibit 19–6   Cash Flow Financing Activities Section

	(Dollars in millons)		
Cash flows from financing activities	2004	2003	2002
Issuance of long-term debt	$2,980	$1,037	$3
Net change in bank borrowing	(500)	200	(2,514)
Repayment of long-term debt	(2,058)	(1,572)	(147)
Issuance (repurchase) of common stock, net	(677)	(1,884)	8
Payment of cash dividends	(44)	(44)	(52)
Other	(37)	8	3
Net cash used in financing activities	**($336)**	**($2,255)**	**($2,699)**

Exhibit 19–7   Cash Flow Investing Activities Section

	(Dollars in millions)		
Cash flows from investing activities	2004	2003	2002
Purchase of property and equipment	($1,155)	($1,287)	($1,255)
Acquisitions of hospitals and health care entities	(350)	0	(215)
Spin-off of facilities to stockholders	0	886	0
Disposal of hospitals and health care entities	327	805	2,060
Change in investments	106	565	(294)
Investment in discontinued operations, net	0	0	677
Other	(15)	(44)	(3)
Net cash provided by (used in) investing activities	**($1,087)**	**$925**	**$970**

Exhibit 19–8	Summary of Cash Flows and Changes in Cash and Cash Equivalents		
(Dollars in millions)			
	2004	2003	2002
Net case provided by continuing operating activities	$1,547	$1,223	$1,916
Net cash provided by (used in) investing activities	($1,087)	$925	$970
Net cash used in financing activities	($336)	($2,255)	($2,699)
Change in cash and cash equivalents	124	(107)	187
Cash and cash equivalents at beginning of period	190	297	110
Cash and cash equivalents at end of period	$314	$190	$297

An increase in investments is shown as having a decrease in cash. A summary of these activities is presented in Exhibit 19–7 to indicate the change in cash and cash equivalents.

Adding each category, continuing operating, financing, and investing provides the change in cash and cash equivalents. Added to or subtracted from (if cash flow is negative as in 2003) cash and cash equivalents at the beginning of the period provides the amounts found on the balance sheet. The cash and cash equivalents account increased in both 2004 and 2002 and decreased in 2003, as shown in **Exhibit 19–8**, which provides a summary of all activities.

Schedule of Changes in Equity

The *Schedule of Changes in Equity* is required for all publicly reporting companies (governed by stock markets such as those sold on the New York Stock Exchange) and presents information for the reader to evaluate all changes in the owner's portion of the balance sheet.

Internal Accounting Information

Cost/Managerial Accounting

Although public-reporting, for-profit healthcare entities must issue financial statements to external users, not-for-profit entities are not required to report to the general public. Accounting information used for internal or management decisions is not available to the general public but is used by management and others working within an organization. This information may be as specific as the pay rate for individual employees or the costs to operate a function of the firm such as laboratories. For many healthcare workers, this is the area where management asks for employee input. This information is also used to evaluate the current operations of the organization and to solicit employee input to improve future operations. As previously mentioned, the amount of payments from third-party payers has declined in recent years. Healthcare facilities used to receive reimbursements based on costs of operation. However, with the advent of prospective payment systems, these amounts have generally been reduced. Thus, input from employees is needed to reduce costs and to improve customer services. As one nurse stated to the author, "I know the technical part of my job, but I am being asked to serve on committees that are looking at changing and improving business operations." Thus, the nurse needs to understand accounting information and how it can be used to support these changes.

Costs

Costs to be considered in making management decisions include differentiating between fixed and variable, direct and indirect, and marginal costs. Included in the discussion of costs is the term *relevant range*. To most, relevant range refers to the likely operating activity level expected to be incurred by a healthcare entity. For example, current staff can handle between 100 and 150 patients per day, which is the average use of the facilities. If the number of patients is either higher or lower than these numbers, costs must be reconsidered (i.e., reduce or add employees to provide services).

From a revenue perspective, previous discussion centered on correct coding and use of diagnosis-related groups and resource utilization groups. Discussion also centered on the collection of these revenue items and the impact on financial statements. When healthcare facilities were forced to more carefully evaluate their operations, they found many services offered were losing money. Because revenues were capped, cost containment became the issue.

Fixed Versus Variable Costs

Evaluating operations begins with the evaluation of the costs involved. First is the distinction between fixed and variable costs. *Fixed costs* do not change with levels of services. If you are dealing with a facility that has 100 beds, building costs such as depreciation will be the same regardless of whether there is 1 patient or 100 patients occupying a bed or beds. *Variable costs* do change with the increase of facility use. As more patients occupy the facility, costs such as food, medicines, and staff increase. These costs are variable because they change as the volume (number of patients or procedures) changes.

Direct Versus Indirect Costs

The second cost distinction is indirect versus direct costs. For an example, let's use the costs of laboratory services. The cost of the lab assistant who draws blood for analysis is a direct cost. Likewise, needles and other supplies are *direct costs*. The staff person who manages the facility, handles the paperwork for the patient upon arrival, or files the claim is an *indirect cost*.

Marginal costs are those costs related to providing additional services. Again, using the laboratory example, assume that the lab can handle 20 patients a day. If the lab is currently offering services to 15 patients, how much will it cost to provide additional services to one more patient? There will be no additional costs for the person drawing the blood sample; thus, there is no marginal cost associated with this service. There will be additional costs associated with the use of needles, bandages, and testing supplies. These are marginal costs. As long as revenue for these services increases more than the costs, services should be expanded.

Average costs are those costs divided by the total number of services provided. Let us assume that it costs $500 per day to maintain the lab. If the lab performs only one test on this day, then the average cost will be $500. However, if the lab performs five tests today, the average cost will be $100 per test. You can operate up to a certain point without expanding facilities, personnel, or equipment. As the number of tests increases, the average cost decreases (this is the relevant range). Let us assume that the facility expands these services to reach 40 tests per day but can process only 20 per day with the current number of employees. The relevant range would be up to 20 tests. More than 20 tests would require the addition of personnel or equipment.

Activity-Based Costing

Once the types of costs are identified, they need to be allocated to the specific services performed. With the limitations on cost recovery (revenue) imposed by third-party payers, healthcare entities must be aware of the costs to provide these services. Why should a facility pay $1.5 million for a magnetic resonance imaging machine and incur the other costs to maintain and staff the center when the revenues will not cover the costs? Recently, one area of thought in accounting has been introduced to help users of accounting information focus on the specific costs of providing services. This is called *activity-based costing (ABC)*.

ABC requires that you identify the cost drivers behind an activity. It requires that you break all services into specific functions and identify the costs associated with each activity. Assume you work in a physician's office and you need to determine the costs of a patient visit for a general exam. What activities are associated with the cost of providing these services? Let us assume the following, which is not a comprehensive example, for purposes of illustration:

- A general practitioner is paid $80,000 per year and spends on the average 15 minutes with each patient, seeing 24 patients per day. The physician works 45 weeks per year.
- A nurse is paid $35,000 per year and also spends 15 minutes with the patient.
- The receptionist is paid $24,000 and spends 5 minutes per patient in taking appointment calls and answering patient questions in the reception area.
- The cashier is paid $24,000 and spends 5 minutes per patient recording doctor information and verifying information for billing.
- All claims are entered electronically, and it takes a data recorder 10 minutes to fill out the electronic filing version. This person is paid $20,000.
- A bookkeeper is paid $25,000 per year to capture accounting information for the facility. The bookkeeper spends 10 minutes per patient on the average collecting and reporting data for management of the facility.
- A stethoscope costs $100 and lasts 2 years.
- Each tongue depressor costs $0.01.
- Each pair of latex gloves costs $0.01.
- Each of the previously mentioned individuals in the physician's office has a computer that costs $2000 and is used for 2 years.
- Utility service per patient is $1.00.
- The cost per patient for building (facility) in the form of depreciation is $1.50.

Based on this information, the following provides an analysis of the cost of providing patient services for a general physical examination. In the example shown in **Exhibit 19–9**, the patient is the cost driver.

The diagnosis-related group code for medium intervention activity is billed at $50.00. A third-party payer remits, on the average, 56% of billed amount, yielding a payment of $35.60. Additional amounts may be collected from the patient, but that is not assumed in this case. (As mentioned earlier, this is true for coinsurance, deductibles, and what is above the reasonable and customary costs with regular insurance. However, with Medicaid and with Medicare, other than billing the deductible and coinsurance, it is illegal to bill the patient for the amount of reimbursement not paid by the government.) Given the cost of the service at $41.21, there is a loss of $5.61 for each patient seen by the physician. This is where decision making using accounting data can improve the profitability of services, whether this is done by a single physician, nursing home, or hospital. What would you suggest to reduce the costs or improve the revenue? The physician and nurse spend 15 minutes per patient, but the others spend less time. Could the time the physician spends with each patient be reduced to increase the number of patients examined per year? Could there be additional physicians or nurse practitioners employed to increase the workload of others such as the receptionist and bookkeeper, thus reducing the costs of others such as the receptionist and cashier? If the number of patients seen increases, the building and computer cost per patient would be

Exhibit 19-9 Activity-Based Costing Example

Cost Driver	Cost	(Dollars in millions) Cost Per Patient	Comments
Physician	$80,000	$14.81	15 minutes per patient/24 patients per day/45 weeks
Nurse	$35,000	$6.48	15 minutes per patient/24 patients per day/45 weeks
Receptionist	$24,000	$4.44	5 minutes per patient/24 patients per day/45 weeks
Cashier	$24,000	$4.44	5 minutes per patient/24 patients per day/45 weeks
Data Recorder	$20,000	$3.70	10 minutes per patient/24 patients per day/45 weeks
Bookkeeper	$25,000	$4.62	10 minutes per patient/24 patients per day/45 weeks
Utility Services		$1.00	
Computers	$12,000	$.19	6 computers/$2,000 per computer cost/life of 2 years
Gloves		.01	
Tongue Depressor		.01	
Building Depreciation		$1.50	
Stethoscope	$100	.01	$100/lasts 2 years
Total		**$41.21**	

decreased. Another alternative is to either expand the nurse's responsibilities or to hire additional nurses to reduce the physician's time with patients.

One solution would be to evaluate the use of each part of the cost structure. In the previous example, the physician was limited to seeing 5400 patients per year. This is also the limitation for each of the other members of the physician's organization and is the cost driver. If the time spent with patients can be reduced to 10 minutes per patient, then the number of patients the physician can examine will be increased to 36 patients per day, or 8100 per year. This causes a decrease in the physician cost per patient to $9.88, and receptionist cost per patient to $2.96. The overall effect causes cost to be reduced to a level below the third-party payment that now exceeds cost.

Previously, different types of costs were defined. Using the example, we can now illustrate the costs. Fixed costs are those that do not change in total as volume (number of patients) increases. All costs except utilities, gloves, and tongue depressors are fixed. These costs are variable in that they change as the number of patients increases. As seen in the revenue and cost comparison, the physician's salary is fixed and as the number of patients increased, the physician's cost per patient decreased (average cost decreases). As with any fixed costs, you want to maximize the use and lower the costs to the lowest level.

Direct costs are those related to the generation of revenues. In this case, the physician and nurse are considered direct costs of providing services, as are the gloves and tongue depressors. The other costs are considered indirect because they are not directly related to production of revenue. Why is this distinction needed? If you are trying to determine whether or not to expand services, you might want to look at the direct costs. Can you cover the direct costs of providing services? If so, then each patient or procedure will add to the profitability of the healthcare entity. For example, in the original illustration, if you can cover the direct costs (physician, nurse, gloves, and tongue depressor—$21.31), then additional amounts received can be applied to the indirect costs. The fixed costs will remain if a facility operates or closes for the weekend or vacations. If you can cover the direct cost, then any excess amount would be used to help cover fixed costs.

Marginal costs are those that increase as additional services are provided. Which costs in the illustration change as additional patients are added? Only the costs of the gloves and tongue depressor are marginal costs. What will it cost to provide service for one additional patient? When evaluating whether or not to accept additional patients, you need to consider the impact on the organization. If no new costs are added for providing additional services, as long as the additional revenue exceeds the additional cost, then the service should be provided. To clarify this point, assume that a third-party insurer approaches your organization offering a new client base consisting of local county employees. However, the insurer will pay a lower amount than that provided by other insurers. If you can determine the marginal costs of the services to be provided, the marginal costs may be less than the revenue received, increasing the contribution to firm profitability. This would benefit the organization.

Conclusion

Employees of healthcare facilities are being asked to improve patient services by generating additional revenue and becoming a valuable member of the management team. Correctly identifying services before filing claims with third parties can improve revenue collection. Additionally, making recommendations for more efficient use of services to minimize costs of these services is important for continuing organizational success. Can the healthcare entity substitute services for those currently being offered? Can someone in an organization provide the same quality services as others? For example, can I use a licensed practical nurse in place of a registered nurse? (This decision would be best only if the work performed by the person was appropriate at the licensed practical nurse level.) This is one of the major issues affecting health care today.

Discussion Questions

1. Why should you be familiar with the balance sheet? Why is it important to the organization? And what area of the balance sheet would you consider the most critical?
2. Comparing costs in this chapter, which costs do you have little control over and why? Which costs would be most important if you are expanding your services?
3. How would you know if the organization is a for-profit or a not-for-profit based on the information available from the balance sheet and the income statement?
4. Goodwill and patents are considered what types of assets?
5. Which asset is considered the lifeblood of the organization, and why?

Glossary of Terms

Accounts (Patients) Receivable—these may be represented by amounts owed by either patients to whom the organization has provided services or by claims filed with third-party providers such as insurance companies.

Accounts Payables—claims on assets. These are short term in nature and are generally expected to be paid in 30–120 days based on the type of claim, but can be unpaid up to 1 year.

Accumulated Depreciation—the sum of the annual depreciation charges subtracted from the plant and equipment balance providing a net figure.

Activity-Based Costing (ABC)—a costing system that requires that you break all services into specific functions and identify the cost drivers associated with each activity

Assets—those items that provide future cash flow or have future economic benefit.

Average Costs—those costs divided by the total number of services provided.

Balance Sheet—a form that consists of the assets, liabilities, and equity.

Buildings—the physical facilities in which patient services are provided.

Cash Flow Statement—a form that provides information explaining why cash changed. Financial statement items causing changes in cash are identified as operating, financing, and investing activities.

Construction in Progress—an account indicating buildings that have not been completed but are being built. The account indicates progress toward completion.

Costs and Expenses—in the income statement, those items used up or incurred in the generation of revenues.

Current Assets—those items that will be used to generate revenue in either 1 year or the operating period, whichever is longer (most often this is 1 year).

Deferred Taxes—the differences between income reported in financial statements and that paid to the U.S. Treasury.

Depreciation—an accounting charge wherein the balance of the equipment and buildings is systematically written off over a period of time.

Equipment—may be items such as X-ray or CT machines or less complex items such as patient beds.

Financial Activities—long-term liabilities (obligations have a due date of longer than 1 year) or equity in the form of common or preferred stock.

Fund Balance—section of the stockholder's equity of a not-for-profit organization.

Goodwill—when an entity purchases another organization and there is an excess amount paid for the net assets of the purchased entity that exceeds market value. This excess amount is goodwill.

Income Statement—a financial statement that captures information about revenue sources, expenses, and costs of doing business during a period of time.

Intangible Assets—generally, those items that have no physical presence but do have value in the form of legal rights to use or sell an asset.

Inventory—items such as drugs in the pharmacy, surgical supplies, items maintained in nursing stations, and drinks and/or food in the cafeteria.

Investment Activities—the long-term assets of an organization.

Investments—classified as long-term in nature in that they are held for income purposes. These may be a result of using excess cash to invest in items such as other organizations, joint ventures, stocks, or bonds of other organizations or donations received from external parties.

Liabilities—claims on the assets of an organization. The claims are those of creditors who have provided resources such as buildings and equipment but have not been fully paid.

Long-Term Debt—such items as mortgages and bonds issued to borrow money. This debt will not be paid in the current year or operating period.

Marginal Costs—those costs that are related to providing additional services.

Net Assets—in not-for-profit organizations the result of subtracting liabilities from assets.

Net Worth—difference between the assets and liabilities of an organization is the equity, or in the personal loan application example, net worth.

Operating Activities—the cash inflows and outflows from events that occur in the current operating period.

Preferred or Common Stock—for-profit corporate firms raise funds by issuing these stocks. These stocks represent ownership shares in an organization.

Provision for Doubtful Accounts—the adjustment for patient services that are expected not to be collected.

Relevant Range—the likely operating activity level expected to be incurred by a healthcare entity.

Retained Earnings—an account used by the accounting function to balance the books at the end of the year.

Schedule of Changes in Equity—required for all publicly reporting companies, information for the reader to evaluate all changes in the owner's portion of the balance sheet.

Tangible Assets—the largest item on a for-profit health care entity's balance sheet, probably buildings and equipment.

Temporary Investments—cash equivalents because they can be sold quickly with little or no loss in value.

Appendix

(All amounts are dollars in millions, except per share amounts.)

Hospital Anywhere USA Consolidated Balance Sheets, December 31, 2004 and 2003		
Assets	**2004**	**2003**
Current Assets:		
Cash and cash equivalents	$314	$190
Accounts receivable, less allowance for doubtful accounts of $1,583 and $1,567	2,211	1,873
Inventories	396	383
Income taxes receivable	197	178
Other	1,335	973
Total Current Assets	**4,453**	**3,597**
Property and equipment at cost:		
Land	793	813
Buildings	6,021	6,108
Equipment	7,045	6,721
Construction in progress	431	442
Total Property and Equipment	**14,290**	**14,084**
Accumulated depreciation	(5,810)	(5,594)
	8,480	8,490
Investments of insurance subsidiary	1,371	1,457
Instruments in and advances to affiliates	779	654
Intangible assets, net of accumulated amortization of $785 and $644	2,155	2,319
Other	330	368
Total assets	**$17,568**	**$16,885**
Liabilities	2004	2003
Current Liabilities:		
Account payable	693	657
Accrued salaries	352	403
Other accrued expenses	1,135	897
Government settlement accrual	840	
Long-term debt due within one year	1,121	1,160
Total Current Liabilities	**4,141**	**3,117**
Long-term debt	5,631	5,284
Professional liability risks, deferred taxes, and other liabilities	2,050	2,104
Minority interests in equity of consolidated entities	572	763
Forward purchase contracts and put options	769	
Total Liabilities	**13,163**	**11,268**
Stockholders equity:		
Common stock $.01 par; authorized 1,600,000,000 voting shares,		
50,000,000 nonvoting shares; outstanding 521,991,700 voting shares		
and 21,000,000 nonvoting shares—2004 and 543,272,900 voting shares		
and 21,000,000 nonvoting shares—2003	5	6
Capital in excess of par value		951
Other	9	8
Accumulated other comprehensive income	52	53
Retained earnings	4,339	4,599
Total Stockholder's Equity	**4,405**	**5,617**
Total Liabilities and Stockholder's Equity	**$17,568**	**$16,885**

Appendix
(All amounts are dollars in millions, except per share amounts.)

Hospital Anywhere USA Consolidated Statement of Cash Flow for the Years Ended December 31, 2004, 2003, and 2002

Cash Flows from Continuing Activities:	2004	2003	2002
Net Income	$219	$657	$379
Adjustments to reconcile net income to net cash provided by continuing operating activities:			
Provision for doubtful accounts	1,255	1,269	1,442
Depreciation and amortization	1,033	1,094	1,247
Income taxes	(219)	(66)	351
Settlement with Federal government	840	0	0
Gains on sales of facilities	(34)	(297)	(744)
Impairment of long-lived assets	117	220	542
Loss from discontinued operating assets	0	0	153
Increase (decrease) in cash from operating assets and liabilities:			
Accounts receivable	(1,678)	(1,463)	(1,229)
Inventories and other assets	90	(119)	(39)
Accounts payable and accrued expenses	(147)	(110)	(177)
Other	71	38	(9)
Net case provided by continuing operating activities	**$1,547**	**$1,223**	**$1,916**
Cash flows from financing activities:	**2004**	**2003**	**2002**
Issuance of long-term debt	$2,980	$1,037	$3
Net change in bank borrowing	(500)	200	(2,514)
Repayment of long-term debt	(2,058)	(1,572)	(147)
Issuance (repurchase) of common stock, net	(677)	(1,884)	8
Payment of cash dividends	(44)	(44)	(52)
Other	(37)	8	3
Net cash used in financing activities	**($336)**	**($2,255)**	**($2,699)**
Cash flows from investing activities:	**2004**	**2003**	**2002**
Purchase of property and equipment	($1,155)	($1,287)	($1,255)
Acquisitions of hospitals and health care entities	(350)	0	(215)
Spin-off of facilities to stockholders	0	886	0
Disposal of hospitals and health care entities	327	805	2,060
Change in investments	106	565	(294)
Investment in discontinued operations, net	0	0	677
Other	(15)	(44)	(3)
Net cash provided by (used in) investing activities	**($1,087)**	**$925**	**$970**

	2004	2003	2002
Net cash provided by continuing operating activities	1,547	1,223	1,916
Net cash provided by (used in) investing activities	(1,087)	925	970
Net cash used in financing activities	(336)	(2,255)	(2,699)
Change in cash and cash equivalents	124	(107)	187
Cash and cash equivalents at beginning of period	190	297	110
Cash and cash equivalents at end of period	**$314**	**$190**	**$297**
Interest payments	$489	$475	$566
Income tax payments, net of refunds	$516	$634	($139)

Hospital Anywhere USA Consolidated Income Statement for the Years Ended December 31, 2004, 2003, and 2002

	2004	2003	2002
Revenues	$16,670	$16,657	$18,681
Salaries and benefits	6,639	6,694	7,766
Supplies	2,640	2,645	2,901
Other operating expenses	3,085	3,251	3,816
Provision for doubtful accounts	1,255	1,269	1,442
Depreciation and amortization	1,033	1,094	1,247
Interest expense	559	471	561
Equity in earnings of affiliates	(126)	(90)	(112)
Settlement with Federal government	840	0	0
Gains on sales of facilities	(34)	(297)	(744)
Impairment of long-lived assets	117	220	542
Restructuring of operations and investigation related costs	62	116	111
Total expenses	**16,070**	**15,373**	**17,530**
Income from continuing operations before minority interests and income taxes	66	1,284	1,151
Minority interests in earnings of consolidated entities	84	57	70
Income from continuing operations before income taxes	516	1,227	1,081
Provision for income taxes	297	570	549
Income from continuing operations	219	657	532
Discontinued operations:			
Loss from operations of discontinued businesses, net of income tax benefit of $26			(80)
Loss of disposals of discontinued businesses			(73)
Net income	$219	$657	$379
Basic earnings per share:			
Income from continuing operations	$0.39	$1.12	$0.82
Discontinued operations:			
Loss from operations of discontinued businesses			(.12)
Loss on disposals of discontinued businesses			(.11)
Net income	**$0.39**	**$1.12**	**$0.59**
Diluted earnings per share:			
Income from continuing operations	$0.39	$1.12	$0.82
Discontinued operations:			
Loss from operations of discontinued businesses			(.12)
Loss on disposals of discontinued businesses			(.11)
Net income	**$0.39**	**$1.12**	**$0.59**

Financial Analysis: Improving Your Decision Making

Paul Bayes, DBA Accounting, MS Economics, BS Accounting

OBJECTIVES

- Provides qualitative analysis examples using the financial statements.
- Identifies key financial ratios used to improve your decision-making process.
- Explains major ratio categories that include: Liquidity, Activity, Leverage, Profitability, and Net trade cycle.
- Discusses ratio categories, why they provide useful information for the organization, and how they affect the company's financial performance.

Numbers by themselves are data, not information. To be an informed and effective decision maker you must be able to convert raw data (numbers) into information. Putting financial data in a format that allows comparisons whether within your organization or between firms makes the information meaningful.

Benchmarking is a process that provides comparisons with the best practices of other organizations. These firms do not have to be within the same industry, but traditionally comparisons are based within specific industries. This is a limiting factor in identifying best practices but simplifies the comparisons.

The purpose of this chapter is to introduce you to financial analysis and to improve your understanding of the accounting information presented earlier. An improved understanding of financial information leads to better future policies and strategic plans. Analysis may be either qualitative (nonfinancial) or quantitative (financial). Most of this chapter focuses on quantitative analysis because this information is more readily available. Qualitative analysis examples are provided within the text of quantitative examples. All examples use the financial statements of Hospital Anywhere USA, a for-profit entity. Selected information from Children's Hospital, a not-for-profit entity, is provided as a contrast to that of Hospital Anywhere USA. The financial statements of Retirement Homes, Inc., facility, a not-for-profit firm, are also provided as an example of a different type of not-for-profit facility. Differences in operating not-for-profit entities versus for-profit are noted.

Qualitative analysis requires a search of not only information in financial statements but also information from external sources. Stockholders' annual reports, not included in this text, along with financial statements, provide information. For example, the section on Management Discussion and Analysis provides information not found elsewhere in the financial statements, including strategic impetus and changes in the market structure. Other parts of the annual reports yield information as to accounting practices (footnotes), segment information, and risk. If an organization has subsidiaries (parts of the firm either partially or wholly owned by the parent company), information on segment information reveals reliance on operations of certain products, services, or geographic areas.

The Securities and Exchange Commission (SEC) for publicly traded stock companies requires supplementary information. Additional information at the SEC Edgar Database can be found at www.sec.gov/edgarhp.htm. Information in Form 10-K and Form 10-Q reports is more comprehensive than the annual reports. In 10-Q (quarterly) reports, you can find information reported for each quarter of a firm. Rather than waiting until annual reports are issued, analysts can better track a firm's progress using these quarterly reports. Although the financial statements are the main focus of annual reports, they only make up a small portion. To illustrate, the annual report of Hospital Anywhere USA totals 51 pages of which the basic financial statements, including summaries, equal 7 pages.

Common Size Balance Sheets

Most of the focus in this chapter is quantitative and based on financial statements and the standard ratios found in both accounting and finance literature. One example of financial analysis is the use of *common size financial statements*. In the balance sheet and income statement, analysts select one number and then divide into all other numbers in the statement. Total assets (balance sheets) are used as the baseline figure in balance sheets. Either gross revenue (sales) or net revenue (sales) (income statement) is used as the basis for income statements. Gross revenue is the total sales made by a firm. The difference with the net figure is deductions such as discounts and returns have been removed. Dividing all items in this set of financial statements and comparing several years provide a quick method to evaluate trends (changes). The caveat is that a 2-year time frame may not be long enough to fully evaluate changes in operations (**Exhibit 20–1**).

Exhibit 20–1   Hospital Anywhere USA Consolidated Balance Sheets, December 31, 2004 and 2003

Assets	Dollars in Millions 2004		2003	
Current Assets				
Cash and cash equivalents	$314	1.79%	$190	1.13%
Accounts receivable, less allowance for doubtful accounts of $1,583 and $1,567	2,211	12.59%	1,873	11.09%
Inventories	396	2.25%	383	2.27%
Income taxes receivable	197	1.12%	178	1.05%
Other	1,335	7.6%	973	5.76%
Total Current Assets	**4,453**	**25.35%**	**3,597**	**21.30%**
Property and equipment at cost:				
Land	793	4.51%	813	4.81%
Buildings	6,021	34.27%	6,108	36.17%
Equipment	7,045	40.10%	6,721	39.80%
Construction in progress	431	2.45%	442	2.62%
Total Property and Equipment	**14,290**	**81.34%**	**14,084**	**83.41%**
Accumulated depreciation	−5,810	−33.07%	−5,594	−33.13%
	8,480	48.27%	8,490	50.28%
Investments of insurance subsidiary	1,371	7.8%	1,457	8.63%
Investments in and advances to affiliates	779	4.43%	654	3.87%
Intangible assets, net of accumulated amortization of $785 and $644	2,155	12.27%	2,319	13.73%
Other	330	1.88%	368	2.18%
Total Assets	**$17,568**	**100%**	**$16,885**	**100%**
Liabilities				
Current Liabilities				
Accounts payable	693	3.94%	657	3.89%
Accrued salaries	352	2.00%	403	2.39%
Other accrued expenses	1,135	6.46%	897	5.31%
Government settlement accrual	840	4.78%		
Long-term debt due within one year	1,121	6.38%	1,160	6.87%
Total Current Liabilities	**4,141**	**23.57%**	**3,117**	**18.46%**
Long-term debt	5,631	32.05%	5,284	31.29%
Professional liability risks, deferred taxes, and other liabilities	2,050	11.67%	2,104	12.46%
Minority interests in equity of consolidated entities	572	3.26%	763	4.92%
Forward purchase contracts and put options	769	4.38%		0%
Total Liabilities	**13,163**	**74.93%**	**11,268**	**66.73%**

(*continues*)

Exhibit 20–1 Hospital Anywhere USA Consolidated Balance Sheets, December 31, 2004 and 2003 *(continued)*

Assets	Dollars in Millions 2004		2003	
Stockholders equity				
Common stock $.01 par; authorized 1,600,000,000 voting shares; 50,000,000 nonvoting shares; outstanding 521,991,700 voting shares and 21,000,000 nonvoting shares—2004 and 543,272,900 voting shares and 21,000,000 nonvoting shares—2003	5	.03%	6	.04%
Capital in excess of par value			951	5.63%
Other	9	0%	8	0%
Accumulated other comprehensive income	52	.30%	53	.31%
Retained earnings	4,339	24.07%	4,599	27.24%
Total Stockholders' Equity	4,405	25.07%	5,617	33.27%
Total Liabilities and Stockholders Equity	**$17,568**	**100%**	**$16,885**	**100%**

Exhibit 20–1 illustrates some minor changes in the assets, liabilities, and stockholders' equity from 2003 to 2004. The cash and cash equivalents increased from 1.13% in 2003 to 1.79% in 2004. This trend indicates that Hospital Anywhere USA had more cash and cash equivalents as a percentage of total assets in 2004 than it had in 2003. This increase may be the result of management anticipation of a need for more cash or a better job of collecting patient accounts. Management may have also reduced expenses, thus improving cash flow. However, the accounts receivable percentages increased from 11.09% to 12.59%, indicating an increase in the amount of "paper" held and collection slowed. This point illustrates that the person doing the financial analysis may have to perform further evaluations rather than look at one piece of information. Total current assets also increased as a percentage of total assets, indicating that Hospital Anywhere USA was holding more liquid assets (ones that can be converted into cash quickly) in 2004 than in 2003.

Three changes occurred in the items defined as long-term assets. First, the buildings account decreased from 36.17% to 34.27% of total assets, which indicates that Hospital Anywhere USA may have sold off some of its buildings. As this account illustrates, the dollar value of buildings in fact declined from $6,108 to $6,021. Footnotes accompanying the financial statements state that three properties were sold. The second change indicates construction in progress decreased slightly, which might provide evidence of some building projects either being completed or abandoned. The third change in these assets occurred in intangible assets, which showed a decrease of 1.46% from the previous year. This could be to the result of the following:

• Selling off parts of the organization, thereby reducing goodwill
• Selling off some patents
• Expired patent rights
• A more aggressive manner used to write off existing patents or other intangible assets

One item that appears in conjunction with this account is that the amortization, systematic writing off of intangible assets, increased from $644 to $785. This explains, at least in part, the decrease in intangible assets but does not provide evidence as to the reason for the increase in write-offs. This would come with additional research in the schedules and notes accompanying the statements.

Current liabilities show one item changing drastically. The government settlement accrual went from zero in 2003 to $840 in 2004, indicating the settlement with the government over billing charges that cost the firm $840. The percentage change was from zero to 4.78%. Long-term debt, forward purchase contracts, and put options also went from zero to $769, making a percentage change from zero to 4.38%. A *forward purchase contract* is where one party agrees to buy a commodity at a specific price on a specific future date and the other party agrees to make the sale. In this case, the agreement was for the repurchase of a limited number of common shares of Hospital Anywhere USA. A *put option* provides the right to sell stock at a specified price in the future. This again was related to the repurchase of the stock from a third party. In both instances a third party purchased shares of Hospital Anywhere USA stock in the market, and the hospital entered into a contract to purchase a set number of shares at a specified price from this third-party entity. Total liabilities also increased from 66.73% to 74.93%, indicating that a larger proportion of the business was financed using debt.

Analysis of stockholders equity indicates that the capital in excess of par values declined from $951 to zero, going from 5.63% to zero. Although no information is directly available, a schedule that accompanies the financial statements provides information concerning this issue. Hospital Anywhere USA repurchased 21,281,200 shares of stock. Part of that repurchase plan would eliminate this account. A second item that negatively impacted the capital in excess of par value account was the reclassification of forward purchase contracts and put options to temporary equity. This was a result of action taken by the Financial Accounting Standards Board, which regulates reporting practices. Retained earnings declined from 27.24% to 24.70% as a result, partially, of the aforementioned reclassification.

Common Size Income Statements

Information in income statements is calculated in the same manner. The baseline number for analysis is either the gross revenue or net revenue. All items in the income statement are divided by this base figure, which converts the information into a common basis to detect trends (changes) in operations (**Exhibit 20–2**).

Salaries and benefits decreased slightly, which indicates that Hospital Anywhere USA may have undertaken some cost control or containment measures during the 2004 reporting period. Other operating expenses also decreased from 19.52% to 18.51%. These would include items such as utilities, property taxes, professional fees (legal and accounting), maintenance, rent, and lease expenses. Interest expense and settlement with the federal government increased during this time period. With the aforementioned increase in debt financing, from the balance sheet analysis, there may be an increase in interest expenses. Unless a firm can negotiate a lower rate than that used in previous financing arrangements, the increased use of debt raises the risk to creditors, which causes the interest rate to increase. A simple explanation is that as more debt is issued, even at the same rate, there will be an increase in interest cost. The settlement with the federal government went from zero to 5.04%. This had a major impact on the profitability of the firm. The only remaining item that had a major change, other than summative categories, such as income from continuing operations before taxes and income from continuing operations, was provision for income taxes. This amount decreased from 3.42% to 1.78%. This may be a result of lower income or having either tax credits or deferred taxes that can be used to reduce the current year's taxable income.

Exhibit 20–2   Hospital Anywhere USA Consolidated Income Statements for the Years Ended December 31, 2004, and 2003

	Dollars in Millions			
	2004		2003	
Revenues	$16,670	100.00%	$16,657	100.00%
Salaries and Benefits	6,639	39.83%	6,694	40.19%
Supplies	2,640	15.84%	2,645	15.88%
Other operating expenses	3,085	18.51%	3,251	19.52%
Provision for doubtful accounts	1,255	7.53%	1,269	7.62%
Depreciation and amortization	1,033	6.20%	1,094	6.57%
Interest expense	559	3.35%	471	2.83%
Equity in earnings of affiliates	−126	−0.76%	−90	−0.54%
Settlement with Federal government	840	5.04%	0	0.00%
Gains on sales of facilities	−34	−0.20%	−297	−1.78%
Impairment of long-lived assets	117	0.70%	220	1.32%
Restructuring of operations and investigation related costs	62	0.37%	116	0.70%
Total Expenses	**16,070**	**96.40%**	**15,373**	**92.29%**
Income from continuing operations before minority interests and income taxes	66	0.40%	1,284	7.71%
Minority interests in earnings of consolidated entities	84	0.50%	57	0.34%
Income from continuing operations before income taxes	516	3.10%	1,227	7.37%
Provision for income taxes	297	1.78%	570	3.42%
Income from continuing operations	219	1.31%	657	3.94%
Discontinued operations:				
Loss from operations of discontinued businesses, net of income tax benefit of $26				
Loss of disposals of discontinued businesses		0.00%		
Net Income	$219	1.31%	$657	3.94%
Basic earnings per share:				
Income from continuing operations	$0.39	0.00%	$1.12	0.01%
Discontinued operations:				
Loss from operations of discontinued businesses				
Loss on disposals of discontinued businesses				
Net income	**$0.39**	**0.00%**	**$1.12**	**0.01%**
Diluted earnings per share:				
Income from continuing operations	$0.39	0.00%	$1.12	0.01%
Discontinued operations:				

| | Dollars in Millions | | | |
	2004		2003	
Loss from operations of discontinued businesses				
Loss on disposals of discontinued businesses				
Net income	$0.39	0.00%	$1.12	0.01%

Tax credits are provided in the tax laws and allow firms to carry losses incurred in any year back for 2 years and forward for 20 years. Deferred taxes are a result of differences between financial reporting tax requirements and those used for reporting taxes to local, state, and federal government units. In some cases, alternative inventory and depreciation may be used for reporting, thus creating a difference in the amounts owed and the payments may be deferred (postponed).

Financial Ratio Analysis

Key financial ratios can be classified into five categories:

1. Liquidity ratios
2. Activity ratios
3. Leverage ratios
4. Profitability ratios
5. Net trade cycle

Each category provides an analysis of different aspects of the organization and indicates how well the firm is managed. The following ratios are limited in number, and use varies by type of organization. The ones presented here are considered the more standard ratios for most businesses. Industry-specific ratios would be used to provide additional information. The names used are the standard ones, and those used by different firms and professional organizations may be different. To provide a more complete analysis, the calculated ratios should be compared with industry averages. Several services provide this information on a for-fee basis. When making the comparisons, you must evaluate each firm by both size and type. For hospitals, the data are provided by size and geographic regions. The information can be obtained from sources for other types of not-for-profit organizations.

Liquidity Ratios

Liquidity ratios are concerned with short-term (current) items. The two most frequently used liquidity ratios are the current ratio and quick or acid-test ratio. The *current ratio* divides the current assets by current liabilities. This provides one measure of a firm's ability to pay short-term obligations, which arise in the course of operations or within one operating cycle (usually 1 year). For example, if the calculated ratio is two, this is interpreted to mean that you have 2 dollars in current assets for every 1 dollar in current liabilities. The limitation is that this ratio does not measure the true ability to pay obligations. A skewed example might be useful for improved understanding of this limitation. If current assets are $2 million and current liabilities are $1 million, then there are twice as many dollars in assets as there are in liabilities. However, let us assume that the current assets consist of $1 in cash and inventories make up the remainder. All current liabilities are due tomorrow. The original answer shows that obligations can be met, but, as the skewed example shows, the current debt cannot be met.

Now let's figure the actual liquidity ratio:

Ratio	How Calculated	2004	2003
Current ratio	Current assets/Current liabilities	$4,453/$4141 = 1.08	$3,597/$3,117 = 1.15
Quick ratio	Current assets – Inventories/ Current liabilities	$4,057/$4141 = .98	$3,214/$3,117 = 1.03

The current ratio declined from 1.15 to 1.08 in the preceding results, indicating the ability to pay short-term obligations has weakened since 2003. Either current liabilities grew faster than current assets or current assets declined more rapidly than current liabilities. The common size balance sheet shows that current liabilities increased faster than current assets did.

The *quick or acid-test ratio* provides additional information to evaluate the ability to meet short-term obligations. To compute this ratio, inventory must be subtracted from current assets. Sometimes items defined as "prepaid" may also be subtracted. The reason for the elimination of inventory from the numerator is that these items cannot be converted into cash quickly without a loss in value.

In the previous example, the current and quick ratio both decreased. However, most current assets of Hospital Anywhere USA can be defined as quick assets (91.1% and 89.3%, respectively, for 2004 and 2003), so the current assets are highly liquid. If items other than cash and cash equivalents plus accounts receivable are eliminated, the quick ratio becomes 0.61 and 0.67, respectively, for 2004 and 2003. Two years is not enough time to make a completely informed judgment about the trends, but the trend is showing a decline. This is one indication of a decline in the ability of the hospital to meet its current obligations.

Activity Ratios

Activity ratios measure the liquidity and efficiency of asset management. The *accounts receivable collection period* measures the average time it takes a firm to collect its accounts (patient/insurance) receivables. The quicker a firm can convert the receivables to cash, the quicker it can pay its obligations or have cash for opportunities that may arise. This ratio is calculated by dividing the accounts receivable by the average daily revenue. Average daily revenue is calculated by dividing the revenue from the income statement by 365. This measures on the average how many times the organization has converted the receivables into cash.

Inventory turnover is found by dividing the cost of goods sold by inventory (accounting) or revenue by inventory (finance). This measures how quickly inventory is sold and is important for firms with products that deteriorate or have a short shelf life (drugs, surgical supplies).

Ratio	How Calculated	2004	2003
Accounts	Accounts receivable/ Receivable collection period	$2,211/($16,670/ 365) = (Revenue/ 365) = 45.67 days	$1,873/($16,657/365) = 45.63 days
Inventory	Cost of goods sold/ Turnover inventory or Revenue/Inventory	$16,670/$396 = 42.09	$16,657/$383 = 43.49

The preceding ratios for Hospital Anywhere USA indicate that the collection of accounts receivable takes an average of approximately 45 days. Once a patient leaves a facility after receiving medical services, the hospital is waiting for money from either the patient or a third-party payer 45 days before the claim is settled. Inventory turnover, from an accounting perspective, cannot be calculated for this hospital because cost of goods sold is not separately reported and cannot be calculated. This ratio is usually provided as supplemental information to the financial statements. If it had a subsidiary that sold medical items or the information was provided in the income statements, then the accounting ratio could be calculated. This is a standard ratio in all accounting literature. Finance literature supports a different calculation. As indicated previously, revenue is divided by the inventory. The turnover has increased slightly. For similar firms to Hospital Anywhere USA, this number would be quite high compared with standard manufacturing organizations.

Management's effectiveness in using assets to generate revenues can be measured by using two ratios. First, *fixed asset turnover* measures how well management is using the long-term assets of the organization to generate revenue. As the balance sheet for this firm shows, this asset consists primarily of buildings and equipment used for providing patient services. For a healthcare organization, this is important in that supplying beds and using equipment creates billable revenue. Fixed asset turnover is found by dividing net revenues by net property, plant, and equipment (cost of property, plant, and equipment minus accumulated depreciation). *Total asset turnover* measures how management is using all assets of the organization to generate revenue. The measure is found by dividing net revenues by all assets.

Ratio	How Calculated	2004	2003
Fixed asset turnover	Net revenue/Net property, plant, and equipment	$16,670/$8480 = 1.966	$16,657/$8490 = 1.96
Total asset turnover	Net revenue/Total assets	$16,670/$17,568 = .949	$16,657/$16,885 = .986

Evaluation of the preceding indicates a minor change in the use of assets to generate revenue. Fixed asset turnover was relatively stable, whereas total asset turnover has declined slightly. However, this may be caused by the increase in current assets as previously discussed.

Leverage Ratios

Leverage ratios, also called *capital structure ratios*, are one measure of how an organization is financed. For-profit firms can either borrow funds using a debt instrument (notes payable or bonds) or sell shares of stock (equity financing). Creditors look at this important ratio to determine if they will provide more funds to an organization or if the cost of funds (interest) will be changed. Remember that A = L − K. If an organization fails to continue in business because of financial setbacks (bankruptcy), the assets of the organization will be sold and distributed first to the creditors. If there is a remainder, the owners (those holding shares of stock) receive this amount. Thus, the more debt that you have, the more risk you take on. This risk limits the amount of debt that creditors are willing to extend and raises the cost to finance projects.

However, on the positive side, debt can be used to improve the investment of stockholders (owners) of an organization. For instance, if you can borrow funds at 6% and invest at 10%, then the stockholders receive the differential. Profits are increased, and these are reinvested in the firm. For Hospital Anywhere

USA, the following three ratios provide an analysis of how much debt is used to finance the organization and the amount of debt compared with equity used to fund the operations and long-term projects of the firm:

Ratio	How Calculated	2004	2003
Debt ratio	Total liabilities/Total assets	$13,163/$17,568 = .749	$11,268/$16,885 = .667
Long-term debt to total capitalization	Long-term debt/ (Long-term debt – Stockholders' equity)	$9,022/($9,022 – $4,405) = .672	$8,151/($8,151 – $5617) = .592
Debt to equity	Total liabilities/ Stockholders' equity	$13,163/4405 = 2.988	$11,268/$5617 = 2.006

The *debt ratio* measures how much of the total assets have been financed using debt (obligations to pay a future amount of funds). The trend from 2003 to 2004, up from 66.7% to 74.9%, shows an increase, which indicates that more of the operations were financed using debt and a future outflow of funds either in interest costs or repayment of debt will be required. This debt may also increase the interest rate charged on these funds based on the increased risk. Remember that analysis of the common size income statement revealed that interest costs were higher in 2004 than in 2003. The other ratios confirm this trend in that debt has increased in relation to total funding (L − K) and compared with the use of equity financing (stocks).

Long-term debt to total capitalization (long-term debt divided by long-term debt plus stockholders' equity) shows that more long-term debt is being used for financing (67.2% up from 59.2%). This number ($9,022 for 2004) is found by subtracting total current liabilities from total liabilities and dividing by long-term debt ($9,022) plus $4,405.

Debt to equity also indicates a larger use of debt financing in the business. This ratio indicates that debt was used approximately twice as often as equity in 2003 and almost three times as much in 2004. Firms with stable revenues can borrow more (increase their debt) than others with revenues that fluctuate. However, there is generally a limitation on the amount of funds that will be provided for operations.

Profitability Ratios

Profitability ratios measure how well a firm is doing in its basic operations. These ratios measure the percentage that revenues minus certain costs exceed the revenues. They also determine how well the assets of the organization and owner's investment are being used. These ratios are the gross profit margin, operating profit margin, net profit margin, return on total assets, and return on equity.

Because Hospital Anywhere USA does not engage in selling physical assets, such as beds and drugs, and these items are not reported separately, the gross profit margin is not applicable. The gross profit amount is determined by subtracting from revenues the cost of goods sold. However, there is no cost of goods sold for this hospital—thus, this amount cannot be calculated.

The *operating profit margin* is found by looking at the net revenues from the normal course of business, providing healthcare services, and subtracting all expenses of operations necessary to generate these revenues. This measure, sometimes called EBIT (earnings before interest and taxes), indicates whether the firm is covering its costs of operations. This amount is then divided by net revenues. Both 2004 and 2003 indicate a reasonable operating profit margin. For 2004, this means that Hospital Anywhere USA is covering operating costs and has approximately 12 cents on the dollar left to cover all other costs, including interest paid on debt and income taxes. The government settlement negatively impacted the earnings, but because of costreduction measures in 2004, other costs such as salaries were reduced, helping to alleviate impact on earnings.

The remaining three measures indicate that expenses were covered but that there was little, percentage-wise, left over to reinvest in the firm. Without knowing how others in the industry are doing, it becomes difficult to make a conclusion about the effectiveness of operations. The results presented indicate a decline in profitability of operations.

Ratio	How Calculated	2004	2003
Gross profit margin	Gross profit/Net revenue	N/A	N/A
Operating profit margin	Operating profit/Net revenue	$2,018/$16,670 = 12.1%	$1704/$16,657 = 10.2%
Net profit margin	Net earnings/Net revenue	$219/$16,670 = 1.31%	$657/$16,657 = 4.18
Return on total assets or Return on investment	Net earnings/Total assets	$219/$17,568 = 1.24%	$657/$16,885 = 3.89%
Return on equity	Net earnings/ Stockholders' equity	$219/$4405 = 4.97%	$657/$5617 = 11.69%

Trade or Cash Conversion Cycle Ratio

The final group of standard ratios, the *trade or cash conversion cycle ratio*, used to analyze a firm's operations evaluates the trade or cash conversion cycle. These ratios measure, on the average, how long it takes to collect from either the patient or third-party providers or how long we are taking to pay our short-term obligations. The number of days in revenue is calculated as accounts receivable turnover previously discussed:

Ratio	How Calculated	2004	2003
Number of Days Revenue	Accounts receivable/ (Revenue/365)	$2,211/($16,670/365) = 48.41	$1,873/($16,670/365) = 41.01
Number of Days Payable	Accounts payable/ (Revenue/365)	$693/($16,670/365) = 15.17	$657/($16,657/365) = 14.38

If creditors provide 30 days in which to pay an obligation and your organization takes 40 days, a cash flow problem may exist. For Hospital Anywhere USA, the number of days in payables, accounts payable divided by average daily revenues, increased from 14.38 to 15.17, which indicates that the hospital took longer to pay current obligations. This is a minor change, and anyone doing an evaluation would have to know the terms for payment that the hospital has with its creditors. This does, however, increase cash flow in that you retain cash longer by postponing the payment (cash outflow). A variation of this ratio is current liabilities divided by operating expenses minus depreciation divided by 365.

Not-for-Profit Comparisons

Not-for-profit entities have some differences that make comparisons more difficult than for for-profit entities. Because profitability is not a mission of not-for-profit organizations, profitability ratios may not be calculated in the same manner. Healthcare organizations must provide an alternative performance indicator. This is normally in a footnote but must be clearly distinguished from other notes. It may take

Exhibit 20–3 Children's Hospital Operating Revenues and Expenses June 30, 2004 and 2003

	2004	2003
Net Patient Services and Revenue	$238,736,833	$228,094,450
Other Sources of Revenue		
Government Research Grants	45,160,159	36,757,430
Support Provided to Cover Operating Expenses	100,137,765	82,342,438
Total Operating Revenues	**$384,034,757**	**$347,194,318**
Operating Expenses		
Salaries and Benefits	$195,621,776	$172,757,651
Services, Supplies, Other	146,371,984	131,094,528
Depreciation	28,116,508	24,262,840
Interest	5,899,845	5,492,360
Bad Debt Expense	3,048,592	6,182,778
Total Operating Expenses	**$383,268,634**	**$339,790,157**
Income (Loss) from Operations	**$769,123**	**$7,404,161**

the form of either revenue over expenses, revenues and gains over expenses and losses, earned income, or performance income.

As the financial statements in **Exhibit 20–3** illustrate, there are differences between hospitals—especially between for-profit and not-for-profit firms. First, the dates of the statements are for June rather than December. The selection of a date is arbitrary. Second, other sources of revenue consist of government research grants and support provided to cover operating expenses. The latter is probably a result of donations by outside persons or organizations. The remaining accounts on the income statements are standard and would be expected to be found on both for-profit and not-for-profit organizations.

The balance sheet has one major difference from that of a for-profit entity. Instead of having stockholders (owners) of the firm, the accounts become unrestricted and temporarily restricted fund balances. *Unrestricted fund balances* are provided by others to support the mission of the hospital. *Temporarily restricted fund balances* are used for projects having a specific purpose and then returned to use for unrestricted purposes (**Exhibit 20–4**).

The four ratios presented in the following table are variations of those used in the analysis of Hospital Anywhere USA but are applied to that of Children's Hospital:

Ratio	How Calculated	2004	2005
Long-Term Debt to Total Capitalization	Long-term debt/ (Long-term debt + Fund balances)	$234,213,357/ $502,059,690 = .4665	$143,476,762/ $400,372,493 = .3584
Debt to Fund Balances	Total liabilities/ Fund balances	$283,587,276/ $267,846,333 = 1.058	$191,239,673/ $256,895,731 = .744
Reported Income Index	Net Income/Changes in Fund Balance	$786,123/ $10,950,602 = .072	N/A
Long-Term Debt to Fund Balances	Long-term debt/ Fund balance	$234,213,357/ $267,846,333 = .874	$143,476,763/ $256,895,731 = .558

Exhibit 20–4 Condensed Balance Sheets as of June 30, 2004 and 2003		
	2004	2003
Assets		
Cash and Temporary Investments	$6,084,671	$3,767,117
Patient Accounts Receivable, Net of Allowances for Uncollectible Accounts	55,084,671	49,121,350
Other Current Assets	36,059,481	27,737,663
Current Assets	$97,388,219	$80,626,130
Plant and Equipment, Net of Accumulated Depreciation	$261,633,535	$223,695,756
Funds Held in Trust	82,118,866	42,568,303
Long-Term in Trust	110,292,993	101,245,215
Total Assets	**$551,433,613**	**$448,135,404**
Liabilities and Fund Balance		
Accounts Payable and Accrued Expenses	$44,489,716	$43,222,493
Current Portion of Long-Term Debt	4,884,203	4,540,418
Current Liabilities	**$49,373,919**	**$47,762,911**
Long-Term Debt	$212,548,645	$119,007,882
Other Long-Term Liabilities	21,664,716	24,468,880
Unrestricted Fund Balance	213,986,611	207,562,498
Temporarily restricted Fund Balance	53,859,722	49,333,233
Total Liabilities and Fund Balances	**$551,433,613**	**$448,135,404**

All three previously used ratios are smaller than those of Hospital Anywhere USA and declined in this time period, indicating this hospital does not use as much debt to finance operations as does Hospital Anywhere USA. The reported income index was not directly applicable to Hospital Anywhere USA but is somewhat equivalent to profitability ratios that used net earnings computed for Hospital Anywhere USA. Again, a direct comparison should not be made with Hospital Anywhere USA, but this hospital could be compared with other not-for-profit hospitals.

A further problem in comparing not-for-profit entities is the lack of standardized terminology or presentation formats. Some of these same problems exist with for-profit entities, but the differences are not as glaring as that of not-for-profits. The last consideration in analyzing different not-for-profit firms is that information is not as readily available as that for publicly reporting firms.

The consolidated balance sheets and statement of activities (equivalent to for-profit income statements) of Retirement Homes, Inc., are introduced in **Exhibits 20–5** and **20–6**. Selected financial ratios follow the financial statements.

Retirement Homes, Inc., shows several differences between the previously reported organizations. In addition to being a smaller entity, it has permanently restricted funds; Children's Hospital does not. It also has gift fees and long-term obligations from advance payments from persons entering the facility. Patients may pay in advance, but until the retirement facility provides the services the income is not earned. The income statement format for Retirement Homes, Inc., also includes fund balance changes that were not included in previously presented income statements.

Exhibit 20–5   Retirement Homes, Inc. Consolidated Balance Sheet

	2000	1999
Assets		
Current Assets		
Cash and equivalents	$1,343,467	$557,494
Investments held by bond trustee	50,653	254,572
Accounts receivable, net of allowance for doubtful accounts of $166,200 and $45,200 in 2000 and 1999	444,396	371,746
Contributions and grants receivable	88,127	
Inventories	56,705	54,597
Prepaid expenses and other	62,133	90,567
Total current assets	**2,045,481**	**1,328,976**
Investments		
Held by bond trustee, net of amount requires to meet current obligations	4,845,585	4,562,685
Board designated funds	869,603	823,758
Foundation	1,832,579	1,637,170
	7,547,767	7,023,6 13
Property and equipment		
Land and improvements	2,630,999	2,537,686
Buildings and improvements	34,046,631	33,359,106
Equipment	1,679,668	1,513,251
Furniture and equipment	1,440,448	1,385,729
	39,797,746	38,795,772
Less accumulated depreciation	12,289,748	11,173,504
	27,507,998	27,622,268
Construction in progress	593,335	521,608
	28,101,333	28,143,876
Beneficial interest in charitable remainder trusts	72,250	
Net deferred charges:		
Marketing and consulting costs	1,568,833	1,758,238
Financing costs	2,437,811	2,774,112
Prepayment in lieu of taxes	210,000	280,000
	4,216,644	4,812,350
Other assets	21,500	21,500
Total assets	**$42,004,975**	**$41,330,315**
Current liabilities		
Accounts payable	$308,493	$399,480
Salaries, wages, and related liabilities	164,551	130,589
Accrued compensated absences	130,843	120,501

	2000	1999
Accrued interest	81,580	83,561
Current portion of long-term debt	904,031	854,212
Other current liabilities	12,012	49,860
Total current liabilities	1,601,510	1,638,203
Other liabilities:		
Long-term obligations	33,247,449	34,163,586
Entrance fees received in advance and deposits	308,124	202,288
Gift annuities payable	377,079	254,184
Deferred entry fee revenue	23,022,153	22,865,940
	56,954,805	57,485,998
Net assets (deficit):		
Unrestricted	(18,014,253)	(19,176,458)
Temporarily restricted	1,415,676	1,382,572
Permanently restricted	47,237	
Total net assets (deficit)	(16,551,340)	(17,793,886)
Total liabilities and net deficit	**$42,004,975**	**$41,330,315**

Exhibit 20–6 Retirement Homes, Inc. Consolidated Statements of Activities Year Ended December 31

	2000	1999
Revenue and other support		
Resident services:		
Monthly service fees	$8,340,317	$8,111,191
Amortization of deferred revenues	3,345,893	3,075,632
Patient revenue from nonresidents	2,217,990	1,629,027
Interest income	258,845	322,954
Medicare and other	804,211	615,273
Net assets released from restriction	132,171	
Total revenue and other support	**15,099,427**	**13,754,077**
Expenses		
Salaries and wages	5,059,124	4,728,354
Employee benefits	733,960	691,892
Total employment expenses	5,793,084	5,420,246
Purchased services	1,534,747	1,082,729
Supplies	1,247,315	1,286,860

(*continues*)

Exhibit 20–6   Retirement Homes, Inc. Consolidated Statements of Activities Year Ended December 31 (*continued*)

	2000	1999
Provision for bad debts	123,404	5,000
Utilities	637,598	624,457
Rent	4,815	4,515
Insurance	204,503	42,417
Interest	2,410,079	2,426,461
Program expenses-foundation	116,924	
Foundation operating expenses	66,282	
Miscellaneous	369,046	
Depreciation and amortization	1,672,950	1,765,252
Total expenses	**14,180,747**	**13,073,233**
Excess of revenue over expenses	918,680	680,844
Net asset reclassification	172,018	
Net assets released from restriction for capital	78,896	
Net unrealized holding losses on investments	(7,389)	1,817
Increase in unrestricted assets	1,162,205	682,661
Temporarily restricted net assets:		
Net asset reclassification	(187,018)	
Contributions	308,263	127,066
Net unrealized holding losses on investments	(168,582)	(54,993)
Investment income	291,508	244,550
Net assets released from restrictions	(211,067)	(50,443)
Increase in temporarily restricted net assets	33,104	266,180
Permanently restricted net assets:		
Net Asset Reclassification	15,000	
Contributions	32,237	
Increase in permanently restricted net assets	47,237	
Increase in net assets	1,242,546	948,841
Net deficit, beginning of year	**(17,793,886)**	**(18,742,727)**
Net deficit, end of year	**$(16,551,340)**	**$(17,793,886)**

Current Ratios

Retirement Homes, Inc., shows an improvement in its ability to meet current obligations. In 2003, both ratios were below 1, whereas both improved to above 1 in 2004. How does this compare with the ratios presented for Hospital Anywhere USA? The ratios for Hospital Anywhere USA deteriorated, whereas those of Retirement Homes, Inc., improved. The trends can be compared, but a direct comparison cannot be made because the firms are in two different industries and operate as two different types of organizations (for-profit vs. not-for-profit).

Ratio	How Calculated	2004	2003
Current ratio	Current assets/Current liabilities	$2,045,481/ $1,601,510 = 1.28	$1,328,976/ $1,638,203 = .81
Quick ratio	Current assets – Inventories/Current liabilities	$1,926,643/ $1,601,510 = 1.20	$1,183,812/ $1,683,203 = .70

Activity Ratios

Notice in the following table that the number of days in the accounts receivable collection period increased, as did the inventory turnover. This indicates that the firm has slowed the time to make collections, whereas inventory was being used faster. Again, a direct comparison cannot be made with Hospital Anywhere USA data. However, you can purchase industry comparison data (*benchmarking*) from either national services or associations and determine how well you are doing compared with others.

Ratio	How Calculated	2004	2003
Accounts Receivable Collection Period	Accounts Receivable/ [(Revenue)/365]	$444,396/ [($15,099,427)/ 365] = 10.7 Days	$371,746/ [($13,754,077)/ 365] = 9.86 Days
Inventory Turnover	Cost of Goods Sold/ Inventory or Revenue. Inventory	$15,099,427/ $56,705 = 266.3	$13,754,077/ $54,597 = 251.9

Notice again that both ratios improved, but assets are not used as well to generate revenue for Retirement Homes, Inc., as they were for Hospital Anywhere USA. You are cautioned again not to make direct comparisons.

Ratio	How Calculated	2004	2003
Fixed asset turnover	Net revenue/Net property, plant, and equipment	$15,099,427/ $28,101,333 = .587	$13,754,077/ $28,143,876 = .488
Total asset turnover	Net revenue/Total assets	$15,099,427/ $42,004,975 = .359	$13,754,077/ $41,330,315 = .382

Leverage Ratios

In each case, the amount of debt, long term and total, is greater than total assets and long-term debt plus net assets. Net assets, equivalent to for-profits' stockholders' equity, are negative. This negative figure is probably a result of losses in previous years of operation. As a result of this negative figure, the calculation is not applicable.

Ratio	How Calculated	2004	2003
Debt Ratio	Total liabilities/Total assets	$56,954,805/ $42,004,975 = 1.356	$57,485,998/ $41,330,315 = 1.39
Long-Term Debt to Total Capitalization	Long-term debt/ (Long-term debt + Net assets)	$55,353,295/ $38,801,955 = 1.43	$55,847,795,/ $38,053,909 = 1.47
Debt to Equity	Total liabilities/Net assets	$56,954,805/ ($16,551,340) = N/A	$57,485,999/ ($17,793,886) = N/A

Profitability Ratios

Two of the following ratios cannot be calculated either because of a lack of available data or because one part of the equation has a negative (deficit) balance. Two of the ratios (indicated with *) are variations of those presented previously for Hospital Anywhere USA. These ratios use the increase in net assets because a not-for-profit does not report profits but rather looks at increases or decreases in assets. All three ratios that were calculated improved in year 2004 over that of 2003.

Ratio	How Calculated	2004	2003
Gross Profit Margin	Gross profit/Net revenue	N/A	N/A
Operating Profit Margin*	Excess of revenue over expenses/Net revenue	$918,680/ $15,099,427 = 6%	$680,844/ $13,654,077 = 4.95%
Net Profit Margin*	Increase in net assets/ Net Revenue	$1,242,546/ $15,099,427 = 8.2%	$948,841/ $13,754,077 = 6.89%
Return on Total Assets or Return on Investment	Increase in Net assets/ Total assets	$1,242,546/ $15,099,427 = 8.22%	$948, 841/ $13,754,077 = 6.89%
Return on Equity	Increase in net assets/ Total net assets	$1,242,546/ ($16,551,340) = N/A	$948, 841/ ($17,793,881) = N/A

Additional Financial Ratios

One ratio that can be applied to both not-for-profit and for-profit entities is the number of day's *cash on hand*. This is the amount of cash necessary to meet actual daily cash operating expenses. This measure excludes both bad debt and depreciation expenses from operating expenses. Remember, these are estimates and are a "paper and pencil" item only. They do not cause cash outflows. The calculation for this ratio follows:

$$\textit{Days of cash on hand} = \frac{\textit{Cash + Marketable securities}}{\textit{(Operating expenses − Bad debts − Depreciation) / 365}}$$

One healthcare organization maintains 200 days of cash on hand. However, this amount is probably high for most firms. The more cash on hand, the less a firm has to invest in assets that have higher returns. A variation of the preceding ratio is the cash flow coverage. This measures how well you are able to cover required payments such as interest, rent, and debt payments. Information for calculation of this ratio would be found in the cash flow statements. Calculation of this ratio follows:

$$\textit{Cash flow coverage} = \frac{\textit{Cash from operations + Interest + Rent}}{\textit{Interest + Rent + Debt payments}}$$

If the previous ratio is less than 1, it indicates that you are only able to make that percentage of required payments. For example, if the ratio is 0.8, you are only able to make 80% of required payments.

A ratio unique to not-for-profit organizations and one that only recently has been calculated is the *program service ratio*. This ratio is designed to determine what proportion of a firm's expenditures goes directly into its program services (core business). This ratio is calculated by dividing program service expenses by total expenses. A firm should be spending a large proportion of its cash inflows on its mission.

$$Program\ service\ ratio = \frac{Program\ services\ expenses}{Total\ expenses}$$

Other financial ratios that might be computed for either for-profit or not-for-profit entities are as follows:

- Revenue per employee: Net revenue/Number of employees
- Net income per employee: Net income/Number of employees
- Price earnings ratio: Market price of stock/Earning per common share
- Growth rate of revenue: Percentage change in revenue from previous time period

Ratios that are more applicable to not-for-profit and healthcare entities are these:

- Percentage of deductibles: Deductibles/Gross patient service revenue
- Reported income index: Net income/Changes in fund balance
- Long-term debt to fund balance: Long-term debt/Fund balance

In any of the previously calculated ratios where stockholders' equity numbers were used, the not-for-profit sector would use the fund balance as a replacement number for calculations. Deductibles are unique to the healthcare industry. The industry is affected negatively by third-party payment systems. Once a claim is filed, deductions based on contracted rates are removed from the expected payment. The actual amount received varies from amounts as low as 25 cents on the dollar to a high of around 60 cents on the dollar.

Conclusion

As with any comparisons that use ratios or common size financial statements, caution must be used. Comparisons must be made for a longer period than 2 years. Past results may not be indicative of future performance. Differences in management, risk aversive or risk taking, for one can affect how a firm is managed. Competition, geographic differences, and other factors can affect operations. Nonetheless, ratios and common size comparisons can provide indications of action that needs to be undertaken. Benchmarking allows a firm to judge how well it is doing in relation to other organizations in the same industry and in other industries. Recall that benchmarking is looking at best practices, not just in firms in your industry but in all firms.

Discussion Questions

1. Which ratios would you consider most important in the daily and monthly operation of the organization? Why?
2. If you were analyzing an organization's ability to borrow money, which ratios would be most helpful?
3. Why is the accounts receivable turnover ratio important to the organization?
4. What process do organizations use to compare themselves with other organizations and how effective is this process?
5. When using common size financial statements, what number do analysts use for the balance sheet and what number is used for the income statements?

Glossary of Terms

Accounts Receivable Collection Period—the average time it takes an organization to collect its accounts (patient/insurance) receivable.

Activity Ratios—the liquidity and efficiency of asset management.

Benchmarking—a process that provides comparisons with the best practices of other organizations. These firms do not have to be within the same industry, but traditionally comparisons are based within specific industries. This is a limiting factor in identifying best practices but simplifies the comparisons.

Cash on Hand—applies to both not-for-profit and for-profit entities; the number of days of cash on hand. This is the amount of cash necessary to meet actual daily cash operating expenses. This measure excludes both bad debt and depreciation expenses from operating expenses.

Common Size Financial Statements—in the balance sheet and income statement, one number is selected and then divided into all other numbers in the statements.

Current Ratio—the current assets divided by current liabilities. This provides one measure of a firm's ability to pay short-term obligations.

Debt Ratio—how much of the total assets have been financed using debt (obligations to pay a future amount of funds).

Fixed Asset Turnover—how well management is using the long-term assets of the organization to generate revenue.

Forward Purchase Contract—where one party agrees to buy a commodity at a specific price on a specific future date and the other party agrees to make the sale.

Inventory Turnover—how quickly inventory is sold; a measure that is important for firms with products that deteriorate or have a short shelf life (drugs, surgical supplies).

Leverage Ratios, or Capital Structure Ratios—one measure of how an organization is financed.

Liquidity Ratios—concerned with short-term (current items). The two most frequently used liquidity ratios are the current ratio and quick or acid-test ratio.

Operating Profit Margin—found by looking at the net revenues from the normal course of business, providing healthcare services, and subtracting all expenses of operations necessary to generate these revenues. This measure, sometimes called EBIT (earnings before interest and taxes), indicates whether the firm is covering its costs of operations.

Profitability Ratios—measures of how well a firm is doing in its basic operations.

Program Service Ratio—a ratio unique to not-for-profit organizations and one that only recently has been calculated. This ratio is designed to determine what proportion of a firm's expenditures go directly into its program services (core business).

Put Option—the right to sell stock at a specified price in the future.

Quick or Acid-test Ratio—additional information to evaluate the ability to meet short-term obligations.

Total Asset Turnover—how management is using all assets of the organization to generate revenue. The measure is found by dividing net revenues by all assets.

Trade or Cash Conversion Cycle Ratio—a measure of, on the average, how long it takes to collect from either the patient or third-party providers or how long the organization is taking to pay short-term obligations.

INDEX